FRENCH'S
Index of
Surgical
Differential
Diagnosis

Edited by

Harold Ellis CBE DM MCh FRCS

Emeritus Professor of Surgery, University of London;
Clinical Anatomist, King's College (Guy's Campus), London

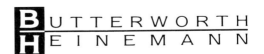

BUTTERWORTH
HEINEMANN

OXFORD AUCKLAND BOSTON JOHANNESBURG
MELBOURNE NEW DELHI

Butterworth-Heinemann
Linacre House, Jordan Hill, Oxford OX2 8DP
225 Wildwood Avenue, Woburn, MA 01801-2041
A division of Reed Educational and Professional Publishing Ltd

A member of the Reed Elsevier plc group

First published 1999

British Library Cataloguing in Publication Data
A catalogue record for this book is available from the British
Library

Library of Congress Cataloguing in Publication Data
A catalogue record for this book is available from the Library of
Congress

ISBN 0 7506 2763 8

Composition by Genesis Typesetting, Rochester, Kent
Printed and bound in Spain

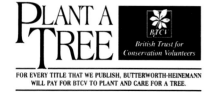

Preface

In 1912, Herbert French, Physician at Guy's Hospital, published the first edition of an 'index of differential diagnosis of main symptoms'. It became an immediate success and its popularity has continued unabated under a series of distinguished editors over the rest of this century. The thirteenth edition was published in 1996.

As a young surgeon in training, I myself used 'French's' as a useful revision for my higher examinations, but I have found that, in contrast to its widespread use among physicians, it is relatively little known or employed by surgeons. Presumably this is because a good deal of the book is taken up by what are regarded as mainly medical topics; neurological, chest, dermatological and psychological problems, for example.

With the intention of making so much of 'French's' that is valuable to the surgeon easily available, I have selected the topics covering surgery in its widest sense, including orthopaedics, ophthalmology, diseases of ear, nose and throat and gynaecology, from the main volume. I hope this edited surgical version will prove of value both to the trainee surgeon and to the established practitioner in providing encyclopaedic cover of the wide range of symptoms that may be encountered in surgical patients.

Harold Ellis

Acknowledgements

I would like to thank my expert contributors to *French's Index of Surgical Differential Diagnosis*. My colleague Mr Lynn Edwards has sadly died and it fell to me to see his sections through to press. Mr Joe Dawes provided excellent illustrations from the Gordon Museum Collection at Guy's. I owe much to the skilled help at Butterworth-Heinemann from Dr Geoffrey Smaldon, Cathy Staves, Claire Hutchins and Chris Jarvis.

Contributors and their subjects

Paul M. Aichroth MS, FRCS
Consultant Orthopaedic Surgeon, Chelsea & Westminster Hospital, and The Wellington Knee Surgery Unit, London
Bone, swelling of
Contractures and deformities of the upper and lower limbs
Foot and toes, deformities of
Spine, curvature of

Michael Baum ChM, FRCS
Professor of Surgery, Royal Marsden Hospital and Past Professor of Surgery, Kings College School of Medicine and Dentistry
Breast lumps
Breast, pain in
Nipple, abnormalities of
Nipple, discharge from

Peter T. Blenkinsopp FRCS, FDS, RCS
Consultant Oral and Maxillofacial Surgeon, Kingston and St Helier Hospitals
Gums, bleeding
Gums, hypertrophy of
Gums, retraction of
Jaw, deformity of
Jaw, pain in
Jaw, swelling of
Mouth, pigmentation of
Mouth, ulcers in

Ian A.D. Bouchier CBE, MD, FRCP, FRCPE, FFPHM, HonFCP(SAF), FRSA, FIBiol, FRSE
Professor of Medicine, University of Edinburgh, Honorary Consultant Physician, Royal Infirmary, Edinburgh
Appetite, disorders of
Flatulence
Indigestion
Nausea
Regurgitation
Succussion sounds
Tongue, discoloration of
Vomiting

N.E.F. Cartlidge MBBS, FRCP
Senior Lecturer in Neurology, Consultant Neurologist, Royal Victoria Infirmary, Newcastle upon Tyne
Pupils, abnormalities of

Graham Clayden MD, FRCP
Reader in Paediatrics, UMDS of Guys and St Thomas's Hospital, London
Enuresis

Lynn Edwards MChir, FRCS (deceased)
Formerly: Consultant Urological Surgeon, Westminster Hospital, London
Dysuria
Micturition, frequency of
Micturition, hesitancy
Pyuria
Urine, incontinence of
Urine, retention of

Harold Ellis CBE, DM, MCH, FRCS, FRCOG
Emeritus Professor of Surgery, University of London
Abdominal pain, acute, localized
Abdominal pain (general)
Abdominal pulsation
Abdominal rigidity
Abdominal swellings
Axillary swelling
Back, pain in
Borborygmi
Constipation
Face, swelling of
Gallbladder, palpable
Gangrene
Kidney, palpable
Leg, ulceration of
Nasal regurgitation
Neck, stiff
Neck, swelling of
Penile sores
Penis, pain in
Perineal pain
Perineal sores
Peristalsis, visible

Contributors and their subjects

Pilimiction
Pneumaturia
Popliteal swelling
Priapism
Pruritis ani
Ptyalism
Salivary glands, pain in
Salivary glands, swelling of
Scrotum, ulceration of
Spine, tenderness of
Stomach, dilatation of
Stools, mucus in
Stools, pus in
Strangury
Testicular pain
Testicular swelling
Thyroid, pain in
Tongue, swelling of
Tongue, ulceration of
Urethra, faeces passed through
Urethral discharge
Veins, varicose abdominal

Peter R. Fleming MD, FRCP
*Formerly: Senior Lecturer in Medicine,
Charing Cross and Westminster Medical
School, London and Consultant
Physician, Westminster Hospital, London*
Haematuria
Leg, oedema of
Oliguria
Urine, abnormal colour of

William M. Haining MB, ChB, FRCSEd,
FRCOph
*Emeritus Head of Department of
Ophthalmology, University of Dundee*
Eye, pain in
Eyelids, disorders of

F. Dudley Hart MD, FRCP
*Consulting Physician, Chelsea Hospital
for Women, The Hospital of St John and
St Elizabeth, and Westminster Hospital,
London*
Face, abnormalities of appearance and
movement

Robert C. Heading BSc, MD, FRCP
*Reader in Medicine, Royal Infirmary,
Edinburgh*
Dysphagia
Heartburn

M.M. Henry FRCS
*Consultant Surgeon, Central Middlesex
Hospital and Honorary Consultant
Surgeon, St Mark's Hospital for Diseases
of the Colon/Rectum, London*
Anorectal pain
Faeces, incontinence of
Rectal bleeding
Rectal discharge
Rectal mass
Rectal tenesmus
Rectal ulceration

Edward Housley MB, ChB, FRCPE, FRCP
Royal Infirmary, Edinburgh
Fingers, dead (white, cold)

Andrew Keat MD, FRCP
*Reader in Rheumatology, Charing Cross
and Westminster Medical School,
Honorary Consultant Physician, Charing
Cross Hospital, London*
Arm, pain in
Joints, affections of
Leg, pain in

Christopher A. Ludlam BSc, PhD, FRCP,
FRCPath
*Consultant Haematologist, Director of
the Haemophilia Centre, Royal Infirmary,
Edinburgh*
Bleeding
Splenomegaly

Ian Mackenzie TD, MD, FRCP (deceased)
*Formerly: Consulting Physician to the
Department of Nervous Diseases, Guy's
Hospital, London*
Face, paralysis of
Trismus (lockjaw)

Charles N. McCollum MD, FRCS
*Professor of Surgery, University Hospital
of South Manchester*
Groin, swellings in

A.G.D. Maran MD, FRCS, FRCS(Ed),
FRCP(Ed), FACS, FDS(Hon)
*Professor of Otolaryngology, University of
Edinburgh, Consultant Otolaryngologist,
Royal Infirmary, Edinburgh, President
Royal College of Surgeons of Edinburgh*
Deafness
Earache

Epistaxis
Nasal deformity
Nasal discharge
Nasal obstruction
Otorrhoea
Tinnitus
Tonsils, enlargement of
Vertigo
Voice, disorders of

K.R. Palmer MD, FRCP(Ed)
Consultant Gastroenterologist, Western General Hospital, Edinburgh
Jaundice
Liver, enlargement of

Naren Patel MB, ChB, PRCOG
Consultant Obstetrician, University of Dundee, Ninewells Hospital, Dundee
Amenorrhoea
Dysmenorrhoea
Dyspareunia
Infertility
Menorrhagia
Metrorrhagia
Pelvis, pain in
Vagina and uterus, prolapse of
Vagina, discharge from
Vagina, swelling in
Vulva, swelling of
Vulva, ulceration of

Ian D. Ramsay MD(Edin), FRCP, FRCP(Edin)
Consultant Endocrinologist, North Middlesex Hospital NHS Trust, London
Gynaecomastia

S.T.D. Roxburgh FRCS(Edin) FRCOph
Head of Department of Ophthalmology, University of Dundee
Exophthalmos
Eye, blindness of
Eye, inflammation of
Ptosis

Robin I. Russell MD, PhD, FRCP
Head of Department of Gastroenterology, Royal Infirmary, Glasgow and the University of Glasgow
Diarrhoea
Faeces, abnormal consistency and shape
Faeces, abnormal contents
Faeces, colour
Haematemesis
Melaena

Richard Staughton MA, FRCP
Consultant Dermatologist, Chelsea and Westminster Hospital, London
Angioma and telangiectasia
Face, ulceration of
Flushing
Foot, ulceration of
Keloid
Lips, affections of
Skin tumours

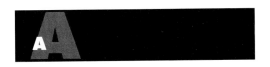

Abdominal pain, acute, localized

A common and extremely important clinical problem is the patient who presents with acute abdominal pain. This may be referred all over the abdominal wall (*see* ABDOMINAL PAIN, general, p. 3) but here we shall consider those patients who present pain localized to a particular part of the abdominal cavity.

The causes are legion and it is a useful exercise to summarize the organs that may be implicated together with the pathological processes pertaining to them so that the clinician can consider the possibilities in a logical manner:

1. Gastroduodenal
Perforated gastric or duodenal ulcer
Perforated gastric carcinoma
Acute gastritis (often alcoholic)
Irritant poisons

2. Intestinal
Intestinal trauma
Small-bowel obstruction (adhesions etc)
Regional ileitis (Crohn's disease)
Intussusception
Sigmoid volvulus
Acute colonic diverticulitis
Large-bowel obstruction due to neoplasm
Strangulated external hernia (inguinal, femoral, umbilical)
Acute mesenteric occlusion due to arterial embolism or thrombosis or to venous thrombosis

3. Appendix
Acute appendicitis

4. Pancreas
Pancreatic trauma
Acute pancreatitis
Recurrent pancreatitis

5. Gallbladder and bile ducts
Calculus in the gallbladder or common bile ducts
Acute cholecystitis
Acute cholangitis

6. Liver
Trauma
Acute hepatitis

Malignant disease (primary or secondary)
Congestive cardiac failure

7. Spleen
Trauma
Spontaneous rupture (in malaria or infectious mononucleosis)
Infarction

8. Urinary tract
Renal trauma
Renal, ureteric or vesical calculus
Pyelonephritis
Pyonephrosis

9. Female genitalia
Salpingitis
Pyosalpinx
Ectopic pregnancy
Torsion of subserous fibroid
Red degeneration of fibroid
Twisted ovarian cyst
Ruptured ovarian cyst

10. Aorta
Ruptured aneurysm
Dissecting aneurysm

In addition to causes from intra-abdominal, retroperitoneal and pelvic organs, it is important to remember that acute localized pain may be referred to the abdomen from other structures:

11. Central nervous system
Herpes zoster affecting the lower thoracic segments
Posterior nerve root pain (e.g. from a collapsed vertebra from trauma or secondary deposits)

12. The heart and pericardium
Myocardial infarction
Acute pericarditis

13. Pleura
Acute diaphragmatic pleurisy

Occasionally patients are seen, who are often well known in the Casualty Department, presenting with simulated acute abdominal pain due to hysteria or malingering.

Patients with acute abdominal pain present one of the most testing trials to the clinician. In the first place, diagnosis is all important since a decision has to be made whether or not the patient requires urgent laparotomy, e.g. for a perforated peptic ulcer, acute appendicitis or acute intestinal obstruction. The history and examination are often difficult to elicit, particularly in a small child or a very ill patient who is in great pain and hardly wishes either to answer a lot of questions or to submit to prolonged examination. Finally, there are very few laboratory or radiological aids to diagnosis. Acute appendicitis, for example, has no specific tests. A raised white blood count suggests intraperitoneal infection but something like a quarter of the cases of acute appendicitis have a white count below 10 000. Plain X-rays of the abdomen may indicate free gas when there is a perforated hollow viscus but this is not invariably so. Intestinal obstruction may be revealed by distended loops of bowel on a plain X-ray of the abdomen but in some 10 per cent of small-bowel obstructions the X-rays are entirely normal, since the distended loops of bowel are filled with fluid only so that the typical gas-distended loops of bowel are not present.

One of the few investigations that the surgeon relies upon heavily is a raised serum amylase. When this is above 1000 units it is almost pathognomic of acute pancreatitis, although every now and then a fulminating case of pancreatitis is seen in whom the amylase is not elevated.

Every effort must therefore be made to establish the diagnosis on a careful history and examination.

One of the important aspects in the assessment of the acute abdomen is the establishment of a trend. Increasing pain, tenderness, guarding or rigidity indicates that there is some progressive intra-abdominal condition. This is also suggested by a rising pulse-rate on hourly or half-hourly observations and it is also suggested by progressive elevation of the temperature. In a doubtful case, repeated clinical examination, together with sequential recordings of the temperature and pulse, will enable the clinician to decide whether the intra-abdominal condition is subsiding or progressing.

GENERAL FEATURES

General inspection of the patient is all important and must never be omitted. The flushed face and coated tongue of acute appendicitis, the agonized expression of the patient with a perforated ulcer, the writhing colic of a patient with ureteric stone, biliary colic or small-bowel obstruction are all most helpful. The skin is inspected for the pallor suggestive of haemorrhage and for the jaundice which may be associated with biliary colic with a stone impacted at the lower end of the common bile duct. In such a case there will also be bile pigment which can be detected in the urine.

ABDOMINAL EXAMINATION

The patient must be placed in a good light and the entire abdomen exposed from the nipples to the knees. The abdomen is inspected. Failure of movement with respiration may suggest an underlying peritoneal irritation. Abdominal distension is present in intestinal obstruction and visible peristalsis may be seen from rhythmic contractions of the small bowel under these circumstances. Retraction of the abdomen may occur in acute peritonitis so that the abdomen assumes a scaphoid appearance, e.g. following perforation of a peptic ulcer.

Guarding, a voluntary contraction of the abdominal wall on palpation, denotes underlying inflammatory disease and this is accompanied by localized tenderness. Rigidity is indicated by an involuntary tightness of the abdominal wall and may be generalized or localized. Localized rigidity over one particular organ suggests local peritoneal involvement, for example in acute appendicitis or acute cholecystitis.

Percussion of the abdomen is useful. Dullness in the flanks suggests the presence of intraperitoneal fluid (e.g. blood in a patient with a ruptured spleen). A resonant distended abdomen is found in obstruction and loss of liver dullness suggests free gas within the peritoneal cavity in a patient with a ruptured hollow viscus.

In intestinal obstruction the bowel sounds are increased and have a particular 'tinkling' quality. In some cases borborygmi may be audible without using the stethoscope. Complete absence of bowel sounds suggests peritonitis.

Examination of the abdomen is not complete until the hernial orifices have been carefully inspected and palpated. It is easy enough to miss a small strangulated inguinal, femoral or umbilical hernia which, surprisingly enough, may have been completely overlooked by the patient.

Rectal examination is then performed. In intestinal obstruction the rectum has a characteristic 'ballooned' empty feel although the exact mechanism of this is unknown. In pelvic peritonitis there will be tenderness anteriorly in the pouch of Douglas. A tender mass suggests an inflamed or twisted pelvic organ and this can be confirmed by bimanual vaginal examination.

THE URINE AND SPECIAL INVESTIGATIONS

The presence of blood, protein, pus or bile pigment in the urine may help to distinguish a renal or biliary colic from other causes of intra-abdominal pain. In obscure cases of abdominal pain, the urine should be examined for porphyrins to exclude porphyria, particularly when the attack appears to have been precipitated by barbiturates.

The clinical assessment of the patient with acute localized abdominal pain, based on a careful history and examination together with examination of the urine, may be supplemented by laboratory and radiological investigations. A full blood count, plain X-ray of the abdomen, estimation of the serum amylase in suspected pancreatitis may all be helpful although, as mentioned above, must be interpreted with caution. Ultrasound of the pelvis may be helpful if a twisted ovarian cyst or some other pelvic pathology is suspected. Ultrasonography is also valuable in demonstrating gall stones in acute cholecystitis, the presence of free intra-abdominal fluid and of a leaking abdominal aneurysm. In a difficult case, computerized tomography (CT) may give valuable information; for example, of a swollen oedematous pancreas in pancreatitis or of a localized collection of pus in acute colonic diverticulitis. An emergency intravenous urogram is indicated when ureteric stone or some other renal pathology is suspected. An electrocardiogram and appropriate cardiac enzyme estimations are performed if it is suspected that the upper abdominal pain is referred from a myocardial infarction and a chest X-ray may demonstrate a basal pneumonia. It must be stressed, however, that the clinical features take precedence over all other diagnostic aids.

Nothing can be simpler nor more difficult than diagnosing a patient with the so-called 'acute abdomen'. Particular difficulties will be encountered in infants (where the history may be difficult and examining a screaming child most demanding) and in the elderly, where again it is often difficult to obtain an accurate history and where physical signs are often atypical. The grossly obese patient and the pregnant patient are two other categories where particular difficulties may be encountered.

When faced with a patient with severe abdominal pain the main decision that must be taken, of course, is whether or not a laparotomy is indicated as a matter of urgency. If careful assessment still makes the decision difficult, then repeated observations must be carried out over the next hours to observe the trend of the particular case and this will nearly always enable a definite decision as to whether laparotomy or further conservative treatment is indicated.

Harold Ellis

Abdominal pain (general)

(*See also*) ABDOMINAL PAIN, acute, localized, p. 2)

Most abdominal pain is localized, for example that due to a renal stone or biliary stone, acute appendicitis, peptic ulceration, and so on. There are, however, a number of causes of generalized abdominal pain, the commonest of which are peritonitis and intestinal obstructions.

ACUTE GENERAL PERITONITIS

Peritonitis must be secondary to some lesion which enables some clue in the history to suggest the initiating disease. Thus the patient with established peritonitis may give a history of onset which indicates acute appendicitis or salpingitis as the source of origin. Where the onset of peritonitis is sudden, one should suspect an acute perforation of a hollow viscus. The early features depend on the severity and the extent of the peritonitis. Pain is always severe and typically the patient lies still on its account, in contrast with the restlessness of a patient with abdominal colic. An extensive peritonitis which involves the abdominal aspect of the diaphragm may be accompanied by shoulder-tip pain. Vomiting often occurs early in the course of the disease. The patient is obviously ill and the temperature frequently elevated. If initially the peritoneal exudate is not purulent, the temperature may be normal. It is a good aphorism concerning the two common causes of this condition that peritonitis due to appendicitis is usually accompanied by a temperature above 38°C (100°F), whereas the temperature in peritonitis due to a perforation of a peptic ulcer seldom reaches this level. The pulse is often raised and tends to increase from hour to hour. Examination of the abdomen demonstrates tenderness, which may be localized to the affected area or is generalized if the peritoneal cavity is extensively involved. There is marked guarding, which again may be localized or generalized, and rebound tenderness is present. The abdomen is silent on auscultation, although sometimes the transmitted sounds of the heart beat and respiration may be detected. Rectally, there is tenderness of the pelvic peritoneum. As the disease progresses, the abdomen becomes distended, signs of free fluid may be detected, the pulse becomes more rapid and feeble. Vomiting is now effortless and faeculent, and the patient, still conscious and mentally alert, demonstrates the Hippocratic facies with sunken eyes, pale, cold and sweating skin, and cyanosis of the extremities.

X-ray of the abdomen in the erect position may reveal free subdiaphragmatic gas in peritonitis due to hollow viscus perforation (e.g. perforated peptic ulcer), but its absence by no means excludes the diagnosis.

The main differential diagnoses are the colics of intestinal obstruction or of ureteric or biliary stone. Intraperitoneal haemorrhage, acute pancreatitis, dissection or leakage of an aortic aneurysm, or a basal pneumonia are also important differential diagnoses.

TUBERCULOUS PERITONITIS

In Great Britain this is now a rare disease. When it is encountered in this country, the patient is usually an immigrant from the Third World. Usually there is a feeling of heaviness rather than acute pain. The onset of symptoms is gradual, with abdominal distension, the presence of fluid within the peritoneal cavity, and often the presence of a puckered, thickened omentum, which forms a tumour lying transversely across the middle of the abdomen.

INTESTINAL COLIC (*see also* ABDOMINAL PAIN, ACUTE, LOCALIZED)

INTESTINAL OBSTRUCTION

This is a common cause of generalized abdominal pain. In peritonitis there is no periodic rhythm, whereas waves of pain interspersed with periods of complete relief or only a dull ache are typical of obstruction. In contrast to the patients with peritonitis who wish to remain completely still, the victim of intestinal obstruction is restless and rolls about with the spasms of the colic. Usually there are the accompaniments of progressive abdominal distension, absolute constipation, progressive vomiting, which becomes faeculent, and the presence of noisy bowel sounds on auscultation. X-rays of the abdomen usually reveal multiple fluid levels on the erect film together with distended loops of gas-filled bowel which are obvious on the supine radiograph.

LEAD COLIC

Inquiry about the patient's occupation may well be the first clue to the diagnosis. Lead colic may cause extremely severe attacks of general abdominal pain. There may be preceding anorexia, constipation and vague abdominal discomfort. The severe pain is usually situated in the lower abdomen radiating to both groins and may sometimes be associated with wrist-drop (due to peripheral neuritis) and occasionally with lead encephalopathy. There may be a blue 'lead line' on the gums if oral sepsis is present, due to the precipitation of lead sulphide. Frequently there is a normocytic hypochromic anaemia with stippling of the red cells (punctate basophilia).

GASTRIC CRISES

Gastric crises, today extremely rare in the Western World, may cause general abdominal pain. The patient has other evidence of tabes dorsalis, with Argyll Robertson pupils, optic atrophy and ptosis, loss of deep sensation (absence of pain on testicular compression or squeezing the tendo Achillis), and loss of ankle- and knee-jerks. The pain is severe and lasts for many hours or even days. There may be accompanying vomiting and there may also be rigidity of the abdominal wall. The visceral crisis may be the sole manifestation of tabes. The mere fact that a patient has tabes dorsalis does not, of course, mean that his abdominal pain must necessarily be a gastric crisis. The author has repaired a perforated duodenal ulcer in a patient with all the classic features of well-documented tabes dorsalis.

ABDOMINAL ANGINA

Abdominal angina occurs in elderly patients as a result of progressive atheromatous narrowing of the superior mesenteric artery. Colicky attacks of central abdominal pain occur after meals and this is followed by diarrhoea. Confirmation of the diagnosis requires arteriography. Complete occlusion with infarction of the intestine is often preceded by attacks of this nature. Occlusion of vessels to small or large intestine as is seen in a number of vasculopathies, such as systemic lupus erythematosus or polyarteritis nodosa, may cause generalized abdominal pain and proceed to gangrene, perforation and general peritonitis.

FUNCTIONAL ABDOMINAL PAIN

One of the most difficult problems is the patient, female more often than male, who presents with severe chronic generalized abdominal pains in whom all clinical, laboratory and radiological tests are negative. Inquiry will often reveal features of depression or the presence of some precipitating factor producing an anxiety state. In some cases the abdomen is covered with scars of previous laparotomies at which various organs have been reposited, non-essential viscera removed, and real or imaginary adhesions divided. Some of these patients prove to be drug addicts, others are frank hysterics, others seek the security of the hospital environment, but in still others the aetiology remains mysterious. This forms one type of the so-called 'Munchausen syndrome', described by the late Dr Richard Asher.

ABDOMINAL PAINS IN GENERAL DISEASE

Acute abdominal pain may occur in a number of medical conditions not already considered. These include sudden and severe pain complicating malignant malaria, familial Mediterranean fever, and cholera, or may accompany uncontrolled diabetes with ketosis, that rare condition known as porphyria, and any of the blood dyscrasias; the best example is Henoch's purpura in children. Bouts of abdominal pain may occur in the hypercalcaemia of hyperparathyroidism.

Harold Ellis

Abdominal pulsation

A pulsatile swelling in the abdomen may be due to:
(1) a prominent aorta—normal or arteriosclerotic;
(2) an abdominal aortic aneurysm; (3) transmission of
aortic pulsations through an abdominal mass; or (4) a
pulsatile enlarged liver.

1. Prominent aorta

The pulsations of the normal aorta may be felt in
perfectly normal but thin subjects along a line extending from the xiphoid to the bifurcation of the aorta at
the level of the fourth lumbar vertebra, about 2 cm
below and a little to the left of the umbilicus. In the
arteriosclerotic and hypertensive subject, it may be
difficult to decide whether or not the aorta is merely
thickened and tortuous or whether it is aneurysmal. If
the two index fingers are placed parallel, one on either
side of the aorta, the distance between the fingers can
be measured. According to the size of the patient, a gap
of 2–3 cm between the fingertips may be considered
normal, but any measurement above this is suspicious
of aneurysmal dilatation. If in doubt, visualization of
the aorta by means of ultrasound or computerized
tomography enables accurate measurement of the
aorta to be made.

2. Abdominal aortic aneurysm

There is no doubt that arteriosclerotic abdominal
aneurysms are becoming more frequently encountered, as is the serious emergency of leakage or rupture
of such an aneurysm. The majority of patients are more
than 60 years of age and the great majority are men.
The aneurysm may be entirely symptomless or the
patient may complain of epigastric or central abdominal discomfort which frequently radiates into the
lumbar region. The patient himself may actually detect
the pulsating mass in the abdomen.

The pulsation may be visible in the upper
abdomen, above the umbilicus and, if large enough,
may actually appear as a pulsating mass. On palpation,
the aneurysm is a midline swelling which bulges over
to the left side. If the mass extends below the level of
the umbilicus it suggests implication of the iliac
arteries. The characteristic physical sign is that the
mass has an expansile pulsation. The index fingers are
placed one on either side of the mass, which enables
the diameter to be assessed. If the diameter is more
than 3 cm, this certainly suggests aneurysmal dilatation
of the aorta and if above 5 cm, the clinical diagnosis is
all but certain. Typically, the fingers are pushed apart
with each pulse and not up and down. The latter sign
suggests *transmission* of the pulsation (*see section
below*).

Usually the aneurysm is resonant to percussion
due to overlying loops of intenstine. However, an
extremely large aneurysm will displace the bowel
laterally to reach the anterior abdominal wall and will
then give a dull percussion note. Auscultation may
reveal bruits over the lower extremity of the aneurysm.
This suggests turbulent flow of blood caused by
relative stenosis at the aorto-iliac junctions.

Rectal examination may reveal a pulsatile mass
when one or both of the internal iliac arteries are
involved in the aneurysmal process.

Leakage or rupture of the aneurysm is an acute
abdominal emergency. The patient presents with the
features of massive blood loss (pale, sweating,
clammy skin, a rapid pulse and low blood pressure)
together with severe abdominal pain, lumbar pain
and marked abdominal tenderness and guarding.
Because of the low blood pressure and the associated
peri-aneurysmal haematoma, as well as the overlying
guarding, the aneurysm may be quite difficult to
palpate and, unless sought for carefully, is easy
enough to miss.

The diagnosis of aortic aneurysm is readily
confirmed by means of a plain abdominal X-ray
(*Fig.* A.1) which frequently delineates the aneurysm
because of the associated calcification in its wall.
Typically the aneurysm is seen to bulge over to the left
side of the abdomen. More accurately, an ultrasound or
computerized tomogram of the abdomen visualizes the
aneurysm and enables its length and diameter to be
measured accurately.

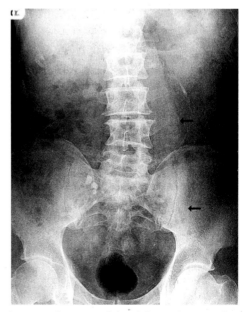

Fig. A.1. Plain X-ray of the abdomen showing a large
calcified aortic aneurysm. The outline of the calcified left
margin of the sac is indicated by the two arrows.

3. Transmission of aortic pulsations through an abdominal mass

A large intra-abdominal or retroperitoneal solid mass, pressing against the aorta, may exhibit transmitted aortic pulsation. Typical examples are a large carcinoma of the body of the stomach, a carcinoma or cyst of the pancreas and a large ovarian cyst. Indeed, when the whole abdomen is filled by a cystic mass it may be quite difficult to distinguish between such a mass and extensive ascites. Percussion, of course, is helpful since ascites gives dullness in the flanks as compared with the central dullness of a large intra-abdominal mass. The two index fingers, placed on the mass, will perceive that the pulsation is transmitted *directly forwards* from the aorta and is not expansile as would be found in an aneurysm.

4. Pulsatile liver

It is unlikely that an enlarged pulsatile liver will be mistaken for any other kind of pulsatile tumour. It occurs in cases of chronic failure of cardiac compensation, generally from mitral stenosis or tricuspid stenosis. There is associated cyanosis, oedema of the legs and ascites. It is not, however, every liver which seems to pulsate that really presents expansile pulsation. An impression of pulsation may be given by the movements transmitted directly to the liver by the hypertrophied right heart.

Harold Ellis

Abdominal rigidity

Rigidity of the abdomen is a sign of the utmost importance, since in most cases it indicates serious intra-abdominal mischief requiring immediate operation. It is the expression of a state of tonic contraction in the muscles of the abdominal wall. The responsible stimulus may be in the brain or basal ganglia, or in the territory of the six lower thoracic nerves that supply the abdominal wall, but not in the visceral sensory fibres of the sympathetic system. The extent of the rigidity will depend on the number of nerves involved, and its degree on the nature and duration of the stimulus. The analysis in the table on page 7 may be considered.

The patient should be examined lying on the back with the whole abdomen and lower thorax exposed, but the shoulders and legs well covered. The room must be warm. The examiner, seated on a level with the patient, should first watch the abdomen to see whether it moves with respiration or not, and whether one part moves more than another; at the same time he may observe other things which will help in the diagnosis, such as asymmetry of the two sides, local swelling, or the movement of coils of bowel. While watching and later when examining he should engage the patient in conversation, encouraging him to talk in order to allay nervousness and to remove any part of the rigidity which is due to a voluntary contraction. Some nervous patients, especially if the room is cold, hold their abdomens intensely rigid, and can be induced to relax only after gentle persuasion; a request to take a few deep breaths, or to draw their knees up and keep their mouths open, will often help. During this preliminary examination one hand, well warmed, may be laid gently on the abdomen and passed over its surface with a light touch that cannot possibly hurt; this manoeuvre will help to allay the patient's anxiety still further and give the examiner an idea of the extent, intensity, and constancy of the rigidity which he must later investigate in more detail.

For more exact examination the observer should sit at the patient's side facing his head, and place both hands on the abdomen, examining comparable areas of both sides, simultaneously, and taking in turn the epigastrium, right and left hypochondria, umbilical region, both flanks as far back as the erector spinae (for the rigidity of a retrocaecal appendix may only affect the posterior part of the abdominal wall), the hypogastrium, and both iliac fossae. First, the whole hand should be applied with light pressure; next, the fingers held flat should be pressed more firmly to estimate the extent of the rigidity and to discover deep tenderness; lastly, detailed examination may be made in suspected areas with the firm pressure of one or two fingers. Evidence is not complete without percussion and auscultation. A rectal examination is indispensable.

After a leisurely examination with warm hands in a warm room, during which the physician has also been able to sum up the patient, his temperament, and whether he is really ill or not, the rigidity of anxiety or cold will have been dispelled or recognized. The abdominal rigidity due to a lesion in the chest or chest wall usually involves a wide area limited to one side—a distribution most unusual with intra-abdominal mischief, which, if it has spread widely but not everywhere, tends to be limited to the upper or lower half. The extent and degree of rigidity in chest affections also vary widely during examination. Other things such as a flushed face, rapid respiration, movement of the alae nasi, or a temperature of more than 39°C (102°F), may suggest that the lesion is not abdominal, and a friction rub may be felt or heard in the chest.

Auscultation and rectal examination dispel any remaining doubts, for in chest conditions peristaltic sounds remain normal, and there is no tenderness in Douglas's pouch. Examination of the blood may show

Site of stimulus	Causative agent	Characters of rigidity
Cerebral cortex or basal ganglia	Nervousness, anticipation of pain, cold	Affects the whole abdominal wall; varies in intensity, can be abolished by appropriate means
Thoracic nerve trunks	Pleurisy; infections of the chest wall	Limited to one side of abdomen; varies in extent and degree
Nerve-endings in abdominal wall	Injury or infection of soft tissues and/or muscles of the abdominal wall	Limited to injured or infected segment
Nerve-endings in peritoneum	Irritation by any intraperitoneal foreign substance: infection, chemical irritant, or blood	Degree varies with nature of irritant and suddenness with which stimulus has arrived. Extent corresponds to area of peritoneum involved. Both degree and extent remain approximately constant during the period of examination

The extent of abdominal rigidity

a high leucocytosis, up to 30 000 or 40 000, whereas in peritonitis the count is seldom over 12 000. Chest X-rays (including a lateral film) will demonstrate the intrathoracic lesion.

Injuries of the abdominal wall, particularly those caused by run-over accidents, lead to very marked rigidity of the injured segment. Here the rigidity is not necessary to establish a diagnosis, for the injury is already known, but its degree and extent should be carefully noted. There must always be a doubt as to whether abdominal viscera are damaged as well as the walls, and this point can only be settled by careful observation. The patient is put to bed and kept warm, the pulse is charted every quarter of an hour, and the abdomen is re-examined from time to time. In the case of a mere contusion, collapse will soon disappear, the abdomen will become less rigid, and the pulse-rate will fall. If the contents of a hollow viscus have escaped, rigidity will extend beyond the area of the damaged muscles, and the signs of peritonitis will develop rapidly. An X-ray of the abdomen, in the erect position, will demonstrate free gas beneath the diaphragm. If there is internal bleeding, for example from a ruptured spleen or liver, there is pallor and progressive elevation of the pulse, together with a falling blood pressure. Dullness in the flanks (especially on the left side, in rupture of the spleen) is often detected, as blood collects in the paracolic gutters.

Peritonitis

The commonest and the most important cause of general abdominal rigidity is peritonitis, and it is a safe rule when meeting true rigidity to diagnose peritonitis till it can be excluded. Actually rigidity means no more than that the peritoneum lining the abdominal cavity is in contact with something differing from the smooth surfaces which are its normal environment. The *presence of rigidity* therefore announces a change in the coelomic cavity that is probably infective in origin. When gallstone colic is followed by rigidity of the right rectus, it means, not only that a stone is blocking the cystic duct, but that the wall of the gallbladder is inflamed. Intestinal obstruction of mechanical origin (such as that due to a band or adhesion) gives colic referred to the umbilicus, but no guarding of the muscles; local rigidity accompanying the clinical picture of intestinal obstruction indicates that there is also a local inflammatory focus such as a strangulated loop of bowel, while a more diffuse rigidity suggests changes such as a thrombosis of the superior mesenteric artery, affecting a large segment of bowel. In appendicitis, rigidity denotes that infection has spread beyond the coats of the appendix.

The *degree of rigidity* varies with the nature of the irritant, the rapidity with which the peritoneum is attacked, and the area involved. At one extreme is the rigidity of a duodenal perforation, where the abdomen is suddenly flooded with gastric contents. Here the whole abdominal wall is fixed in a contraction that can best be described as board-like: there is no respiratory movement, and no yielding to the firmest pressure. At the other extreme is the relatively minor degree of rigidity which accompanies the presence of small amounts of blood or urine in the peritoneal cavity; there is perhaps only a slightly increased resistance when the hands are pressed on the abdomen. Perforation of a gastric or duodenal ulcer produces the most intense rigidity; the escape of pancreatic enzymes in acute pancreatitis leads to less; escape of other sterile fluids, urine for instance, or blood, still less. Bacterial invasion of the peritoneum produces marked rigidity.

The degree of muscle contraction also alters during the development of a case. The board-like abdominal wall of a perforation is considerably softer after 3 or 4 hours when the peritoneum has recovered from the shock of the first insult. The slight resistance apparent when sterile urine escapes from a ruptured bladder rapidly increases as infection supervenes.

The *extent of the rigidity* usually corresponds to the area of peritoneum affected. The whole abdomen may be rigid, the upper or lower part only, one side, or a restricted part. Total rigidity should mean a total peritonitis, but because the peritoneum reacts immediately to invasion by forming adhesions which localize the mischief, a general peritonitis is only seen when an irritant or infected fluid is suddenly discharged in large quantities – as in duodenal perforation, pancreatitis, or the bursting of a large abscess or distended viscus – or when the infection is brought by the bloodstream and reaches all parts simultaneously. Occasionally, particularly in children, the reaction to a sudden infection may be excessive and the muscles contract over a wide area in response to a purely local infection, for instance of the appendix, but this exaggerated response rapidly disappears. Conversely the aged, with atrophic abdominal muscles, may exhibit only slight rigidity, even in generalized peritonitis. Local peritonitis starts around some site of infection, and as it spreads is guided by certain peritoneal watersheds, of which the most important is the attachment of the great omentum to the transverse colon, dividing the abdomen into supra- and infra-colic compartments: rigidity accompanies the infection. Thus localized rigidity is found over any inflamed organ, and as the infection and the guarding spread, they tend to involve the upper or the lower half of the abdomen as a whole. When we have mapped out the extent of the rigidity, we should, from a knowledge of the organs at that site and of the watersheds that guide the spread of infection, be able, in conjunction with the history, to make a diagnosis.

The influence of natural subdivisions in guiding intraperitoneal extension must always be taken into account. Infections in the right supracolic compartment tend to pass down between the ascending colon and the right abdominal wall, while one in the pelvis is guided by the pelvic mesocolon to the left side of the abdomen as it ascends. Thus rigidity in the right iliac fossa may indicate a leaking duodenal ulcer, and in the left may be due to a pelvic appendix.

Since the diagnosis of peritonitis in most cases means immediate operation, every endeavour must be made to confirm the diagnosis, particularly by the simple tests of percussion, auscultation and rectal examination. Percussion may reveal the outline of some dilated hollow organ, such as the caecum; it may disclose free gas escaped from a perforation as a shifting circle of resonance or a tympanitic note where liver dullness should be; it may map out an abnormal area of dullness where there is an abscess or a collection of blood; or it may indicate free fluid in the peritoneum. Auscultation is even more important, for with peritonitis peristalsis ceases: in a normal abdomen peristaltic sounds can be heard every 4–10 seconds; in obstruction they are increased in loudness, pitch and frequency; in peritonitis there is complete silence. Rectal examination nearly always reveals tenderness when there is intra-abdominal infection, even if it is distant and localized.

Other signs must be mentioned: the patient lies still, sometimes with the knees drawn up, and resists interference. The abdomen gradually becomes distended, tense and tympanitic. The tongue is brown and dry. Vomiting is to be expected at the onset of any abdominal catastrophe, but except in intestinal obstruction it usually ceases; with advancing peritonitis it reappears, and the vomit becomes first bile-stained, later brownish and faecal smelling, and is allowed to dribble from the corner of the mouth in contrast to the projectile vomiting of obstruction. There may be diarrhoea at first, but absolute constipation soon succeeds it. The temperature tends to fall; the pulse is small and rapid, rising progressively. In late stages the sunken cheeks, wide eyes and anxious expression of the patient form a characteristic feature – the Hippocratic facies.

These signs are indications of a peritonitis discovered too late, and are the heralds of approaching death. Abdominal rigidity, abdominal silence, rectal tenderness and a rising pulse are a tetrad that calls for immediate definitive treatment.

A more detailed diagnosis is usually possible when the history and other signs are taken together, but a consideration of all the alternatives is out of the question in this section. Abdominal paracentesis with a fine needle may clinch the presence of pus, blood or urine in the peritoneal cavity, but a false negative tap may delay rather than aid diagnosis. A list of the more common conditions associated with rigidity may, however, help the inquiry:

STOMACH OR DUODENUM
Perforation of peptic ulcer

GALLBLADDER
Acute cholecystitis
Rupture of gallbladder

PANCREAS
Acute pancreatitis

SMALL INTESTINE
Strangulation of a loop
Traumatic perforation
Mesenteric vascular thrombosis or embolism
Meckel's diverticulitis
Acute ileitis

LARGE INTESTINE
Appendicitis
Volvulus
Diverticulitis with perforation

PERITONEUM
Acute blood-borne peritonitis:
Streptococcal
Pneumococcal
Gonococcal

FEMALE GENERATIVE ORGANS
Twisted or perforated ovarian cyst
Ruptured ectopic pregnancy
Acute salpingitis
Torsion or red degeneration of fibroid
Perforation of uterus or posterior fornix of vagina in
attempted abortion

SPLEEN AND/OR LIVER
Traumatic rupture

AORTA
Ruptured aneurysm

Perforation of a peptic ulcer is characterized by the most sudden onset, the worst agony and the most extreme abdominal rigidity that the physician is ever likely to see. Radiation of pain to the right shoulder tip (referred pain from diaphragmatic irritation) may be experienced. Immediately afterwards the patient is motionless and speechless, in a state of obvious collapse. A few hours later pain, rigidity and shock have all diminished, and only the dramatic history and persistent abdominal and rectal tenderness may remain to indicate the seriousness of the condition.

Acute pancreatitis is seldom accompanied by the severe pain described in textbooks, or indeed by pain as bad as that of gallstone colic. The abdominal rigidity is more marked in the upper abdomen but is not profound. On the other hand, the patient shows a degree of toxaemia out of all proportion to the physical signs in the abdomen. The diagnosis is confirmed by a considerable rise in the serum amylase.

A *ruptured ectopic pregnancy* may simulate a lower abdominal peritonitis, but the signs of bleeding predominate and rigidity is not well marked. If the patient is a woman of child-bearing age who is known to have missed a period, the onset of abdominal pain and pallor suggest the diagnosis. Extravasated blood will be felt in the pelvis, together with acute tenderness on vaginal and rectal examinations.

Blue discoloration of the skin around the umbilicus, Cullen's sign, may be associated with rigidity. This discoloration is due to extravasated blood coming forwards from the retroperitoneal space. The sign is seen in ruptured kidney, leaking abdominal aneurysm and acute pancreatitis. Occasionally it is seen in ruptured ectopic pregnancy, when the blood gains entry to the subperitoneal space through the broad ligament. Although pancreatitis may produce this sign,

it is more common to see a green discoloration in the loins (Grey Turner's sign).

Harold Ellis

Abdominal swellings

(*See also* Varicose veins, Abdominal.)

This may be acute or chronic, general or local, and caused by abdominal accumulations that are gaseous, liquid or solid. They may arise in the abdominal cavity itself or in the abdominal wall.

A. Swellings in the abdominal wall

Swellings situated in the abdominal wall itself can be recognized by their superficial position, by their adherence to the skin, subcutaneous fascia or muscles, or by their failure to follow the movements of the viscera immediately underlying the abdominal wall (*Fig.* A.2).

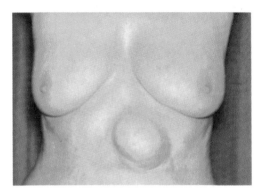

Fig. A.2. Large subcutaneous lipoma in the epigastrium. This moved freely on the abdominal wall even when the underlying muscles were tightly contracted.

It may be impossible to differentiate, for obvious reasons, an intra-abdominal mass that has become attached to the abdominal parietes either as an inflammatory or malignant process. A simple test which should be applied to all abdominal masses is to ask the patient to raise either his legs or shoulders from the couch. This procedure tightens the abdominal muscles; if the lump is intraperitoneal it disappears, but if it is situated in the abdominal wall itself it persists.

Inflammatory swelling of the abdominal wall most commonly complicates a laparotomy incision and the diagnosis is obvious. A superficial cellulitis may complicate infection of a small abrasion or hair-follicle infection. Inflammation of the abdominal wall may be secondary to an extension of an intraperitoneal abscess, particularly an appendix abscess in the right iliac fossa or, on the left side, a paracolic abscess in relation to diverticular disease of the sigmoid colon or to perforation of a carcinoma of the large bowel.

Inflammatory swelling of the umbilicus in newborn infants is rare except in primitive communities where the cord is not divided with the niceties of modern aseptic practice. Suppuration at the umbilicus in adults is not uncommon if the navel is deep and narrow.

A tender haematoma in the lower abdomen may result from rupture of the rectus abdominis muscle or tearing of the inferior epigastric artery which may occur as the result of violent cough.

Tumours of the abdominal wall are usually subcutaneous lipomas. These may be multiple and may be a feature of Dercum's disease (adiposa dolorosa). Lipomas should be carefully differentiated from irreducible umbilical or epigastric hernias containing omentum.

A desmoid tumour may arise in the lower part of the abdominal wall and occasionally malignant fibrosarcomas or melanomas may be encountered. A neoplastic deposit may occasionally be palpated at the umbilicus and represents a transcoelomic seeding, usually from a carcinoma of the stomach or large bowel (Sister Joseph's nodule; named after a Sister at the Mayo Clinic).

B. General abdominal swellings

Every medical student knows the mnemonic of the five causes of gross generalized swelling of the abdomen: Fat, Fluid, Flatus, Faeces and Fetus.

In *obesity* the abdomen may swell either in consequence of the deposit of fat in the abdominal wall itself or as the result of adipose tissue in the mesentery, the omentum, and in the extraperitoneal layer. In very obese persons it is rarely possible to diagnose the exact nature of an intra-abdominal mass by the usual clinical methods. Indeed, tumours of quite remarkable size, including the full-term fetus, may remain occult to even the most careful examiner.

Distension of the intestines with gas occurs in *intestinal obstruction* and is particularly marked in cases of volvulus of the sigmoid colon, chronic large bowel obstruction and megacolon. It also occurs in adynamic ileus. The whole of the abdomen, or, in special cases, some part of it, is distended and gives on percussion a highly resonant or tympanitic note. The outlines of the gas-distended viscera are often visible; loops of dilated small bowel, one above the other, may produce a characteristic 'ladder pattern'. The increased size of the inflated intestine may produce displacement of the other viscera; the dome of the diaphragm

is pushed up into the chest, shifting the apex beat of the heart upwards. The liver is similarly displaced. The distended *stomach* may occasionally be gross enough all but to fill the abdomen in very advanced cases of pyloric stenosis and in acute gastric dilatation.

The causes producing an accumulation of liquid in the peritoneal cavity can be listed as: congestive cardiac failure, cirrhosis, the nephrotic syndrome, carcinomatosis peritonei and tuberculous peritonitis.

In severe cases of *chronic constipation*, abdominal distension may result from accumulation of faeces in the large intestine, particularly where megacolon exists. The scybala may be felt, usually soft and plastic in the region of the ascending colon, and hard and nodular in the descending and sigmoid colon. Rectal examination often reveals an enormous accumulation of faeces. In some cases of tuberculous peritonitis semisolid inflammatory masses may bring about a general swelling of the abdomen. General swelling of the abdomen may occur in *malignant disease involving the peritoneum* due to the growth of numerous secondary nodules in addition to a concomitant ascites. *Pseudomyxoma peritonei* may follow rupture of a pseudomucinous cystadenoma of the ovary or of a mucocele of the appendix. The whole abdominal cavity becomes distended with gelatinous material.

C. Local intra-abdominal swellings

These may be due to some general cause or to a mass arising in a specific viscus.

1. Due to general causes

Causes which ordinarily produce general swelling of the abdomen may sometimes give rise to only a local swelling. Thus with *encysted ascites* left after an acute diffuse peritonitis or accompanying tuberculous peritonitis, an accumulation of fluid bounded by adhesions between the adjacent viscera may be found in any part of the peritoneal cavity, most often in the flanks or pelvis. A reliable history may be a clue to the nature of such a mass although its cause may not be revealed until a laparotomy has been performed.

Abdominal swellings may occur in *tuberculous peritonitis* resulting from the rolled-up, matted and infiltrated omentum, doughy masses of adherent intestine, or enlarged tuberculous mesenteric lymph nodes. The amount of ascites in such cases varies considerably from a gross degree to almost complete absence (the obliterative form). Discovery of a tuberculous focus elsewhere in the body is support for the diagnosis.

Hydatid cysts may occur in any part of the abdominal cavity. They are usually single. The liver, particularly the right lobe, is the most common situation; more rarely the spleen, omentum, mesentery or peritoneum. The cyst grows slowly and is spherical except in so far as it is moulded by the pressure of adjacent structures. It contains a clear fluid in which may be found hooklets, scolices and secondary or daughter cysts detached from the walls of the parent cyst. Unless large enough to cause mechanical pressure, the single hydatid cyst gives rise to little pain or indeed to any complaint of any kind. It may produce a smooth, rounded, tense bulging of the overlying abdominal wall. It is dull on percussion, and it may yield a 'hydatid thrill' as may any other cyst; this thrill is the vibratory sensation experienced by the rest of the hand when, with the whole hand laid flat over the tumour, a central finger is percussed. Occasionally there may be pain and fever due to inflammation within these cysts, and rupture into the peritoneal cavity may cause a severe anaphylactic reaction. Rupture of a hydatid cyst of the liver into a bile duct may cause jaundice due to biliary obstruction by daughter cysts. Hydatid disease is rare except in countries where the inhabitants live in close association with dogs that are the hosts of *Taenia echinococcus* (Australasia, South America, Greece, Cyprus, and, in the British Isles, North Wales). About one-quarter of patients demonstrate eosinophilia. A complement fixation test gives a high degree of accuracy. X-rays of the abdomen may reveal calcification of the cyst wall in long-standing cases. Ultrasonography and computerized tomography will delineate the cysts with accuracy even if they are not calcified.

Any part of the abdomen may swell from the formation of an *abscess*. A subphrenic abscess following a general peritonitis is occasionally large enough to produce an upper abdominal swelling. The patient is usually seriously ill with a swinging fever, rapid pulse, leucocytosis and all the general manifestations of toxaemia. However, in this antibiotic era, more and more examples are being seen of a more insidious and chronic progress of the disease, with onset delayed weeks or even many months after the initial peritoneal infection. X-ray examination together with screening of the diaphragms is extremely useful and at least 90 per cent of patients with subphrenic infection have some abnormality on this investigation. On the affected side the diaphragm is raised and its sharp definition is lost. Its mobility on screening is diminished or absent. There is frequently a pleural effusion, collapse of the lung base or evidence of pneumonitis. About 25 per cent of patients have gas below the diaphragm, frequently associated with a fluid level. This gas is usually derived from a perforated abdominal viscus but occasionally is formed by gas-producing organisms. On the left side, gas under the diaphragm may be confused with the gastric bubble. An important differential feature is that the gas shadow of the stomach rarely reaches the lateral abdominal wall, but if there is doubt, a mouthful of barium is given in order to demarcate the stomach. Ultrasonography and/or computerized tomography usually clinch the diagnosis.

Pus may localize in either the right or left paracolic gutter or iliac fossa. On the right side this commonly follows a ruptured appendix or occasionally a perforated duodenal ulcer. On the left, a perforation of an inflamed diverticulum or carcinoma of the sigmoid colon is the usual cause. A large pelvic abscess frequently extends above the pubis or into one or other iliac fossa from the pelvis and can be palpated abdominally as well as on pelvic or rectal examination. About 75 per cent result from gangrenous appendicitis and the rest follow gynaecological infections, pelvic surgery, or any general peritonitis.

2. The regional diagnosis of local abdominal swellings

For clinical purposes the abdomen may be subdivided into nine regions by two vertical lines drawn upwards from the mid-inguinal point midway between the anterior superior iliac spine and the symphysis pubis, and by two horizontal lines, the upper one passing through the lowest points of the 10th ribs (the subcostal line), the other drawn at the highest points of the iliac crests (*Fig.* A.3).

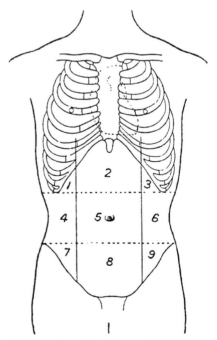

Fig A.3. The regions of the abdomen, for the significance of the numerals, *see* the adjoining table.

The three median areas thus mapped out are named, from above downwards, the epigastric, umbilical and hypogastric (or suprapubic) regions; the six lateral areas are, from above downwards, the right and left hypochondriac, lumbar and iliac regions.

The viscera, or portions of viscera, commonly situated in the areas thus demarcated are given in the accompanying table.

The abdominal swellings that may be felt in and about these nine regions, excluding the tumours situated in the abdominal wall itself that have already been described, are as follows:

A.   RIGHT HYPOCHONDRIAC REGION

Most tumours in this area are connected with the liver or gallbladder and their differential diagnosis is discussed under Liver, Enlargement of (p. 251) and Gallbladder, Palpable (p. 132)

A mistake easily made is to regard the firm and rounded swelling produced by the upper segment of the right rectus abdominis muscle, especially in a well-developed subject, as a tumour of the liver or gallbladder.

Tumours in connection with the hepatic flexure of the colon, scybalous collections in the hepatic flexure region, or the head of an intussusception may present as masses in this area.

B.   EPIGASTRIC REGION

Enlargement of the *liver* may be felt in this area, and indeed it is common to feel the normal liver in this region, especially in infants and in adults with an acute costal angle. The dilated *stomach* produced by pyloric stenosis in either children or adults may present as a visible swelling demonstrating waves of peristalsis travelling from left to right. A succussion splash is usually elicited. Tumours of the stomach, apart from malignant growth, are rare. At the turn of this century a hair ball or trichobezoar was frequently encountered as an epigastric mass in hysterical girls who chewed and swallowed their hair, which then formed an exact mould of the stomach. Hairballs are only rarely encountered these days and modern textbooks hardly mention them; however, as fashions and hair styles change they may reappear on the clinical scene (*Fig. A.4*). Other foreign bodies are sometimes ingested by mental defectives and form a palpable mass. In congenital pyloric stenosis a tumour the size of a small marble is palpable at the right border of the right rectus.

The *transverse colon* usually passes across the upper part of the umbilical area and may be palpated when it is the site of a carcinoma, when it is impacted

The normal contents of the abdominal regions

1. *Right hypochondriac*	2. *Epigastric*
Liver	Liver
Gallbladder	Stomach and pylorus
Hepatic flexure of colon	Transverse colon
Right kidney	Omentum
Right suprarenal gland	Pancreas
	Duodenum
	Kidneys
	Suprarenal glands
	Aorta
	Lymph nodes

3. *Left hypochondriac*	4. *Right lumbar*
Liver	Riedel's lobe of the liver
Stomach	Ascending colon
Splenic flexure of colon	Small intestine
Spleen	Right kidney
Tail of pancreas	
Left kidney	
Left suprarenal gland	

5. *Umbilical*	6. *Left lumbar*
Stomach	Descending colon
Duodenum	Small intestine
Transverse colon	Left kidney
Omentum	
Urachus	
Small intestine	
Aorta	
Lymph nodes	

7. *Right iliac fossa*	8. *Hypogastric*
Caecum	Small intestine
Vermiform appendix	Sigmoid flexure
Lymph nodes	Distended bladder
	Urachus
	Enlarged uterus and
	adnexa

9. *Left iliac fossa*
Sigmoid flexure
Lymph nodes

with faeces, or when it is distended by a large-bowel obstruction placed distal to it.

Swellings in connection with the *omentum* may be due to tuberculous peritonitis or, more commonly, due to infiltration with secondary malignant deposits.

Swellings arising from the *pancreas* push forward from the depths of the abdominal cavity towards the epigastric and the upper part of the umbilical areas, and present themselves as vaguely palpable deeply seated masses. They have the stomach, or the stomach and colon, in front of them and are fixed to the posterior abdominal wall, thus moving but little on

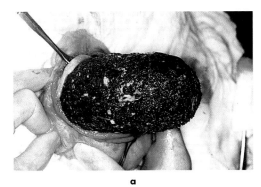

a

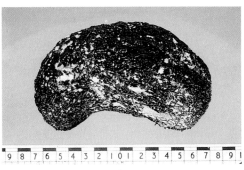

9 8 7 6 5 4 3 2 1 0 1 2 3 4 5 6 7 8 9 1

b

Fig. A.4. Gastric hairball. This formed a large, mobile epigastric mass in a young married woman with long hair, *a*, shows the mass being removed at gastrotomy. *b*, Demonstrates the specimen.

respiration. They may transmit a non-expansile pulsation from the subjacent aorta. Unless extremely large, such swellings are resonant on percussion, due to the overlying air-filled gut. A pancreatic swelling may be carcinomatous, in which case wasting, anaemia, and jaundice are likely to be observed. There may be clay-coloured stools and dark urine and it is important to note that frequently the onset of jaundice is preceded by deeply placed abdominal pain, or pain in the back. Glycosuria of recent origin in an elderly patient also raises suspicion of a pancreatic carcinoma. In about half the patients with jaundice due to carcinomatous obstruction the gallbladder is palpably distended (Courvoisier's law). Occasionally the mass may result from chronic pancreatitis; the swollen pancreas of acute pancreatitis has only exceptionally been palpated before laparotomy.

Pancreatic cysts are the pancreatic swellings which are most commonly palpable. Only 20 per cent are true cysts; these are either single or multiple retention cysts which usually result from chronic pancreatitis, neoplastic cysts (cystadenoma and cystadenocarcinoma) and the rare congenital polycystic

disease of the pancreas and hydatid cyst of the pancreas. Far more often the cysts are not in the pancreas itself but comprise a collection of fluid sealed off in the lesser sac due to closure of the foramen of Winslow (pseudocyst of the pancreas). This may occur after trauma to the pancreas, following acute pancreatitis, or, less commonly, resulting from perforation of a posterior gastric ulcer. They may reach an enormous size and fill the whole upper part of the abdomen.

Retroperitoneal cysts are rare. The majority arise from remnants of the mesonephric (Wolffian) duct and occur in adult women. Others are teratomatous, lymphangiomatous or dermoid.

Retroperitoneal tumours (apart from those arising in the pancreas, suprarenal or kidney) originate in the mesenchymal tissues, the sympathetic chain and the para-aortic lymph nodes.

Swellings in connection with the *duodenum* are excessively rare. They may result from an inflammatory mass developing around a penetrating duodenal ulcer or be due to a duodenal malignant tumour, but the latter is a pathological curiosity. Those in connection with the *kidneys* and *suprarenal glands* are found in the epigastrium only if very large. Their diagnosis is considered below.

Enlargement of the *spleen* may bring its notched anterior edge into the epigastric area; a splenic swelling always lies in contact with the anterior wall of the abdomen (*see* SPLENOMEGALY).

Lymph nodes, which are numerous in the para-aortic retroperitoneal tissues and in the mesentery, may become palpable in the reticuloses, tuberculous peritonitis, or secondary malignant disease as nodulated chains or masses.

C.   LEFT HYPOCHONDRIAC REGION

An abnormal lobe or a tumour in the left lobe of the *liver* may appear as a superficial tumour in this area.

Much of the *stomach* normally lies in the left hypochondrium; the diagnosis of gastric swelling has been considered above and a gastric tumour is commonly felt in this region. On physical signs alone it must be differentiated from a swelling of the adjoining *spleen*. A barium-meal X-ray examination, ultrasound or CT scan help considerably in differentiating between a gastric and a splenic swelling.

The diagnosis of a tumour of the splenic flexure of the *colon*, whether scybalous or malignant, is arrived at in the same way as a case of a tumour of the hepatic flexure or transverse colon (*see* (A) and (B)).

The diagnosis of the various causes of enlargement of the *spleen* is discussed under SPLENOMEGALY. The distinguishing features are that it comes down from under the left costal margin in direct contact with the anterior abdominal wall (and is therefore dull on percussion), descends on inspiration, has a smooth surface, and a notch may be palpable on its inner margin. A splenic swelling may be identified on a plain X-ray of the abdomen and differentiated from a renal mass by means of pyelography. A barium-meal examination may show displacement and indentation of the adjacent stomach. Ultrasound or CT scan will clinch the diagnosis.

Tumours of the *pancreas* may project into the left hypochondrium as may retroperitoneal tumours and cysts (*see* (B)).

Tumours of the left *kidney* and *suprarenal gland* have the stomach and colon in front of them and therefore, unless extremely large, are resonant on percussion. Since they arise in the loin, these masses can usually be balloted by bimanual palpation.

D.   RIGHT LUMBAR REGION

Occasionally a congenital projection of the *liver*, known as Riedel's lobe, may appear as a superficial tumour continuous with the liver above it in this zone. It may be mistaken for a dilated gallbladder.

The *ascending colon* may be palpable due to contained faecal masses, owing to thickening as a result of long-standing colitis, Crohn's disease or hyperplastic tuberculosis, or due to malignant disease.

The ascending colon can be felt in acute or chronic *ileocaecal and ileocolic intussusception* as a sausage-shaped tumour, at first situated in the right flank, then moving across the abdomen above the umbilicus and finally down the left flank into the pelvis. The vast majority of these cases occur in infants or young children commonly aged between 3 and 12 months. Boys are affected twice as often as girls. The history is of paroxysms of abdominal colic typified by screaming and pallor. There is vomiting and usually the passage of blood and mucus per rectum, giving the characteristic 'red-currant-jelly stool'. Rectal examination nearly always reveals this typical feature and rarely the tip of the intussusception can be felt. In infants there is usually no obvious cause, but the mesenteric lymph nodes in these cases are invariably enlarged. In adults a polyp, carcinoma or an inverted Meckel's diverticulum may form the apex of the intussusception.

Tumours in connection with the *right kidney* and *suprarenal gland* usually appear deep down in this region, having the ascending colon and small intestine in front of them. They can be lifted forwards *en masse* from behind by a hand placed at the back of the loin and thus palpated bimanually. For their diagnosis *see* KIDNEY, PALPABLE. The lower pole of the right kidney can

be felt in many normal persons on deep abdominal palpation, especially in thin females. When abnormally low and mobile, the whole of the otherwise normal kidney may be palpable. Its shape and consistency are characteristic. Renal swellings move on respiration and, unless very large, are resonant on percussion due to the anteriorly related gut. However, Riedel's lobe of the liver, an enlarged gallbladder, masses in the ascending colon and secondary deposits in the omentum have all been mistaken for it, although they are more superficially placed and lie in contact with the anterior abdominal wall. Other wandering masses, e.g. those arising from the ovary, Fallopian tube and mesentery, as well as hydatid cysts, are all liable to the same error of identification.

Imaging, by means of ultrasound or CT scanning, is invaluable in assistance with the differential diagnosis.

E.   UMBILICAL REGION

The grossly dilated *stomach* resulting from long-standing pyloric obstruction may occupy the umbilical region; indeed it may descend below it down into the pelvis.

Tumours in connection with the *transverse colon* have been considered in (B) and (D) above.

Tumours in connection with the *omentum* are common in this region; those arising from the *small intestine* are much rarer, although the thickened small bowel in Crohn's disease may form a palpable mass.

Swellings arising from the *kidneys*, *suprarenals*, *pancreas*, *retroperitoneal tissues*, *para-aortic nodes* and *mesentery* may all present themselves in the deeper parts of the umbilical region, usually as more or less fixed masses arising from or connected with the posterior wall of the abdomen.

The *aorta* bifurcates half an inch below and to the left of the umbilicus (at the level of the 4th lumbar vertebra). In thin patients, pulsation of the normal aorta can often be felt and indeed seen in this region and may lead to the incorrect diagnosis of an abdominal aneurysm. Careful examination, however, will show that this pulsation is no more than a throbbing, up-and-down movement, and is not laterally expansile. Aneurysm of the abdominal aorta forms an expansile mass situated above the umbilicus itself and may be accompanied by pain in the back from erosion of the bodies of the lumbar vertebrae. Often X-rays of the abdomen in such cases will reveal calcification in the aneurysmal wall. Ultrasound and computerized tomography enable accurate delineation of the size and extent of the aneurysm. They are also valuable in the visualization of the other retroperitoneal masses enumerated above.

F.   LEFT LUMBAR REGION

An enlarged *spleen* (*see* (C)) may protrude into this area. It forms a firm mass in contact with the abdominal wall and its dullness to percussion continues with its thoracic dullness which extends back up into the axilla along the line of the 9th or 10th ribs. Tumours in connection with the *right kidney*, the *right suprarenal gland* and the *descending colon* give similar features to those considered in (C) above.

G.   RIGHT ILIAC FOSSA

An inflammatory mass in this region is most commonly associated with an *appendix abscess*. Less commonly there may be a *paracaecal abscess* in relation to a perforated carcinoma of the caecum or a solitary caecal benign ulcer. A *pyosalpinx* may result from salpingitis and rarely, inflammatory swellings may arise in connection with suppurating *iliac lymph nodes* or a *psoas abscess*.

An important differential diagnosis is between an appendix mass and a carcinoma of the caecum. Usually in the former there is a preceding episode of an acute abdominal pain, typical of appendicitis, with fever and leucocytosis. The inflammatory mass subsides progressively over 2 or 3 weeks and the occult blood test in the stools is negative. A carcinoma of the caecum may be suspected if there is a preceding history of bowel disturbance in a middle-aged or elderly patient, if the mass fails to resolve rapidly, and if the occult blood test in the stools is repeatedly positive. If there is any clinical doubt, a barium-enema X-ray examination should be carried out and, if necessary, resort made to laparotomy.

It is not at all rare for a soft 'squelchy' caecum to be palpable in a perfectly normal thin, usually female, subject.

Occasionally a grossly distended *gallbladder* may project down as far as the right iliac fossa and a low-lying *kidney* may form a palpable mass in this region. An *ovarian tumour* or *cyst* or a pedunculated *fibroid* of the *uterus* may project into this area.

H.   HYPOGASTRIC REGION

The commonest mass to be felt in this region is the distended *bladder*. This may reach as high as, or slightly above, the umbilicus. Not uncommonly this midline structure tilts over to one or other side. A distended bladder has been tapped as ascites, operated upon as an ovarian cyst or fibroid, or mistaken for the pregnant uterus. No diagnostic opinion should be advanced, and no operative procedure undertaken respecting a tumour in this situation, until the bladder has been emptied, either by voluntary micturition or by the passing of a catheter.

Abdominal swellings arising from the *uterus*, *ovaries*, *Fallopian tubes* and *uterine ligaments* may all rise up out of the pelvis and present themselves as swellings in this region; as they grow larger they may be spread into any part of the abdomen. While they remain comparatively small and are manifestedly connected with some intrapelvic organ, their origin, is not difficult to determine. However, when they have extended into the abdomen or have acquired a long pedicle, or have become fixed by adhesions to some distant part of the abdominal wall or to some other viscus, these pelvic tumours may give rise to signs and symptoms which bear no relation to pelvic disease. In such cases they may only be correctly diagnosed at laparotomy. The discerning clinician will always remember the possibility of pregnancy in every female patient between the menarche and menopause.

Tumours of ileal Crohn's disease arising in the *small intestine* may be felt in the hypogastric area.

The *urachus* is a fibrous cord running in the middle line in front of the peritoneum from the fundus of the bladder to the umbilicus. Occasionally it becomes the seat of cyst formation, more often in women than in men. The urachal cyst is a rounded tumour lying between the umbilicus and the pubic symphysis, which occasionally becomes infected.

I.   LEFT ILIAC FOSSA

The *pelvic colon* can often be felt in normal subjects as a tube-like cord either when empty and in spasm or else when distended with faecal masses. This region is a common site for carcinoma of the colon and there are usually symptoms of chronic intestinal obstruction, or bowel disturbance with the passage of blood and mucus in the stools. It is clinically impossible to differentiate between such a mass and that associated with diverticular disease of the sigmoid colon. Similarly a paracolic abscess in this region may equally well be associated with suppuration of an inflamed colonic diverticulum or a perforating carcinoma. Rarely such an abscess may be due to perforation of the tip of a long *appendix* passing over the left iliac fossa, or as an extreme rarity due to local perforation of a left-sided appendix in transposition of the viscera. The diagnosis would be suggested by finding the cardiac apex beat to lie on the *right* side.

Harold Ellis

Amenorrhoea

The age at which menstruation first appears is variable, being influenced by climatic and racial peculiarities; in UK about 13 years may be taken as the average. About one girl in a hundred does not menstruate until the age of 16 years and it is usual to wait until then before becoming concerned. When the menstrual flow has not become established it is usual to speak of 'primary amenorrhoea', while premature cessation of the flow after it has once been regularly established is known as 'secondary amenorrhoea'. From the table of the causes of amenorrhoea below it will be seen that some of them must of necessity give rise to the primary variety, while others more commonly produce the secondary. In investigating a case one should ascertain first whether the condition is primary or secondary, and next whether it is real or only apparent. The latter condition, known as *cryptomenorrhoea*, implies that the menstrual flow takes place but is unable to escape externally because there is some closure of a part of the genital canal. The congenital form of cryptomenorrhoea is the only variety met with commonly, acquired closure of a part of the genital canal being very rare. Stenosis of the vagina may result from injury or infection, but a small sinus is usually left which suffices for the escape of the menstrual fluid. We are led to suspect cryptomenorrhoea when the patient volunteers the statement that she has pelvic pain, headache, and possibly vomiting, of monthly occurrence – in fact the usual menstrual symptoms, unaccompanied by any visible flow. Secondary sexual development is normal. A not uncommon deciding symptom is the occurrence of acute retention of urine, the result of elongation and stretching of the urethra by a haematocolpos. A physical examination should be made, including abdominal palpation, inspection of the vulva and a recto-abdominal bimanual examination. The common form is that in which the lower end of the vagina is imperforate, the hymen usually being visible on the outer side of the occluding membrane through which a dark blue cystic swelling protrudes. The complete examination will reveal a fluctuating swelling reaching from the vulva to the pelvic brim, above which the uterus can often be palpated and moved about. Distension of the vagina or *haematocolpos* is complete in this case, but may be partial where the lower part of the vagina is absent, and then is likely to be accompanied by distension of the uterus (haematometra) and haematosalpinx. It is important to make out whether the uterus and Fallopian tubes are distended with menstrual products along with the distended vagina, for in the presence of haematosalpinges the uterus and tubes may take longer to recover following surgical drainage. Congenital absence of the vagina can only be inferred from local physical examination. Since the vulva is normally formed and a slight depression is present, only a careful examination, if necessary under anaesthesia, will reveal absence of the vagina. Very often the patient only presents at the time of marriage, complaining of dyspareunia. Complete absence of the vagina is nearly always associated with the absence also of the uterus which means that amenorrhoea will be permanent and there is no hope of child-bearing.

Acquired cryptomenorrhoea produces the same symptoms and requires the same kind of investigation as the congenital cases. Acquired closure of the vagina following the vaginitis of specific fevers may occur in infancy, and then produces primary amenorrhoea.

Causes of apparent amenorrhoea

CONGENITAL
Imperforate vagina
Imperforate hymen
Absence of the vagina
Imperforate cervix
Double uterus with retention
Haematocolpos
Haematometra
Haematosalpinx

ACQUIRED
Closure of the vagina
Due to specific fevers
Due to injury

Closure of the cervix
Due to injury
Following operations

Causes of real amenorrhoea

PHYSIOLOGICAL
Before puberty
After the menopause
During pregnancy
During lactation

PATHOLOGICAL
Generative system
Congenital absence of uterus
Congenital absence of ovaries (rare)
Uterine hypoplasia of infantile type
Uterine hypoplasia of adult type
Ovarian agenesis
Gonadal dysgenesis (Turner's syndrome)
Destruction of both ovaries by double ovarian growths, pelvic inflammation, operation, irradiation
Hysterectomy

Circulatory system
Anaemia
Leukaemia
Hodgkin's disease

Wasting conditions
Malignant growths
Tuberculosis

Prolonged suppuration
Diabetes
Late stages of nephritis
Late stage of some forms of heart disease
Late stage of cirrhosis of the liver

Nervous system
Cretinism
Various forms of insanity
Suggestion-fear of pregnancy (pseudocyesis)
Anorexia nervosa or loss of weight

Altered internal secretions
Primary hypothalamic-pituitary failure
Following oral contraceptives (post-pill)
Anterior pituitary failure (Simmond's disease)
Absence of ovarian hormones
Certain rare functioning tumours of the ovary: arrhenoblastoma; granulosa-cell tumour
Stein-Leventhal syndrome (polycystic ovary)
Myxoedema
Addison's disease
Thyrotoxicosis
Adrenal hyperplasia
Adrenal cortical tumours
Acromegaly
Obesity
Dystrophia adipose-genitalis (Fröhlich's syndrome)
Change of habits and environment causing emotional strain
Climatic changes
Dietetic deficiencies, the result of attempts to slim

Toxic
During and after specific fevers
Chronic poisoning by lead, mercury, morphine, alcohol

Real amenorrhoea may be: (1) Primary with delayed onset; (2) Primary and permanent; (3) Secondary. If menstruation has once been established regularly, it is clear that there cannot be any serious congenital anomaly of the generative system; the uterus and ovaries must at least have been present and functioning. We must then make a systematic examination of the generative, circulatory, nervous and endocrine systems, in order to learn by a process of exclusion which group of causes we have to deal with. If, however, the amenorrhoea is primary and real, that is, the patient has no symptoms, our examination must first be directed towards finding out whether the essential organs, namely uterus and ovaries, are present, and are normal in size and shape as far as a bimanual examination can ascertain. If necessary, an anaesthetic may be given for this purpose. In doubtful cases laparoscopy with ovarian biopsy may by helpful.

Certain rare inter-sex cases may present with primary amenorrhoea. They include Turner's syndrome (gonadal dysgenesis) in which there is also dwarfism, web-neck, cubitus valgus (increase in the carrying angle of the elbows), and an XO sex-chromosome pattern; testicular feminization (which is in reality androgen insensitivity) in which the form is female with well-developed breasts but absent or sparse pubic and axillary hair and the gonad, which may be found in the groin or in the abdomen, is a testicle that should be removed because of the risk of malignancy; and ovarian dysgenesis in which there are streak ovaries, an infantile uterus and absent secondary sexual characteristics (*Figs*. A.5–A.8). In these cases a buccal smear for sex chromatin and a chromosome analysis on a sample of peripheral blood are indicated. In ovarian dysgenesis there is a chromatin negative smear but only 45 chromosomes, a single X chromosome (XO); in testicular feminization the smear is also chromatin negative but there are 46 chromosomes, XY. Gonadal biopsy is also helpful in diagnosis. When the secondary sexual development is absent or very poor and there is no chromosome abnormality, further investigation becomes necessary. This includes assay of gonadotrophin and suprarenal excretion and of thyroid function.

Apart from congenital anomalies remarkably few lesions of the generative organs produce amenorrhoea; only those diseases which destroy both ovaries completely or render the uterus functionless can cause amenorrhoea, and under this heading we find only bilateral malignant ovarian growths and complete removal of the endometrium by too vigorous curetting (Asherman's syndrome). A tumour destroying one ovary has no effect on menstruation, provided the other is present and functioning. The presence of two tumours in the abdomen symmetrically arranged with regard to the uterus will sometimes permit of the diagnosis of double ovarian destruction if there is amenorrhoea in addition, especially in the case of malignant growths, but commonly one tumour is much larger than the other and the double nature of the lesion cannot be established on clinical examination. Pelvic ultrasonography or CT scan will visualize the situation, which may then be confirmed at laparoscopy and/or laparotomy. The common benign tumours, cystic adenomas, even if bilateral, do not destroy the ovarian tissue and consequently do not produce amenorrhoea. On rare occasions bilateral fibromas of the ovaries may destroy all ovarian tissue and therefore be the cause of amenorrhoea.

In the absence of the above-mentioned gross lesions, which are rare causes of amenorrhoea, most cases, other than those due to pregnancy, will be found to be the result of deficient secretion of gonadotrophins by the anterior pituitary lobe or failure of the ovaries to secrete oestrogen and progesterone (ovarian failure). Pituitary failure may be due to a tumour but is more commonly due to inhibition of hypothalamic releasing factor from extreme loss of weight as the result of severe dieting or anorexia nervosa, from emotional disturbances, or from taking the combined oestrogen-progestagen contraceptive pill. The thy-

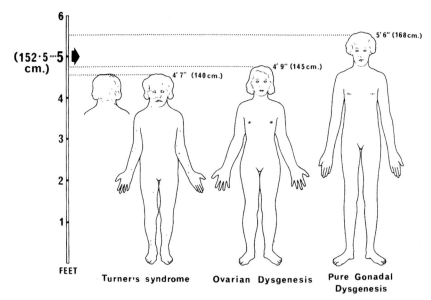

Fig. A.5. (*Professor Paul Polani.*)

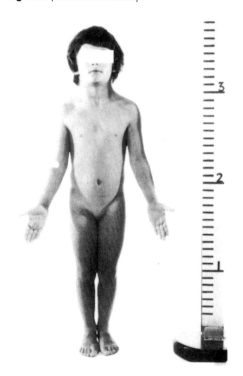

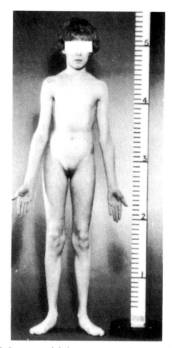

Fig. A.7. Pure gonadal dysgenesis. (*Professor Paul Polani.*)

Fig. A.6. Turner's syndrome. (*Professor Paul Polani.*) Note the webbing of the neck and the increased carrying angle at the elbows.

roid, or more rarely the suprarenal glands, may be at fault. In some cases the evidence of the failure of certain glands is clear, in others it is difficult to be sure. Such investigations as endometrial biopsy, blood and urine hormone estimations, basal temperature charts, vaginal smear tests, the basal metabolic rate estimation, sugar tolerance tests and X-ray examination of the pituitary fossa may all be useful in determining the main gland at fault.

Gonadotrophin estimations in the urine indicate premature ovarian failure when the gonadotrophins

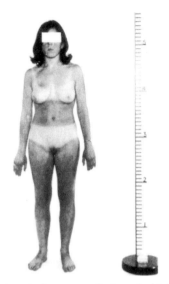

Fig. A.8. Testicular feminization. (*Professor Paul Polani.*)

(particularly FSH) reach menopausal levels. If gonado-trophin excretion is low or normal, the ovaries are probably still responsive and induction of ovulation is likely to be successful. Although severe loss of weight is associated with amenorrhoea, young women who are subjected to emotional strain may suffer temporarily from amenorrhoea and suddenly gain in weight. Women who have long intervals between periods (oligomenorrhoea) from puberty are particularly liable to have prolonged amenorrhoea, and therefore inability to conceive, when they stop taking the contraceptive pill, which, for them, is contra-indicated (post-pill amenorrhoea).

Amenorrhoea may be associated with galactor-rhoea. Typically the syndrome occurs postpartum but it may follow the contraceptive pill or arise without an apparent cause. Raised serum prolactin levels are found, probably because of a lowered secretion by the hypothalamus of prolactin-inhibiting factor.

Simmonds' disease (or Sheehan's syndrome) is a rare cause of pituitary failure. It commonly follows very severe postpartum haemorrhage causing necrosis of most of the anterior pituitary gland through venous thrombosis. It is accompanied by failure of lactation, loss of body hair, wasting and lowered basal metabolism, and the periods fail to be re-established.

An arrhenoblastoma is a very rare ovarian tumour causing virilism in the female, often a young adult woman. In addition to amenorrhoea and atrophy of the breasts, there is growth of hair on the face, chest and abdomen, deepening of the voice and enlargement of the clitoris. 17–Ketosteroid excretion is normal. Granulosa cell tumours of the ovary secrete oestrogen

which gives rise to bouts of amenorrhoea interpersed with prolonged irregular vaginal bleeding.

The various disorders of the circulatory, nervous and other systems that may be associated with amenorrhoea are discussed under the headings of other symptoms. With regard to pregnancy, which is the commonest of all causes of secondary amenorrhoea, it may be formulated as an axiom that an otherwise healthy woman who has had perfectly regular menstruation is probably pregnant if she suddenly gets amenorrhoea. Nevertheless, the presence of pregnancy must never be assumed without careful consideration of the history, combined with a complete physical examination. The diagnosis of pregnancy is made upon a complex of symptoms rather than upon any one; but the combination of amenorrhoea, secretion to be squeezed from the breasts, morning sickness, vaginal discoloration and uterine enlargement can only mean pregnancy in the majority of cases; the addition of fetal movements and the fetal heart sounds makes the diagnosis absolute. Immunological pregnancy tests and ultrasound examination are essential when the diagnosis is in doubt.

Summary of the investigation in a case of amenorrhoea

Amenorrhoea may arise in any one of four levels in the body. They are: (1) the hypothalamus; (2) the anterior pituitary; (3) the ovary and (4) the uterus and vagina. To discover at which level lies the cause a careful history and thorough clinical examination should first be done. Next the endogenous blood oestrogen and the serum prolactin levels should be measured. A progestational agent which has no oestrogenic activity, such as 200 mg progesterone in oil, should be given intramuscularly or 10 mg medroxyprogesterone acetate (Provera) by mouth for 5 days. If bleeding occurs within 2–7 days after cessation of the treatment it shows that there is a functional uterus with reactive endometrium and a patent cervix and vagina. Providing there is no galactorrhoea and the serum prolactin is normal (100–620 mU/1) no further investigation is necessary. Galactorrhoea or a raised serum prolactin means that a CT scan should be taken or that the sella turcica should be X-rayed for evidence of prolactinoma. If bleeding does not follow the giving of progestagen, there may be an abnormality of the uterus or vagina, such as congenital absence, vaginal atresia, testicular feminization or Asherman's syndrome. Confirmation of these conditions is obtained by priming the endometrium with oestrogen (20 μg ethinyl oestradiol daily for 21 days) before adding progestagen and no bleeding will occur. If bleeding takes place with oestrogen and progestagen, but not with progestagen alone, the fault may lie in the ovary, pituitary or hypothalamus. Now the serum gonadotrophins should be measured by radio-immunoassay. The normal range of FSH is 0.5–5 U/1 and for LH 3–12 U/1. A raised FSH and LH level indicates ovarian failure with absent follicles from a premature menopause, Turner's syndrome, other forms of ovarian dysgenesis, ovarian agenesis (very rare) or the resistant ovary syndrome, a rare condition in which the gonadotrophins are raised, there is amenorrhoea and the ovary contains follicles which do not react to gonadotrophins. The most common situation is that in which the pelvic organs, prolactin level, skull X-ray and gonadotrophins are normal, the condition then being hypothalamic in origin. This commonly follows weight loss or the contraceptive pill. No treatment is needed. Ovulation can be induced in order to produce pregnancy, but not otherwise.

N. Patel

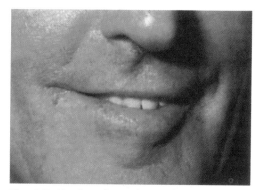

Fig. A.9. Hereditary haemorrhagic telangiectasia (Osler-Rendu-Weber syndrome). (*King Edward VII Hospital, Windsor.*)

Angioma and telangiectasia

An angioma is a proliferation of blood vessels and occurs as a developmental or an acquired vascular abnormality (*see Table* A.1).

Table A.1. Angioma and telangiectasia

Developmental
Vascular birthmarks
  Naevus flammeus
  Cavernous haemangioma (strawberry naevus)
  Capillary haemangioma (port wine stain)
Blue rubber-bleb naevus syndrome
Hereditary haemorrhagic telangiectasia (*Fig.* A.9)
Generalized essential telangiectasia
Ataxia-telangiectasia
Acquired
Cherry angiomas (Campbell de Morgan spots)
Venous lakes
Angiokeratoma
  of Fordyce (scrotum and vulva)
  Anderson–Fabry disease
Pyogenic granuloma
Glomus tumour
Kaposi's sarcoma
Acquired telangiectases (spider naevi)
  Pregnancy
  Hyperthyroidism
  Liver disease
  Carcinoid
  Systemic mastocytosis
  X-radiation skin damage
  Topical corticosteroid abuse
  Rosacea
  Poikiloderma
  Scleroderma (matt telangiectases)
  Dermatomyositis
  Lupus erythematosus

Developmental vascular abnormalities

Vascular birthmarks. Transient small salmon-pink macular birthmarks—naevus flammeus—are remarkably common and are thought to occur in over 50 per cent of live births, affecting the sexes equally. They are most commonly on the nape of the neck, forehead or eyelids. Those on the face usually resolve within months, but the flame naevus on the nape of the neck more often persists into adult life. More significant and disfiguring vascular malformations are also common. They are often not apparent at birth but develop during the first month of life. Further classification is made depending on the size of blood vessels affected (capillary or cavernous haemangiomas) but in practice the lesions are often of mixed type.

Cavernous haemangioma (*Fig.* A.10) or 'strawberry naevus' comprises large vessels proliferating in the dermis and protruding, sometimes alarmingly, from the skin surface. The overlying epidermis may ulcerate with minor trauma, causing brisk bleeding. A strawberry naevus may become very large and disfiguring. It

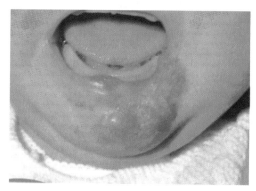

Fig. A.10. Cavernous haemangioma. (*Westminster Hospital.*)

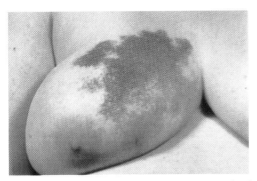

Fig. A.11. Port wine stain over the breast. (*Dr Richard Staughton.*)

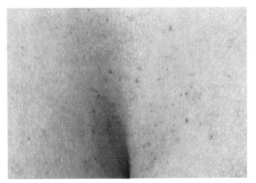

Fig. A.12. Anderson–Fabry disease involving skin above the natal cleft. (*Westminster Hospital.*)

usually appears within or just after the first month of life and undergoes a growth phase for 6–12 months and thereafter gradually shrinks. By the age of 8 a white redundant skin fold is usually all that remains. If sited near the eye a large strawberry naevus may interrupt the development of binocular vision. Rarely a massive cavernous haemangioma may sequestrate platelets and lead to a bleeding tendency (Kasabach–Merritt syndrome).

The *capillary haemangioma* (port wine stain) (*Fig*. A.11) is less frequent, but more significant, as the lesions show little tendency to fade with time. They vary in colour from pale pink to deep purple and in size from a few millimetres to lesions which cover very large areas. They seldom cross the midline, and localized tissue hypertrophy may accompany large lesions. A port wine stain in a trigeminal nerve distribution may signal underlying intracranial angiomatosis, especially where ipsilateral ocular abnormalities are also present — the *Sturge–Weber* syndrome.

In the *blue rubber-bleb naevus syndrome* large rubbery cutaneous angiomas of the extremities are associated with bleeding, vascular ectasia in the respiratory and gastrointestinal tracts, beginning with recurrent epistaxis in early adult life. In *generalized essential telangiectasia* the mucosae are spared but the body is more widely affected with telangiectases, which are arborizing rather than spider. *Ataxia-telangiectasia* (Louis–Bar syndrome) is a recessively inherited immunodeficiency syndrome. Affected children are small of stature, and develop progressive cerebellar ataxia from the age of 2; telangiectases appear on conjunctivae, ears and cheeks from the age of 3.

Acquired vascular abnormalities

Cherry angiomata (Campbell de Morgan spots) develop on the trunks of almost all persons past middle age. They are usually small, from 1 to 3 mm in diameter, bright red, globular and soft. They are of no systemic significance but are said to involute spontaneously should the 8th decade be reached. Larger cavernous lesions, especially on the lower lips, are common in old age (*venous lakes*). Small angiomas surmounted by a variable amount of hyperkeratosis (angiokeratoma) are common on the scrotum (angiokeratomas of Fordyce) but also occur scattered in the bathing trunk area in the extremely rare *Anderson–Fabry disease* (*Fig*. A.12). This is an important diagnosis to make, often delayed due to the inconspicuous nature of the angiokeratomas, because internal organ involvement can lead to early death.

Pyogenic granuloma has a characteristic morphology, growing on a stalk surrounded by a collarette of normal skin. These rapidly growing angiomas are seen on the chest and extremities of young people and because of their tendency to bleed they are often the cause of alarm. A *glomus tumour* (glomangioma) also occurs on the extremities, often beneath a nail, and is composed of a bluish-red, rounded firm papule a few millimetres in diameter. Lesions can be excruciatingly painful on pressure. *Kaposi's sarcoma* (*Fig*. A.13) is a form of angiosarcoma, which in its classical form

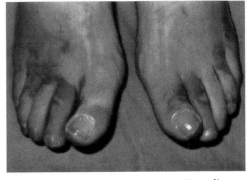

Fig. A.13. Kaposi's sarcoma. (*Westminster Hospital.*)

grows indolently on the extremities of elderly Jewish or Southern Italian persons. An *endemic* form, more aggressive and metastasizing, was described in younger people in subequatorial East and Central Africa in the 1950s. The *epidemic* of similarly aggressive Kaposi's sarcoma in homosexuals, chiefly though not exclusively with HIV infection, has spread alarmingly from the U.S.A. since the late 1970s. It has been seen in occasional transplant recipients. The sarcoma waxes in people with decreased immunity, and wanes should this improve.

Acquired telangiectases are common. Isolated spider naevi appear on children's faces, and during late pregnancy over half of the mothers develop several scattered over the face, upper chest, arms and hands. These usually disappear within 6 weeks of delivery. Similar lesions appear in *hyperthyroidism and liver disease*, and also in two conditions where vasodilatory chemicals are released into the circulation intermittently—the *carcinoid syndrome* and *systemic mastocytosis*. Telangiectasia on exposed skin is related to the gradual disappearance of support tissue that occurs with age and more particularly with cumulative sun exposure. This is extremely rare in older blacks. Similar mechanisms cause telangiectasia after X-radiation, and abuse of *topical corticosteroids*. They are also seen in localized skin disorders such as *rosacea*, and *poikiloderma*, as well as in collagen-vascular disorders, e.g. *scleroderma* (matt-telangiectases), *dermatomyositis* and *lupus erythematosus*.

Richard Staughton

Anorectal pain

Where there is an evident cause, the history of anorectal pain is usually of relatively short duration and treatment is frequently successful in relieving symptoms. A small subgroup exists, however, in whom symptoms are longstanding and no organic cause is found; these patients present a major therapeutic challenge to the clinician.

Anorectal pain: classification of major causes

ACUTE CAUSES
Anal fissure
Anal haematoma/thrombosis
Infection
  Perianal abscess
  Intersphincteric abscess
CHRONIC CAUSES
Proctalgia fugax
Coccygodynia
Idiopathic

Sometimes associated with descending perineum syndrome
Gynaecological disorders
  Ovarian cyst or tumour
  Endometriosis
Anorectal malignancy
Presacral tumours or cysts
Cauda equina lesions
  Trauma
Chronic perianal sepsis
  Anal fistula
  Crohn's disease
  Anorectal tuberculosis

Short history of pain

Acute disorders in the perianal region usually give rise to severe pain because of the profusion of sensory nerve endings prevalent in the squamous epithelium at and below the level of the dentate line. A sudden onset of pain in association with a dark blue oedematous perianal swelling are the characteristic features of either a *perianal haematoma* or *perianal thrombosis*. The two conditions are now generally considered to have the same cause, which is thrombosis of a large venous dilatation in the external venous plexus. A history of anal pain initiated by defaecation and lasting for a variable period up to an hour afterwards is usually diagnostic of an *acute anal fissure*. The lesion is observed on inspection of the anus usually in either the anterior or posterior midline positions and may be associated with an oedematous 'sentinel' skin tag at its more caudal margin. Digital examination or instrumentation of the anal canal causes severe pain and tenderness associated with marked spasm of the internal anal sphincter. Chronicity or multiplicity of a fissure observed in unusual sites around the circumference of the anal canal should arouse suspicions of underlying *Crohn's disease*.

The association of a short history of pain with fever and purulent anal discharge usually signifies *perianal sepsis*. The primary source is usually an infected anal gland and if the sepsis remains localized an intersphincteric abscess is the result. The diagnosis can be notoriously difficult because there may be no overt signs of infection; exquisite tenderness on digital examination of the anal canal may be the only physical finding. Usually pus in the infected anal gland extends to the surface (i.e. to the perineum or buttock) in which case a fistula opening will be clearly visible and an area of induration corresponding to the fistula track will be palpable.

Pain of chronic duration

Patients with chronic perineal pain may be found to have organic disease but in many, after exhaustive investigation, no cause is apparent. *Proctalgia fugax* is a common source of perineal pain in which no structural abnormality is apparent. The pain is spasmodic with episodes lasting up to 30 minutes and is probably the consequence of paroxysmal contraction of the levator ani musculature. *Coccygodynia* is a rather loose term applied to a history of vague tenderness and ache in the region of the sacrum and coccyx. Sometimes the pain radiates to the back of the thighs or buttocks and is usually provoked by sitting. Symptoms, without any convincing evidence, have been considered to arise from the coccyx. Idiopathic perineal pain is sometimes associated with the *descending perineum syndrome*, a disorder of the pelvic floor in which the pelvic floor becomes denervated and on examination the perineum is seen to 'balloon' well below the bony pelvis as represented by the level of the ischial tuberosities. The pain, in these patients, may arise from stretching of the pudendal nerves or alternatively from the mucosal prolapse which occurs secondarily to loss of muscle tone. Characteristically the pain is provoked by prolonged standing or walking and is relieved by lying flat.

Of the treatable underlying disorders, malignancy in the rectum or anus must be excluded early on by digital examination and sigmoidoscopy. Gynaecological and presacral pathology should be excluded by ultrasound and CT scanning of the pelvis. If the history of pain accompanies motor disorder of the anorectum and bladder, a cauda equina lesion should be suspected and excluded by lumbar myelography or MRI examination. Finally, chronic perianal sepsis should always suggest a possible inflammatory disorder such as Crohn's disease or anorectal tuberculosis.

M. M. Henry

Appetite, disorders of

Loss of appetite

Loss of appetite is so common and non-specific that its presence is rarely of assistance in making a diagnosis. It can be a feature of many physical or psychological disorders, as well as a transient phenomenon in stress or even ordinary living. When a patient complains of diminished appetite, a useful pointer to the importance and clinical significance is the presence and amount of accompanying weight loss. Without confirmed weight loss or other evidence of illness it is inappropriate to pursue investigations of loss of appetite.

Gastrointestinal disorders which are characteristically associated with loss of appetite include the *prodromal stage of viral hepatitis, gastric carcinoma,*

gastric ulcer and *coeliac disease*. In coeliac disease, however, the patient may occasionally compensate for the malabsorption with an increase in appetite and under these circumstances, loss of weight is not a problem. Patients with *roundworm* infestation may also have a loss of appetite but, uncommonly, the patient may have an increase in appetite.

Anorexia may be a prominent feature of chronic diseases such as *advanced malignant disease, chronic alcoholism, uraemia, severe congestive heart failure, chronic pulmonary disease*, and *cirrhosis of the liver. Suprarenal insufficiency* is constantly associated with anorexia and loss of weight. On the other hand, both *hyperthyroidism* and *diabetes mellitus* may have marked loss of weight in the absence of any impairment of appetite.

Anorexia may feature prominently in patients with psychiatric illness including *anxiety, stress,* and *depression*. However, there are two psychiatric illnesses in which a disorder of eating features prominently, *anorexia nervosa* and *bulimia*, which may affect as many as 5–10 per cent of adolescent girls and young women with a significant morbidity and mortality. It is rare for these syndromes to occur in males. *Anorexia nervosa* usually begins in teenage in a girl who is either overweight or believes herself to be so. There is a refusal to maintain normal body weight, a loss of more than 25 per cent of original body weight, a disturbance of body image, an intense fear of becoming fat, and there is no associated medical illness leading to weight loss. There are many accompanying physical abnormalities in the patient with established anorexia nervosa. These include amenorrhoea, osteoporosis, abnormal temperature regulation, bradycardia and hypotension, decreased glomerular filtration rate, renal calculi, oedema, constipation, and abnormalities of liver biochemistry. The patient will become anaemic with leucopenia and thrombocytopenia.

Increased appetite

An increase in appetite will occur normally in individuals exercising strenuously and transiently in those recovering from an illness. An increased appetite can occur in *mania* and *hyperthyroidism. Hypoglycaemia*, such as occurs with an insulinoma, may be associated with an increased appetite but this is an uncommon manifestation of the disease. Occasionally the *depressed* or *hysterical* patient may eat to excess.

Bulimia is characterized by recurrent episodes of binge eating. There is consumption of high calorie easily ingested foods taken in a binge and terminated by abdominal pain, sleep or vomiting. In between binges, there are repeated attempts to lose weight and weight can fluctuate rapidly over short periods of time by more than 5 kg. The patient usually is aware that there is an abnormal eating pattern but she fears that she will not be able to stop voluntarily. After the eating binge the patient becomes depressed. Physical features in bulimia include menstrual abnormalities, hypokalaemia, acute gastric dilatation, parotid gland enlargement, dental-enamel erosion, the risk of Mallory–Weiss tears, and aspiration pneumonia.

Perverted appetite (pica)

A perverted appetite may be a striking manifestation of *iron deficiency anaemia*. Affected individuals may crave earth or clay (geophagia), starch (amylophagia) or ice (pagophagia). Perversion of the appetite is also seen in other psychiatric disorders. Pica may also occur in the course of *pregnancy* and is of no special significance.

Ian A.D. Bouchier

Arm, pain in

This section deals primarily with pain referred into the arm from the neck and thorax. In addition, pain arising in the brachial plexus and peripheral nerves is included as also are lesions at the shoulder, elbow, wrist and hand which specifically or characteristically affect the upper limb. The causes of such pain are summarized in *Table* A.2.

Lesions which may arise at any site such as arthritis, bone tumours, injuries and skin disease are excluded.

Pain referred into the arm falls into two major categories. Sharp, well localized neuralgia often associated with paraesthesiae is usually attributed to nerve root or trunk compression. Dull diffuse discomfort in the limb, which is often difficult for the patient to describe and which may be accompanied by changes in skin temperature, vascularity and sweating is often ascribed to involvement of autonomic pathways. In the case of this 'cylindrical' limb pain an origin within the thorax or the thoracic spine should be considered.

Lesions in the neck

X-ray changes of cervical spondylosis are a normal finding after the age of 40. Over the age of 60, neurological symptoms and signs referred from the cervical roots are common. Great care must be taken, therefore, before ascribing patients' symptoms to spondylosis.

Cervical spondylosis can produce three clinical syndromes which may occur alone or in combination. First, pain and stiffness of the neck, which is often recurrent and may be aggravated by tension, anxiety and posture. Secondly, radicular pain radiating down

Table A.2. Causes of pain specific to the arm

Lesions in the neck
Disc prolapse
Spondylosis
Syringomyelia
Fracture dislocations
Post-herpetic neuralgia
Radiculitis—paralytic/viral
(Neuralgic amyotrophy)
Spinal abscess—Tuberculous
—brucella
—pyogenic
Epidural abscess
Pachymeningitis cervicalis
Tumours—spinal cord
meninges
nerve roots
vertebrae—primary
—secondary

Lesions of the brachial plexus
Cervical rib
Malignant infiltration
Costoclavicular compression
Subclavian aneurysm
Scalenus anterior syndrome

Lesions of the thorax and thoracic spine
Cardiac ischaemia
Syphilitic aortitis
Thoracic disc
Spondylosis
Tumour
Oesophagitis

Lesions at the shoulder
Periarthritis/capsulitis
Subacromial bursitis
Calcific tendonitis
Bicipital tendonitis
Shoulder-hand syndrome
Lesions at the elbow
Epicondylitis
Olecranon bursitis

Lesions of the forearm, wrist and hand
Carpal tunnel syndrome
Tenosynovitis
Ulnar neuritis
Trigger finger
Algodystrophy
Hypertrophic osteoarthropathy
Pachydermoperiostitis
Repetitive strain injury (RSI)
Writer's cramp

one or both arms and which may or may not be associated with muscle wasting, weakness and reflex changes referred to as brachial neuralgia. Thirdly, compression of the cervical cord may produce three sets of symptoms and signs:

1. Weakness, wasting and fibrillation in the upper limbs with reduction or loss of the tendon reflexes at the level of the compression.

2. Paraesthesiae in the arms and legs with or without impaired sensation in the hands and feet.

3. Pyramidal involvement with weakness, spasticity, hyperreflexia and extensor plantar responses in the legs.

The combination of weakness and wasting in the arms and spastic weakness in the legs resembles amyotrophic lateral sclerosis; spondylosis may usually be distinguished from this by the history of paraesthesiae, evidence of sensory impairment and radiographic or MRI evidence of cord compression.

Disc herniation at the C5/6 and C6/7 intervertebral spaces is a common cause of pain in the upper limb. Onset may be acute with well localized pain radiating from the back of the neck across the back of the shoulder down the arm and forearm to the wrist or fingers; more commonly onset is less dramatic, often after a period of recurrent aching and stiffness in the neck. Pain may be aggravated by movements of the neck, by downward pressure on the head and by changing position of the arm. Pain may radiate downwards into the scapular region and to the upper chest. Sensory disturbances are uncommon though may be detected in a dermatomal distribution (*Fig. A.14*) and muscle weakness may be detected in the appropriate muscles. The clinical signs associated with the most common root lesions are indicated in *Table A.3*. Depression of the biceps jerk may indicate a lesion of the C5 root, paraesthesiae in the thumb and index finger with depression of the supinator jerk indicate a lesion at the C6 root and paraesthesiae in the index and middle fingers with loss of the triceps jerk are associated with a lesion of the C7 root. Paraesthesiae in the feet with spasticity in the legs and extensor plantar responses indicate pyramidal damage associated with cord compression. X-rays of the cervical spine may show disc space narrowing especially at the C5/6 or C6/7 levels with lipping of the adjacent margins of the vertebral bodies. In the acute stage X-rays may not

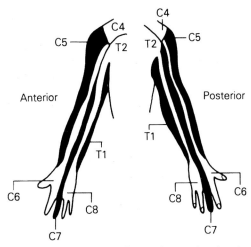

Fig. A.14 Dermatomal distribution of pain referred to the arms. (Redrawn with permission from Doherty, MacFarlane and Maddison (1985), *Rheumatological Medicine*, Churchill Livingstone, Edinburgh.)

reveal a relevant abnormality, disc space narrowing in the lower cervical spine being an extremely common appearance in normal individuals over the age of 40. Protrusion of a disc may be demonstrated by contrast myelography, CT or MRI examination, MRI being especially helpful in the demonstration of herniation into the lateral recess. Spinal fluid examination is usually normal though with large herniations the protein content may be raised, especially in the presence of cord compression.

Other causes of brachial neuralgia are uncommon. Viral, bacterial and fungal infections should be considered. Herpes zoster may give rise to persistent pain in the arm, especially in the elderly. The history of a vesicular rash and residual pigmented scars in dermatomal distribution is usually diagnostic; weakness of one or more muscles in the limb with cutaneous hyperalgesia or hypoaesthesia may also be

Table A.3. Signs and symptoms associated with common nerve root lesions affecting the arms

Root	Paraesthesiae/numbness	Muscle weakness	Reflex change
C5	Radial aspect of forearm	Shoulder abduction Elbow flexion	Biceps jerk diminished
C6	Thumb and index finger	Wrist extension and pronation	Supinator jerk diminished
C7	Middle finger, back of hand	Elbow extension and finger extension	Triceps jerk diminished
C8	Little finger, ulnar border of hand	Finger and wrist flexion	
T1	Ulnar border of forearm (see *Fig.* A.14)	Intrinsic muscles of hand	

present in a minority of cases. Acute viral radiculitis (paralytic brachial radiculitis, neuralgic amyotrophy) produces severe pain in the shoulder and upper arm, often with rapid onset of muscle wasting and weakness. Symptoms usually subside after a few days though there may be some persisting weakness and ache. Vertebral and paravertebral abscesses may result from tuberculosis or brucellosis or be caused by more common pyogenic organisms such as *Staphylococcus aureus*. In drug addicts and immunocompromised individuals, including those with AIDS, fungal or parasitic lesions may occasionally develop. Such lesions may or may not be accompanied by fever and initial symptoms may closely resemble cervical disc prolapse. Occasionally there are no other pointers to a septic lesion so that severe root symptoms in the arms in the absence of clear radiographic abnormalities should prompt CT or MRI examination of the neck. Pachymeningitis cervicalis hypertrophica is a rare condition, sometimes syphilitic in origin, which causes diffuse pain in both arms together with paraesthesiae, widespread atrophy, loss of reflexes and variable sensory loss; more than one root is implicated. Positive syphilitic serology should not be taken to indicate this rare condition in the absence of other diagnostic features. Primary or secondary neoplasms of the vertebral bodies may give rise to root pain with or without motor, sensory and reflex changes. X-ray examination is usually diagnostic though isotope bone scanning may also be helpful. Spurious hot spots may be seen in the presence of marked degenerative disease of the spine and it is important to bear in mind that plasmacytomas and myeloma deposits may not be detected by this technique. CT scanning may be helpful in early lesions. Tumours of the meninges and roots usually cause symptoms in the legs, from compression of the pyramidal and sensory tracts, as well as pain in the arm. Root lesions in the presence of multiple cutaneous neurofibromata (von Recklinghausen's disease) should raise the possibility of the development of a neurofibrosarcoma. Specialized spinal imaging is necessary for diagnosis. Where a neural tumour is suspected MRI scanning may provide the most sensitive diagnostic information. *Syringomyelia* occasionally causes pain in the arm but only as a late feature. By this stage the classical features of dissociated sensory loss, muscle wasting and hyporeflexia in the arms with pyramidal signs below the level of the lesion are likely to be apparent. Fracture dislocations of the cervical spine are especially likely in the presence of rheumatoid arthritis or ankylosing spondylitis. In the former atlanto-axial and/or subaxial subluxation of the spine may lead to upper and lower limb symptoms and fused segments of spondylitic spine are particularly at risk of fracture with or without displacement. Fractures of cervical vertebrae due to osteoporosis are unusual.

Lesions of the brachial plexus

Compression of the neurovascular bundle including the brachial plexus may occur at several sites giving rise to characteristic features classified as thoracic outlet syndromes. Symptoms include paraesthesiae of the fingertips, especially in the night or early morning; the ulnar border of the hand is typically affected (in contrast to carpal tunnel syndrome which affects the radial border) but numbness on waking may extend to the distal forearm. Symptoms may be aggravated by carrying heavy weights, though this is not diagnostic. The diagnosis is usually based on induction of paraesthesiae and numbness by abduction of the arm to 90° with external rotation, detection of an arterial bruit in the supraclavicular fossa during this manoeuvre and disappearance of symptoms and bruit with return of the arm to the neutral position. Finding a position of the arm in which the radial pulse is obliterated has been considered a key diagnostic finding. However, this may be demonstrated in normal subjects and symptoms may be due to compression of the brachial plexus without involvement of the subclavian artery. The diagnosis is not, therefore, dependent on demonstration of arterial compression. When chronic or recurrent subclavian artery compression is present this may lead rarely to the development of aneurysmal dilatation of the subclavian artery; such aneurysms may lead to emboli producing digital infarcts.

Compression of the neurovascular bundle may be due to the position of the scalenus anterior muscle, presence of a cervical rib and stretching of the plexus over a normal first rib by drooping of the shoulder, which may occur in middle life. Typically pain is felt behind the clavicle and down the inner aspect of the arm and there may be atrophy of the hypothenar eminence and interossei. Paraesthesiae and hypoaesthesia in the C8 and T1 dermatomes with associated vasospastic features are common findings. In a few patients the accessory rib may be palpable and visible on X-ray (*Fig.* A.15); not infrequently the rib is vestigial, occuring as a fibrous band which cannot be detected. In the majority of instances in which the diagnosis of thoracic outlet syndrome is considered an alternative cause such as cervical spondylosis, cervical disc lesion or peripheral nerve lesion will be detected.

Pain in the arm is occasionally due to pressure on, or infiltration of, the brachial plexus by malignant tumours. Lymphadenopathy associated with lympho-

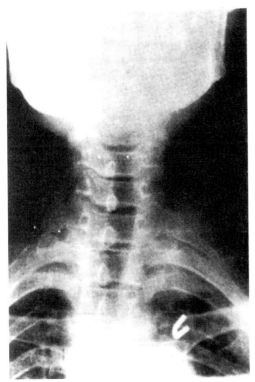

Fig. A.15. Radiograph of cervical ribs in an adult. These are bilateral but more fully developed on the left.

Pain associated with myocardial infarction and the exercise or stress-related pain of angina pectoris is usually readily recognized and confirmed by ECG or exercise testing. Syphilitic aortitis may induce similar referred pain. Oesophagitis may also produce cylindrical arm pain with or without more classical 'heartburn'. Such pain may also be accompanied by ECG abnormalities so that accurate distinction from myocardial ischaemia may rest upon exercise testing, trial of glyceryl trinitrate and visualization of the upper GI tract. Referral from the thoracic spine is a major but little recognized cause of aching in the arm or 'fibrositis'. Thoracic disc prolapse usually leads to benign thoracic pain though it may also cause referral to the upper limb. Onset is usually insidious and back pain may not be present. However, physical examination of the spine usually reveals local thoracic spine tenderness, often with rib and sternal tenderness and pain on thoracic rotation. Other causes of stiffness of the thoracic spine including spondylosis and secondary malignant deposits or myeloma may lead to similar symptoms.

In a minority of instances myocardial infarction leads to the development of pain and stiffness at one shoulder with varying degrees of pain, swelling, osteoporosis and vasomotor disturbance more distally in the limb. This 'shoulder-hand syndrome' is discussed further below.

mas or carcinoma will usually be detectable by palpation of the axilla and of the posterior triangle of the neck though infiltration of the plexus by metastatic carcinoma, especially from the breast, may take a long time to become detectable. Involvement of the plexus by upward spread of an apical bronchial carcinoma (Pancoast tumour) or more rarely by apical inflammatory lung disease may produce unilateral Horner's syndrome in addition to arm pain. Such lesions can usually be detected on a chest X-ray and confirmed by CT scanning of the apical thorax. In each of these conditions pain may be very severe without any accompanying signs in the early stages. Further infiltration usually leads to paralysis with relative sparing of sensation.

Lesions of the thorax and thoracic spine

In contrast to the characteristically searing localized pain of nerve root involvement, pain in the arm originating in the chest has a dull poorly localized quality, sometimes described as cylindrical. Such pain may also be associated with alterations in autonomic functions including temperature of the limb and sweating.

Lesions around the shoulder, elbow and wrist

In the absence of swelling, many painful lesions in the arm are referred from the spine even in the presence of local tenderness. Thus even apparently discrete lesions of the shoulder and elbow may originate from spinal lesions.

Degenerative arthritis at the shoulder joint is unusual. Pain around the shoulder radiating to the outer aspect of the upper arm with pain and reduction of glenohumeral movement in all planes is referred to as capsulitis or peri-arthritis. A painful arc on abduction of the shoulder, especially with tenderness at the shoulder tip is typical of supraspinatus tendonitis or subacromial bursitis. Transient calcification around the supraspinatus tendon may be seen on X-ray (*Fig.* A.16). Similarly, tenderness of the long head of biceps (bicipital tendonitis) may be noted usually in association with capsulitis of the shoulder. The pain of tendonitis at the shoulder is usually exacerbated by resisted movement of the appropriate muscles: (a) Supraspinatus—abduction; (b) Infraspinatus—external rotation; (c) Subscapularis—internal rotation; (d) Biceps—supination and flexion of elbow. MRI examination of the shoulder region can delineate these lesions with anatomical accuracy.

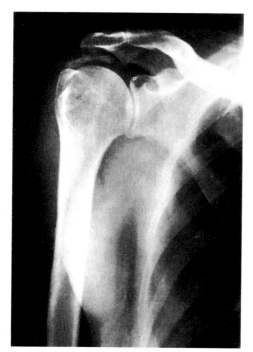

Fig. A.16. Calcific supraspinatus tendonitis. The calcification is seen on a plain AP radiograph of the shoulder.

minority, trauma may play a part. Tenderness over the lateral epicondyle sometimes extending to involve the superior radioulnar joint is referred to as 'tennis elbow' and over the medial epicondyle as 'golfer's elbow'. Swelling of the olecranon bursa, due to trauma, gout or infection, may produce pain over the extensor aspect of the elbow with limitation of movement.

Inflammatory or traumatic lesions at the medial aspect of the elbow may lead to ulnar neuritis with characteristic pain, tingling and numbness radiating down the ulnar border of the forearm and hand with impaired intrinsic muscle function. This is especially common after prolonged bed rest where prolonged pressure is applied to the elbows. Radial nerve injury, producing wrist drop with pain, numbness or tingling over the back of the hand is more likely to result from pressure or trauma above the elbow where the nerve runs around the posterior aspect of the humerus in the radial groove. Median nerve dysfunction produces characteristic pain, numbness and tingling in the thumb, index and middle fingers. Symptoms are often worse at night and first thing in the morning. This is most commonly caused by carpal tunnel syndrome, especially in the presence of hypothyroidism, pregnancy or inflammatory arthritis at the wrist. Pressure may also be exerted on the median nerve where it passes between the two heads of pronator teres in the forearm. A positive Tinel's sign with wasting and weakness of abductor pollicis

Epicondylitis is a misnomer for a group of non-inflammatory conditions at the elbow. The cause of such lesions is not usually established, though in a

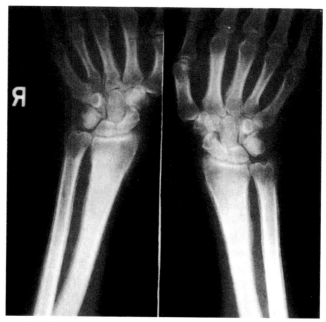

Fig. A.17. Pseudohypertrophic pulmonary osteoarthropathy of the radius and ulna showing new periosteal bone deposition. (*Dr T.H. Hills.*)

brevis and slowed median nerve conduction on electromyography confirm the diagnosis.

A variety of repetitive strain syndromes are now described. These soft tissue syndromes relate to repeated or sustained actions of the upper limb and produce local pain, fatigue and decline in performance. Symptoms are commonest in young adults especially keyboard workers and a variety of factors including poor posture, stress, inadequate rest periods, poor training and worker's compensation may contribute to their development. Both work and recreational activities may be implicated. Writer's cramp, with pain in the wrist and shoulder associated with an excessively tight grip of the pen and a tense posture whilst writing may be a related condition.

Tenosynovitis of flexor tendons in the hand may occur as part of generalized arthropathies but also in isolation and in association with diabetes mellitus. The combination of nodular degeneration of a flexor tendon and stenosing tenosynovitis usually at the level of the metacarpophalangeal joint gives rise to 'trigger finger' with pain on flexing the finger followed by inability to extend the finger actively.

miscellaneous conditions

Reflex sympathetic dystrophies may affect the upper limb being usually referred to as shoulder-hand syndrome, causalgia or algodystrophy. This condition is characterized by pain, swelling, vasomotor disturbances and trophic skin changes usually affecting the distal part of the limb. This may follow peripheral nerve injury or myocardial infarction, though in at least 50% of cases no cause is demonstrable. In the later stages contractures may also develop.

Hypertrophic (pulmonary) osteoarthropathy (HPOA) may affect many sites but in particular the elbows, wrists, and fingers. Onset of joint pain is often acute with stiffness and weakness and there may be marked tenderness of distal long bones associated with radiographic appearances of periostitis (*Fig.* A.17). Clubbing of the fingers is also present. HPOA is usually associated with malignancy of the lung, pleura or diaphragm though may occasionally be benign or hereditary; it is usually bilateral and symmetrical. Only the upper limbs are affected in association with Pancoast's syndrome and aortic aneurysms. Similar changes of periostitis and clubbing associated with thickening of the skin, especially in the scalp, may develop soon after puberty in the syndrome of pachydermoperiostitis. The condition is benign and gradually becomes inactive after a few years.

Andrew Keat

Axillary swelling

Swelling in the axilla is due in the great majority of cases to enlargement of the lymph nodes. If the enlargement is inflammatory, a subsequent abscess, either acute or chronic, is frequent. Any form of tumour other than involvement of the nodes by secondary deposits is distinctly rare, but unfortunately it is common to find the axillary nodes to be the seat of metastases from carcinoma of the breast.

Acute abscess

Acute abscess may be recognized at once by the well-marked signs of local inflammation and the general febrile disturbance. There is one form of acute abscess that may not be obvious, namely one situated in the upper part of the axilla and covered by the pectoral muscles. On account of its distance from the surface the local signs of inflammation may not be great, though the general signs are marked. There will be great disinclination to move the arm on account of pain, and there is usually some cause, such as a whitlow on the finger, to account for the trouble. It must be remembered, however, that the abscess may be 'residual'; that is to say, the original source of infection, such as the whitlow, may have healed completely 2, 3 weeks or even longer before the axillary abscess declares itself. Rarely an empyema points in the axilla; there are generally, but not always, abnormal lung signs to suggest the diagnosis.

Chronic or tuberculous abscess

Chronic or tuberculous abscess (*Fig.* A.18) forms a single fluctuating swelling which, if large, may extend upwards under the pectoralis major. Owing to the fact that few, if any, of the local signs of inflammation may

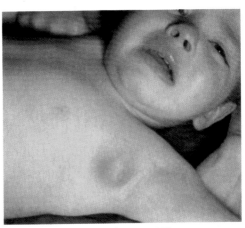

Fig. A.18. Tuberculous abscess in a child.

be present, difficulty may arise in distinguishing this form of abscess from a soft lipoma. The duration and the rapidity of growth of the swelling are good guides, for though the duration of a chronic abscess may run into months, it does not exist for years, as does a lipoma. Aspiration will settle the difficulty.

Enlargement of the lymph nodes

Next, supposing that examination proves that the swelling is not an abscess, attention should be directed to ascertain whether it arises from lymph nodes, which may present as a single enlarged node, a number of discrete individual nodes or as a mass of matted glands. For the differential diagnosis of nodular swelling. It is sufficient here to enumerate the principal causes. These are: acute infection, chronic infection with tuberculosis; rheumatoid arthritis, lymphatic leukaemia, Hodgkin's disease and non-Hodgkin's lymphoma; malignant glandular metastases. The first and the last are far the most common in the axilla (*Fig.* A.19).

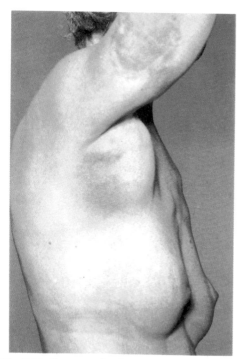

Fig. A.19. Huge mass of melanotic deposits in the axillary nodes following previous resection of malignant melanoma of the upper arm (note the skin graft at this point).

Occasionally a node or group of nodes in the axilla appears malignant and on being removed for histological section is found to be infiltrated with metastatic carcinoma, and yet no source for the primary can be found. The most likely site for such a hidden primary is undoubtedly the breast and, next to this, the lung, so that an energetic search should be instituted by clinical examination, chest X-ray and mammography (in the female), as well as by bronchoscopy to incriminate or exculpate these two organs. Other less common possibilities are the stomach and the ovary, and if all investigations have so far been negative, expert pelvic examination and a complete investigation of the gastrointestinal tract are called for. If, after careful search in this way, no primary can be detected it may be assumed that this is within the breast. The introduction of mammography has helped to reveal very small breast carcinomas presenting as enlarged axillary nodes.

Primary tumours of the axilla

Primary tumours of the axilla are distinctly rare, but it is a possible site for an accessory breast, the nipple of which will provide the diagnosis.

LIPOMA is the most common tumour (*Fig.* A.20). It may attain a large size and extend up under the pectoral muscles. It should be diagnosed by its long history, slow growth, definite outline and free mobility. When very soft, the tumour may give the feeling of fluctuation, and so be mistaken for a chronic tuberculous abscess, and as it consists of large lobules of fat, some degree of translucency may be present. The skin wrinkles when one attempts to raise it away from the tumour.

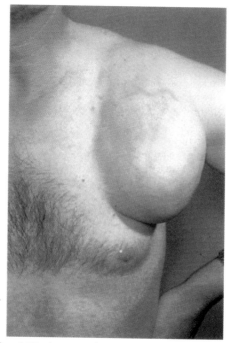

Fig. A.20. A massive but entirely benign lipoma of the axilla.

CYSTIC HYGROMA of the axilla is rare. It is usually congenital, but apparently similar cystic swellings may appear in adult life. It forms a soft, fluctuating, quite translucent and painless swelling, which sometimes grows rapidly. It may be mistaken for a lipoma, and the diagnosis may not be certain until excision and microscopical examination are completed.

PRIMARY MALIGNANT TUMOURS may arise, but are of extreme rarity.

ANEURYSM OF THE AXILLARY ARTERY does occur, but is very uncommon. It is recognized easily because it is comparatively superficial and it gives an expansile pulsation synchronous with the heart's beat; the veins of the forearm may be distended on account of pressure on the axillary vein, and the radial pulse on the affected side is diminished in size and delayed. There may be a definite history of local injury, or in cases of apparently spontaneous aneurysm there may be signs or symptoms of bacterial endocarditis.

Harold Ellis

Back, pain in

Pain in the back is one of the commonest complaints in general and specialist practice, and no specialty is immune from it. The differential diagnosis therefore covers most of medicine. The first important subdivision is into acute and chronic back pain.

ACUTE SELF-LIMITING PAIN IN THE BACK

This may occur in any febrile condition. A striking, though rare, example is dengue or 'break-bone fever'. It may also result from soft-tissue injury: any gardener, spring-cleaning house-cleaner or horse rider knows how common such minor insults are. Such pains usually rapidly settle either when the cause is removed or as the injured tissues heal. Only when the back aches and pains persist after several days does one look further into the possible causes.

CHRONIC BACKACHE

In any backache lasting more than 2–3 weeks the conditions listed in the table below should be considered. By far the commonest are the first four mentioned (1(*a*)–(*d*)), sometimes associated with depression or anxiety.

THE CAUSES OF CHRONIC BACKACHE

1. *Traumatic, mechanical or degenerative:*
(*a*) Low back strain; fatigue; obesity; pregnancy. (*b*) Injuries of bone, joint or ligament. (*c*) Degenerative disease of the spine (osteo-arthritis) including ankylosing hyperostosis. (*d*) Intervertebral disc lesions. (*e*) Lumbar instability syndromes, e.g. spondylolisthesis. (*f*) Scoliosis: primary and secondary. (*g*) Spinal stenosis

2. *Metabolic:*
Osteoporosis. Osteomalacia. Hyper- and hypoparathyroidism. Ochronosis (*Figs* B.1, B.2). Fluorosis. Hypophosphataemic rickets

3. *Unknown causes:*
Inflammatory arthropathies of the spine, such as ankylosing spondylitis and the spondylitis of Reiter's syndrome, psoriasis, ulcerative colitis, Whipple's and Crohn's diseases. Rarely polymyositis and polymyalgia rheumatica. Paget's disease of bone. Osteochondritis—(Scheuermann's disease)

4. *Infective conditions of bone, joint and theca of spine:*
Osteomyelitis. Tuberculosis. Undulant fever (abortus and melitensis). Typhoid and paratyphoid fever and other *Salmonella* infections. Syphilis. Yaws. Very rarely Weil's disease (leptospirosis icterohaemorrhagica). Spinal pachymeningitis. Chronic meningitis. Subarachnoid or spinal abscess

5. *Psychogenic:*
Anxiety. Depression. Hysteria. Compensation neurosis. Malingering

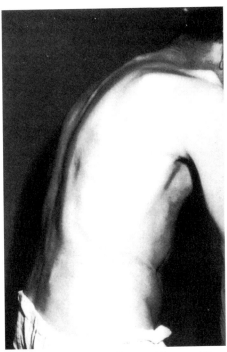

Fig. B.1. Rigid spine due to ochronosis. (*Courtesy of General Raji Al-Tikriti of Baghdad.*)

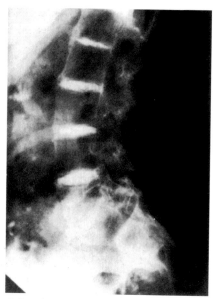

Fig. B.2. Radiograph showing calcification of intervertebral discs in ochronosis. (*Courtesy of the Arthritis and Rheumatism Council.*)

13. *Normality:*
(Non-disease)
With depression or anxiety

The list is probably incomplete but covers most of the likely causes. In eliciting the cause a full history is essential, with particular reference to factors operating at the time of onset and factors known to ease or aggravate the condition. On examination the way a patient moves, walks, sits or lies, and how he rises from sitting and lying positions may be highly informative. Spinal range of movement may be measured by various instruments such as Dunham's spondylometer (*Fig.* B.3) or Loebl's inclinometer. Another method is that of Schober, which depends on stretching of the skin over the lumbar spine in spinal flexion. More sensitive and accurate is Macrae's modification of the same method which measures stretching of the skin in spinal flexion between a point 10 cm above the lumbosacral junction and a spot 15 cm below over the sacrum. Ability to touch the toes is a poor measure of spinal movement as it depends greatly on hip flexion; these methods eliminate the hip component. They also

6. *Neoplastic—benign or malignant, primary or secondary:*
Osteoid osteoma. Eosinophilic granuloma. Metastatic deposits from primary carcinoma of bronchus, breast, prostate, kidney, thyroid and rarely, from other primaries. Direct invasion from carcinoma of the oesophagus. Myeloma. Primary and secondary tumours of spinal canal and nerve roots: ependymoma; neurofibroma; glioma; angioma; meningioma; lipoma; rarely chordoma. Reticuloses, e.g. Hodgkin's disease

7. *Cardiac and vascular:*
Subarachnoid or spinal haemorrhage. Syphylitic, degenerative or dissecting aneurysm. Grossly enlarged left atrium in mitral valve disease. Rarely myocardial infarction

8. *Gynaecological conditions:*
Rarely prolapse or retroversion of uterus. Dysmenorrhoea. Chronic salpingitis. Pelvic tuberculosis. Pelvic abscess or chronic cervicitis. Tumours

9. *Gastrointestinal conditions:*
Perforating posterior gastric or duodenal ulcer. Pancreatitis, acute or chronic. Referred pain from biliary calculi. Retroperitonial neoplasms (particularly pancreatic carcinoma).

10. *Renal and genito-urinary causes:*
Carcinoma of kidney. Calculus. Hydronephrosis. Polycystic kidney. Necrotizing papillitis. Pyelitis and pyelonephritis. Perinephric abscess

11. *Blood disorders:*
Sickle-cell crisis. Acute haemolytic states

12. *Drugs:*
Corticosteroids. Methysergide. Compound analgesic tablets

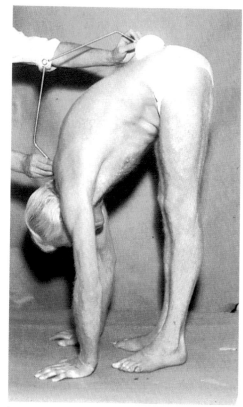

Fig. B.3. Ankylosing spondylitis. The patient can touch the floor easily with his hands as he has very supple hips, but measurement with a spondylometer shows spinal movement to be restricted to 60 per cent of normal.

enable the examiner to give a positive figure for the spinal range of movement, which can be measured repeatedly to assess progression or regression of the spinal disorder. Radiography often helps in diagnosis, but even more often does not. The fact that there are radiological changes does not mean that these are the cause of the symptoms. Radiologically speaking, there is no such thing as a normal spine after middle age is passed. Nevertheless, many diagnoses of chronic backache are dependent on radiography, and computed tomography (CT scanning) also helps in the diagnosis of certain back pains due to trauma, malignancy or spinal stenosis, where the degree of stenosis can be assessed. A virtue of computed tomography is that the vertebrae, spinal cord, subarachnoid space and nerve root sleeves can be shown without the use of a contrast medium given intrathecally. Magnetic resonance imaging, where available, gives extremely accurate visualization of this region.

1. Non-infective traumatic and degenerative disorders

Non-infective traumatic and degenerative disorders arising in the bones, joints and soft tissues of the spine are extremely common. In a structure of such complexity as the human spine, with so many joints, ligaments and cartilages at risk, it is no wonder that aches and pains are commonplace. Too-easy chairs at home, badly placed and badly shaped car seats, and unsatisfactory chairs at work are often the cause of postural strain. Fixed unnatural positions held for hours on end are highly productive of symptoms. Bad posture and fatigue act together to produce one of the most common of backaches. The postural back pain of pregnancy usually goes soon after childbirth but is sometimes replaced by one of lumbosacral origin due to the childbirth itself. Obesity is an aggravating factor rather than a sole cause, but chronic backaches may not infrequently be improved or cured by the loss of 30-90 kg (1-3 stones) or more in weight.

Degenerative changes of the spine are almost always present after the age of 45 years, but only sometimes are they accompanied by symptoms, and these in turn are often due to some of the factors mentioned above. *Ankylosing hyperostosis*, a condition often associated with diabetes mellitus, is characterized by coarse bridging along the anterior borders of the lower dorsal vertebrae, seen well in lateral radiographs. Degenerative changes in the *intervertebral cartilages* may be associated with chronic backache, and such changes may be localized, usually to lower cervical and lumbar areas, or may extend widely throughout the entire spine. More severe symptoms of compression may occur when a disc herniation protrudes through a tear of the posterior longitudinal ligament and presses on root and/or cord causing symptoms and signs of sciatica, femoral neuropathy or brachialgia, depending on the site of the lesion. Such lesions can cause severe and prostrating pains which may be aggravated by coughing and straining. A sudden strain, such as lifting a heavy weight with the spine flexed, is often the precipitating cause. Paraesthesia in the distribution of the affected nerve is common and the appropriate reflex may be diminished or absent (*see Table B.1*).

In lumbar lesions the normal lumbar lordosis may be lost; stooping causes great pain but lateral spinal movement may be painless. The so called 'sciatica scoliosis' is a lumbar scoliosis with a limping gait in an

Table B.1. Neurological signs of lumbar disc lesions

Root	Pain reference	Motor weakness	Sensory changes	Reflex changes	Muscle wasting
L2	Anterior upper thigh	Flexion and adduction of hip	None or upper thigh lateral and anterior	None or reduced knee reflex	None
L3	Anterior thigh and knee	Knee extension. Hip flexion and adduction	None or lower thigh medial and anterior	Reduced knee reflex	Thigh
L4	Lateral thigh. Median calf	Foot inversion and dorsiflexion. Knee extension	Antero-medial calf and shin	Reduced or absent knee reflex	Thigh
L5	Buttock, back and side thigh. Lateral lower leg	Extension and abduction of hip. Flexion knee. Dorsiflexion foot and toes. Foot eversion	Lateral calf, dorsal and medial foot, especially hallux	None or (rarely) reduced ankle reflex	Calf
S1	Buttock. Back of thigh and calf to heel	Flexion knee, foot eversion and plantar flexion	Lateral foot, ankle and lower calf, back of heel and sole of foot	Reduced or absent ankle reflex	Calf

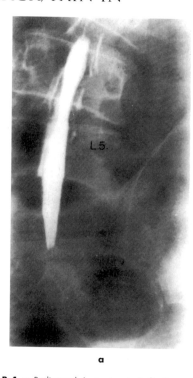
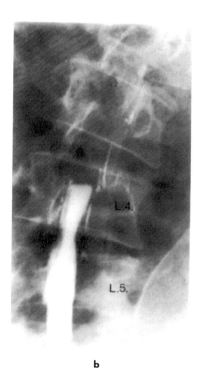

a
b

Fig. B.4. *a.* Radiograph (patient supine) after intraspinal injection of lipiodol showing narrowing of the oil column at the level of the interspace between the 4th and 5th lumbar vertebrae and scoliosis due to muscular spasm. A protruded portion of disc was removed with complete relief of pain in the back and sciatica. (*Dr H.M. Worth.*) *b.* Radiograph in same case with the patient prone.

attempt by the patient to avoid pain. The back is held stiffly and painfully, the patient feeling the need to press it on to a hard, flat surface for support and pain relief. Stiffness and pain are often worst in the morning when rising from bed and may be agonizing. Straight-leg raising may cause pain. But not always; pulling the bent knee backwards while pushing the buttocks forwards with the other hand, the patient lying half prone with his back to the examiner, may give a more positive result as it stretches the femoral nerve and puts tension on the upper lumbar roots. A large disc protrusion may not only press directly on nervous tissue but also interfere with its blood supply. Cerebrospinal fluid may show an increase of protein, often with an increase of lymphocytes and perhaps some red blood cells, and the fluid pressure may be altered. Radiographs of the spine after introduction of a contrast medium may occasionally be necessary to localize the obstruction, as is shown in *Fig.* B.4, although CT scans and MRI are more appropriate as non-invasive investigations (*Fig.* B.5).

Many disc protrusions are posterior rather than posterolateral. In the former case they cause back pain only, rarely root compression. There may be tenderness over the affected area, in some cases referred to paravertebral muscles or buttocks.

Spondylolisthesis, usually in the lower lumbar spine, occurs as a result of the bilateral lesion in the pars interarticularis, i.e. that bony bridge which unites the superior articular facet and pedicle to the lamina and inferior articular process. A forward or backward (retrospondylolisthesis) displacement may also occur as a result of the degeneration of an intervertebral disc ('pseudospondylolisthesis') resulting in instability of the upper vertebra and narrowing of the intervertebral foramina. Well-centred radiographs taken in full flexion and extension will show the lesion. There may be no symptoms in some cases, others have low backache and aches extending round into the groins; unilateral or bilateral sciatica is rare, as is a cauda equina lesion. This (cauda equina) lesion, partly due to compression, partly due to traction, the severest of the syndromes associated with spondylolisthesis, is more often seen in adolescent children. Physical signs are often non-existent, but the visible and palpable prominence of the spine of the affected vertebra may become more obvious as the patient flexes his spine. Cervical spondylolisthesis is much less common than lumbar.

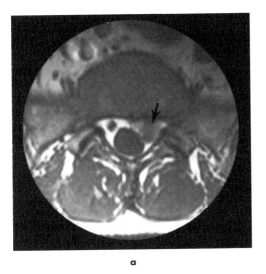
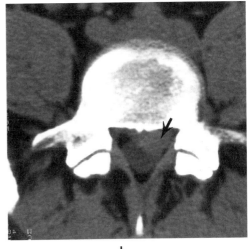

a   b

Fig. B.5. *a.* CT scan. *b.* MRI scan. Both scans demonstrate prolapsed L5/S1 disc (arrowed). (Films supplied by Prof. Adrian Dixon, Addenbrookes Hospital, Cambridge.)

Scoliosis is a lateral deviation of the spine from a straight line. When the subject flexes his spine a functional scoliosis will disappear but a structural one will persist or even increase. A scoliosis may be compensatory to a short leg, painful hip or knee or any other cause of a pelvic tilt, but if the iliac crests are level the cause of the 'scoliosis' is in the spine itself. Pain may arise from an idiopathic adolescent scoliosis but in most adults arises from factors outside the spine.

Spinal stenosis. The spinal canal can be narrowed by degenerative changes and/or developmentally either centrally or laterally, damaging nervous tissue directly or by leaving less space for a prolapsed disc or osteophyte. Narrowing of the spinal canal may also interfere with the blood supply to the cauda equina causing weakness, burning or numbness on exertion which is eased by resting, a kind of intermittent claudication without muscle cramps and with normal peripheral pulses. This claudication is present, however, only in a minority of cases and degenerative (acquired) cases are more common than developmental, though both factors may be present. Lumbar stenosis often presents as a nerve root compression distinguished from root compression by a disc by the absence of abnormal straight-leg raising and spinal stiffness. Spinal stenosis may be: (1) congenital—idiopathic or associated with achondroplasia; (2) acquired—degenerative (osteo-arthritic, discogenic, spondylolytic or spondylolisthetic); (3) postoperative or post-traumatic; (4) due to Paget's disease; or (5) fluorosis, but may be due to combinations of the above.

2. Crushed or wedged vertebrae

Crushed or wedged vertebrae due to osteoporosis are seen in radiographs to be part of a diffuse thinning of the texture of the bone without lytic lesions or condensation. There is often wedging of several vertebrae from previous crushes and the back is usually rounded. The patient is in most cases an elderly woman. Blood chemistry (serum alkaline phosphatase, calcium and plasma phosphate) is typically normal, though hypocalcaemia often occurs. In a spine painful from malignant deposits there is actual destruction of bone tissue in the radiographs and porosis is patchy and not generalized; if due to carcinoma of the prostate the bone shadow may be denser and dead-white in the radiographs in the affected areas. The serum alkaline phosphatase is elevated in metastatic malignant disease but normal in myelomatosis. In both cases the sedimentation rate is raised, usually in carcinomatosis, invariably and to a high figure around 80–100 mm in 1 hour (Westergren) in myelomatosis; marrow biopsy and electrophoretic studies clinch the diagnosis. The commonest source of spinal malignant deposits today is carcinoma of the breast in the female and the bronchus and prostate in the male, but multiple myeloma should always be kept in mind in any unexplained backache. Deposits in the spine from prostatic carcinoma are usually associated with a raised serum acid phosphatase. Prostate specific antigen is also raised although it may be elevated in benign prostatic disease, especially in the elderly. Radiologically the prostatic secondary deposits are often sclerotic, unlike the usually lytic lesions of other tumours.

Osteomalacia differs from osteoporosis in that there is often a history of dietetic and/or intestinal insufficiency or of chronic disease and sometimes of a previous gastrectomy. The serum alkaline phosphatase is often elevated, serum calcium and plasma phosphate normal or decreased. Urinary 24-hour calcium output is low. The aches are more diffuse and are not centred on the crushed vertebra, as in osteoporosis; they are nagging and unremitting, are eased by rest, and aggravated by activity. Pain in osteoporosis appears to be due to local fracture of a brittle non-tender vertebral body, in osteomalacia to strain of the tender soft bones of the spine. Radiographs may show stress fractures (pseudo-fractures) and Milkman's lines or Looser zones in pelvis or ribs, rarefied areas consisting of uncalcified osteoid. In *hyperparathyroidism* there may be generalized osteoporosis in the radiographs. Bone cysts may occur; subperiosteal resorption of phalanges and of the distal ends of the clavicles is characteristic. There may be generalized backache and tenderness. Serum calcium is raised, but repeated estimates over a period of time may have to be done to demonstrate this. Plasma phosphorus may be low, though it rises with renal failure, and the alkaline phosphatase is usually but not invariably raised. There may be other features of hypercalcaemia, such as nausea and vomiting, muscle weakness or a true myopathy, corneal calcification (band keratitis) and nephrocalcinosis. Peptic ulceration and pancreatitis may occur. The syndrome is usually due to primary hyperparathyroidism, from hyperplasia or adenoma of the parathyroid gland, but it can occur as secondary to renal and other diseases, in which case the serum calcium may be normal. The finding of plasma chloride levels consistently less than 100 mmol/l in the presence of hypercalcaemia virtually excludes the diagnosis of primary hyperparathyroidism. Back pains may also rarely occur in *idiopathic hypoparathyroidism* associated with the hypocalcaemia, cataracts, fits, tetany and rashes.

Paget's disease of bone is often an incidental radiological finding in a patient with no symptoms. It can occasionally, however, cause quite severe backache. Diagnosis is made on X-rays and an elevated serum alkaline phosphatase. The disease may extend throughout the pelvis and spine or involve one or two vertebral bodies only. A small number of the lesions become sarcomatous, and severe pain should arouse suspicions of malignant change.

Scheuermann's osteochondritis is a condition of unknown aetiology predominantly affecting adolescent males. There is irregular ossification of the vertebral epiphysial end-plates of the lower dorsal but also the upper lumbar spine, the disc spaces becoming narrowed and the vertebral bodies wedged anteriorly,

the patient developing rounded shoulders, a smoother dorsal kyphosis and flat chest.

3. Inflammatory arthropathies of the spine

The best example is idiopathic ankylosing spondylitis (*Fig.* B.6). Here the patient is usually a male aged between 16 and 36, and in the large majority of cases he is of tissue type HLA-B27 (*see Figs* B.3, B.6, B.7). His spine is stiffened and restricted in movement *in all planes*. Neck movements are often restricted and intercostal expansion at nipple level reduced from the normal 5–7.5 to 2.5 cm or less. This intercostal restriction occurs early in the course of the disease and is not a late complication but an essential and early part of the clinical picture. Diaphragmatic movement is normal. Evidence of active or old iridocyclitis is present in over 20 per cent of the patients, in most cases seen as iritic adhesions or dark spots in the anterior chamber on the posterior surface of the cornea. Tender heels or tender areas over the pelvic brim, ischial tuberosities, or greater trochanters are not uncommon. Peripheral arthritis occurs in some 25 per cent of cases initially and hydrarthrosis of knees in about 7 per cent of cases. The sedimentation rate is elevated in almost all cases, but sheep-cell agglutination and latex tests are negative. Nodules do not occur, nor does lymphadenopathy or splenomegaly. The commonest initial symptom is aching in the buttocks,

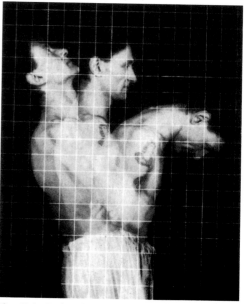

Fig. B.6. Triple-exposure photograph showing restricted spinal extension and flexion in a young man with ankylosing spondylitis.

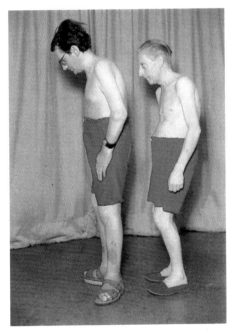

Fig. B.7. Two patients with severe ankylosing spondylitis both of whom have had wedge lumbar osteotomies to straighten the previously grossly flexed spine.

the patient drawing his hand down the back of the buttocks and thighs at the site of discomfort, but lumbar backache and stiffness soon occur and may be the initial symptoms. Two radiographs help in early diagnosis, a postero-anterior view of the sacro-iliacs and an anteroposterior of the dorsolumbar spine D 8–L 3, but X-ray changes may not be present until symptoms have been present 2–3 years or more. The earliest radiological sacro-iliac changes are blurring of the joint outlines with para-articular iliac sclerosis, erosions and apparent widening, gradually giving way over the years to narrowing and obliteration of the joint. Small syndesmophytes, resembling bony 'stalagmites and stalactites', are usually seen first along the edges of the intervertebral cartilages between the vertebral bodies of D 10 and L 2; this is where the 'bamboo spine' usually first becomes evident. Lytic lesions with periosteal elevation and 'whiskering' may be seen in the pelvis or in the spine, most commonly in the ischial tuberosities. Ankylosing spondylitis affects the spine primarily (*Fig.* B.7), girdle joints (hips and shoulders) secondly, and peripheral joints least often, in contrast to the distribution of joint involvement seen in rheumatoid arthritis, where initial involvement is usually feet, hands and wrists. The spondylitic pattern of disease may also be seen occasionally in Reiter's syndrome, or in association with psoriasis, ulcerative colitis, Crohn's disease, and

occasionally Whipple's disease and Behçet's disease and, very rarely, polymyalgia rheumatica. Some male cases of juvenile chronic polyarthritis progress to the spondylitic picture. In the diagnosis of ankylosing spondylitis these variants should always be considered.

4. Infective conditions

Infective conditions of bones and joints are uncommon and the history will often give a lead to the diagnosis. The *Staphylococcus aureus* is the most common causative organism. The lesions tend to be lytic and abscesses may form and discharge. The final picture may resemble osteoarthritis or even ankylosing spondylitis. *Tuberculosis* of sacro-iliac joint or spine is more painful than these conditions, however, and more incapacitating. The dorsal spine is the most commonly affected portion of the spine, the vertebral bodies being most commonly involved though the disease may start in the intervertebral disc. Collapse of vertebral bodies leads to angulation of the spine. Cold-abscess formation and paresis are much less common today than in the pre-antibiotic era. There is pain and weakness in the back and tenderness and muscle spasm in the affected area, the spine being held rigidly. Sacro-iliac disease is usually unilateral in tuberculous disease, bilateral in ankylosing spondylitis.

In brucellosis contracted from *Br. abortus* in cattle, *melitensis* in goats and *suis* in pigs, generalized aches, fever, sweats, anorexia and other features of a febrile infective process may coexist with backache and joint and bone pains; signs of actual joint inflammation are rare. The lesion is essentially an osteomyelitis of the spine or pelvis; both bone and disc may be involved, only occasionally with pus formation. Localization in the spinal column may occur many weeks or months after the original infection, which may have been overlooked and undiagnosed at the time. The same delay of months, or even years, before the advent of spinal symptoms is also seen with typhoid and paratyphoid fevers. *Weil's disease* (leptospirosis icterohaemorrhagia), characterized by fever and high leucocytosis, haemorrhagic manifestations and jaundice, may give rise at the time to acute backache and later to destructive and degenerative changes in the spine with chronic symptoms.

5. Psychogenic

The essence of hysteria is the theatrical nature of the symptoms it causes. This is true of the hysterical spine. The spine is held elaborately bent (camptocormia), all attempts at movement being resisted with great drama and much expression of suffering. The back, nevertheless, straightens out readily on bed, couch or floor. The patient may be able to flex his spine painlessly, but will not straighten it. Palpation or attempts at movement by the examiner may produce much louder groans, grimaces and excessive reactions than in a patient with a true acute inflammatory spondylitis. It is this 'over-reaction' which is typical of the hysteric. Watched closely, movements previously impossible are later made without discomfort and areas previously acutely tender touched without complaint. *Malingering* may give a similar picture though usually less dramatic. In both cases spinal movements are often more grossly restricted than in severe spinal disease. *Compensation neurosis* tends to improve when the case is settled, whatever the legal decision. The history and features of *anxiety* and *depression* are usually apparent in a well-taken history. Backache may be entirely due to either or both, or features of these disorders may become superimposed on an organic cause. Such a picture is common in the overworked, harassed, anxious housewife.

6. Spinal tumours

Spinal tumours may be divided into extradural and intradural, the latter being further subdivided into those outside and those within the cord, i.e. extra- or intramedullary. Meningiomas and neurofibromas are the commonest extramedullary growths, the latter usually arising from spinal roots, the posterior more often than the anterior. They may be single or multiple and may or may not be part of a generalized neurofibromatosis.

Benign tumours of the spine are uncommon. Bone cysts, giant-cell tumours, osteochondroma and chondroma may occur but more common are haemangiomas, aneurysmal bone cysts and osteoid osteomas. Not all haemangiomas are benign; some lead to extensive destruction of bone. X-rays show vertical striations in the vertebral body which may be partially crushed. Aneurysmal bone cysts form large paraspinal masses, usually posteriorly, with scattered calcific deposits. The osteoid osteoma is a painful lesion in which new bone is formed leading to considerable surrounding bony sclerosis. Tomograms may be necessary to demonstrate the lesion well, a zone of dense bone encircling a small radiolucent centre. The pain is often severe and worse at night.

7. Backache caused by cardiovascular and intrathoracic disorders

Backache may be caused by cardiovascular and intrathoracic disorders, of which a good example is the intense, demoralizing, boring pains of an aneurysm invading the spine. Features of syphilitic aneurysm of the arch and early descending aorta will probably be present with signs of an aortic reflux, collapsing

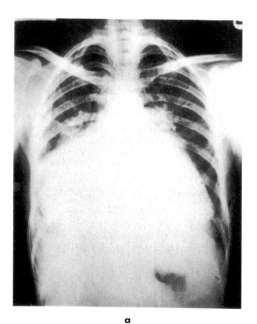

a

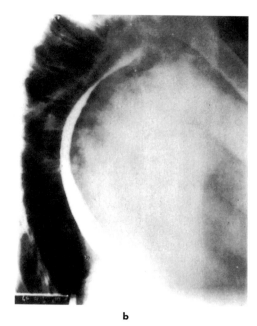

b

Fig. B.8. *a.* A case of backache due to enormous enlargement of the left atrium in mitral stenosis. The heart shadow to the right of the spine is due to superimposed right and left atrium. *b.* The same case showing scythe-shaped oesophagus (on a barium swallow, lateral view) from left atrial pressure. (*Dr A. Schott.*)

arterial pulses, and possibly signs of neurosyphilis also. Dissecting aneurysms of the descending aorta below the arch are less apparent; unequal or delayed pulses in arms and legs should be noted. An arteriosclerotic aneurysm of the abdominal aorta may cause pain in the lower part of the back as well as in the upper abdomen, the groin, and occasionally in the testicles; a pulsating mass may be felt in the abdomen. A carcinoma of the bronchus or oesophagus may cause backache, myocardial infarction only rarely. *Fig.* B.8 shows a rare cause, enormous enlargement of the left atrium in mitral disease. The pain in such cases is usually relieved by leaning forwards and to the left.

8. Gynaecological conditions

Gynaecological conditions are, on the whole, a rare cause of low lumbar and sacral backache. Disease of the ovaries and tubes may be responsible in a few cases, prolapse or retroversion of the uterus occasionally, but the cause commonly lies elsewhere and correcting the gynaecological condition leaves the backache in most cases unrelieved. If backache worsens during the menses this may suggest a gynaecological cause, but may also suggest a change in pain threshold at this time. Tuberculous endometritis may cause backache which is relieved by appropriate therapy.

9. Gastrointestinal conditions

There are gastrointestinal conditions from which backache may be referred. Chronic pancreatitis and carcinoma of the pancreas may cause a dull, persistent, upper lumbar ache, usually but not always associated with upper abdominal pain and discomfort. Relief of pain may be obtained by leaning forwards. A penetrating ulcer on the posterior wall of the stomach or first part of duodenum quite characteristically gives a boring pain in the upper lumbar region which is related to meals and which may be relieved by antacid therapy. Enlargement of the liver from any cause may give a dull ache felt to the right of the lower dorsal spine, but aches are usually felt also elsewhere in the abdomen and lower chest. The pain of cholecystitis or cholelithiasis may be experienced posteriorly over the liver, or a little higher, classically the lower pole of the right scapula, in addition to the upper abdomen.

10. Renal and genitourinary causes

Renal and genitourinary causes are not uncommon. Pyelitis and pyelonephritis may cause lower dorsal and lumbar backaches; the diagnosis is usually evident. It is less obvious with renal tumours such as carcinoma, which may remain largely silent since haematuria and the finding of a palpable mass in the flank may only occur late in the course of the disease. Prostatic neoplastic disease with secondary spinal and sacral deposits may be associated with backache, usually low lumbosacral, but occasionally higher.

Renal papillary nacrosis occurs as a complication of pyelonephritis, particularly in diabetics and particularly if there is urinary obstruction: it is also a feature of analgesic nephropathy.

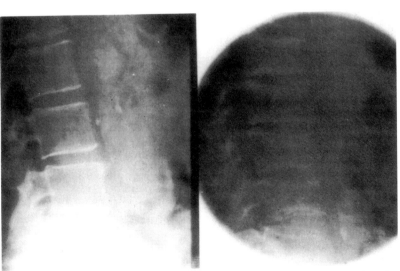

Fig. B.9. Rapid advance of spinal osteoporosis over a 1-year period in a rheumatoid patient on prolonged corticosteroid therapy.

11. **Blood disorders**

Severe attacks of backache, often with fever, may occur in sickle-cell disease and haemolytic crises in other disorders. Backache may also be a manifestation of acute or chronic leukaemia.

12. **Drugs**

Corticosteroids may increase osteoporosis due to other causes and help to precipitate crush factures (*Fig.* B.9). Methysergide taken over long periods to prevent migraine may cause backache from retroperitoneal fibrosis.

13. **Normality** (*non-disease*)

A chronic backache may be an expression of frustration, unhappiness, or strain and fatigue. The back is a sounding-board for many persons' dissatisfaction with their lives, and no organic or psychiatric disease need be present.

Harold Ellis

Bleeding, excessive

Excessive haemorrhage may be observed in many different circumstances. In the presence of a normal haemostatic system it may arise secondary to a structural lesion, e.g. peptic ulcer, and if recurrent bleeding is observed predominantly from a single locus a local pathological lesion may be present. More generalized bleeding may arise either due to an isolated coagulation defect, e.g. haemophilia, or platelet disorder, e.g. thrombocytopenia. Many medical disorders, e.g. liver disease, are often associated with a haemorrhagic state which is usually multifactorial in origin. The severity of the haemorrhagic diathesis is usually proportional to the severity of the underlying disorder.

The maintenance of blood within the vascular system depends upon the integrity of the coagulation mechanism, the presence of a reasonable number of functional platelets as well as endothelial-lined vessels capable of constriction when severed.

Platelets are responsible for controlling the initial onset of haemorrhage by adhering to subendothelial components, e.g. collagen and microfibrils, and forming a plug in the severed vessel. After release from bone marrow megakaryocytes, platelets circulate for 7–10 days. They have a complex structure which is adapted to responding rapidly to breaches in vascular integrity. In addition to cell surface receptors for various activated components of the coagulation cascade, e.g. thrombin, they possess delta granules which contain vascoactive amines e.g. ATP and 5-HT, as well as alpha granules containing proteins which are components of the haemostatic system, e.g. vWF and factor V. Failure of either platelet function or the presence of thrombocytopenia may result in characteristic bleeding e.g. purpura, easy bruising; epistaxis, gastrointestinal haemorrhage or menorrhagia.

The von Willebrand factor is an important plasma protein, secreted by endothelial cells, which promotes adhesion of platelets to damaged vessel walls. It also acts as a carrier protein for factor VIII; hence in von Willebrand's disease the plasma level of factor VIII is often reduced because without its carrier it is unstable and has a reduced plasma half-life. In von Willebrand's disease bleeding is similar to that in individuals with platelet functional disorders, e.g. mucosal haemorrhage, because the von Willebrand factor is essential for the adhesion of platelet to traumatized vessels.

The coagulation cascade consists of a series of proenzymes; each acts initially as an enzyme substrate and after activation itself has enzymic activity and activates a subsequent proenzyme in the cascade (*Fig.* B.10). Although the reactions can take place in plasma the rates of many of the individual steps can be greatly enhanced if they occur on the platelet surface. This procoagulant property of platelets is due to their possession of specific receptors for components of the coagulation cascade.

Conventionally the coagulation system is considered to be composed of two parts, the intrinsic and extrinsic components, although recent research has revealed that the system is considerably more complicated than is illustrated in *Fig.* B.10.

Deficiencies in the coagulation system may be either single, e.g. haemophilia (Factor VIII deficiency), or multiple, e.g. warfarin therapy. Bleeding can occur due to the presence of an inhibitor (usually an IgG antibody) against one or more of the coagulation factors or platelets, e.g. idiopathic thrombocytopenic purpura (ITP).

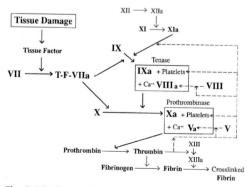

Fig. B.10. The coagulation cascade.

	Platelet count	Bleeding time	APTT	Prothrombin ratio	Fibrinogen	D-dimer
Thrombocytopenia	↓	↑	N	N	N	N
von Willebrand's disease	N	↑	N or ↑	N	N	N
Haemophilia A or B	N	N	↑	N	N	N
Warfarin/liver disease	N	N	N	↑	N	N
Disseminated intravascular coagulation	↓	↑	↑	↑	↓	↑

Bleeding manifestations of isolated deficiencies tend to cause haemarthrosis or muscle haematoma but multiple abnormalities may cause almost any bleeding manifestation. As the primary haemostatic mechanism involving platelets is normal in haemophilia the bleeding often stops immediately after trauma; however haemorrhage may start several hours later because the platelet plug is not consolidated by the deposition of fibrin.

When clinically assessing a patient presenting with possible excessive bleeding it is important to know the following:

1   The duration of symptomatology may indicate whether the possible haemorrhagic predisposition is congenital or acquired.
2   The sites of bleeding may allow assessment of the component of the haemostatic system which is deficient; thrombocytopenia and platelet disorders give rise to purpura and bleeding into mucosal surfaces. A coagulation defect usually results in muscle and joint haemorrhage.
3   Bleeding that starts at the time of trauma, e.g. dental extraction, indicates failure of platelet plug formation due to a platelet disorder or von Willebrand's disease.
4   Haemorrhage which occurs spontaneously is indicative of a more severe bleeding disorder than that which is only provoked by trauma.
5   Dental extractions, tonsillectomy and circumcision are all potent stresses of the haemostatic mechanism. A patient that has had any two of these procedures without loss of excessive blood is unlikely to have a clinically significant bleeding problem.
6   A family history is important as many congenital conditions have a familial predisposition.
7   A drug history is essential because almost all medicines can, by one mechanism or another, predispose to bleeding. Ingestion of warfarin or aspirin are often overlooked. Exposure to toxins or solvents at work or with hobbies may result in hypoplastic anaemia.
8   A general medical history is also essential because many disorders can result in thrombocytopenia or coagulation disturbances, e.g. liver disease or renal failure.

On examination it is important to assess fully the sites of haemorrhage. Examination of the buccal cavity and optic fundi should be carried out in all individuals as superficial bleeding at these sites is indicative of severe platelet dysfunction. It may be necessary to use imaging procedures, e.g. CT scanning or ultrasound to document fully the extent of internal haematoma formation.

Initial screening tests include a complete blood count, examination of a blood film, bleeding time, activated partial thromboplastin time (APTT) (intrinsic system), prothrombin time (extrinsic system), fibrinogen and D-dimers (measure of fibrinolysis).

If a coagulation deficiency is suspected because of a prolongation of either the APTT or PT it is essential to repeat the test after addition of normal plasma when the test time will become normal. Failure to normalize the clotting time should raise the suspicion of the presence of an inhibitor.

Any patient with thrombocytopenia for which the cause is not immediately and unequivocally apparent should have a bone marrow aspirate and/or trephine performed. This will allow assessment of megakaryocytic numbers; reduced in conditions of under production of platelets, e.g. hypoplastic anaemia, or increased when there is increased destruction and/or pooling of platelets in the circulation, e.g. splenomegaly. A trephine biopsy is particularly useful, for assessing whether the bone marrow is infiltrated with carcinoma cells.

C. A. Ludlam

Bone, swelling of

A simple emuneration of the more important conditions to be considered will indicate the complexity of this subject:

(a) *Trauma*
Subperiosteal haematoma (calcified or ossified)
Callus following fracture

(b) *Infection*
Acute osteomyelitis
Chronic osteomyelitis (including Brodie's abscess)
Tuberculous disease of bone
Syphilitic disease of bone
Typhoid (periostitis)

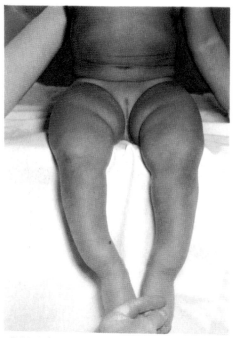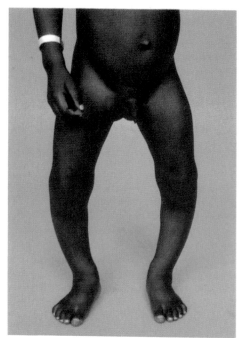

Fig. B.11. Rickets: Note bow legs and swelling in the region of the epiphyses at the knee of both these children from developing countries. (*Courtsey of the Gordon Museum, Guy's Hospital.*)

(c) *Metabolic etc.*

Rickets (*Fig.* B.11)

Scurvy

Leontiasis ossea

Acromegaly

Generalized fibrocystic disease
    (von Recklinghausen)

Paget's disease of bone

(d) *Tumours*

Chondroma

Osteoma

Localized fibrocystic disease (or solitary bone cyst)

Giant-cell tumour (osteoclastoma)

Aneurysmal bone cyst

Non-osteogenic fibroma

Benign chondroblastoma

Osteosarcoma

Fibrosarcoma

Chondrosarcoma

Angiomas and angiosarcoma

Ewing's tumour

Myeloma

Metastatic tumours

Joint conditions such as Charcot's disease and osteoarthritis give rise to swelling of the ends of the bones involved, but these lesions are more properly considered in the discussion on joints.

This list includes diseases which are prevalent at certain ages and it can be simplified for diagnostic purposes by sifting the conditions into approximate age-groups:

From birth until 5 years

Intra-uterine fracture with callus, including those due to osteogenesis imperfecta

Battered baby syndrome

Rickets (*Fig.* B.11)

Scurvy

Congenital syphilitic epiphysitis

Acute osteomyelitis

From 5 until 15 years

Fracture

Calcified subperiosteal haematoma

Acute osteomyelitis

Tuberculous disease

Congenital syphilitic periostitis

Localized fibrocystic disease

Multiple exostoses usually come under observation at this age

Ewing's tumour

Aneurysmal bone cyst

Non-osteogenic fibroma

Benign chondroblastoma

Osteosarcoma

From 15 until 25 years

Fracture

Calcified subperiosteal haematoma

Chronic osteomyelitis

Tuberculous rib and cold abscess

Osteoma, osteochondroma, chondroma
Chondrosarcoma
Angioma
Osteosarcoma
Ewing's tumour

From 25 until 40 years

Fracture
Onset of acromegaly
Tuberculous rib and cold abscess
Acquired syphilitic disease of bone
Osteoclastoma
Fibrosarcoma
Chondrosarcoma
Generalized fibrocystic disease (von Recklinghausen)

From 40 onwards

Fracture
Acquired syphilitic disease of bone
Paget's disease (in the upper years of age-group)
Acromegaly
Myeloma
Metastitic tumours

Although these groups are obviously very elastic there are only a certain number of possibilities at any given age and the field is therefore restricted a little. The difficulties of diagnosis lie not only in distinguishing the varieties of bone swelling, but also in deciding whether the condition is arising from the bone or not, which may be particularly difficult in the case of inflammatory lesions where there is surrounding oedema of soft parts and very little enlargement of the bone itself. If careful palpation fails to reveal alteration in the normal bony contour in a patient where a bone lesion is suspected, the character of any overlying soft-tissue swelling that may be present will sometimes act as a guide. If present it involves all layers, arising from the deep tissues and radiating more or less symmetrically outwards. A central bone lesion will result in swelling of the whole contour of the limb in the area at fault. Pain originating in bone is deep and boring in character and often very intense.

Special investigations

In all cases a radiograph is essential and the differential diagnosis of many of these conditions often resolves itself into a question of interpreting the radiograph. The definite diagnosis of a bone abnormality is now frequently made on isotope bone scanning. In acute osteomyelitis the radiographic evidence of infection is not revealed until the 10th–12th day. An isotope scan, however, will show at the earliest stage an increased bone blood flow and this is indicated by an increased uptake of the isotopic material. Isotopic technetium and gallium are used and both these indicators will show tumours (*Fig.* B.12) and infections in bone.

Computerized tomography (CT) is able to show clearly the gross anatomy and the detailed architecture

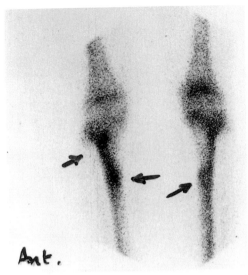

Fig. B.12. Radio-isotope bone scan showing increased uptake in both tibial shafts in a patient with metastic bone disease.

of bone in transverse section. The surrounding soft tissues are also demonstrated (*Fig.* B.13). With the appropriate computer software, these CT sections may be brought up into a three-dimensional reconstruction and this is of great help to the surgeon in planning operative procedures.

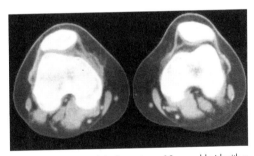

Fig. B.13. CT scan of the knees in an 18-year-old girl with a history of recurrent bilateral subluxation of the patellae.

Magnetic resonance imaging (MRI) will show sections in any plane of altered anatomy of the bone and surrounding soft tissues. Enhanced signals are also seen where there is alteration of blood flow and also of chemistry (*Fig.* B.14). The combination of several of these investigations may be necessary in order to elucidate fully the nature of an obscure bone swelling.

It must be stressed that biopsy of the swelling is the only technique that will give the definitive histological diagnosis.

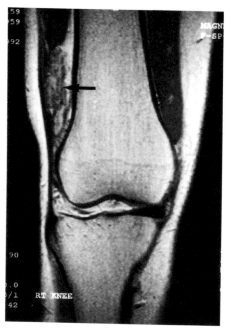

Fig. B.14. Coronal view of magnetic resonance image in a 32-year-old patient, showing cavernous haemangioma in the inferior part of the vastus lateralis muscle (arrowed).

Bone swellings prevalent in infancy

Fractures rarely occur at the time of birth. In breech deliveries, fractures of the lower limbs may be sustained with the usual signs of fracture—swelling, pain, tenderness and loss of function. In oestogenesis imperfecta, rickets, scurvy and syphilis the bone lesions are multiple and in scurvy and rickets they are symmetrical.

INTRA-UTERINE FRACTURE

This occurs in osteogenesis imperfecta. The disease may be familial and is characterized by blue sclera, multiple fractures which result in limb deformity, broadness of the skull base and poor and retarded dentition. In severe cases the child may be stillborn. If the child lives then deformity may be very severe in the overt case but in the 'tarda' variety fractures will be less problematic and later surgical treatment by means of internal fixation rods will control the bone fragility.

THE BATTERED BABY

The battered baby may have multiple fractures and there is usually evidence of repeated external injury in association. Whole body X-rays are required, for multiple fractures in various healing phases may be seen.

RICKETS (*Fig.* B.11)

Rickets is rarely recognized before the age of 6 months and more usually at a year to 18 months. General backwardness often calls attention to the disease, the child being late in sitting up and in dentition, and making little attempt to walk. Restlessness, fretfulness, sweating of the head and abdominal distension are other features. The bone swellings occur in the region of the epiphyses and are often most marked in the lower end of the radius. The ribs are another situation where the deformity occurs, with resulting 'rickety rosary'. Bossing of the frontal and parietal bones leads to the 'hot-cross bun' head. Bowlegs, sinking in of the ribs at the costochondral junctions, and other bending deformities are due to softening of the bones. The history may reveal that the diet has been inadequate in vitamin D and that there has been a lack of fresh air and sunlight. Radiographic examination shows general osteoporosis with considerable broadening and cupping of the metaphyses, which have a hazy irregular margin as if the bone had melted away. The lower end of the radius is usually the best area to choose to obtain a good radiograph. The diagnosis is not difficult except in the mildest cases.

SCURVY

Scurvy is commonly manifest about the age of 12 months or later. The child is restless and irritable and develops extreme tenderness of the affected bones. These are usually the lower end of the femur and upper end of the tibia, and to touch them or even to approach the infant results in paroxysms of screaming. The bone lesion is one of subperiosteal haemorrhage, to which the swelling is due. The overlying skin may become glossy although signs of inflammation are absent. The gums may become swollen and dusky, and haematuria is an occasional feature. In the radiograph the bones show loss of cancellous structure and extreme thinning of the cortex. The haematoma calcifies, beginning at the deep surface of the periosteum; as soon as this has occurred the haemorrhages can be delineated on the radiograph. Here as in rickets a history of inadequate nutrition (vitamin C deficiency) may be obtained.

CONGENITAL SYPHILITIC EPIPHYSITIS

This appears earlier than rickets or scurvy and can sometimes be demonstrated radiographically as early as the second month. The bones of the knee- and wrist-joints are the commonest to show the characteristic changes, and the pain of the lesion is such that the affected limb is often held quite still (syphilitic pseudo-paralysis). The pseudo-paresis which accompanies syphilitic epiphysitis can be distinguished from that occurring in rickets or scurvy by the younger age of onset in the syphilitic form and by other stigmata of congential syphilis (*see below*). The radiograph shows broadening and irregularity of the metaphysis which is quite different from rickets in that the outline, although irregular, is dense and sclerosis is predominant, whereas in rickets the outline is hazy and ill defined and osteoporosis is marked. Typically the layer of dense irregular bone capping the metaphysis is bounded on the shaft side by a thin layer appearing translucent in the radiograph, while the cortical region of this part of the bone shows punched-out areas of subperiosteal erosion. Other bone manifestations present in syphilis of infancy include areas of periosteal new-bone formation, syphilitic dactylitis, and also Parrot's nodes. These last are bosses on the bones of the vertex of the skull which results in a 'hot-cross bun' head often of more exaggerated shape than in rickets. Syphilitic dactylitis is discussed with tuberculous dactylitis in the next section. Other signs of syphilis will of course aid the diagnosis. Pemphigus and other skin eruptions, snuffles, condylomas, mucous patches and fissures at the corners of the mouth are all stigmata to be looked for, while in any suspicious case the VDRL reaction will be tested both in the infant and the parents.

NEONATAL SEPTIC ARTHRITIS OF HIP (TOM SMITH'S DISEASE)

The hip of an infant may become infected at the 7th–10th day of life. The infection is blood-borne with the portal of entry usually being an infected umbilical remnant. The diagnosis is frequently made late, as there are no external signs. However, the child becomes ill, feverish and fretful and is in obvious pain. The affected hip becomes immobile and then, after a day or two, there is a marked swelling around the hip and upper femoral region. There are no early radiological signs but later the joint becomes distended and the femoral head may actually dislocate. Early surgical treatment is imperative.

Bone swellings prevalent in childhood and early adolescence: 5–15 years

Fractures and subperiosteal haematoma are considered in the next age group.

ACUTE OSTEOMYELITIS

This occurs in this period in the great majority of cases. The diagnosis does not present itself as a bony swelling of doubtful nature, but as an acute inflammatory condition whose anatomical origin is the matter for decision. A history of sepsis such as boils or tonsillitis is frequently obtained. The lesion is usually found at one end of a long bone and the severe pain with which it is accompanied causes the child to cry when the limb is touched or moved. There is hot tender brawny oedema of the part, with subsequent reddening and glossiness of the skin; the temperature and the leucocyte count and the ESR are high and the patient is very toxic. The differential diagnosis is from cellulitis of soft parts and from an acute joint lesion. Cellulitis does not usually result in such severe toxaemia as does osteomyelitis and there may be a skin lesion such as a septic abrasion over the area of cellulitis to indicate its origin, in which case the diagnosis will be rendered much easier. The swelling of a cellulitis tends to be localized, at least in the early stages, to one aspect of the limb and its limits can be approximately gauged, whereas the swelling over an osteomyelitis is more generalized and less defined. Furthermore, cellulitis is usually accompanied by lymphangitis and lymphadenitis, whereas osteomyelitis, unless it has extended through the periosteum and invaded the soft tissues around, is not commonly associated with these complications. The diagnosis from a joint lesion such as an acute infective arthritis is made more difficult by the frequent presence of a sympathetic effusion into the joint in cases of oestomyelitis. The maximum swelling in the bone lesion, however, is not over the joint but over the end of the bone, and gentle passive movements of the joint are just possible; in the primary arthritic condition movement is exquisitely painful and the maximum swelling is confined to the joint. Rheumatic fever is differentiated by the unusually rapid pulse-rate as compared with the rise in temperature, by the 'flitting' nature of the pains, and by the response to salicylate therapy.

Osteomyelitis is diagnosed by these clinical features in the early stage together with a positive blood culture. The early X-ray is negative but the gamma scan is intensely positive. A combination antibiotic therapeutic course of high dose is started as soon as the blood culture has been taken. This antibiotic is changed to the appropriate drugs as soon as the culture and sensitivity is available. If the antibiotic regime is not successful in reducing the fever and the acute symptoms within 48 hours, then surgical decompression must be undertaken without further delay.

CHRONIC OSTEOMYELITIS

This may follow acute osteomyelitis, the infection persisting and chronic discharging sinuses developing as a result of sequestra still present. A subacute or chronic abscess may also form as a metastasis in another bone or may arise as a chronic infection from the beginning. A Brodie's abscess, as it is called, is usually found near the end of a long bone and is evidenced by palpable thickening of the bone. Radiographs show a central area of rarefaction with more or less surrounding sclerosis, with a deposition of subperiosteal new bone and sometimes with a sequestrum in the cavity. The diagnosis is chiefly from a tuberculous lesion. This may be impossible without exploration, although sclerosis and subperiosteal new bone are in favour of pyogenic infection. On opening a Brodie's abscess, pus and granulation tissue, usually not exuberant, are found. A tuberculous abscess contains caseous material and the granulations are thick and juicy. If microscopy does not reveal tubercle bacilli in a suspicious case, bacteriological culture is essential. It may not be possible to distinguish radiologically a Brodie's abscess in an older patient from a central gumma. Other signs of syphilis and the serological reactions will give help in this direction.

There are two likely situations for *tuberculosis* to present itself as a bony swelling of doubtful origin. One is the digits, when one or more of the phalanges, metacarpals or metatarsals may be the subject of tuberculous dactylitis; and the other is the ends of the long bones, where a focus may remain localized for some time before spreading, as eventually it frequently does, into the joint. Tuberculous dactylitis begins early in life, usually before the age of 5, and results in a spindle-shaped swelling of the affected segment of the digit. Radiography shows central erosion with deposition of subperiosteal new bone with consequent expansion (*Fig.* B.15). The erosion may spread outwards, destroying the new bone laid down, and finally breaking through the skin already red and shiny. At the stage when the original cortex has been destroyed and there is just a shell of the new bone left the appearance in the radiograph is of the shaft distended as if by gas bubbles, to which the term 'spina ventosa' has been applied. Pain is not a marked feature of the disease. The diagnosis is from syphilitic dactylitis. This latter condition occurs at an even earlier age than tuberculosis, usually before 12 months. Other signs of syphilis (skin rashes, snuffles, thick mop of coarse hair, oral fissures, etc.) and positive serological tests of infant and parents will in most cases aid the diagnosis. Locally the distinction is difficult; there is not the same tendency in syphilis to erosion of the bone or the formation of sinuses, and the new bone is usually thicker and denser, but these slight differences are unreliable. Sarcoidosis of the phalanges may produce a similar radiographic appearance and only biopsy will confirm. Enchondromas should not enter into the differential diagnosis as they

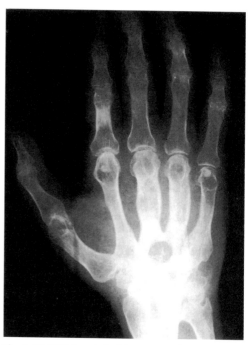

Fig. B.15. Old tuberculosis of the carpus and metacarpus. (*Dr T.H. Hills.*)

occur in adult life, rarely in childhood, never in infancy; and the radiograph shows clear-cut central rarefaction without erosion, and expansion without new bone formation. The only other site of bone tuberculosis where periosteal new bone formation is common is in the ribs. This is a disease of adult life and is not usually presented as a bony swelling but as a cystic swelling, the result of abscess formation. Tuberculosis of the ends of long bones results in an ill-defined swelling with slight pain and some evidence of loss of function, for example a persistent slight limp if the lower limb is involved. Clinically some thickening can be detected, but the diagnosis really rests on the radiograph, which shows an area of rarefaction sometimes containing an ill-defined sequestrum and with little or no new bone formation. The differential diagnosis is from a lesion due to nonspecific pyogenic organisms and is discussed under *chronic osteomyelitis* above. Tuberculosis of bone is a condition insidious in onset and chronic in progress: there may be slight pyrexia, there is no increase in polymorph leucocytes, but usually a slight lymphocytosis. Abscess formation is common in the late stages; the abscess is of the cold variety and tends to break down through an indolent undermined opening on to the skin. Wasting, reflex guarding and starting pains are marked only when the adjacent joint is invaded.

SYPHILITIC PERIOSITIS

At about the age of 9 or 10 congenital syphilitics are liable to develop local or diffuse deposition of dense periosteal bone. This typically occurs in the tibias, which also undergo some elongation resulting in the well-known sabre shape. Other signs of congenital syphilis appear at this age, including Clutton's joints, interstitial keratitis and Hutchinson's teeth (affecting the permanent incisors), and these, together with signs present since infancy (rhagades, saddle-shaped nose, etc.), and the positive serology will give the diagnosis.

LOCALIZED FIBROCYSTIC DISEASE OR SOLITARY BONE CYST

Commonly occurs between the ages of 10 and 15 and usually arises in the upper ends of the humerus, femur or tibia, the patient most often coming under observation for a pathological fracture. The fracture is notably caused by comparatively slight violence, and the radiograph shows the well-defined outline of a cyst with cortical thinning but no erosion. There are usually trabeculae running across the cyst cavity which may lead to confusion with a giant-cell tumour, but the simple cyst occurs at a younger age, does not invade the epiphysis, and does not expand to the same extent as an osteoclastoma and therefore does not perforate the cortex. The clear-cut margins and the absence of erosion or melting away of the bone differentiate the condition from a sarcoma. Following a fracture, healing may occur.

FIBROUS DYSPLASIA (*Figs* B.16, B.17)

Fibrocystic disease may extend through much of the diaphysis and metaphysis of a long bone in a child of this age. The extension of the fibrous infiltration continues up to maturity and again the commonest presenting feature is a pathological fracture. The mechanical weakness produced by this fibrous lesion may require exploration of this area of bone, curettage of the fibrous area, cancellous bone grafting and sometimes strengthening by internal fixation. This will also allow adequate biopsy material to be taken.

MULTIPLE CARTILAGE-CAPPED EXOSTOSES (DIAPHYSIAL ACLASIA)

A hereditary disease where multiple bony outgrowths may be accompanied by dwarfing and by curved and deformed limbs. The radiographs are typical (*Fig.* B.18).

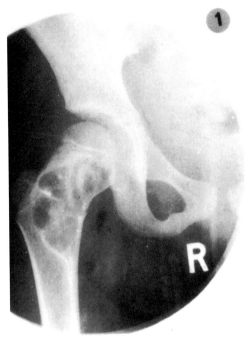

Fig. B.16. Fibrous dysplasia of the femoral neck.

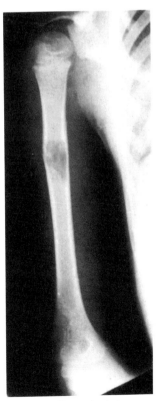

Fig. B.17. Bone cyst in fibrous dysplasia.

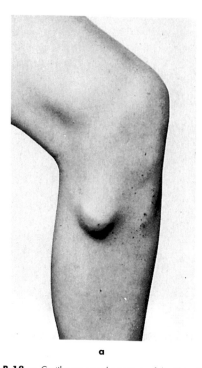

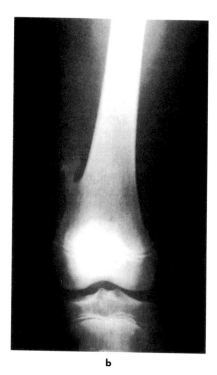

a
b

Fig. B.18. *a.* Cartilage-capped exostosis of the tibia. *b.* Exostosis of the lower end of the femur. *(Dr T.H. Hills.)*

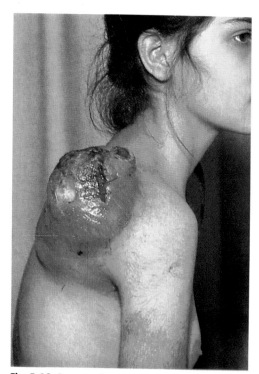

Fig. B.19. Fungating Ewing's tumour of the scapula.

EWING'S TUMOUR *(Fig. B.19)*

This is a sarcoma of small, round progenitor cells in the bone. The characteristic site of this tumour is the diaphysis of a long bone but no area of the skeleton is exempt. The tumour classically metastasizes to bone and it is highly malignant. The clinical presentation is frequently one of an inflamed area of the bone with localized tenderness, swelling, heat and redness. The child may become systemically ill. Radiographs show increased density and width of the cortex with some mottling of the medulla and later some erosion and destruction of bone. The characteristic feature of the radiological diagnosis is, however, the multiple periosteal layers of new bone which are built up around this mid-diaphysial region and the classic radiological appearances are often described as resembling 'onion skins'. As the tumour metastasizes to other bones a full skeletal survey must be undertaken together with an isotope scan. Biopsy is necessary and this is best undertaken through a small puncture with a trocar and cannula and appropriate biopsy forceps. In the past there has been some confusion between this tumour and secondary deposits from a medulloblastoma, but it is now accepted that this is a sarcoma, primarily from bone and it is not a metastasis.

ANEURYSMAL BONE CYSTS

These may occur in any bone but mainly in the axial skeleton. The affected bone is expanded, the cyst thinning and distending the cortex. Pathological fractures may occur through this lesion which frequently requires biopsy for its final diagnosis. The gross appearance of the aneurysmal bone cyst resembles that of the giant-cell tumour in later life and the histological features are very similar, including many giant cells. The aneurysmal bone cyst, however, only occurs in the immature skeleton and remains benign.

NON-OSTEOGENIC FIBROMA

This lesion is usually an incidental X-ray finding in the long bones, particularly of the lower limb. However, it may affect any area of the immature skeleton and is seen incidentally on radiographs as a 'bubble' in the cortex. At the time of skeletal maturity these fibromas disappear but their site may be marked by a little sclerosis, sometimes called a 'bone island'. Non-osteogenic fibromas may become large and again may be the site of a pathological fracture.

BENIGN CHONDROBLASTOMA AND OSTEOBLASTOMA

These are rare, benign tumours affecting the epiphysis. The osteoblastoma resembles the osteoid osteoma when it affects the spine and particularly its lamina and pedicle. Diagnosis is made on radiological features with a rarefied zone in the epiphysis; final biopsy is essential.

OSTEOSARCOMA

Although the osteosarcoma is the most common of the primary malignant bone tumours, it is still seen as a rare event and it is calculated that in Britain each general practitioner will see one new case in his professional lifetime. The tumour affects the young person between the age of 5 and 25, but it may be seen *de novo* in the elderly person in an area of Paget's disease (Paget's osteosarcoma). It is a highly malignant tumour with early metastases to the lungs. It develops in the metaphysis of the long bone, but again no area of the skeleton is exempt. The most common sites are around the knee, where the lower femur and upper tibial metaphyses are involved (*Fig.* B.20). The lower forearm and upper arm are again the most specific sites in the upper limb. The clinical presentation is frequently insidious and the symptoms and signs may be those of an inflammatory condition. The area around the knee joint may become a little swollen, inflamed, red, hot and somewhat painful. Differential diagnosis

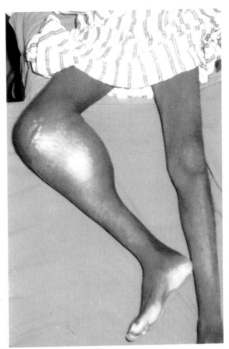

Fig. B.20. Osteosarcoma of the upper tibia.

at this early stage may be that of a cellulitis, an inflammatory arthropathy or even an internal derangement of the knee, and for this reason the diagnosis may be sadly delayed. The radiological appearance, however, is characteristic and is characterized by new bone formation with sclerosis of the metaphysical region and osteogenic bone spreading out in a radial fashion (sun-ray spicules) (*Fig.* B.21). Periosteal new bone at the end of the tumour area may form a small triangle known as 'Codman's triangle'. Radiologically there is a soft tissue mass in continuity and the tumour may produce bone rarefaction in its destructive area.

A full radiological review of the patient's skeleton should be made together with detailed radiographs of the lungs, to include either tomography or CT scanning. An isotope bone scan of the body is also required to determine 'skip' lesions in the same bone or rarely distant metastases to other bones.

The final diagnosis is by biopsy. Although the material submitted to the pathologist must be adequate, it should be remembered that a puncture over the tumour is ideal and a longer incision may be regretted for this highly malignant sarcoma may rapidly fungate through such a wound. Through a small puncture wound a trocar and cannula is inserted under image intensification X-ray control and appropriate biopsy forceps are inserted to take representative portions of this tumour for histological assessment.

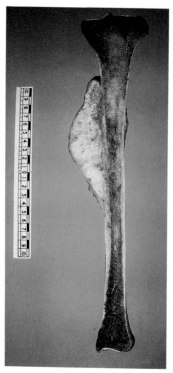

Fig. B.21. Operative specimen of tibia split longitudinally to show osteosarcoma.

Bone swellings seen from 15 until 25 years

FRACTURE

That *fracture* is a possible diagnosis can usually be suspected from the history. It is uncommon for patients to present themselves with a bony swelling without having had pain dating from definite trauma. Occasionally, however, a fracture has occurred without very much being noticed at the time and as the lack of immobilization may cause excessive formation of callus, the consequent swelling, possibly associated with some continued slight weakness or discomfort, is the symptom for which the patient seeks advice. Likely situations for this to occur are in a metatarsal ('march fracture') and at the upper end the tibia ('recruits' fracture'). Both these fractures are stress fractures and the radiological diagnosis may be delayed. At a later stage (after 3 weeks) a little sclerosis of the cortex may be seen and the only way to make a diagnosis before this time is to undertake an isotope bone scan which clearly shows increased bone blood flow. There is also some possibility of confusing the mass of callus with a bone sarcoma but it is only rarely necessary to biopsy this area if doubt persists. A spontaneous pathological fracture is more properly considered with the appropriate cause. Radiologically there is usually some abnormal rarefaction around the fracture site and on isotope scanning other multiple deposits may be detected.

A SUBPERIOSTEAL HAEMATOMA

This is formed as the result of a blow. Calcification and subsequent ossification may follow, leaving a small permanent thickening. Such nodes are found not infrequently on the shins of football players. The diagnosis should present no difficulty, the swelling is quite localized and the radiograph shows normal dense bone causing a slight increase in the thickness of the cortex.

OSTEOCHONDROMAS (CANCELLOUS EXOSTOSES)

These are found most commonly in the bones forming the knee joint, the upper end of the tibia and the lower end of the femur. The upper ends of the femur and humerus and the small bones of the foot are the other common sites. Typically the outgrowth is pedunculated and projects from the metaphysis overhanging the shaft away from the epiphysis (*see Fig.* B.18). The base is osseous and is capped by cartilage—the extent of each and the degree of pedunculation being variable. The patient usually seeks advice because he has noticed the swelling, there may be some discomfort, or some injury may have drawn attention to the outgrowth. The only likely cause for confusion is myositis ossificans, particularly if the lesion is found around the elbow or hip, but differentiation should not be difficult as it can be demonstrated on the radiograph that the bony swelling of traumatic myositis is not continuous with the bone.

OSTEOMAS (IVORY EXOSTOSES)

These are hard sessile growths, densely opaque to X-rays, which occur in the membrane bones, notably the vertex of the skull and the maxillae. On the inner surface of the skull bones they may give rise to signs resembling a cerebral tumour.

PURE CHONDROMAS

These occur in the great majority of cases in the fingers, the only other common sites being the toes and the chondrosternal junctions (*Fig.* B.22). They cause a painless expansion of the bone and the patient again

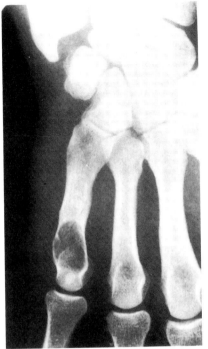

Fig. B.22. Enchondroma of 5th metacarpal. (*Dr John D. Dow.*)

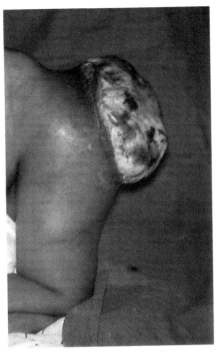

Fig. B.23. Fungating chondrosarcoma of the scapula.

comes for advice for the tumour. Radiographs (*Fig. B.23*) show a clear-cut translucent central space with thinned cortex predisposing to pathological fracture. Trabeculae traverse the cavity and the general picture somewhat resembles a giant-cell tumour or a bone cyst, but neither of these conditions occurs in the small bones of the hand or foot or in the sternum.

CHONDROSARCOMA

This is the commonest primary malignant tumour of bone. Any age between 20 and 60 may be affected. The pelvis, ribs, sternum, scapula and femur are common sites. A useful aphorism is that 'the nearer a cartilaginous tumour is to the axial skeleton and the larger it is, the more likely it is to be malignant'. Macroscopically it is a bulky tumour which extends away from the bone to invade adjacent soft tissues (*Fig. B.23*). Blood spread occurs to the lungs. X-rays of the tumour reveal an expanding lesion with irregular mottling and calcification, often with frank destruction of cortical and trabecular bone.

Microscopically, the tumour shows cellular atypical cartilage with irregular cells, many of which have double nuclei. There may be areas of cystic change and calcification or ossification is frequently seen in the stroma.

ANGIOMA

Angioma is a very rare condition, as a rule only diagnosed by microscopy. The skull and vertebrae are occasionally subject to this tumour. Radiography shows a spongy honeycombed appearance at the site of the lesion.

OSTEOID OSTEOMA

This is a rare tumour of the adolescent and young adult. It is considered to be a primary bone tumour arising from osteoblasts, usually in the cortex of a bone. Osteoid is laid down within this cortex and soon comes under substantial pressure, producing severe pain. Although it is considered to be a neoplasm there has been considerable debate over the past few years as to the exact nature of this lesion. The symptoms are those of severe pain both day and night. The night pain is frequently so disturbing as to make the patient haggard and ill and the most effective analgesic is aspirin. The specific relief of painful symptoms with pure aspirin may be considered a diagnostic feature. There is usually an area of tenderness of the bone at the site of this osteoid osteoma but if the lesion is hidden in an inaccesible part of the skeleton, pain may be present over a much wider area.

Radiologically the features are those of a peaked-up area of sclerotic cortical bone with a central translucent nidus. At the early stages in the life of this lesion the minor radiological changes may be missed but an isotope bone scan is again characteristic, showing the localized hot spot. Tomography may assist the localization of the nidus when X-ray changes are present. Simple local excision of the lesion is curative.

Bone swellings from 25 until 40 years

ACROMEGALY is a general disease affecting the skeleton symmetrically, particularly the bones of the head, face and hands, which undergo together with the adjacent soft tissues a tremendous hypertrophy. The condition is unlikely to be presented as a doubtful bony swelling.

Leontiasis ossea is of unknown aetiology. Here again there is a generalized overgrowth of the bones of the head and face, but without changes in the soft tissues or in other areas.

ACQUIRED SYPHILITIC DISEASE OF BONE

Most commonly presents in the form of circumscribed gummas, which may appear in the cancellous tissue or subperiosteally. The skull is a common site, the bone being eroded by gummatous infiltration, leaving a worm-eaten defect of serpiginous outline with areas of dense sclerosis and irregular sequestra. The ulceration involves the scalp, and the typical 'wash-leather' base to the ulcer is observed. The sternum, clavicle and ribs are the subject of subperiosteal lesions of bone which tend to be accompanied by dense sclerosis, limiting the outline of the punched-out area of gummatous formation and piling up under the periosteum at the edges of the lesion. Central gummas may appear at the end of a long bone in the form of localized areas of rarefaction. The diagnosis is aided by the presence of other signs of tertiary syphilis, including skin lesions, scarring and perforations of the palate, testicular swelling and loss of sensation, and sometimes the presence of cerebrospinal syphilis or rarely tabes and general paralysis of the insane, and in all cases of bone lesions the serological reaction should be tested. This rule has saved needless amputations, although of course syphilis and malignant disease can be present together, but in the case of a purely syphilitic lesion the administration of anti-syphilitic treatment will cause regression of signs (*Fig.* B.24).

GIANT-CELL TUMOUR OR OSTEOCLASTOMA

This occurs, as do so many bone lesions, most commonly around the knee joint, but a second

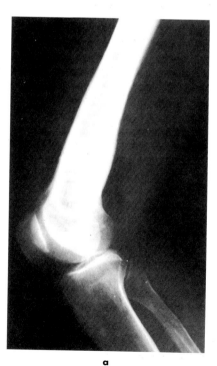 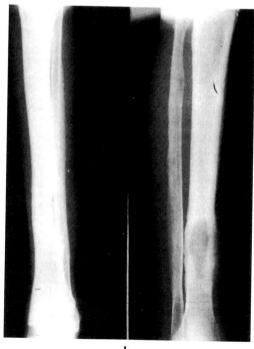

a   b

Fig. B.24. *a.* Syphilitic osteitis of the femur, showing sclerosis and periosteal new bone formation. *b.* Gumma of the tibia, showing dense sclerosis around area of rarefaction. (*Dr T.H. Hills.*)

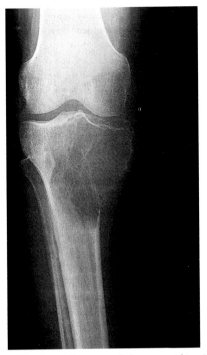

Fig. B.25. Giant-cell tumour of the upper tibia, X-ray appearance.

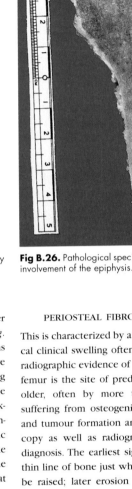

Fig B.26. Pathological specimen from the same patient. Note involvement of the epiphysis.

common site, not so frequently shared with other conditions, is the lower end of the radius (*Fig.* B.25). Pain and tumour formation are the symptoms for which the patient seeks advice, and these are often preceded by a history of injury. The swelling is usually easily palpable and in advanced cases the shell of bone becomes so thin that 'egg-shell crack-ing' can be elicited. Early perforation of the expan-ded cortex is common. This is seen on radiographic examination (*Fig.* B.26), the radiograph showing the trabeculated translucent growth so typical of the condition, expanding the cortex asymmetrically at first and later generally. The epiphysis is involved in the process but the articular cartilage is seldom perforated. There is complete absence of new bone formation, which helps to distinguish the condition from sarcoma. The characteristic radiograph does not usually suggest confusion with a malignant lesion but rather with simple bone cysts. In the latter case the age of onset is earlier and the bone expansion and destruction much less marked. Microscopy of a giant-cell tumour shows the typical picture of a round celled stroma densely packed with giant cells each with a large number of crowded nuclei. However, careful histology is nee-ded for differentiation from the three other giant-cell tumours.

PERIOSTEAL FIBROSARCOMA

This is characterized by a very large usually asymmetri-cal clinical swelling often out of all proportion to the radiographic evidence of disease. The lower end of the femur is the site of predilection and the patients are older, often by more than a decade, than those suffering from osteogenic sarcoma. Once more pain and tumour formation are the symptoms and micros-copy as well as radiography may be necessary for diagnosis. The earliest sign on a radiograph is a little thin line of bone just where the periosteum begins to be raised; later erosion of the bone gradually takes place from without inwards.

GENERALIZED FIBROCYSTIC DISEASE (VON RECKLINGHAUSEN)

A rare condition sometimes associated with hyper-parathyroidism due to adenoma or hypertrophy of these glands. There is widespread resorption of the skeleton resulting in softening and bending of the bones. X-ray shows diminished density, areas of fibro-cystic formation (*Fig.* B.27), and the presence of bone cysts in varying numbers and sizes. The diagnosis is clinched by the increased serum-calcium and urinary-calcium output, the diminished plasma-phosphorus and the increased plasma-phosphatase (normals—

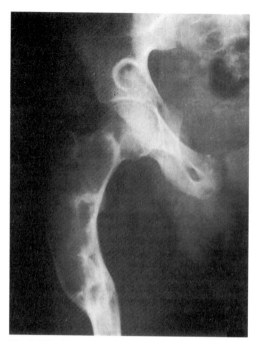

Fig. B.27. Fibrocystic disease of the upper end of the femur and ilium. (*Dr T.H. Hills.*)

serum calcium 9–11 mg per cent (2·25–2·75 mmol/l), often raised to 12–15 mg (3–3·75 mmol/l); phosphate 3·5 mg per cent (1·15 mmol/l), often lowered to below 2 mg (0·65 mmol/l).

Bone swelling prevalent in advancing years

PAGET'S DISEASE

Paget's disease (osteitis deformans) is a generalized condition occurring in old age and resulting in progressive enlargement of the long bones and the skull. The normal architecture is lost and there is deposition of soft porous bone both inside and outside the cortex, the whole bone becoming very much broadened. The skull may show the most marked increase in size, rendering necessary the wearing of a progressively larger size in hats. The long bones tend to bend and the femurs to become bowed, which, together with the kyphosis which develops, causes the hands to hang at a very low level; the large head is thrust forward and the whole attitude is 'simian'. Radiography show a genarlized thickening of the cortical bone without increased density. The tibia, femur, pelvis, skull and spine are the bones most commonly affected, occasionally asymmetrically, while

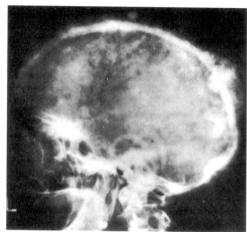

Fig. B.28. Paget's disease of the skull with sarcomatous change.

in rare cases one bone is affected for a long period before any others. Sarcoma may develop in a bone affected by Paget's disease (*Fig.* B.28).

MULTIPLE MYELOMA

Multiple myeloma is a disease of older life, being commonest in males between the ages of 40 and 60. The outstanding symptom is pain, beginning inter-

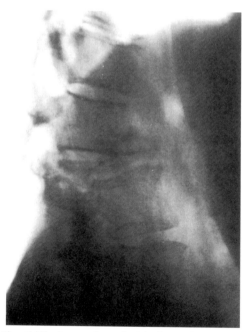

Fig. B.29. Destroyed vertebral bodies with secondary deposits.

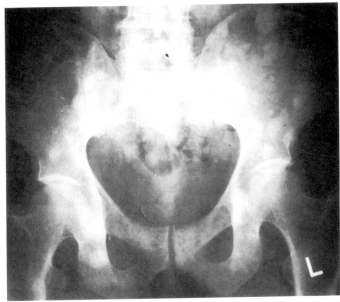

Fig. B.30. Secondary deposits of carcinoma of the prostate, showing discrete osteoblastic areas. (*Dr T.H. Hills.*)

mittently and wandering and becoming so severe as to cause the patient to shrink back as the clinician approaches to carry out his examination. A severe bout of pain may leave the patient exhausted and collapsed. The ribs and vertebrae and skull are the most frequent sites, followed by the upper end of the femur, the upper end of the humerus and the pelvic bones. The lesions are almost without exception multiple, and therefore in any suspicious case the ribs, spine and skull should all be radiographed. There is frequently a palpable mass, fairly often a pathological fracture. Radiography shows the typical lesions as rounded, punched-out holes occurring in the marrow, varying in size greatly, but usually between 0·5 and 2·5 cm. In their characteristic form they are unmistakable. Microscopy shows the majority of the cells to be oval with eccentric nuclei, so-called plasma cells. Another diagnostic point is the presence in about 60 per cent of cases of Bence-Jones protein in the urine. A light cloud of protein is precipitated as the urine is heated between the temperatures of 50 (122°F) and 60°C (140°F); as the temperature is raised the cloud goes into solution again, to reappear on cooling. Bence Jones protein is also present in a number of other conditions involving bone marrow, as for example malignant metastases, which is the only condition likely to be confused with multiple myeloma. Electrophoretic study of the serum shows a 'spike' close to the gamma position and this is highly distinctive of multiple myeloma.

METASTATIC TUMOURS

These are liable to occur in the bones when the primary lesion is in the breast, lung, prostate, kidney, thyroid and uterus. The appearance of the secondary tumours varies according to the primary conditions (*Fig.* B.29). The three liable to produce multiple lesions are the breast, lung and prostate; in the former particularly the appearances can simulate those of multiple myeloma, but fortunately the breast being so easily accessible the primary (or an operation scar) is usually readily detectable to suggest the diagnosis. Metastates from a prostatic carcinoma tend to be osteoblastic and the radiograph shows diffuse mottling, usually of the pelvic bones, with general increase in density (*Fig.* B.30).

Paul Aichroth

Borborygmi

'Borborygmi' is the term applied to rumbling noises of varying quality and intensity produced by peristaltic movements of the bowel propelling mixed gaseous and liquid contents.

These sounds, although normally inaudible to the patient or to other persons, and detected only by auscultation by means of a stethoscope, may occasionally be annoyingly obtrusive. They may occur in perfectly normal people, especially when the alimentary canal is relatively empty, for instance when a meal is overdue, and they may occur as a result of nervous air-swallowing. They may be due to excessive ingestion of aperients or may complicate the excessive fermentation within the bowel that may occur in steatorrhoea. In other cases they may be due to the powerful peristaltic waves of a bowel that is hypertrophied and dilated above a slowly developing obstruction of the large bowel; here there will usually be accompanying progressive constipation, colicky abdominal pains and distension. Some people are able to produce a loud sound by forcibly contracting the muscles of the anterior abdominal wall and splashing the fluid content of the stomach. Avery Jones reports one patient who could be heard the whole distance across a large outpatient clinic.

The *carcinoid syndrome* may feature loud borborygmi as well as flushing of the face, trunk and limbs, pulmonary stenosis, cramping abdominal pains and diarrhoea. In the *Peutz–Jeghers* syndrome (adenomatosis of the small intestine) borborygmi are common, the intenstinal polyps causing increased peristalsis and sometimes intussusecption. This syndrome is characterized by melanotic spots of great profusion around the lips and usually extending onto the buccal mucosa.

The absence of borborygmi, resulting in complete silence in the abdomen on auscultation for several minutes, is seen in adynamic ileus and peritonitis.

Harold Ellis

Breast lumps

(*See also* Nipple, Abnormalities of)

Method of examination

The patient should sit stripped to the waist, so that a clear view of both breasts, the thorax, axillae and supraclavicular fossae may be obtained. The surgeon should sit with his eyes level with the nipples. Both breasts should first be looked at as a whole, to see whether they are symmetrical in size, contour and level, and whether the two nipples are in the same site and of the same circumference, prominence and inclination. One breast may always have been smaller or one nipple inverted, but any recent change is highly significant. The patient should then lie on a couch and the breasts be studied in detail for the evidence of local enlargement or shrinking, and for abnormalities such as redness of the skin, dilatation of veins, tumour or ulcer. If no difference is at first noticed, the patient should be asked to raise both arms slowly above the head and bring them down again to the side, since differences previously invisible, particularly dimpling of the skin from attachment of a lump, may come into

view as the breast glides over the chest wall. Next the breasts are felt, using first the flat of the hand, passingly systematically over all parts, examining comparable sectors on the two sides simultaneously; afterwards the fingers are used for more detailed examination of any irregularity that may have been discovered or suspected. The axillae should also be palpated carefully for enlarged nodes, particular attention being paid to the inner wall, along the pectoralis minor and to the apex. In cases of suspected cancer the supra and infraclavicular fossae should also be examined for fullness or enlarged nodes, and the chest and liver should be investigated for signs of secondary growth. Examination from behind with the patient sitting may be used to check any abnormalities seen, felt or suspected in the lying position.

ALTERNATIVE POSTURE FOR DIFFICULT OR PENDULOUS BREASTS

When dealing with a woman with large, obese or pendulous breasts, the conventional posture for examination is often unsatisfactory. An alternative posture is to arrange the woman in a semi-recumbent position, rotated obliquely with a pillow behind the scapula of the side under examination and the shoulder fully abducted, with the hand tucked behind the head. This fixes the pectoralis major and allows the breast disc to 'float' over a rigid base (*Fig.* B.31).

Classification

SWELLINGS OF THE WHOLE BREAST
Bilateral
Pregnancy
Lactation
ANDI (abnormalities of normal development and involution)
Hypertrophy
In males from stilboestrol administration
Acute mastitis

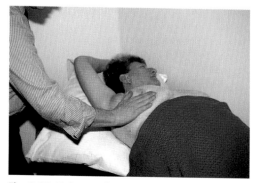

Fig. B.31. Technique of examining the breast in an obese subject.

Unilateral
Fibro-adenosis of the newborn
Puberty
Unilateral hypertrophy

DISCRETE LUMPS IN BREAST
Benign
Fibro-adenoma
Simple cyst
Galactocele
Lipoma
Plasma cell mastitis
(Rare fat necrosis
　Tuberculous abscess)
　Phylloides tumour

Malignant
Carcinoma
(Rare sarcoma
　Lymphoma)

MULTIPLE SWELLINGS, USUALLY INVOLVING
BOTH BREASTS
ANDI
Multiple cysts

SWELLINGS THAT ARE NOT OF THE BREAST
Retromammary abscess:
　From disease of rib
　Chronic empyema
Chondroma of chest wall
Deformities of the ribs
Mondor's disease

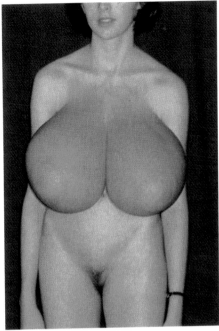

Fig. B.32. Enormous bilateral breast hypertrophy in a teenaged girl.

Swelling in pregnancy and lactation

Swelling in these cases is normal, and only liable to cause confusion when the patient is unaware of her condition. Both breasts are enlarged equally and feel tense and nodular. The superficial veins are usually prominent, and on gentle squeezing a few drops of milk are discharged from the nipple. Montgomery's tubercles will be evident.

True hypertrophy

True hypertrophy is rare. The enlargement is of two types; the commoner where multiple fibro-adenomas cause a bilateral enlargement of varying consistency, and the less common consisting in a diffuse lipomatosis of both breasts sometimes attaining prodigious proportions (*Fig.* B.32). The condition is usually bilateral, but may be one-sided, in which case it is very disfiguring.

Unilateral enlargements

These are usually found in the undeveloped breast. In the *newborn* one breast is often enlarged to the limits of its infantile size, and may discharge a little serous fluid from the nipple. The enlargement used to be attributed to the manipulation of midwives, but it is more probably due to an endocrine imbalance consequent on the withdrawal of the maternal hormones in the fetal circulation, and subsides rapidly. In girls at *puberty* one breast may enlarge several months before the other, and may distress a solicitous mother; unless there are obvious signs of an inflammatory change, no notice need be taken of unilateral enlargement of the breast in girls from 10 to 13. Uniform enlargement of one breast also occurs in *men* usually after the age of 40, and nodular plaques may appear in both sexes at puberty as a result of endocrine disturbance.

On no account should the breast disc of an adolescent girl be biopsied, as this may cause failure of either a quadrant or the whole breast to develop and would be a legitimate reason for litigation.

Acute mastitis

Actue mastitis usually occurs during lactation, occasionally during pregnancy, and is most often due to infection with pyogenic organisms which have gained entrance through cracks in the nipple. At the beginning of the illness there is shivering, followed by fever and a feeling of weight and pain in the breast; the pain soon becomes very acute. In the early stages the swelling is limited to one part of the breast, which feels more resistant than normal; the skin is not reddened at first, nor are the lymphatic nodes enlarged. Pressure over the swelling may cause extrusion of a drop of pus from the nipple, and this is distinguished from milk by its viscidity and yellow colour. Later, fluctuation may become evident and, as the inflammation approaches the skin, this becomes red and oedematous, and ultimately an abscess may point and burst through it; at the same time other foci of suppuration form, until the breast may be a bag of pus. The presence of fever and the intense tenderness of one portion of the breast are sufficient to distinguish acute mastitis from physiological engorgement.

It is not uncommon to find a small *areolar abscess*, which represents an infected gland of Montgomery.

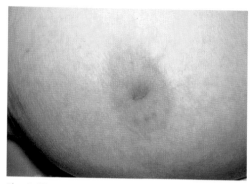

Fig. B.33. Duct ectasia of the nipple.

Duct Ectasia/Plasma Cell Mastitis (Periductal Mastitis)

There is a common group of diseases which are generally poorly recognized, that cluster together under this heading. Their aetiology is unknown. For example, it is even uncertain whether the inflammatory process comes first, followed by ectasia of the duct, or whether ectatic ducts are the primary phenomena with sloughing duct epithelium responsible for initiating the process of periductal mastitis. Assuming the latter sequence of events, then the cycle of clinical features may develop in the following way. The terminal lactiferous ducts dilate and often become hugely ectatic. As a consequence of this, the epithelial lining loosens and liquifies, causing plugs of cellular debris to fill up the ectatic ducts. The first clinical symptom of this condition is the extrusion of viscous multicoloured discharge from multiple duct orifices on the nipple surface. The milk ducts then become permeable to cellular and lipid contents normally contained within the lumina and these then excite a chemical periductal inflammatory process, which is characterized by infiltration with plasma cells and foreign body giant cells. At this stage, a hard indurated mass with overlying inflammation may appear at the areolar margin. Commonly this condition resolves spontaneously within a week or two. Less often, the inflammatory mass becomes secondarily infected with anaerobic organisms, liquifying to produce a peri-areolar abscess. This may point at the areolar margin and spontaneously discharge. If the condition is not recognized and treated appropriately, then a pathological communication between the ducts of the nipple and the skin develops, forming a so-called mamillary duct fistula. Over the years, a series of clinical or subclinical episodes of periductal mastitis produces fibrosis along the ducts, causing them to shrink and pull in the nipple, producing a typical slit-like indrawing at the centre (*Fig.* B.33). Ultimately the condition burns itself out with age. This complex of conditions is most common postmenopausally but, if it occurs in premenopausal women, tends to be more florid, often bilateral, leading to multiple abscesses and fistulae. The mammillary duct fistula should be treated by laying open the fistula track and excising the chronic inflammatory tissue. Recurrent episodes of periductal mastitis and troublesome nipple discharge should be treated by removing surgically the whole of the subareolar system, according to Hadfield's procedure.

Tuberculous abscess

Tuberculous abscess is rare, but a certain number of cases of chronic mastitis and chronic abscess are really tuberculous, particularly in developing countries. The disease is insidious, starting as a painless irregular swelling, the periphery of which is hard and the centre soft. Later, the skin becomes reddened, and an abscess forms which may burst and leave a sinus. It differs from an acute abscess in that the duration is much longer, there is little or no pain or fever, and the pus, if examined, reveals no organisms on culture unless there has been secondary infection; direct examination of stained films of the pus may show tubercle bacilli. The facts that the history is a long one, that the swelling or the edges of it are hard, and that the axillary nodes may be enlarged, render this condition liable to be confounded with carcinoma of the ordinary form, or one in which suppuration has occurred.

Local fat necrosis

If this follows a blow on the breast it may give rise to a tumour almost indistinguishable from cancer. It is hard, irregular in outline, and fixed to the skin. Points of distinction are the previous history of severe injury at the exact spot where the swelling lies, the impression given on palpation that the lump is *on* rather than *of* the breast, and the absence of hard nodes in the axilla. Sometimes a period of 2 to 3 weeks observation is justifiable, in which time a traumatic swelling should decrease in size, but if there is any real doubt about its nature it should be excised and submitted to section.

Contrary to popular myth this is a rare condition of the breast. It is usually wise to ignore a history of trauma to the breast and fully investigate the lump with mammography and biopsy.

Galactocele

A cyst containing milk, this is formed by dilatation of one of the larger ducts owing to obstruction. Galactoceles occur only during lactation and very rarely in the later months of pregnancy; they form oval fluctuating swellings lying in the central zone of the breast just outside the areola, and on pressure milk can sometimes be squeezed out of the nipple. Aspiration both confirms the diagnosis and cures the condition.

Single cysts

These usually lie on the deep surface of the breast, so that their outline is obscured and they bear a considerable resemblance to carcinoma. The absence of skin dimpling and of any alteration in the size or shape of the breast as a whole or in the appearance of the nipple, and a sensation of elasticity when the swelling is pressed firmly, suggest the diagnosis.

Innocent tumours

A fibro-adenoma is the only common innocent tumour of the breast. It is an encapsulated tumour, generally single, but sometimes multiple, and varying in size. It is more common (and often multiple) in Afro-Carribean women. It is firm, with the consistency of hard rubber, rounded, or with irregular rounded projections, and clearly outlined. Most characteristic is the ease with which it can be moved under the skin and in the substance of the breast, to neither of which does it appear to have any attachment, hence the term 'breast mouse' which is applied to this lesion. These tumours generally occur between the ages of 18 and 30 and, though they are quite painless, they are so firm that they are usually discovered by the patient. Although a carcinoma of the breast is rare in this age group, it is wise practice to remove all such lumps for urgent microscopic examination. A *lipoma* may occur in the breast as elsewhere, and has the same characters.

However, always beware the 'pseudolipoma' which may be the earliest sign of a small invasive duct

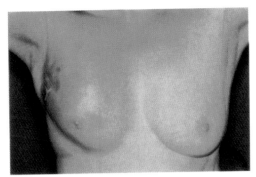

Fig. B.34. Massive carcinoma of the right breast. Note incipient skin ulceration and the elevation and retraction of the nipple.

cancer, which by infiltrating Cooper's ligaments may extrude fatty lobules forming a mushroom-like umbrella over the primary focus.

Malignant tumours

Malignant tumours of the breast are nearly always primary. Sarcoma is very rare, but *carcinoma* is common and the most important tumour that affects the breast. It is essentially a disease of the female breast, only about 1 per cent of the cases occurring in males. It is common in both married and unmarried women, and may occur at any age after puberty, though the majority are in women between 35 and 60. In advanced cases the disease is obvious (*Fig.* B.34); the tumour is large and hard, attached to and ultimately, if not removed, fungating through the skin and becoming fixed to the chest wall; the axillary nodes are enlarged and hard; at this stage the patient is often cachectic. Such cases are beyond any but palliative treatment, and the importance of diagnosis lies in the recognition of the early case, where the only sign is a small lump which the patient has probably discovered accidentally. Usually there is no pain and the patient looks and feels perfectly well. The lump may lie in any part of the breast, but typically is intermediate between the nipple and the periphery, and is more commonly in the upper and outer quadrant than in the other three. It can usually be felt with the flat of the hand. These lumps may be stony hard, but any consistency may be met with. Its outline is usually not sharply defined. In the early stage it is freely movable over the pectoral muscles and under the skin, but it is not so movable in the breast substance as is a fibro-adenoma. Very soon bands of fibrous tissue that connect the breast with the skin become involved, and by their contraction prevent free movement of the skin over the swelling, and cause first dimpling when the tumour is displaced, later puckering visible all the

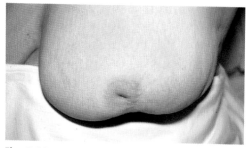

Fig. B.35. Recent nipple inversion in carcinoma of the breast.

time. If the tumour is anywhere near the centre of the breast, the nipple becomes retracted (*Fig.* B.35); a nipple may have been always depressed, but if one previously well formed becomes retracted the sign is of serious import. Fixation to the deep fascia, which usually comes later, can be demonstrated by making the patient press her hands on the iliac crests to fix the pectoralis major, when the involved breast will be found to move less on the muscle than the normal one. Many cancerous tumours, even when extensive infiltration has occurred, cause shrinkage, so that the affected breast may appear smaller than the healthy one, and in the atrophic form it may almost disappear (*Fig.* B.36). In the ordinary form it will be rare to find any discharge from the nipple. After a while the axillary nodes become enlarged and hard. Too much attention should not be given to the absence of palpable nodes; in a fat patient they may be enlarged but impalpable, and in any case it is hoped to recognize cancer before the nodes are involved.

DUCT CARCINOMA IN SITU

The earliest premalignant condition affecting the breast ducts is referred to as duct carcinoma-in-situ (DCIS). Rarely the condition starts within the lobules, where it is referred to as lobular carcinoma-in-situ. In most cases the condition is impalpable and may only be discovered at a chance biopsy of a coincidental benign lump. More commonly these days DCIS may be discovered as a result of a breast screening programme, where the condition shows itself as a cluster of microcalcifications on mammography. Rarely a large mass of duct carcinoma *in situ* of the comedo variety may present as a clinical mass or, if the *in situ* disease is close to the nipple, may present as a bloody nipple discharge or Paget's disease (*see* NIPPLE, ABNORMALITIES OF).

Sarcoma of the breast is rare. It generally occurs in women under the age of 40. In the early stages it is not easily distinguishable from a fibro-adenoma, particularly one which is enlarging rapidly on account of a cyst or intracycstic growth. It is soft, vascular, grows quickly, at first seems to push the breast aside, but later infiltrates its tissues and eventually fungates through the skin.

PHYLLOIDES TUMOUR

A phylloides tumour is a rare clinical and pathological entity which presents with all the features of a giant fibroadenoma. In the past this condition was referred to as a cystosarcoma phylloides. However, the majority of these lesions are completely benign. The term phylloides means 'leaf-like'. This refers to the slit-like clefts arranged in a 'botanical' manner when viewed on cut section. Rarely the stromal elements of these tumours become hyperplastic and atypical, adopting some of the features of a sarcoma. This tumour is then referred to as a malignant phylloides tumour. They have a tendency to recur locally if not widely excised at the first attempt and, with each recurrence, their malignant potential is more pronounced.

Abnormalities of normal development and involution (ANDI)

When a woman presents at the clinic complaining of a lump in the breast, the first step on clinical examination is to distinguish between a discrete lump and an area of lumpiness or nodularity. Although these lumpy areas in the breast of a young woman are extremely common (perhaps affecting 30 per cent of the female population), there is enormous confusion amongst the medical profession as to the correct terminology. In the past these lumpy areas have been referred to by a series of terms, such as fibrocystic disease, fibroadenosis, mammary dysplasia, cystic hyperplasia, Schimmelbusch's disease, chronic cystic mastitis, cystic mastopathy, Koenig's disease and mastoplasia. Whatever name is given to these lumpy breasts, there are no consistent pathological

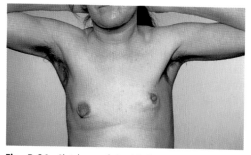

Fig. B.36. Shrinkage of the left breast in an advanced scirrhous cancer.

features which explain the varying textures palpable in different quandrants of the breast. For that reason, a group of clinicians in the University Hospital of Wales headed by Professor Hughes has come up with a rational description of these conditions, which can be grouped together under the catchy acronym ANDI, standing for abnormalities of normal development and involution. These abnormalities vary in extreme from normal physiological processes, which may be considered as benign disorders of little significance, to the other extreme where the pathology can produce particular problems of discomfort or anxiety to the young woman. For example, during the developmental phase of the breast architecture, duct lobular overgrowth can lead to a fibroadenoma, which may cease growing at 2 cm or continue to grow to the extreme of a giant fibroadenoma, reaching sizes of 4 or 5 cm. Normal cyclical changes can produce premenstrual swelling and epithelial hyperplasia. Physiological abnormalities in sensitivity of the duct epithelium to the cyclical hormone changes can lead to cyclical mastalgia, nodularity and intraduct papilloma. Taken to its extreme, the intraduct epithelial hyperplasia can progress to atypia which is known as a risk factor predicting the development of breast cancer. Finally, normal lobular involution may progress to the formation of cysts, sclerosing adenosis and duct ectasia. If a lumpy area of breast tissue is biopsied, almost all these features can be seen under the microscope to one extent or another. Accepting that these conditions are aberrations of normal physiological developments or involution, it can be accepted that in most cases the woman with a lumpy breast or a painful lumpy breast can be reassured. However, if the condition extends beyond the menopause into the cancer age group, clinical diagnosis can be extremely difficult and it is in this area that X-ray mammography is of great value. In younger women, where there is great uncertainty as to the presence of a discrete lump within a diffuse area of nodularity, ultrasound scanning is proving to be a useful complementary investigation.

Multiple cystic disease

Multiple cystic disease of the breast is usually regarded as a variety of ANDI. One breast, sometimes both, becomes filled with cysts, some microscopic, others as large as walnuts, with all intermediate sizes, so that the organ has a bossy appearance. The diagnosis is usually simple but can be confirmed by aspiration of the cysts—a simple outpatient procedure, which is also curative, although several aspirations may sometimes be necessary.

The diagnosis of a single lump in the breast, where cancer must be taken into consideration, may cause considerably difficulty. A lump definite enough to be felt with the flat of the hand and hard enough to resemble cancer is a fibro-adenoma or a tense cyst or a carcinoma. A fibro-adenoma is usually found in women under 30, is less hard than a carcinoma, and is of rounded outline, but its contour may be obscured by surrounding fibro-adenosis. A cyst in fibro-adenosis is usually round and elastic, but if it is deep its outline is obscured, and if it is tense it may feel hard. A carcinoma is undoubtedly solid, and has an ill-defined outline; where these characters are present or where there is the slightest suggestion of skin dimpling, local flattening of the breast or alteration in the nipple, cancer must be diagnosed.

The diagnosis of cancer at this early stage is intensely important, for only then is the prospect of cure high. If there is the possibility that the lump is a cyst this can easily be confirmed by ultrasound scanning, then aspiration is attempted under local anaesthetic. If clear fluid is obtained and the lump disappears, then we can be certain that the diagnosis is one of simple cyst – this can easily be confirmed by ultrasound screening. If no fluid is obtained, or only a few drops of blood, smears should be made for cytological examination, a core-cut biopsy taken or arrangements must be made for urgent excision and microscopic examination of the specimen. Local resection of a doubtful lump is imperative. It is important that this procedure should be carried out in an institution where, should the lump turn out to be a cancer, there will not be delay of more than a day or two before definitive treatment is carried out.

Swellings pushing the breast forwards

There are often mistaken by the patient for breast tumours. *A retromammary abscess* is most commonly tuberculous, arising in an underlying rib or in a mediastinal abscess that has tracked along a branch of the internal thoracic artery. Sometimes an empyema points beneath the breast, usually in the 5th or 6th intercostal space in the midclavicular line. A *chondroma* is a hard nodular swelling springing form one of the ribs and tilting the breast or pushing it aside. More common is a swelling of one or more of the costal cartilages, especially the 2nd and 3rd, which may be bilateral. This condition, *Tietze's syndrome*, is entirely benign and requires no treatment.

Deformities of the ribs may also cause confusion; the commonest is a prominence of the costochondral junction of the 3rd rib, which may be forked and join two cartilages. The condition is often bilateral, and may

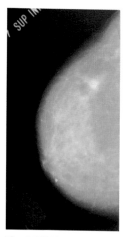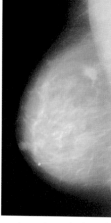

Fig. B.37. Mammogram demonstrating a dense shadow of a carcinoma in the upper outer quadrant of the breast.

be associated with other abnormalities of the ribs or vertebrae.

Role of X-ray mammography and ultrasound scanning

It is now well established that routine X-ray mammography for women over the age of 50 who are otherwise asymptomatic may be of value in preventing premature death from breast cancer by the detection of subclinical cancers (*Fig.* B.37). In addition, no patient with breast cancer should be managed without mammography, as this will define the extent of the disease within the ipsilateral breast and exclude the presence of synchronous contralateral cancers. Ultrasound scanning may help distinguish a solid from a cystic lump and may help define a discrete lump within an area of diffuse nodularity (*see section on* ANDI above).

MONDOR'S DISEASE

Although strictly speaking not a lump in the breast, it is difficult to know how to classify this condition. If a woman presents with characteristic guttering over the surface of the breast, this a pathognomonic sign of Mondor's disease, which is due to spontaneous thrombophlebitis of a superficial vein coursing over the thorax and breast. It has an indurated feel and can be mistaken for the dimpling of an underlying cancer except for its linearity. The author has reported a case where Mondor's disease was the only presenting sign of a cancer, which was detected on mammography. Other such cases have been reported but it is unsure whether this may be coincidental or casual.

Michael Baum

Breast, pain in

Pain in the breast (*mastalgia*) is a common symptom encountered in general surgical practice.

When pain in one breast is the chief symptom the first step is to palpate both breasts with a view to detecting any abnormality which might suggest an early carcinoma. The methods of such examination are described on p. 56. Unfortunately, pain does not occur as an early symptom in carcinoma of the breast, and by the time it is pronounced there may be an obvious stony-hard tumour.

Other causes of pain in the breast are:

Pregnancy
Menstruation (cylical mastalgia)
The onset of puberty
Lactation
Cracked nipple
Inflammation of the nipple
Cyst of the breast
Galactocele
Breast abscess
Submammary abscess
Mastitis, acute mastitis, periductal
Epithelioma of the nipple
Tuberculous disease of the breast
The after-effects of a blow or injury
Anxiety state
Angina
Cervical spondylosis
Herpes zoster

The differential diagnosis of most of these conditions is discussed under the heading of BREAST LUMPS.

Pain in the breast due to intrauterine or to ectopic *pregnancy* will generally be bilateral and will be associated with the other signs of pregnancy. Suggestive indications are the dark brown colour of the nipples, and the broad secondary areola and swollen Montgomery's glands.

The pains in the breast which precede *menstruation* are also bilateral, and their relationship may be indicated by their development synchronously with the first menstruation or their periodic recurrence before each menstrual period. This common condition is best described as pronounced cyclical mastalgia.

Pronounced cylicial mastalgia

Most young women notice some soreness and discomfort in the upper outer quadrants of their breasts in the week preceding a period and this is a normal consequence of cyclical changes in their hormonal environment. In about one in ten women, this condition is sufficiently pronounced to cause anxiety, distress and insomnia. Characteristically the pain is felt in the upper outer quadrants of both breasts, reaching a crescendo 2 or 3 days before the menses. Immediately after this, 2 weeks of comfort are experienced and then the pain starts building up during the luteal phase of the cycle. The cyclical mastalgia may or may not be associated with lumpiness and the two conditions should be considered separately. In the majority of such cases simple reassurance with advice on mild analgesia is all that is needed. However, in severe cases, it is worth asking the woman to keep a diary and if the pattern is clearly cyclical, then a 6-month course of prolactin inhibitors can be prescribed (bromocriptine, danazol). In addition there is some circumstantial evidence that oil of evening primrose and the withdrawal of caffeine may benefit the condition, although it is notorious for this self-limiting disease to respond remarkably well to suggestion or placebo. By common consent, cyclical mastalgia has nothing to do with water retention and therefore diuretics are not indicated. The underlying pathology is thought to relate to a hypersensitivity of the duct epithelium to biologically active prolactin.

Mammography is only indicated in women over the age of 35 or if pain is non-cyclical and localized to one area of the breast.

Michael Baum

| Constipation

A. Acute Constipation

Acute constipation may be: (1) due to acute intestinal obstruction; (2) a symptom of some general disease or of some other acute abdominal disease; or (3) due to a sudden alteration in daily habits, e.g. admission to hospital.

1. Acute intestinal obstruction

The following points help in the distinction between acute intestinal obstruction and severe cases of acute constipation of other origin:

a   In other conditions the constipation is incomplete, in that flatus, and even a small quantity of faeces, may be passed spontaneously. A rectal examination should always be made. In organic intestinal obstruction the rectum is usually empty. If it contains faeces these may be present below an obstruction or, if impacted, may themselves be responsible for the occlusion, but it is exceedingly rare for faecal impaction to produce symptoms quite comparable in severity with those due to acute obstruction. In doubtful cases, it used to be the custom to carry out the two-enema test; the first enema generally brought away a certain amount of faeces even if obstruction was complete; the second, given at an interval of half to one hour, resulted in the passage of faeces or flatus if obstruction was incomplete, whereas, in complete obstruction, the second enema was either retained or expelled unaltered. This test should never be employed; it is exhausting to the patient, time wasting, and the information obtained is often equivocal. Diagnosis can usually be made on clinical grounds supplemented by abdominal radiographs.

b   Vomiting is rarely a feature of constipation, whereas it is frequently present in small-bowel obstruction, and in late cases becomes faeculent.

c   Visible peristalsis, accompanied by noisy borborygmi, is never present except in obstruction.

d   Obstruction is accompanied by progressive distension of the abdomen.

e   Pain is usually the first symptom of intestinal obstruction and is colicky in nature; its severity is out of all proportion to the mild abdominal discomfort that may accompany simple constipation.

Plain radiographs of the abdomen are essential in the diagnosis of intestinal obstruction and in attempting to localize its site. A loop or loops of distended bowel are usually seen, together with multiple fluid levels. Small bowel is suggested by a ladder pattern of distended loops, by their central position, and by striations which pass completely across the width of the distended loop and which are produced by its circular mucosal folds (*Fig.* C.1). Distended large bowel tends to lie peripherally and to show the corrugations produced by the taenia coli (*Fig.* C.2). A small percentage, perhaps 5 per cent of intestinal obstructions, shows no abnormality on plain radiographs. This is due to the bowel being completely distended with fluid in a closed loop and thus without the fluid levels which are produced by coexistent gas.

AETIOLOGY OF ACUTE INTESTINAL OBSTRUCTION

The causes of intestinal obstruction may be classified as:

a. In the lumen—faecal impaction, gallstone ileus, pedunculated tumour and meconium ileus.

b. In the wall—congenital atresia, Crohn's disease, tumours, diverticular disease of the colon and tuberculous stricture.

c. Outside the wall—strangulated hernia (external or internal), volvulus, intussusception, adhesions and bands.

Before considering any other possibility, all the hernial apertures should be examined, even in the absence of local pain, as a small strangulated femoral hernia in an obese woman, for example, may easily be overlooked.

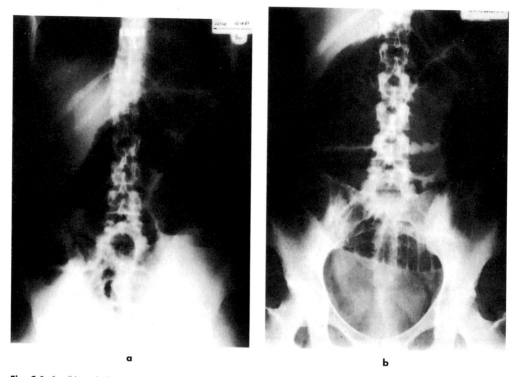

a   b

Fig. C.1. Small bowel obstruction due to a band. *a* Erect: showing fluid levels. *b* Supine: showing ladder pattern of distended small bowel loops, the valvulae conniventes make complete bands across the width of the gut.

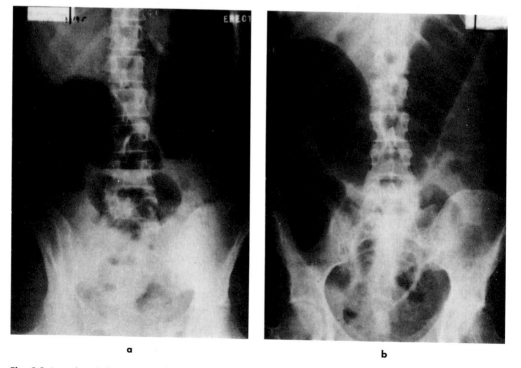

a   b

Fig. C.2. Large bowel obstruction due to carcinoma of sigmoid colon. *a* Erect: showing fluid levels. *b* Supine: gas distend the colon and caecum, the haustrae make incomplete bands across the width of the gut.

The following points should be considered in determining the cause of the acute intestinal obstruction.

i. Age

Intestinal obstruction in the newborn should always be suspected in the presence of bile-vomiting; the rectum should be examined first for the presence of an imperforate anus; other possibilities are congenital atresia or stenosis of the intestine, volvulus neonatorum, meconium ileus and Hirschsprung's disease. In infants the commonest cause of intestinal obstruction is intussusception, but Hirschsprung's disease, strangulated inguinal hernia, and obstruction due to a band from the tip of a Meckel's diverticulum should be considered. In young adults and patients of middle age, adhesions and bands from previous surgery or intraperitoneal inflammation are common, but strangulated hernia and Crohn's disease are also encountered. In older patients strangulated hernias, carcinoma of the bowel and diverticular disease, as well as postoperative adhesions, are all common conditions.

ii. History

The history of a previous abdominal operation, or of inflammatory pelvic disease in females, suggest the possibility of bands or adhesions. A history of biliary colic or of the symptoms which may result from cholecystitis may suggest that obstruction might be due to impaction of a gallstone in the ileum. Obstruction following a period of increasing constipation, perhaps with blood or slime in the stools or spurious diarrhoea, in a middle-aged or elderly patient, suggests cancer or diverticular disease of the colon. The history in an infant or child that blood and mucus have been passed per rectum is suggestive of an intussusception.

iii. Abdominal examination

We have already mentioned the importance of searching specifically for a strangulated hernia. The presence of a recent or old laparotomy scar always raises the possibility of postoperative adhesions. Gross distension generally means that the obstruction is in the colon; if occurring very soon after the onset of symptoms it suggests volvulus of the sigmoid or, less commonly, the caecum. If distension has been present to a less extent for some time before the onset of acute symptoms, a growth is likely. In infants and small children great distension suggests Hirschsprung's disease. Slight distension occurs when the obstruction is in the duodenum or high in the jejunum.

The diagnosis of intussusception can be made with certainty only when the characteristic sausage-shaped tumour situated somewhere in the course of the colon is felt. In acute obstruction due to cancer the tumour is often not palpable as it may be disguised by the dilated intestine; however, large masses are sometimes felt, especially when present in the right or left iliac fossa. On the right side, they are generally due to cancer of the caecum, on the left to cancer of the sigmoid colon or diverticular disease.

iv. Rectal examination

A growth of the rectum should be recognized easily, although this is rather unusual as a cause of obstruction. Sometimes a growth of the pelvic colon can be felt through the front wall of the rectum. In infants, the tip of an intussusception may be felt in the lumen of the rectum and the typical red-current jelly stool (a mixture of blood and mucus) will be seen on the examining finger. Occasionally the mother will report that a sausage-like structure actually prolapses from the child's anal verge during the attacks of colic accompanying the intussusception. I have only seen this on one occasion. A much-ballooned rectum suggests obstruction in the colon; this is an undoubted fact but its cause is obscure.

v. Vomiting

The more frequent the vomiting and the earlier the onset of faeculent vomiting the higher in the intestine is the obstruction likely to be. Its onset is later and its occurrence less frequent in cases of colonic obstruction.

2. Symptomatic

A. In acute general diseases

Constipation beginning acutely is a frequent symptom of a large variety of acute infective and other diseases. It is never so severe as to become a presenting symptom and the other features in the majority of cases are so much more striking that the presence of constipation has little influence on making a diagnosis.

B. In acute abdominal conditions

Constipation is a conspicuous symptom in most acute abdominal conditions. However, once again, other symptoms are often so well marked that the question of intestinal obstruction hardly arises. Thus it frequently accompanies acute appendicitis, salpingitis, perforation of a peptic ulcer, and biliary and renal colic. In lead colic the constipation is not absolute and the occupation of the patient, the blue line on the gums, and the presence of punctate basophilia point to the diagnosis.

3. Changes of daily routine

These may precipitate constipation as in patients admitted to hospital, children going to boarding school, or patients suddenly being confined to bed from illness.

B. Chronic Constipation

Constipation can be defined as delay in the passage of faeces through the large bowel and is frequently associated with difficulty in defecation. Most people empty the bowel once in every 24 hours, but there is a considerable range of variation in perfectly normal individuals; in one study of a large working population this varied from three bowel actions daily to one act every three days.

The abnormal action of the bowel in constipation may manifest itself in three different ways:

1. Defecation may occur with insufficient frequency.
2. The stools may be insufficient in quantity and a certain amount of faeces is retained although the bowels may be opened once daily or more often (cumulative constipation).
3. The bowels may be open daily yet the faeces are hard and dry owing to prolonged retention in the bowel, dehydration, or insufficient residue in the food consumed.

The commoner causes of chronic constipation are as follows:

1. Organic obstructions, for example carcinoma of the colon or diverticular disease.
2. Painful anal conditions, e.g. fissure in ano or prolapsed piles.
3. Adynamic bowel as may occur in Hirschsprung's disease, senility, spinal cord injuries and diseases, and myxoedema.
4. Drugs which decrease peristaltic activity of the bowel— including codeine, probanthine and other ganglion-blocking agents, and morphine.
5. Habit and diet, for example dehydration, starvation, lack of suitable bulk in the diet, and dyschezia.

It is comparatively rare for a patient to consult a doctor on account of constipation without having already attempted to cure himself with aperients. The symptoms generally ascribed to 'auto-intoxication' caused by intestinal stasis are usually really caused by the purgatives themselves, which may produce depletion of sodium and potassium in the resultant watery stools, or from the abdominal colic and flatulence produced by powerful aperients.

In spite of his probable protests, the patient is instructed to see what happens if no drugs are taken for a few days, an attempt being made to open the bowels each morning on a normal diet containing plenty of fruit and vegetables. In most cases he loses his abdominal pains and so-called 'toxic' symptoms. During this test the bowels are often opened daily, in which case a diagnosis of functional pseudoconstipation can be made, the patient having suggested to himself, as a result of faulty education combined with advice of his friends and with the reading pernicious advertisements, that he was constipated and required aperients to keep himself well; whereas a little psychotherapy in the form of explanation of the physiology of his bowels and the origin of his symptoms, and persuasion to try to open his bowels each morning without artificial help results in a cure.

The investigation of constipation entails a careful and accurate history, full examination including, of course, examination of the rectum and sigmoidoscopy, followed, in some cases, by special laboratory tests and a barium-enema X-ray examination.

Organic obstructions

The two common causes of narrowing of the lumen of the large bowel are diverticular disease and carcinoma of the colon. Other non-malignant strictures are rare but include Crohn's disease of the large bowel, stricture complicating ulcerative colitis and tuberculous stricture.

Organic stricture of the colon is most commonly due to carcinoma. The possibility of cancer should always be considered when an individual above the age of 40, whose bowels have been regular previously, without change of diet or habit develops constipation of increasing severity, or when a patient who is habitually constipated becomes more so without obvious reason. The constipation is at first intermittent and may alternate with diarrhoea, or rather with a frequent desire to go to stool without effective evacuation. Aperients become steadily less helpful. There may be colicky pain and episodes of distension and the patient may notice blood, pus, and mucus in the faeces. Examination of the abdomen may reveal a palpable mass due to the presence of the tumour itself or to inspissated faeces which have become impacted above a cancerous stricture which is itself impalpable. Progressive loss of weight and strength, anorexia and anaemia are rather late features of the disease. A rectal examination reveals a usually empty rectum but not infrequently a carcinoma in the sigmoid colon can be felt through the rectal wall as the mass in this loop of bowel prolapses into the pelvis. An occult blood test on any faecal material is often positive. Sigmoidoscopy or colonoscopy may visualize the tumour and its nature can be confirmed by biopsy and histological examination. A barium-enema examination is invaluable (*Fig.* C.3).

DIVERTICULAR DISEASE of the sigmoid colon can mimic carcinoma exactly and indeed the surgeon, even at laparotomy, may not be able to differentiate between

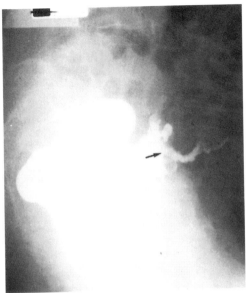

Fig. C.3. Barium enema showing an obstructing carcinoma of the sigmoid colon (arrowed). Note that the patient also has diverticulosis—not an uncommon combination.

the two conditions. The barium-enema examination (*Fig.* C.4) is often helpful, but the radiologist may have difficulty himself in distinguishing a stricture due to one or other cause; indeed not infrequently these two common diseases may co-exist. Again, colonoscopy

will often be useful in making the differential diagnosis.

Occasionally extracolonic masses may press upon the rectum or sigmoid colon with resultant constipation; for example, the pregnant uterus, a mass of fibroids, a large ovarian cyst or other pelvic tumours.

Painful anal conditions

When defecation is painful, reflex spasm of the anal sphincter may be produced with resultant acute constipation. A local cause of the pain such as a fissure in ano, strangulated haemorrhoids or a perianal abscess is obvious on careful local examination of the anal verge and surrounds.

Adynamic bowel

In Hirschsprung's disease there is always a history of constipation dating from the first few months of life. The abdomen becomes greatly enlarged soon after birth and the outline of distended colon can be seen, often with visible peristalsis. The abdomen finally becomes enormous and it is then tense and tympanitic. There may be eversion of the umbilicus and marked widening of the subcostal angle. The condition is due to the absence of ganglion cells in the wall of the rectosigmoid region of the large bowel, although in some cases a more extensive part of the colon may be involved. Males are affected more often than females.

A barium-enema examination reveals gross dilatation of the colon leading down to a narrow funnel in the aganglionic rectum (*Fig.* C.5).

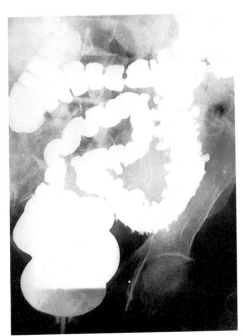

Fig. C.4. Extensive diverticulosis of the descending and sigmoid colon.

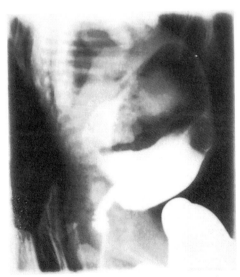

Fig. C.5. Barium enema in a case of Hirschsprung's disease showing enormous dilatation of the pelvic colon proximal to the narrow aganglionic segment of rectum. (*Dr T.H. Hills.*)

Deficient motor activity of the bowel may be due to senile changes in the elderly and may be a prominent feature of myxoedemic patients. Constipation may occur in the course of organic nervous diseases, including tabes dorsalis, spinal compression from tumour, transverse myelitis, and disseminated sclerosis, as well as cord transection in trauma. This is due to disturbance of the motor and sensory pathways responsible for defecation.

Drugs

Many commonly employed drugs have a constipating effect on the bowel; these include codeine, morphine and the ganglion-blocking agents. Constipation accompanied by abdominal pain may be a feature of lead poisoning.

Habit and diet

By far the greatest number of patients complaining of constipation fall into this group. When the faeces are abnormally hard as a result of dehydration, inadequate liquid intake or inadequate cellulose material in the diet, rectal examination will reveal impacted faeces of rocklike consistency. This may occur as an acute phenomenon following barium-meal examination when masses of inspissated barium may lodge in the rectum.

Dyschezia

Dyschezia is the term applied to difficulty in defecation due to faulty bowel habit. The patient ignores the normal call to stool, the rectum distends with faeces with eventual loss of the defecation reflex. The very same patient who gets into this habit is probably one who lives on the modern synthetic diet grossly deficient in roughage. As we have mentioned above, the so-called symptoms of constipation usually result from the purgatives that the patient ingests when he becomes anxious about the scarcity of his bowel actions. Rectal examination in such individuals often reveals large amounts of faeces in the rectum and more scybala may be palpated in the sigmoid colon. Dyschezia is, of course, present in those patients who have to remove faeces from the rectum digitally.

Harold Ellis

Contractures and deformities of the upper and lower limbs

(*See also* FOOT AND TOES, DEFORMITIES OF)

Lower limb

Lower limb contractures occur in:

1   Post-trauma states,
2   Spastic conditions — upper motor neurone lesions
3   Flaccid paralysis — lower motor neurone lesions and peripheral nerve injuries
4   Joint disease and injury
5   Growth disorders
6   Muscle dystrophies and primary muscle disease and damage.

1.   Trauma

Malunion of fractures may leave a deformity. The femur may be left in varus, the tibia may be bowed into any deformity and fractures malunited around the knee and ankle are potent causes of joint deformity.

2.   The spastic lower limb

Cerebral palsy due to birth trauma will produce spasticity in the limbs — quadriplegia, diplegia or a monoparesis. Contractures frequently follow. Treatment is by stretching and physical therapy, splintage with orthoses and sometimes surgical releases. Upper motor neurone lesions producing similar spastic states may occur in postmeningitis syndromes, post-intracerebral haemorrhage, intracerebral tumours and other space-occupying lesions.

3.   Flaccid paralysis

Poliomyelitis is the most common condition producing muscle weakness and subsequent contracture when the world scene is observed. Muscle imbalance will produce contractures of any type and in any area of the body. The most frequent are flexion contractures of the hips and knees, together with equinus deformities of the feet and ankles. There is no associated sensory loss in this disease, since the lesions are confined to the motor anterior horn cells of the spinal cord. Treatment depends upon appropriate surgical correction of deformities with muscle transplants and transfers. Calliper or orthosis splintage is frequently required.

PERONEAL MUSCULAR ATROPHY
(CHARCOT MARIE TOOTH DISEASE)

This produces wasting, particularly below the knee. The lower limbs appear like inverted champagne

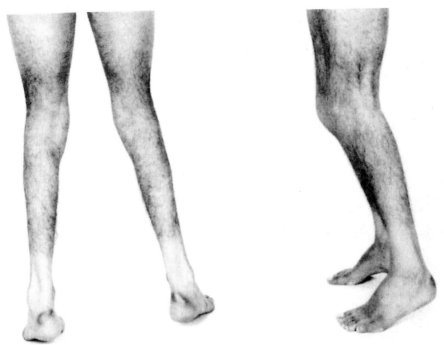

Fig. C.6. Contractures due to peroneal muscular atrophy sent to the author as an old poliomyelitis.

bottles (*Fig.* C.6). Contractures of the feet and ankles occur—equinovarus deformities together with a pes cavus and claw toes (*see Fig.* F.41). The upper limbs show wasting of the hand intrinsic muscles.

SPINA BIFIDA

The neurological abnormality is complex, for although most contractures are due to lower motor neurone paralysis, there is a frequent spastic element due to cord lesion or hydrocephalus. Contractures are often gross and extremely disabling and are resistant to treatment (*Fig.* C.7).

4. Joint disease

Any destructive joint disease will produce contractures if severe. Septic arthritis may leave a contracted articulation with a fibrous ankylosis and may eventually fuse the joint (*Fig.* C.8). Rheumatoid arthritis and other inflammatory arthropathies produce joint contracture of any part of the body (*Fig.* C.9). Degenerative joint disease such as osteoarthrosis may produce contractures or deformity due to bone collapse.

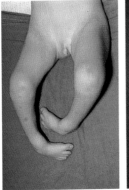
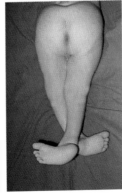

Fig. C.7. *a, b* Lower limb contractures in spina bifida.

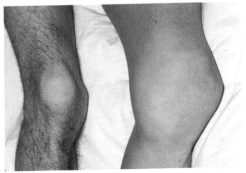

Fig. C.8. Flexion contracture of left knee following septic arthritis.

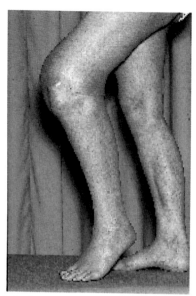

Fig. C.9. Flexion contracture of left knee in rheumatoid arthritis.

5. Growth disorders

These are due to:

1   Primary epiphyseal dysplasia,
2   Metabolic abnormalities such as rickets (*see Fig.* B.11) and
3   Injury to the epiphyseal plate.

6. Muscle dystrophy

Duchenne-type muscle dystrophy produces initially an enlargement of the muscle bulk in the child ('infantile Hercules') but there is progessive weakening of all muscle groups and contractures may eventually develop. Diagnosis is made from the clinical state and increased level of creatinine phosphokinase (CPK).

Muscle injury may occur in severe trauma and acute pyogenic infections may produce a septic myositis.

Muscle Ischaemia

This occurs in the lower limb when traumatized. A closed compartment syndrome with muscle ischaemia may occur in trauma with or without a fracture. The most common deformities are those of an equinus ankle and foot with clawing of the toes and weakness, or frank paralysis of the ischaemic musculature.

Primary muscle contracture

Arthrogryphosis multiplex congenita is a congenital abnormality due to non-differentiation of mesenchymal tissue. There is frequently a neurogenic element (lower motor neurone) with severe weakness. The combination produces gross contracture.

Upper limb

The general causes of upper limb contractures are similar to those described in the lower limb (*see* p. 68).

1   Post-trauma states
2   Spastic conditions—upper motor neurone lesions
3   Flaccid paralysis—lower motor neurone lesions and peripheral nerve injuries
4   Joint disease and injury
5   Growth disorders
6   Muscle dystrophies and primary muscle disease and damage.

Peripheral nerve injuries

THE ULNAR NERVE

The ulnar nerve may be divided or compressed at the elbow, or in the forearm or the wrist. The hand intrinsic muscles are paralysed with gross wasting of the interossei and a claw hand results. The thenar eminence musculature is variably innervated by the median nerve and abductor pollicis brevis is always preserved. There is anaesthesia over the little finger and ulnar border of the hand together variably with the ring finger—part or whole.

THE RADIAL NERVE

The radial nerve may be divided or compressed in the arm, usually in association with a compound fracture of the shaft of the humerus, producing paralysis of the wrist and forearm extensors. A wrist drop develops and anaesthesia is present over the dorsal surface of the hand in an area usually confined to the first web space.

THE MEDIAN NERVE

The median nerve may be divided or compressed at the elbow or above producing a 'pointing hand'. The thenar eminence is wasted due to paralysis of abductor pollicis brevis and, variably, the other short thenar muscles are involved. The index and middle fingers are weak in flexion and are therefore kept extended in repose by the unopposed action of the finger extensors. The ring and little fingers are held in some flexion for the deep flexor muscles to these digits are innervated by the ulnar nerve. Anaesthesia is over the palmar surface of the radial three-and-a-half digits.

Carpal tunnel syndrome

The median nerve at the wrist is compressed within the carpal tunnel which results in wasting of the thenar eminence. There is always abductor pollicis brevis wasting, for this muscle is autonomously supplied by the median nerve and the other short thenar muscles are variably supplied by the ulnar nerve. Anaesthesia may eventually involve the whole radial three-and-a-half digits but initially there is hypoaesthesia together with tingling, numbness and some pain over the tips of the thumb, middle and index fingers. The symptoms are very specific to the night hours or at the time of awakening with exacerbation by hand exercise. The majority of cases are in women at or just beyond the menopause. Compression in the carpal tunnel may occur also in pregnancy, following a Colles' fracture, in myxoedema and in situations where ganglia or other space-occupying lesions are present around the median nerve at the wrist.

The rheumatoid hand

Rheumatoid synovium may produce swelling of the synovial sheath in the hand and this leads to destruction of extensor tendons with the fingers 'dropping'. The metacarpophalangeal joints are involved at an early stage and the fingers drift into ulnar deviation (*Fig.* C.10). As the disease progresses, mutilation and destruction of all finger joints may occur. Swan neck deformities occur due to intrinsic muscle spasm and then contracture. Psoriatic arthropathy produces inflammation of the distal finger joints together with characteristic pitting of the finger nails.

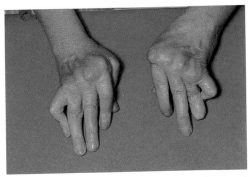

Fig. C.10. Contractures of the hands in severe rheumatoid arthritis.

The osteoarthritic hand

The terminal phalangeal joints are primarily affected. The distal joint osteophytes are nodular and are called 'Heberden's nodes'. There are sometimes small retention cysts in association with these.

Trigger finger

When the flexed fingers are extended one digit may remain flexed. It may be manually extended with a snap and this phenomenon is termed 'trigger finger'. It is due to localized stenosis of the fibrous flexor sheath opposite the metacarpophalangeal joint. The post-stenotic swelling of the tendon is pulled into the sheath in flexion and remains stuck until forcibly extended. It is due to an idiopathic stenosis in most cases. Diabetics may develop one or more trigger fingers. The stenosis may also occur in rheumatoid arthritis.

Snapping thumb

The same triggering phenomenon may occur in the thumb. The child may be affected by a congenital stenosis of the sheath of the flexor pollicis longus. The continued flexion contracture of the thumb interphalangeal joint is rarely noted until the child is a year old. Similar surgical release is required.

De Quervain's stenosing tenosynovitis

The thumb tendon sheaths at the wrist may become inflamed and stenosed. Abductor pollicis longus and extensor pollicis brevis run over the radial styloid, usually in their common sheath, and here there is localized tenderness, severe pain on thumb movement and eventual stenosis, which results in an extension and adduction contracture of the thumb.

Mallet finger

This is otherwise known as a cricket or baseball finger. The distal phalanx of one finger remains flexed following a stubbing injury. The distal insertion of the extensor tendon to the phalanx is ripped and the finger tip drops.

Dupuytren's contracture

A fibrotic nodule in the palmar fascia is frequently felt or seen in the older man. This nodule may then extend and produce skin puckering with subsequent contracture of the palmar aponeurosis. The thickening and contracture then extends to the digits and the little, ring and middle fingers contract in that order. No digit is exempt. The contracture may become severe and disabling and surgical treatment should be undertaken before the deformity becomes gross (*Fig.* C.11). The ideal time for release is when the finger metacarpophalangeal joints present a flexion contracture of some 30 degrees. Garrod's pads occur in Dupuytren's disease

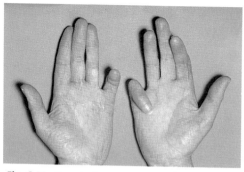
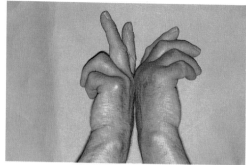

Fig. C.11. Dupuytren's contractures: *a*, affecting the little fingers; *b* severe deformities.

and the lump on the dorsal aspects of the knuckles contains Dupuytren's tissue. In 5 per cent of patients Dupuytren's contracture occurs on the foot with the plantar aponeurosis involved.

The aetiology of Dupuytren's contracture is unknown but there is a very definite genetic association. Although far commoner in men, it does occur in women. Patients with liver disease have a higher incidence and epileptics on Epanutin medication have a predisposition.

Volkmann's ischaemic contracture

Contracture of the hand may occur in unrecognized avascularity of the upper limb after fracture. The supracondylar fracture in the child is the most commonly associated injury. The displacement of the lower humeral fragment compresses, or in some cases lacerates the brachial artery. The large associated

haematoma may similarly compress the vessel which easily goes into spasm.

The damage to forearm muscles and nerves occurs in the first few hours. It is usually identified by the absence of the radial pulse, but this is not always the case. The most important early sign is the inability to extend the patient's fingers without severe pain and the possibility of this diagnosis must be based on this sign. The features of an avascular extremity will then progressively follow and at this stage it is too late to reverse the damage (*Fig.* C.12). In the full Volkmann's contracture the claw fingers become more flexed with the wrist extended and the fingers extend as the wrist flexes. The median, ulnar and sometimes the radial nerves are frequently damaged by this ischaemia.

Paul Aichroth

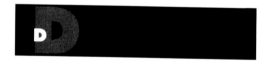

Deafness

Deafness is one of the major handicaps suffered by mankind and is inevitable with the ageing process. There are many causes of deafness in the younger years and, of these causes, 99 per cent are peripheral. If information reaches the acoustic nerve, it is very rare for there ever to be any lesions beyond the acoustic nerve which can cause deafness. Peripheral causes of deafness can be classified as:

Conductive
These are obstructive lesions in the external and/or middle ear which prevent sound from reaching the cochlea.
Sensorineural
These are lesions in the cochlea or acoustic nerve which prevent sound from reaching the brain-stem.
Mixed
Combined conductive and sensorineural lesions.

Fig. C.12. Volkmann's contracture following brachial artery trauma in a 70-year-old man. Note also the obvious cutaneous cyanosis. (*Professor Harold Ellis.*)

Hearing Tests

These are carried out to diagnose the cause of the deafness and also to ascertain its severity. We will list them in ascending order of complexity.

Voice tests

In the clinical situation, a good idea of the severity of the deafness can be gained from these simple clinical tests. The patient sits facing a wall at one end of the room and occludes one ear pressing a finger against the tragus. He is instructed to repeat after the examiner whatever the latter says.

The examiner stands behind the patient and whispers test words. He increases the distance between him and the patient until the patient is no longer able to repeat the words accurately. The same process is repeated with the use of the conversation voice. Someone with normal hearing should be able to hear both a whispered and a conversation voice at 20 ft with each ear. Someone who is able to hear a conversation voice at 20 ft but a whispered voice only at say 6 ft is suffering from a sensorineural deafness. Patients with conductive loss will have a diminished but equal response to both conversation and whispered voice tests. In assessing medicolegal cases, malingerers quite often show a discrepancy between the assessment by voice test and by more complex tests.

It is important that lip-reading is avoided and so the patient should never be allowed to see the examiner's lips.

Tuning-fork tests

These have been used for over a century for the purpose not only of measuring the degree of deafness but also to subdivide it into sensorineural or conductive. The tuning-fork should either by a 256 cps or a 512 cps fork and should be big enough so that its note lasts at least 60 seconds after being sounded.

THE RINNE'S TEST

Someone with normal hearing will hear the tuning-fork better by air-conduction than by bone-conduction. This, unfortunately, is the same in someone with sensorineural deafness and so the test does not have a diagnostic specificity. It can, however, distinguish between sensorineural and conductive deafness because, in conductive deafness, the patient hears bone-conduction better than air-conduction, the so-called Rinne negative test. There is no logical reason why one response is called Rinne positive and the other Rinne negative. It is only by convention that the conductive deafness response is known as a negative Rinne.

The base of the tuning-fork is held on the patient's mastoid process until he says he can no longer hear the sound. The fork is then rapidly transferred so that the vibrating forks are close to the external auditory meatus. If the patient continues to hear the sound then it is considered that he hears better by air-conduction than by bone-conduction.

If there is a big difference between the ears then an extraneous sound should be introduced into the non-tested ear to prevent a false response.

WEBER'S TEST

In the Weber test, the sound is heard either in the better ear if there is a sensorineural deafness present or in the worse ear if it is a conductive deafness. The normal response is to hear the sound equally in both ears. Again, the test does not have a diagnostic specificity unless it is lateralized. The tuning-fork is placed in the middle of the forehead and the patient is asked to signify in which ear he hears the sound clearly.

ABSOLUTE BONE-CONDUCTION TEST

In this test an assessment is made of the patient's ability to hear by bone-conduction. This is a measure of sensorineural deafness and the patient's response is compared to the examiner's response. If the examiner has roughly normal hearing then the patient ought to hear a tuning-fork placed on his mastoid as long as the examiner does. If he hears it for less time then it is considered that his bone-conduction is diminished and, thus, he has a sensorineural deafness.

Audiometry

PURE-TONE AUDIOMETRY

A pure-tone audiometer produces tones of varying intensity (0–100 db) and frequency (250 cps to 8000 cps). The test is carried out by the patient wearing earphones. Test sounds at different intensities and frequencies are introduced via the earphones and the patient is asked to indicate when he hears the sound. The sounds are produced at the threshold of hearing and this is marked on a graph producing an audiogram (*Fig.* D.1). A normal person should hear between 0–10 dB over the full frequency range.

Bone conduction is tested by putting an applicator in contact with the patient's mastoid process. The test is then carried out in the same manner and the threshold of hearing indicated on the audiogram. In

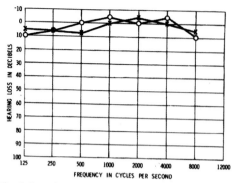

Fig. D.1. Audiogram showing hearing that is within 'normal limits'. It is conventional to represent hearing by air-conduction in the right ear by O—O, and in the left ear by X—X.

this way it can be seen if bone-conduction is better than air-conduction (conductive deafness) or if bone-conduction and air-conduction are roughly equal (normal or sensorineural deafness).

SPEECH AUDIOMETRY

It is possible for a patient to have a normal pure-tone audiogram because for this he only requires to have about half of the acoustic nerve functioning. A more discriminatory test of hearing is a speech audiogram where the patient has to respond to a list of test words played at threshold through earphones. Either a graph can be made of the patient's speech responses or a simple raw speech discrimination score can be recorded.

A difference between the speech audiogram and the pure-tone audiogram is indicative of malingering.

TYMPANOMETRY

This is carried out by an Impedance Meter and two tests are possible with this. In the first, the pressure in the middle ear is measured as is the compliance of the drum. A graph is produced and it is possible to diagnose Eustachian tube obstruction, fluid in the middle ear, otosclerotic fixation and ossicular discontinuity. The stapedius muscle reflexes can also be measured and this is of diagnostic importance in otosclerosis, ossicular discontinuity and in facial palsy.

TESTS FOR RECRUITMENT

In the space available it is not possible to give an explanation of the phenomenon of recruitment. Suffice it to say that this is a very important test of hearing because it can distinguish between lesions of the acoustic nerve and lesions of the cochlea. It is a simple test to do and is carried out with a pure-tone audiometer.

EVOKED RESPONSE AUDIOMETRY

This can be done as cortical evoked response audiometry, electrocochleography or brainstem-evoked audiometry. It is now the main test of hearing after pure-tone audiometry. It is invaluable in assessing medico-legal problems and the brainstem-evoked response audiogram can clearly indicate whether or not there is a lesion in the acoustic nerve.

Evoked response audiometry is of enormous importance in the testing of infants, young children and people with multiple handicaps.

Hearing tests in children

Deafness should be diagnosed in infants as early as possible. The earlier deafness is diagnosed, the more chance there is of the child developing normal lingual language as opposed to sign language.

Every child now born in the UK has a hearing test by specially trained nurses at 6 weeks and at the end of the first year of life. Where the nurse does not receive an unambiguous response indicating normal hearing from her simple clinical tests, the child is referred to special children's speech and hearing clinics. There, further clinical tests will be carried out and probably evoked response audiometry.

If the child is found to be deaf then special education is set in hand at a very early age and amplification devices are fitted to the child, depending on the severity of the deafness.

CONDUCTIVE DEAFNESS

The causes of conductive deafness may be summarized in *Table* D.1.

Conductive deafness is often less severe than sensorineural deafness and it has a maximum of 60 dB. Very frequently medical or surgical procedures can be carried out either to arrest the process or to cure it. In some cases, such as serious otitis media or otosclerosis, there can be a dramatic restoration of hearing with relatively simple surgery.

It is relatively easy to establish whether a deafness is conductive or sensorineural with the tests listed above. In certain cases of conductive deafness, radiography has to be used, especially in the assessment of congenital syndromes or ossicular discontinuity. In this, CT scanning is extremely helpful.

There are a very considerable number of congenital syndromes associated with deafness; mostly sensor-

Table D.1. The causes of conductive deafness

Congenital lesions
1. Atresia of the external meatus and middle ear usually with microtia (*see Fig.* D.2)
2. Atresia associated with other facial defects
3. Middle-ear deformities
   Some syndromes (frequently associated with sensorineural loss in addition to the conductive loss)
      Mandibulofacial dysostosis (Treacher Collins)
      Crouzon deformity
      Marfan's syndrome
      Klippel–Feil syndrome
      Trisomy D and E
      Cretinism
      Cleft palate
      Submucous cleft palate
      Osteogenesis imperfecta (van der Hoeve–de
        Kleyn triad)
      Thalidomide
      Rubella

External auditory meatus
   Wax
   Foreign bodies
   Otitis externa
   Exostoses (Diver's ear) (Wet ear)

Middle-ear lesions
   Trauma
     Blood
     Ossicular disruption
     Perforated tympanic membrane
   Acute otitis media
   Eustachian malfunction
     Atelectasis of middle ear
     Serous otitis ('Glue ear')
   Otitic barotrauma
   Chronic otitis media
   Haemotympanum
   Malignant disease
   Glomus tumour
   Otosclerosis

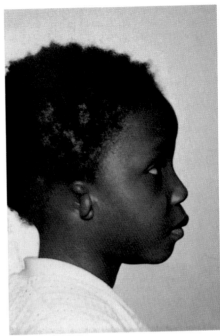

Fig. D.2. Atresia of the right ear showing absent external auditory meatus and deformed auricle.

ineural in character. Where conductive lesions occur there is often an inner ear lesion so that a mixed deafness is the result. It is quite impossible to list all the possible recorded combinations of congenital abnormalities, but the golden rule is that if one abnormality is observed a careful search for others must be made and, during this search, deafness must never be forgotten.

Some of the more common are listed. The Treacher Collins syndrome (*Fig.* D.3) comprises micrognathia, depressed malar bones, eyes sloping downwards and outwards with notched lower lids, ptosis of the auricles and middle-ear abnormalities with deformed ossicles. The Crouzon deformity is craniofacial dysostosis. Marfan's syndrome comprises an inherited collagen disorder—abnormally long extremities, subluxation of the lens, cardiovascular abnormalities

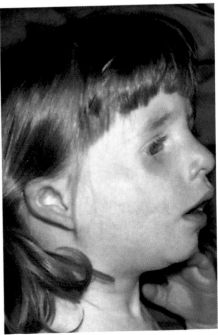

Fig. D.3. Treacher Collins syndrome showing typical appearance of eye, micrognathia, depressed malar bone and ptosis of the ear.

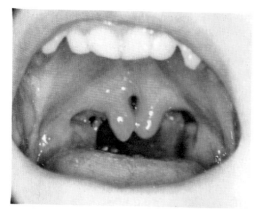

Fig. D.4. Submucous cleft palate with deeply bifid uvula typical of this rare condition.

and deafness. In the Klippel–Feil syndrome there are malformed cervical vertebrae and a webbed neck.

Chromosomal disorders in the trisomy D and E cause very marked ossicular abnormalities. Thyroid deficiency leads more often to cochlear end-organ damage as do rubella and the thalidomide abnormality, but in all these middle-ear deformities are found.

The van der Hoeve–de Kleyn triad of deafness, due to stapedial fixation (otosclerosis), blue sclerotics and fragile bones is uncommon with a frequency of 2–3/100,000. It is a strongly familial disorder.

Cleft-palate (*Fig.* D.4), with a frequency of about 1/1000, is much more common and is an important cause of deafness. Since it is the palatal muscles (tensor palati and levator palati) that control the Eustachian tube it is not surprising that nearly every cleft-palate child before closure of the cleft is deaf to some degree due to failure of tubal opening and atelectasis or fluid in the middle ear. After operation a considerable but reducing number of children are still deaf, often to some 30 dB.

A submucous cleft-palate, where the muscle layer is separated under intact mucosa, has the same effects on the ear but is not easy to recognize. The uvula is deeply bifid and a notch instead of a tubercle may be palpated in the centre of the free border of the hard palate.

Diseases of the external auditory meatus rarely cause deafness as hearing is retained while there is the smallest airway past the obstruction to the drum. Sudden deafness results from closure—often as wax swells on contact with water.

Middle-ear lesions causing deafness are often easily identified by thorough and careful otoscopy with a good light. Two of those listed deserve special mention: serous otitis and otosclerosis.

Serous otitis, otherwise known as 'secretory otitis media' or 'glue ear', is extremely common and is present in 4 per cent of all children between the ages 5 and 15. This means that almost every classroom in the country will contain one child deaf to a level of 20 dB or more. Detection and treatment of deafness in these children is very important because it has been shown that it can hold up progress at school.

The changes in the drum are fairly typical. There can be a dark appearance or a yellowish glaze. Occasionally, fluid levels and bubbles can be seen through the drum membrane but in other instances there may be no observable clinical signs. The diagnosis is primarily by tympanometry where a negative middle-ear pressure is found together with an increased drum compliance.

In adults, serous otitis media may be the first sign of Eustachian tube obstruction by a nasopharyngeal carcinoma. Although not so important in the European, it is of very definite clinical significance in the Chinese where nasopharyngeal carcinoma is the commonest head and neck tumour.

Otosclerosis occurs in young adults with females being more commonly afflicted than males. In females the deafness is often made worse by pregnancy. Patients very often hear better in noisy environments (paracusis). Audiometry shows a conductive loss with bone-conduction being better than air-conduction. Depending on the so-called 'air–bone gap', decisions regarding surgery can be made. When the air–bone gap is more than 30 dB then the patient stands to gain from surgery but, until then, should probably use a hearing aid.

SENSORINEURAL DEAFNESS

Though there may be some overlap it is probably better to separate those conditions chiefly arising in childhood (*Table* D.2) from the adult deaf.

The importance of early testing and the identification of the profoundly deaf child has already been mentioned. Normal development of an infant is greatly dependent upon hearing, the understanding of speech being the one function of human behaviour which sets man apart from animals. Failure to hear speech not only prevents the development of language but inhibits formation of personal and social relationships. Since nearly all deaf children have some residual hearing it is of vital importance to pick out the deaf and maximize the use of the hearing they have as early as possible, at least by 6 months of age, and before they have developed into 'fixed visualizers'.

Infants who have a family history of deafness, maternal infections during the pregnancy or perinatal problems, who are late to talk or who have other

Table D.2. Causes of deafness in children

1. **Prenatal**
   a. Genetic
      Scheibe type
      Bing–Siebenmann type
      Waardenburg's syndrome
      Pendred's syndrome
      Mondini-Alexander type
      Michel type
      Usher's syndrome
      Endemic cretinism
      Klippel–Feil syndrome
   b. Non-genetic
      Diseases occurring in pregnancy
         Rubella and other viral illnesses
         Toxaemia
         Diabetes
         Syphilis
         Nephritis
      Drugs taken in pregnancy
         Streptomycin
         Quinine
         Salicylates
         Thalidomide

2. **Perinatal**
   Prematurity
   Jaundice—haemolytic disease and kernicterus
   Anoxia due to birth trauma

3. **Postnatal**
   a. Genetic
      Familial degenerative deafness
      Otosclerosis
      Alport's syndrome
   b. Non-genetic infectious diseases
      Measles
      Mumps
      Meningitis
         Meningococcal
         Pneumococcal
         Viral
         Tuberculous
      Trauma
      Otitis media
      Ototoxic antibiotics
         Streptomycin
         Neomycin
         Gentamicin

congenital defects, must be considered as being 'at risk' and should be carefully tested. The frequency of sporadic cases of deafness makes testing of all babies important. In this respect the mother's views should never be ignored; if she thinks her child is deaf the diagnosis should be presumed correct until firmly proved otherwise. It must be remembered, also, that mild or moderate conductive deafness may be an additional handicap and even a small amount of additional deafness is significant when the base line is already low.

There are many more genetically determined syndromes involving sensorineural deafness than conductive; a number of examples from the main groups have been listed. The Scheibe abnormality shows a normal vestibular mechanism with failure of sacculo-cochlear development; in the Mondini type of deficiency both vestibular and cochlear structures are deformed. The Bing type has a normal bony labyrinth but the membranous labyrinth is malformed or degenerate in both cochlea and vestibule; in addition there may be central nervous system abnormalities. The fourth member of this group where abnormalities are mainly in the otic capsule, the Michel type, shows almost complete lack of development of the inner ear and often associated mental retardation.

Waardenburg's syndrome is an example of the group of integumentary system disease and deafness. A white forelock and heterochromia of the iris are combined with familial genetic deafness.

Pendred's syndrome comprises a congenital goitre, hypothyroidism with severe abnormalities of the labyrinth, both vestibular and cochlear parts.

A large group of abnormalities is described where hearing loss is associated with eye disease, retinal abnormalities, myopia, optic atrophy and corneal degeneration. Usher's syndrome is deafness combined with retinitis pigmentosa.

Cretinism is associated with deafness which may respond to early and intensive treatment.

The Klippel–Feil syndrome has been mentioned above.

Non-genetic prenatal influences are well known from the rubella story. A careful history may implicate one or other factor. It should be noted that, with regard to rubella, the virus may persist after birth and deafness may develop as a late-onset problem in childhood.

Perinatal causes of deafness are important and preventable. The resulting deafness is in general less severe than that arising from rubella which is characteristically very profound.

Late-onset genetic deafness is now considered to be a much more important cause of deafness in childhood and later life than previously thought. Alport's syndrome is an example of this and is also representative of a group of syndromes where genetic hearing loss is associated with nephritis. Otosclerosis as a cause of mixed deafness is included here as well as elsewhere.

Of the non-genetic group the diagnosis will be arrived at from the history or from consideration of the disease. Mumps deafness is usually very profound but, curiously, is nearly always unilateral and this serves to identify it on occasion.

The proportion of the various groups of conditions causing congenital deafness has been estimated as one-quarter each of genetic, maternal rubella, perinatal causes and unknown. Genetic causes, either alone or as a contributory factor by increasing the liability to other influences, are being increasingly implicated. In areas of the world where consanguinous marriages are common—and in expatriate communities of those peoples—genetic sensorineural deafness is reported to comprise 70–80 per cent. A careful family history is most important in making a probable diagnosis.

A different scheme of classification is appropriate for adults (see Table D.3).

Many conditions in this list of the causes of sensorineural deafness in adults have been considered above. Some, however, require more attention.

Refsum's disease is yet another syndrome combining eye disease (retinitis pigmentosa), polyneuritis, cerebellar ataxia and a genetic late onset deafness. The inheritance is autosomal recessive.

Acoustic trauma from noise is wholly preventable and entirely untreatable. It may be diagnosed from the history and the audiogram which shows a typical curve, sharply falling in the higher frequencies with a dip at 4 kHz. As the lesion is at the end-organ, recruitment of loudness is present and patients are intolerant of amplification and often have little benefit from hearing aids. Noise-induced hearing loss may be demonstrated audiometrically as temporary (Noise-Induced Temporary Threshold Shift—NITTS) or permanent (Noise-Induced Permanent Threshold Shift—NIPTS) and may be caused by sudden loud sounds such as gunfire or by continuous trauma such as traffic noise, industrial noise, agricultural noise or 'pop' music.

Compensation is now being offered on a very large scale to workers exposed to noise in industry. This affects mainly shipyard and railway workers, motor car industry workers and miners. In the early stages these men show a dip at 6 kHz. With long exposure to noise, the dip widens and affects 3, 4 and 6 kHz. It is usually hearing maintained at 8 kHz until the late stages of deafness. Tinnitus is very frequently present in noise-induced hearing loss.

Vascular lesions of the inner ear are the cause, or part cause, of many cases of deafness. Sudden, small vascular accidents in the end-arterioles may cause deafness by damaging part or the whole of the organ of Corti. Immediate treatment with vasodilators may restore the whole circulation, so early diagnosis is important.

The cause of Menière's disease (Fig. D.7) is not fully known and is probably multi-factorial, but failure of vasomotor control and vasoconstriction of the

Table D.3. Causes of deafness in older children and in adults

1. **Cochlear lesions**
   Late-onset genetic deafness
     Familial degenerative
     Alport's syndrome
     Refsum's syndrome
     Otosclerosis (later cochlear effects)
   Inflammatory (labyrinthitis)
     Bacterial
     Late-onset rubella
     Syphilis
     Mumps
     Herpes
     Measles
   Trauma
     Fracture of temporal bone
     Acoustic trauma—temporary
                                permanent
   Vascular lesions
     Atherosclerosis
     Hypertension
     Vascular accident of end-artery
     Menière's disease (labyrinthine hydrops)
     Lermoyez's syndrome
     Leukaemia
     Malaria
   Degenerative (partly vascular)
     Presbyacusis (Figs D.5, D.6)
   Vitamin deficiency
     Vitamin B deficiency
   Dietary
     Tropical ataxic neuropathy
   Hormonal
     Myxoedema
     Pregnancy
   Drug-induced deafness
     Antibiotics
       Aminoglycosides
         Streptomycin
         Neomycin
         Gentamicin
       Others in large doses
     Aspirin (reversible deafness)
     Quinine
     Chloroquine
     Chemotherapeutic agents for malignant
       disease
   Unknown

2. **Retrocochlear lesions**
   a. Neural Acoustic neuroma
                (8th nerve neurilemmoma)
              Cerebello-pontine angle tumour
              Meningitis
                Leptomeningitis
                Syphilitic
                Tuberculous
              Trauma
              Carcinomatous neuropathy
              Vogt–Koyanagi syndrome
              Harada's disease
              Unknown
   b. Central Multiple sclerosis
              Encephalitis
              Meningomyelitis
              Pontine glioma
              Concussion
              Vascular accidents
              Brainstem damage from head injury
              Psychogenic—hysterical
              Unknown

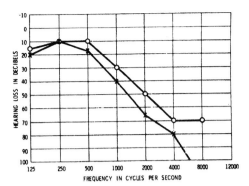

Fig. D.5. Audiogram showing the fairly symmetrical hearing loss for high tones in presbyacusis.

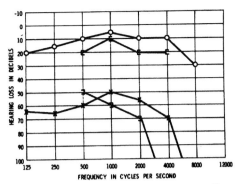

Fig. D.7. Audiogram in a case of Menière's disease affecting the left labyrinth. Careful investigations are required to exclude acoustic neuroma if unilateral sensorineural deafness such as this is found.

vessels of the stria vascularis play an important part. Diagnosis is made from the typical history of fluctuant sensorineural deafness with a gradual increase in severity, combined with tinnitus and prolonged and severe attacks of vertigo with vomiting. The disease shows periods of remission between groups of attacks. There is a psychological component as well. Depressed vestibular function and an end-organ deafness together with the history serve to identify this disease. Lermoyez's syndrome is a variant where the hearing improves very suddenly after an attack of vertigo and tinnitus. It is thought that the membranous labyrinth ruptures releasing the endolymphatic pressure and restoring cochlear function.

Leukaemia causes haemorrhage in the inner ear and in malaria the destruction of the blood cells leaves pigment in the cells. Deafness in this disease may also be caused by antimalarial drugs.

Presbyacusis (senile deafness) is common to mankind and loss of hearing in the higher frequencies

is almost invariable with age, though the rate is dependent upon genetic background, exposure to noise (city dwellers lose their hearing more rapidly than country dwellers) and vascular changes of atherosclerosis. The audiogram shows an increasing depression in the high frequencies. Failure to hear speech ('I can hear you talking but I cannot hear what you say'), in background noise especially, results from the high tone loss and inability to hear the consonants which carry the meaning in speech.

Diet is important. Vitamin B deficiency leads to dermal, mucosal and aural damage. It has been shown that hearing loss stemming from other causes is always worse in those with a B-deficient diet. Cassava, which contains cyanides and is an important part of the diet of Africans and some Caribbeans, allied to genetic factors it is thought, causes tropical ataxic neuropathy, an oto-ophthalmo-neuropathy described in tropical regions.

The deafness of myxoedema, the occasional deafness of pregnancy and aspirin deafness are unusual among the causes of sensorineural loss in that they are reversible.

With regard to drug-induced deafness it must be noted that ototoxicity results not only from systemic treatment but also from the use of antibiotics locally in the ear to treat otitis media—chloramphenicol, neomycin and gentamicin may all act in this manner.

Among the neural and central lesions acoustic neuromas are important because they are silent, slow growing, difficult to diagnose and potentially lethal if not found in a small and easily operable state. They may be solitary or occur as a manifestation of familial neurofibromasosis (von Recklinghausen's disease), when other fibromas will be seen. The presentation is usually with increasing, unilateral, non-recruiting sensorineural deafness often accompanied by tinnitus. Vertigo is not intermittent and severe as in Menière's

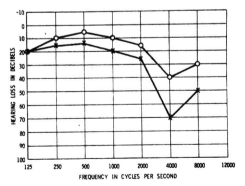

Fig. D.6. Audiogram showing the typical findings in noise-inducing hearing loss. In this case the patient had been shooting for some years with a 12-bore gun and the left ear, being nearer the muzzle, has sustained greater damage than the right.

disease but it is often present in the form of a vague unsteadiness. Vestibular function is affected and there is a canal paresis on the side of the tumour. Fifth nerve symptoms are often early with loss of homolateral pain and temperature sensation on the face due to pressure on the descending tract of the 5th nerve. The best clinical method is to test the corneal reflex as an indicator of pain sensation. Nowadays it is hoped to find these tumours before they have extended beyond the internal auditory meatus to impinge on the brainstem.

Diagnosis of acoustic neuroma, after clinical, audiometric and vestibular tests, requires an MRI to show any enlargement or erosion of the internal auditory meatus, as little as 1–2 mm of difference being significant.

The Vogt–Koyanagi syndrome, from which it is thought that the artist Goya suffered, is a sudden and rare illness with severe headache and malaise which goes on to uveitis, alopecia, vitiligo and deafness. Harada's disease is very similar but with retinal detachment instead of uveitis. The deafness is usually permanent but the uveitis recovers. The depressing effects of sudden complete deafness on a sensitive artist such as Goya explains his change of style from brightly coloured, happy pictures of handsome men and pretty girls to those of his later 'Black Period' and the 'Disasters of War'. This is an indication of the severe psychological effects that deafness may bring.

A.G.D. Maran

Diarrhoea

Diarrhoea is defined as increased frequency, fluidity or volume of bowel motions. It is commonly, but not exclusively, associated with an increase in faecal excretion of water and electrolytes, with consequent increase in faecal weight. In some instances there is frequent passage of bowel motions of normal consistency and weight, or of blood and pus (exudative diarrhoea).

In an assessment of the many differential diagnoses of diarrhoea, it is important to consider the possible mechanisms which may be involved. Diarrhoea may be classified as being due to reduced fluid reabsorption (osmotic effects, mucosal defects, motility abnormalities), increased fluid secretion (bacterial toxins, hormones and neurotransmitters, prostaglandins, bile acids and fatty acids, detergent laxatives, immature enterocytes and secretion), and exudative diarrhoea.

As diarrhoea is a symptom, and not a disease in itself, it is important that in every patient the underlying cause is identified. After routine history and physical examination (including rectal examination),

investigations of importance include examination of the stools by naked eye, by the microscope and by microbiological investigation, sigmoidoscopy and possibly colonoscopy, radiological examination (barium enema and small-bowel enema) and analyses of stools for lipids, bile acids and osmolarity. Tests of absorption, digestion, nutritional deficiency possibly associated with abnormal absorption, and tests such as jejunal biopsy, bacteriological studies of the small and large bowel and intestinal permeability may all be helpful.

Although there is overlap, it is convenient to consider the causes of diarrhoea into those affecting infants and young children and those occurring in adults.

Diarrhoea in infancy and early childhood

Diarrhoea, with or without vomiting, is a presenting feature of a wide variety of conditions which may occur in infancy. The most important of these are: infantile gastroenteritis, systemic infections, unsuitable foods, carbohydrate intolerance, malabsorption, with or without steatorrhoea—coeliac disease, pancreatic disease, giardiasis, protein-losing enteropathy, drugs, ulcerative colitis or Crohn's disease (both rare in childhood), or Hirschsprung's disease.

Diarrhoea may be mimicked by the blood and mucus associated with intussusception (red current-jelly stools) or by pseudo-diarrhoea associated with constipation.

Infantile gastroenteritis, although less common than previously, still remains a serious problem in many parts of the world and is a prominent cause of mortality and morbidity in infants. In developed countries, infantile gastroenteritis still remains a common cause of diarrhoea in infants and young children and is epidemic in some areas. A wide variety of pathogenic organisms may be responsible, including *Salmonella*, *Shigella*, and enteropathogenic *E. coli*. More rarely, other organisms such as *staphylococci*, are involved. In mild cases there may be diarrhoea without systemic disturbance but in more severe cases the infant passes watery green stools, which may be accompanied by vomiting and may rapidly develop a state of shock due to water and electrolyte depletion.

All other causes of diarrhoea in infancy and childhood must be considered in every case of acute or chronic diarrhoea in young children, possibly associated with failure to thrive. Diarrhoea may be the first sign of a disease such as coeliac disease or cystic fibrosis. *Coeliac disease* (gluten-induced enteropathy) may present in early childhood with acute or chronic diarrhoea. Failure to thrive, abdominal pain and distension may occur. The diagnosis is made by jejunal biopsy showing subtotal villous atrophy. The patient generally responds rapidly and effectively to the exclusion of gluten from the diet.

Cystic fibrosis may be manifested by meconium ileus in the neonatal period and thereafter children develop steatorrhoea with pale, bulky and offensive stools, failure to thrive and marked abdominal distension. The condition is associated with frequent respiratory infections. The prognosis of cystic fibrosis has much improved with nutritional support, pancreatic supplementation and control of repeated chest infections.

TODDLER DIARRHOEA

Toddler diarrhoea is defined as recurrent passage of frequent loose stools by a child who is thriving (maintaining a normal growth pattern compared to children of the same age). By thriving, the children can be distinguished, without full investigations, from those suffering from other causes of chronic diarrhoea such as coeliac disease, cystic fibrosis, secondary lactose intolerance, and severe cows' milk protein intolerance. By being healthy and active children, they can be reasonably distinguished from children with giardiasis or inflammatory bowel disease such as Crohn's disease or ulcerative colitis. There is a gradual improvement in the frequency and consistency of the stool with age although the age at which faecal continence is achieved may be significantly delayed.

Diarrhoea in adults

The following causes should be considered:

Specific bacterial or viral infections, e.g. *Salmonella* gastroenteritis, dysentery (amoebic or bacillary), cholera, viral infections, AIDS
Inflammatory bowel disease, e.g. ulcerative colitis, Crohn's disease
Malabsorption/maldigestion, e.g. coeliac disease, loss of damage to the absorptive surface of the small intestine (due to resection and short-bowel syndrome), extensive Crohn's disease of the small intestine, progressive systemic sclerosis, vascular insufficiency, lymphoma, lymphangiectasia, bacterial overgrowth, radiation damage, Whipple's disease
Following gastric resection, gastroenterostomy and vagotomy
Pancreatic dysfunction, e.g. chronic pancreatitis, cystic fibrosis, carcinoma of pancreas, pancreatic resection
Tumours of the intestine, e.g. lymphoma of the small intestine, carcinoma of colon or rectum, Zollinger–Ellison syndrome, carcinoid and other hormone-producing tumours
Diverticular disease of the colon
Irritable bowel syndrome
Anxiety states, associated with generalized diseases
Other systemic disease such as hyperthyroidism, diabetes mellitus

Drugs, antibiotics (including pseudomembranous colitis), cytotoxic agents, abuse of laxatives, alcohol, neomycin, mefanamic acid, magnesium-containing antacids, arsenic, colchicine and others

It is helpful to subdivide the causes of diarrhoea into acute and chronic diarrhoea, although many causes of chronic diarrhoea may have acute episodes.

ACUTE DIARRHOEA

Acute diarrhoea in adults is most likely to be due to infection—bacterial or viral, but a detailed history may elicit dietary indiscretion, or the ingestion of a drug which may be the responsible factor.

In dysentery there are generally symptoms of tenesmus, with blood and mucus in the bowel motions. In *amoebic dysentery*, *Entamoeba histolytica* may be found in the stools, and multiple, small, pitted ulcers may be seen at sigmoidoscopy. An amoebic cyst may be found in the mucosa on rectal biopsy. In *bacillary dysentery* agglutination may be positive and the organism recovered from the stools; the incubation period is 1–5 days. *Salmonella infection* has a shorter incubation period (8–24 hours or at most 2 days) and presents with acute vomiting and diarrhoea, frequently associated with pyrexia.

'*Traveller's diarrhoea*', sometimes also associated with vomiting, may be due to specific *E. Coli* or digestive infections, but is probably caused in many cases by alteration of the normal bacteria of bowel. The diagnosis is generally suggested by a recent history of travel abroad and can be confirmed by the finding of *E. Coli*, or other pathogens including *Giardia lamblia*, campylobacter, salmonella or shigella in the stools.

Infection may trigger an acute exacerbation of ulcerative colitis or Crohn's disease in individuals afflicted by these conditions.

CHRONIC DIARRHOEA

There are many interrelated causes of chronic diarrhoea, associated with a large number of diseases of all parts of the gastrointestinal tract, and sometimes found in non-gastrointestinal conditions.

In *ulcerative colitis* stools are frequent, and often watery, blood is generally present and mucus and pus are often a feature. The disease is confluent and distal, the diagnosis being made in most patients at sigmoidoscopy, which reveals a red, oedematous, friable mucosa. Histological confirmation can be obtained by rectal biopsy.

Crohn's disease affecting small or large intestine, is frequently associated with bouts of diarrhoea. Frequent bowel motions are common, mucus and pus may occasionally be present, but blood occurs in only 10 per cent of cases. It is to be noted that although ulcerative colitis is still commoner than Crohn's disease, Crohn's disease has markedly increased in incidence in Western countries in recent years. Both ulcerative colitis and Crohn's disease may present with acute diarrhoea due to an exacerbation of the disease. Such an episode may be triggered by an acute infection; thus stool cultures should be performed in all patients suspected of having ulcerative colitis or Crohn's disease, or if an exacerbation of these inflammatory bowel diseases is present. Colonoscopy may be of value in confirming the diagnosis, and in determining the extent, and the degree of activity throughout the bowel.

Chronic dysentery may occur in tropical countries and the diagnosis can be made by bacteriological examination of the stools. These conditions may give rise to watery diarrhoea or the passage of pale, white or yellow, bulky, strong-smelling stools, which are often difficult to flush away. There may be abdominal distension and discomfort, and deficiency states leading to anaemias, angular stomatitis, muscle weakness, skin rashes, etc., depending upon the single or multiple deficiencies which may be present. The presence of diarrhoea and/or steatorrhoea may be characteristic of these syndromes, but not diagnostic. It is not possible on clinical grounds to establish the basic cause of these lesions.

Malabsorption may be due to gastric or pancreatic causes; gastric causes include gastric resection, gastroenterostomy and total vagotomy; pancreatic causes include chronic pancreatitis, carcinoma, cystic fibrosis of the pancreas, resection, hypoplasia (Schwachman's syndrome), or congenital enzyme defects. Diarrhoea secondary to pancreatic maldigestion is often associated with marked steatorrhoea, and other aspects of pancreatic disease may be present, such as jaundice.

Diarrhoea associated with malabsorption may be due to a wide range of small intestinal diseases. Damage to the small intestinal mucosa with associated abnormalities of mucosal transport may occur in coeliac disease, dermatitis herpetiformis, tropical malabsorption, Crohn's disease, Whipple's disease, radiation damage to the small intestine, lymphoma, tuberculosis, or damage due to drugs such as neomycin. Other causes include vascular abnormalities of the small intestine, gangrene, abnormalities of the intestinal lymphatics, intestinal resections (tumours, vascular abnormalities, Crohn's disease), endocrine abnormalities, immunodeficiency syndromes, or drug-induced damage. Bacterial overgrowth may also result in malabsorption and diarrhoea, and be due to progressive systemic sclerosis, the short-bowel syndrome

following surgical intervention, strictures or the presence of jejunal diverticulosis. Crohn's disease can also cause small intestinal damage with malabsorption and diarrhoea, or lead to small intestinal resection or bacterial overgrowth following the development of strictures. Disaccharidase deficiency may also be a cause of diarrhoea; this may be primary, or secondary to a range of disorders affecting the small intestine.

If maldigestion or malabsorption is suspected as a cause of diarrhoea, the following investigations are appropriate; jejunal biopsy with disaccharidase assay; small intestinal radiology (small-bowel enema), studies of bacterial status of the small bowel with collection and culture of aspirated fluid, or H_2 breath tests, pancreatic function tests, ultrasound and CT scanning.

Tumours of the alimentary tract can also lead to diarrhoea. Carcinoma of the colon is classically associated with alternating constipation and diarrhoea, or the passage of small frequent narrow stools. Tumours of the small intestine may follow coeliac disease and are most commonly lymphomas. Radiological investigations (barium enema or small-bowel enema) are of most value in diagnosing these lesions, although a suspected lesion in the colon may be diagnosed by colonoscopy and biopsy.

Diarrhoea associated with increased excretion of bile acids (cholerrheic diarrhoea) is generally associated with damage to bile acid absorbing mechanisms in the terminal ileum in Crohn's disease or in tumours. Liver disease may also be associated with diarrhoea due to bile acid abnormalities. The diagnosis is confirmed by measuring faecal bile acid excretion or by assessing bile acid absorption using the Se HCAT test; radiology of the terminal ileum may also be helpful.

Other colonic diseases may be associated with diarrhoea; these include diverticular disease of the colon characterized by watery diarrhoea, sometimes containing blood, and the irritable bowel syndrome in which motility disturbance may occur in both large and small bowel; in this condition, alteration of bowel habit may occur with diarrhoea or constipation, associated with lower abdominal pain.

Some generalized diseases may be accompanied by diarrhoea; these include hyperthyroidism, hypothyroidism and diabetes mellitus. Tumours associated with abnormal production of hormones such as the carcinoid syndrome, vipomas (Verner–Morrison syndrome) or gastrin-producing tumour (Zollinger–Ellison syndrome) may present with diarrhoea. A number of drugs have now been recognized as causing diarrhoea. Abuse of laxatives is perhaps the most common cause of diarrhoea due to drugs; antibiotics such as ampicillin and tetracycline may alter gut flora resulting in diarrhoea; neomycin and PAS cause mucosal damage and diarrhoea and pseudomembranous colitis is commonly associated with the use of antibiotics with the production of clostridium difficile toxin. Ethanol in excess is also a common cause of diarrhoea. An accurate drug history should be sufficient to confirm the drug-related nature of diarrhoea in patients although measurements of chemicals associated with laxatives in faeces or urine may be required.

R. I. Russell

Dysmenorrhoea

The causes of painful menstrual periods may be tabulated as follows:

1 SPASMODIC OR PRIMARY
   Uterine hypoplasia (small, acutely anteflexed uterus, long conical cervix, stenosed os)
   Congenital malformations
   Ovarian dysfunction
   Psychogenic
2 CONGESTIVE OR SECONDARY
   Arising from infection:
   Pelvic peritonitis, salpingo-oophoritis, parametritis, cervicitis
   Arising from endometriosis:
   Chocolate cysts of ovary, adenomyoma
   Retroversion of the uterus
   Uterine fibroids
   If complicated by pelvic infection or endometriosis
   Psychogenic
3 MEMBRANOUS

The distribution of the cases into these three classes is often easy; in the first place, spasmodic cases are practically always *primary*, that is they begin when ovulation first takes place, i.e. within 2 or 3 years of the onset of the periods; while congestive cases are *secondary*, that is, acquired later as a result of some definite lesion. Further, the nature of the pain is often characteristic of the type of case, for in spasmodic cases the pain begins with the flow or only just before. It is aching in character, often with griping or colicky exacerbations felt in the midline above the symphysis pubis and passing down the anterior aspect of the thighs. It is associated with prostration, pallor, headache and vomiting. It usually continues for 6–12 hours until the menstrual flow is well established. In the congestive cases, on the other hand, the pain is continuous and aching, begins some hours or days before the flow, and in typical cases is relieved by the flow. In the membranous cases, which may complicate either primary or secondary dysmenorrhoea, the nature of the pain partakes of the characters of both the former types, being aching and continuous first, then becoming colicky and spasmodic when the uterus is attempting to expel the characteristic membrane or cast, and being finally relieved when this comes away.

Many cases are met with in which the pain partakes of the nature of both the congestive and spasmodic types. This usually means that a woman who originally had spasmodic dysmenorrhoea acquires some lesion which in its turn gives rise also to the congestive type of pain.

Having settled that a case belongs to one of the three main types, it is possible to work out the actual causation. This is more difficult in the spasmodic cases than in the congestive, because the latter depend upon well-defined lesions, and the former do not.

1. Spasmodic cases

The causation of the pain in this type of case is obscure because the physical signs are essentially normal. Not infrequently the uterus may be small with a long conical cervix and an exaggerated anterior bend (the 'cochleate' uterus of Pozzi). A sound may pass with difficulty into such a uterus giving rise to the suggestion that there is a stenosis of the internal os. These findings are common in young adult women, however, and are more likely to be a manifestation of their immaturity than a cause of the spasmodic dysmenorrhoea, because they are found just as often in girls of the same age who do not suffer from dysmenorrhoea.

Many cases with spasmodic dysmenorrhoea, moreover, appear to have a normal uterus. In such cases evidence of degenerative or inflammatory changes in the presacral nerve have been described but their existence is very doubtful. The function of the ovarian hormones in causing spasmodic dysmenorrhoea is also not clear. For the first 2 or 3 years of anovular menstruation the periods do not as a rule cause pain. But when ovulation begins, a corpus luteum is formed and progesterone secreted and the periods become painful. Inhibition of ovulation by the use of the contraceptive pill usually renders the periods painless in such cases unless there is a large psychogenic element. It is tempting to explain spasmodic dysmenorrhoea by saying it is due to an ovarian dysfunction but if this is so its nature is unknown. The psychogenic factor is also emphasized and said to be increased by a doting mother who herself suffered from severe dysmenorrhoea. Marriage and child-bearing may improve or cure spasmodic dysmenorrhoea but this does not prove its psychogenic origin in the first place. Nevertheless, a healthy attitude by the patient to the condition and an assurance that it does not signify disease helps her to put up with it.

2. Congestive cases

It is unnecessary to differentiate the congestive cases as tubal, ovarian or uterine because the underlying cause in all is pelvic congestion accompanying such lesions as are shown in the table above. Their differential diagnosis is made by careful consideration of the history, combined with bimanual examination of the pelvic organs, and if required, laparoscopy. Simple *retroversion and flexion* can be recognized on bimanual examination; the fundus will be felt posteriorly, the cervix looking directly down the vagina in a forward direction. Retroversion of the uterus by itself does not cause dysmenorrhoea and painful periods mean that either pelvic infection or endometriosis coexists. *Salpingo-oophoritis* in its typical chronic form gives rise to irregular tender swellings on either side and behind the uterus, sometimes forming definitely retort-shaped swellings, especially if pus is present in the tubes. Fixation of these swellings and of the uterus is a very definite sign of the disease; while the history of one or more attacks of acute illness, with pelvic pain, will assist to make the diagnosis certain. Small haemorrhagic cysts of the ovary, the contents of which may be 'tarry' or of chocolate-like consistence, are also important causes of premenstrual dysmenorrhoea; they are always fixed, and are of endometrial origin (*endometrioma of the ovary*). Adenomyosis may produce general enlargement of the uterus or there may be a localized adenomyoma in part of the uterus. Then an asymmetrical swelling can be felt in the uterus on bimanual vaginal examination, as in the case of a uterine fibroid.

Any psychogenic factor will naturally accentuate the pain. Often associated with this type of dysmenorrhoea is some constitutional disability, the result of anaemia, overwork, worry, anxiety or other conditions leading to a lowering of the pain threshold.

In nearly all cases of congestive dysmenorrhoea the underlying cause also produces other symptoms such as menorrhagia, dyspareunia, backache and vaginal discharge. It is unusual to find congestive dysmenorrhoea as a symptom by itself.

3. Membranous cases

A cast of uterine endometrium, complete or incomplete, may be passed in either spasmodic or congestive dysmenorrhoea. Its passage through the cervix is likely to cause spasmodic pain because of the colicky uterine contractions. The cast may have to be distinguished from a decidual cast passed following the rupture of an ectopic pregnancy or from the cast of an early miscarriage. In either of these conditions a careful review of the history should lead to the diagnosis but if there is doubt histology of the cast should settle it. In ectopic pregnancy the cast contains the decidua of pregnancy but no chorionic villi and in the case of an early miscarriage there are villi in the decidua.

Cases of dysmenorrhoea may be confused with those of abdominal pain due to other lesions unconnected with menstruation; and the differentiation of such cases may be a matter of considerable importance. It is conceivable that the following conditions may be mistaken for dysmenorrhoea:

Appendicitis
Colic: intestinal, renal or biliary
Ruptured tubal gestation
Torsion of an ovarian cyst pedicle
Haemorrhage from or into a Graafian follicle
Rupture of an ovarian cyst or pyosalpinx
Threatened or actual abortion
Endometriosis

Obviously, some of these lesions are dangerous to life, and therefore it is essential that they are not overlooked. The danger of this occurring is increased if any of these lesions start at or near the expected time of a menstrual period, and would hardly arise if a menstrual period had terminated recently, or was not expected for some days. It will be noted that all these lesions are accompanied by sudden abdominal pain, which might perhaps lead to a suspicion of spasmodic dysmenorrhoea, but hardly of congestive, owing to the character of the pain.

N. Patel

Dyspareunia

Dyspareunia, or painful coitus, may depend on a variety of local lesions, or it may occur when no local lesion can be found. It is associated closely with vaginismus, or painful spasm of the levator ani muscle on attempts at coitus, and the same lesions which cause simple dyspareunia may also give rise to vaginismus; vaginismus is particularly likely to develop if the simple dyspareunia remains untreated for any length of time. In some women a local lesion produces no pain upon attempts at coitus which in others will cause pain accompanied by violent spasm of the levator ani. In some cases pain arises because there is a difficulty of penetration of the vaginal orifice, while in others there is no difficulty, but pain is caused on deep penetration—'deep dyspareunia'. The following lesions commonly give rise to dyspareunia:

Congenital absence of the lower part of the vagina
Unruptured hymen
Inflamed hymeneal orifice
Vulvitis
Bartholinitis
Disparity in size

Vulval dystrophy
—hyperplastic (leucoplakia)
—hypoplastic (atrophic vulvitis)
Healed perineal lacerations giving rise to a narrow introitus
Urethral caruncle
Urethritis
Cystitis
Prolapsed tender ovaries with retroverted uterus
Salpingo-oophoritis
Anal fissure
Thrombosed piles
Endometriosis
Arthritis of the hips
'Functional' causes

The lesions fall into natural groups, according to whether the situation of the lesion is at the vulva, the uterus and ovaries, the urinary passages, or at the anus and rectum; it is necessary to carry out a detailed examination of any case of dyspareunia in order to find out whether any of these well-defined lesions are present. The commonest is *inflamed hymeneal remains*, sometimes gonorrhoeal, accompanied by redness and swelling of the orifice of the duct of Bartholin's gland. The lesion is evident on inspection, and the parts are acutely sensitive to the least touch. Hyperplastic vulval dystrophy is a lesion that is obvious from the white, sodden appearance of the labia, and causes pain on account of the sensitive cracks and fissures which accompany it. Hypoplastic vulval dystrophy causes actual contraction of the vaginal orifice, and consequently penetration is difficult and causes pain. The red projecting growth from the urinary meatus, *caruncle*, is self-evident and acutely tender, while *urethritis* is diagnosed by the issue of pus on squeezing the urethra. *Cystitis* is diagnosed by the presence of pus and bacilli in the urine, accompanied by frequency of micturition, and it causes pain because the bladder is painful and intolerant of the disturbance caused by coitus. *Prolapsed, tender ovaries* and *backward displacements of the uterus* cause no pain on penetration and no difficulty, but coitus with deep penetration gives acute pain at the time or a dull pelvic ache later; the condition is recognized by a bimanual examination, as is also *salpingo-oophoritis*, in connection with which there is usually a history of some acute attack of pelvic peritonitis. Vaginitis due to a trichomonas infection, or a chronic endocervitis with or without erosion, may be responsible. Endometriosis in the pelvis is a common cause of deep dyspareunia. Ovarian and other neoplasms are hardly ever responsible; severe constipation is not an uncommon cause. Disproportion in size is rarely in itself of importance as the vagina is very distensile, but if in addition there is any local lesion the pain will be accentuated. *Anal fissure* and *thrombosed and inflamed piles* are recognized by careful examination of the anus and

rectum by the finger or speculum. Arthritis of the hips or lumbar spine may cause dyspareunia.

In the cases which occur without local lesions the vaginal entrance will be found to be acutely hyperaesthetic and penetration difficult, and there is spasmodic vaginismus. Careful examination fails to demonstrate a lesion, and these cases are usually termed 'neurotic' or 'functional'; sexual desire is not necessarily absent; indeed many such patients are over-desirous of the consummation of marriage. Fear, arising from painful attempts at coitus, is often the cause of the condition. Enlarging the orifice by gradual dilatation, using vaginal dilators, or by a small plastic operation often leads to cure as the patient gains confidence. Child-bearing also cures a case of this nature. These cases must be distinguished from those in which the underlying factor is absence of sexual desire and actual dislike of the sexual act, when the dyspareunia is merely a defence mechanism built up by the woman to avoid coitus. Unhappy and unsuitable marriages or fear of pregnancy conduce to this state of affairs, and the patient is prone to complain of pain when dislike is really what is meant. There is no difficulty in penetration in such cases.

N. Patel

Dysphagia

Dysphagia means difficulty in swallowing. The difficulty may be in the initiation of swallowing, which is of course under voluntary control, or in the later involuntary stages of swallowing, in which no conscious sensation is associated with the normal passage of a swallowed bolus from pharynx to stomach. If this transit is impeded, however, there is a sensation that swallowed food does not progress normally through the oesophagus. The patients then perceive a hold-up to the swallowed food and will complain of 'food sticking'. Dysphagia should be distinguished from painful swallowing, sometimes termed odynophagia, and from the globus sensation—a feeling of a lump in the throat—which does not interfere with swallowing in any way.

Oropharyngeal dysphagia

Neuromuscular disorders which affect oropharyngeal function cause difficulty in swallowing which is associated with a tendency to aspirate swallowed material into the airway, and with nasopharyngeal reflux. Unilateral cerebral lesions, such as cerebrovascular accidents, cause transient dysphagia of this type. Infarction of the brainstem, as in pseudo-bulbar palsy and the posteroinferior cerebellar artery syndrome causes oropharyngeal dysphagia, as will any cause of lower cranial nerve palsies including motor neurone disease, the Guillain–Barré syndrome and poliomyelitis affecting the brainstem. Dysphagia will also occur when the brainstem is affected by multiple sclerosis and with extrapyramidal disorders such as Parkinsonism. The oropharyngeal dysphagia which occurs in rabies, tetanus and botulism is likewise a consequence of neural dysfunction.

Myasthenia gravis and diseases affecting the pharyngeal musculature impair the ability to swallow normally. The inherited muscular dystrophies, including dystrophia myotonica, polymyositis and dermatomyositis may involve the pharynx.

Structural abnormality in the pharynx should be suspected when oropharyngeal dysphagia occurs in the absence of nasopharyngeal regurgitation or a tendency to aspirate into the airway. Pharyngeal carcinoma and lymphoma cause dysphagia of this type. Xerostomia may be responsible for a similar complaint, however, as grossly impaired salivary secretion may be recognized particularly by elderly patients only in terms of difficulty in initiating swallowing. Extrapharyngeal tumours causing pharyngeal compression can give rise to dysphagia, especially when they also invade the pharyngeal wall. Thyroid enlargement, however, seldom does so except when retrosternal extension of the gland compresses the proximal oesophagus.

Partial obstructions of the high oesophagus produce a clinical picture virtually indistinguishable from pharyngeal obstruction. An oesophageal web situated just below the cricopharyngeus and associated with iron-deficiency anaemia (the Plummer–Vinson or Paterson–Kelly syndrome) is now an uncommon cause of high oesophageal obstruction; squamous carcinomas occasionally occur at this level.

Cricopharyngeal spasm is sometimes suggested when a prominent indentation produced by the cricopharyngeus muscle is seen on a radiograph of the barium-filled upper oesophagus. The existence of a relationship between this radiological sign and a complaint of dysphagia or abnormality of cricopharyngeal muscle function is far from certain.

A *pharyngeal diverticulum* (Zenker's diverticulum) (*Fig.* D.8) is a posterior herniation of the pharynx giving rise to a pouch liable to fill with food and saliva. Dysphagia occurs in consequence of compression of the lower pharynx and upper oesophagus. Regurgitation of some of the diverticulum contents may occur long after they have been swallowed. There is a view that disordered contraction of the cricopharyngeus muscle contributes both to the dysphagia of this condition and to the development of the diverticulum itself.

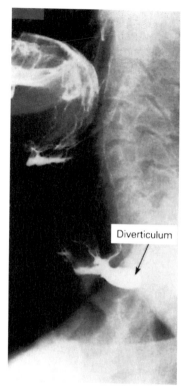

Fig. D.8. Barium radiograph of cervical oesophagus, showing contrast in a pharyngeal diverticulum (see arrow).

Oesophageal dysphagia

A sensation that swallowed food is 'sticking' during its passage from the pharynx to the stomach is readily recognized and described by patients. Many will indicate the level at which the sticking sensation is felt, though this correlates imperfectly with the level at which obstruction actually occurs. Mechanical obstruction of the oesophagus characteristically manifests with dysphagia for solid foods such as meat, fish or bread whereas dysphagia due to disordered motility of the oesophagus is perceived to affect both solids and liquids.

MECHANICAL OBSTRUCTION OF THE OESOPHAGUS

Benign and malignant strictures of the oesophagus are the common causes of mechanical obstruction. *Benign (peptic) strictures* develop in consequence of long-standing gastro-oesophageal reflux and are encountered most commonly in the lower oesophagus, though they may develop at any level. Most, but not all patients with such strictures give a clear history of troublesome heartburn. Benign stricturing of the

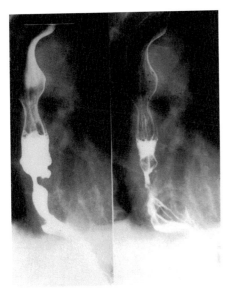

Fig. D.9. Oesophageal carcinoma. There is a constant narrowing on barium swallow in the lower third of the oesophagus.

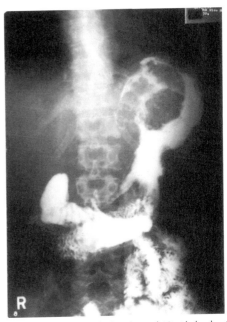

Fig. D.10. Barium meal of a female aged 60 with dysphagia. There is an extensive proliferative adenocarcinoma of the cardia extending into the gastric fundus.

oesophagus may also develop as a consequence of swallowing corrosive substances. Accidental ingestion of such materials occurs particularly in young children. Epidermolysis bullosa affects the squamous epithelium of the oesophagus as well as the skin, and benign oesophageal strictures often develop in patients with this rare disease.

Malignant strictures of the oesophagus characteristically present with a short history of progressively worsening dysphagia, initially for solids but potentially evolving to cause complete oesophageal obstruction (*Fig.* D.9). Squamous carcinoma may develop at any level; adenocarcinomas are less common and usually occur at the lower end of the oesophagus but may develop at any level in an oesophagus lined with Barrett's epithelium. An adenocarcinoma of the gastric fundus is an important cause dysphagia if it invades or obstructs the lower oesophagus (*Fig.* D.10).

A Schatzki ring is a web which occasionally develops at the oesophago-gastric junction, usually in association with a hiatus hernia. Many of these rings cause no symptoms but the minority which narrow the lumen to 12 mm or less present a risk of oesophageal obstruction by impaction of a bolus of solid food.

Extraluminal compression of the oesophagus is an uncommon cause of dysphagia. Mediastinal tumours, however, particularly lymphoma and bronchial carcinoma may encircle and compress the oesophagus sufficiently to cause the symptom.

In older patients, a prominent indentation or even right lateral displacement of the oesophagus at the level of the aortic arch is frequently seen on barium

radiographs. Dysphagia is rare, however, even when there is aneurysmal dilatation of the aorta. Enlargement of the left atrium, as in long-standing mitral stenosis, likewise rarely causes dysphagia even when oesophageal displacement is pronounced. In contrast, compression of the oesophagus by the aorta at the level of the diaphragm may give rise to significant obstruction and consequent dysphagia.

Dysphagia lusoria is a very rare condition in which the oesophagus is compressed by an anomalous right subclavian artery.

OESOPHAGEAL MOTILITY DISORDERS

Motility disorders of the oesophagus are well-recognized causes of dysphagia, but are uncommon. *Achalasia* is a disorder in which there is degeneration or functional failure of the oesophageal myenteric plexus, resulting in loss of all peristaltic contraction in the oesophageal body and failure of the lower oesophageal sphincter to relax in response to swallowing (*Fig.* D.11). Food and fluid thus tend to accumulate in the oesophagus, although most food ingested at each meal does very gradually pass through to the stomach. The patient is aware that ingested food and fluid are 'held-up' and the consequent discomfort is sometimes relieved by self-induced regurgitation. Spasms of more severe retrosternal pain sometimes occur. Fluid retained in the achalasic oesophagus may regurgitate

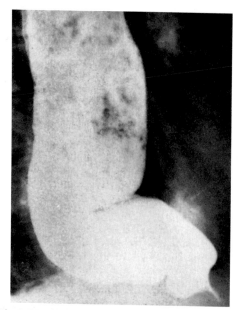

Fig. D.11. Achalasia, showing the 'bird-beak' appearance at the cardia. Many patients with achalasia present before significant oesophageal dilatation has developed, as in this example. (Dr R.C. Heading).

into the pharynx, particularly at night. Aspiration of this fluid into the airway may cause the patient to awaken with a bout of coughing; more commonly the fluid just dribbles from the mouth, resulting in a damp patch on the pillow each morning.

Chagas' disease is a degeneration of the oesophageal myenteric plexus caused by South American trypanosomal infection. The oesophageal manifestations are identical to those of achalasia.

Diffuse oesophageal spasm is even rarer than achalasia. Frequent non-peristaltic contractions of the oesophageal circular muscle cause dysphagia for solids and liquids and may be responsible for severe chest pain resembling that of myocardial infarction. Dysphagia and pain can sometimes be provoked by drinking hot or ice cold fluids, and many patients avoid such drinks.

The endoscopic appearances of the oesophagus may be normal both in achalasia and in diffuse oesophageal spasm. Barium-swallow examination will establish the diagnosis in most cases of achalasia and in some cases of diffuse oesophageal spasm but oesophageal manometry provides a more secure foundation for either diagnosis.

Impaired or absent peristalsis in the distal oesophagus occurs in scleroderma, and in a minority of patients with gastro-oesophageal reflux. Intermittent dysphagia for solids, which is usually mild, may then occur.

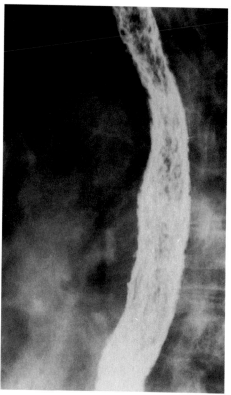

Fig. D.12. Extensive oesophageal candidiasis in a patient receiving chemotherapy for lymphoma.

Dysphagia associated with painful swallowing

Acute inflammatory conditions affecting the mouth, pharynx or oesophagus may cause swallowing to be painful (odynophagia) with a consequent difficulty in swallowing. The clinical history usually makes clear that painful swallowing is the dominant symptom. Ludwig's angina, acute laryngitis and the laryngeal element of angioneurotic oedema are rare causes of painful swallowing; candidiasis of the oesophagus is more often encountered. Patients who are debilitated or immuno-suppressed are at particular risk of oesophageal candidiasis (*Fig.* D.12) but it is occasionally encountered in individuals who are otherwise healthy.

Acute inflammation and ulceration of the oesophagus may be caused by some drugs when an ingested tablet or capsule lodges for some hours in the oesophagus instead of passing promptly to the stomach. This is particularly likely with tablets which are taken last thing at night. Emepronium bromide and doxycycline have been notable for causing oesophageal ulceration in this way. Swallowing is then painful and there may also be an element of dysphagia.

R. C. Heading

Dysuria

Dysuria is pain felt during the act of micturition. It is a urethral pain and relates to irritation of the urethral mucosa. It may, therefore, be experienced by an otherwise normal individual when concentrated or acid urine is passed, for example, when the patient is dehydrated from the excessive fluid loss associated with exercise or hot climate, or from an inability to drink enough fluid, for example during an intercontinental flight. Dysuria under these circumstances is rarely severe, and felt more as a tingling or slight stinging as urine is passed. The symptom is short-lived and corrected as soon as the relative dehydration resolves.

True dysuria is associated with a urinary tract infection. This may have arisen in the upper tract as pyelitis, in which case the bladder is invariably infected secondarily. It may be due to primary cystitis, or due to acute urethritis. True dysuria in women may also be found in the 'urethral syndrome', otherwise known as 'acute abacterial cystitis'. The feeling exactly mimicks a true cystitis but no microbiological evidence of infection can be found. This condition is noted elsewhere under URINE, RETENTION OF.

Pain felt in the bladder area is not true dysuria but may also be present during an acute episode of cystitis. Bladder pain can also be experienced in the presence of a bladder stone, when the stone bounces up and down on the trigone during the act of micturition. The trigone is a particularly sensitive area of the bladder and can therefore cause pain when involved by bladder or prostatic carcinoma and in acute and chronic prostatitis. Prostatitis is a difficult condition to diagnose — acute prostatitis renders digital examination of the prostate per rectum virtually impossible, as the gland is exquisitely tender; the diagnosis of chronic prostatitis is rarely satisfactory although the presence of threads on post-massage urine examination is usually taken as sufficient evidence of the condition. Positive cultures are rarely obtained from cases of 'chronic prostatitis' even when tissue cores of prostate are subject to bacteriological examination. Tuberculous cystitis may not be particularly symptomatic but bladder pain and true dysuria may both occur. When diagnosed, often after prolonged searching for positive cultures of early morning urines, it should be considered as a disease of the whole urinary tract.

Perineal pain during micturition is often indicative of prostatic disease, usually inflammatory. Prostatic carcinoma occasionally presents in this manner.

Acute urethral pain during micturition, associated with sudden cessation of a stream, implies the impaction of a calculus, a retained 'chip' following transurethral resection of the prostate or a dislodged portion of bladder tumour, along the urethra. As the narrowest portion of the urethra is the meatus, examination of the patient under these circumstances may reveal the object responsible protruding in part through the orifice. A stone impacted at the ureteric meatus provokes an intense oedematous reaction around the uretero-vesical junction and this may also cause a severe pain radiated to the distal end of the urethra.

In children, acute cystitis often presents in a non-specific way, the child having a sequence of screaming attacks which are obviously related to pain, the cause of which is not immediately apparent. Meatal ulceration and acute balanitis, both in the male infant, may provoke similar screaming attacks as the affected areas are, in effect, burnt by the ammonia in the urine each time micturition occurs.

Lynn Edwards

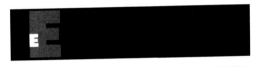

Earache

Earache (otalgia) may be due to a considerable number of diseases of the auricle or pinna, the external auditory meatus or middle ear. It may also be caused, most importantly, by referred pain from structures which share a common nerve supply. It is one of the common symptoms of childhood and may be one of the most deep-seated and unpleasant pains to bear. The causes of earache are listed in *Table* E.1.

Local causes of otalgia

Auricle — causes in the auricle are usually obvious and include direct trauma, haematoma, furuncles and otitis externa which cause pain because of the swelling of the skin which is firmly attached to the underlying cartilage. Perichondritis may occur following infection. 'Chondrodermatitis nodularis chronicis helicis' is the name given to a very painful nodular lesion of the pinna thought to be due to vasoconstriction following exposure to cold. Malignant disease may be painful; rodent ulcers and squamous carcinomas are usually only markedly so during the later stages.

Meatus — the external auditory meatus is the site of many painful conditions; local infection of the skin and small furuncles may be extremely painful, the amount of pain bearing little relationship to the size of the furuncle which may be only the size of a pin's head.

Table E.1. Causes of earache

Local

Auricle
  Trauma
    Direct
    Haematoma
  Furuncle
  Boils
  Otitis externa (*see Fig.* E.1)
  Perichondritis
  Chondrodermatitis nodularis
  Malignant disease
External auditory meatus
  Diffuse otitis externa
    Infective
      Bacterial
      Fungal
      Viral
    Reactive
      Eczematous
      Seborrhoeic dermatitis
      Neurodermatitis
  Malignant otitis externa
  Necrotizing osteitis
  Wax
  Keratosis obturans
  Foreign body—impacted
  Trauma
  Malignant disease
Middle ear
  Acute otitis media
  Chronic otitis media
    Tubotympanic otitis media
    Attic disease
  Serous otitis (rarely)
  Mastoiditis
  Malignant disease

Referred

Dental
  Caries
  Abscess
  Impacted molar
  Costen's syndrome
Pharynx
  Tonsillitis
  Pharyngitis
  Postoperative pain
  Quinsy
  Foreign bodies
  Malignant disease
Cervical spine
  Osteoarthritis
  Spondylosis

Neurological

Herpes zoster
Glossopharyngeal neuralgia
Trigeminal neuralgia (occasional)

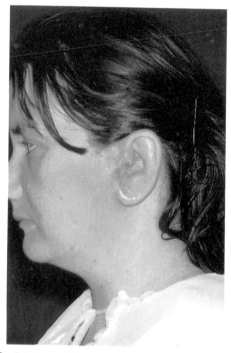

Fig. E.1. Severe otitis externa.

In many cases of diffuse otitis externa there is great swelling of the meatal skin and it may not be possible to see the drum. There is pain on moving the pinna and this is a valuable sign to differentiate the condition from mastoiditis. Fungal infection (otomycosis) is often especially painful (*Fig.* E.1).

In addition to the above, a condition called by Chandler (1968) 'malignant' otitis externa is found usually in diabetics where advancing infection leads to osteomyelitis and mastoiditis. The organism is always *B. pyocyaneus*.

Otitis externa haemorrhagica is described but it is best known as 'bullous myringitis' and is an infection of the middle layers of the tympanic membrane, usually caused by infection by *H. influenzae*. There is considerable pain when the layers of the drum are separated by fluid which causes a bleb within the drum, which must be carefully differentiated from the bulging drum of otitis media. The pain ceases if the bleb discharges its serosanguineous contents.

Finally, among the infections, necrotizing osteitis of the tympanic ring is a chronic condition with low grade aching in the ear. A small ulcer with bare bone exposed at the base may be seen in the deep meatus and this may rarely go on to extensive necrosis around the tympanic plate. The aetiology is obscure.

Impacted wax may cause considerable pain and discomfort especially following swimming and ineffec-

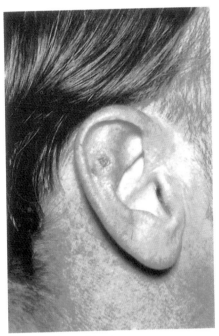

Fig. E.2. Epithelioma of the pinna.

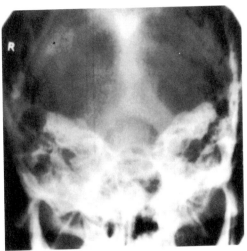

Fig. E.3. Chronic suppurative otitis media with a large cholesteatoma of the right temporal bone. (*Dr Lorna Davison.*)

tive attempts at removal by syringeing. Water may cause swelling of the wax and sudden deafness follows complete occlusion of the meatus. A more severe condition is keratosis obturans, where abnormal desquamation of the epithelium comes to lie in layers together with the wax and is most difficult to move. Pressure of this mass may cause bony necrosis and enlargement of the meatus. There is an association with chronic bronchitis and bronchiectasis, perhaps due to stimulation of the vagus and consequent reflex secretion of wax.

Foreign bodies may cause pain, usually after ineffective and incompetent attempts at removal. Insects are not infrequently found in tropical lands. Trauma, often self-inflicted in attempts to relieve irritation or remove wax, may cause scratches, ulcers or even perforations of the drum.

Malignant disease of the external meatus (*Fig. E.2*) is usually squamous-cell carcinoma. It often follows prolonged suppuration and is locally invasive, causing severe pain in the later stages. Rodent ulcers, common on the pinna, are rare in the meatus.

Middle ear. Acute otitis media is one of the commonest infections in childhood—hardly a child escapes one or more attacks. The infection follows an upper respiratory infection or cold and the pain may come on with great rapidity and usually becomes worse in the evening. It often ceases abruptly as the drum ruptures and the child falls asleep, the discharge

not being noticed by the mother till the following morning. It must be remembered that young children do not localize pain accurately and earache may not be a complaint. Unresolved acute otitis media may go on to acute mastoiditis, where there is severe pain and tenderness behind and above the ear centred over the mastoid antrum. Swelling behind the ear may follow and a subperiosteal abscess may push the pinna forwards. Differentiation from otitis externa is most important. In otitis media and mastoiditis deafness is invariable, while good hearing and pain on moving the pinna indicate otitis externa.

Chronic otitis media (*Fig.* E.3) is not often accompanied by pain though exacerbations of infection in both tubotympanic otitis media and in attic disease causing earache are often of serious import. The intracranial complications of otogenic disease—subperiosteal abscess, extradural abscess and brain abscess—are all accompanied by headache and when this occurs together with pyrexia and vertigo in a patient with chronic otitis media great care should be taken.

Trauma may be direct due to perforation of the drum by foreign bodies (a matchstick used in an ear is a most dangerous weapon) or by water or air pressure changes, diving or a blow on the ear. Otitic barotrauma is not so common now that aircraft are pressurized but it may still occur on descent if the air pressure is increased suddenly or if the patient is suffering from Eustachian tubal dysfunction at the time of the flight.

Secretory otitis media, so common in children, is usually characterized by a symptomless deafness. Dull aching pain or, rarely, stabs of acute pain may be a symptom.

Malignant disease, again usually squamous-cell carcinoma, occurring in chronically infected ears, rare tumours such as the glomus tumour, myelomas and secondary malignant disease all cause pain. Diagnosis is by observation, X-ray studies and biopsy.

Referred pain

Referred pain affecting the ear is very common. Pain is referred through the 5th, 7th, 9th and 10th cranial nerves, the upper cervical nerves and possibly the sympathetic nerve supply. Despite careful examination no abnormality is found in the ear. It has always been taught that 'a swelling in the neck and cottonwool in the ear' is a sign of malignant disease of pharynx or nasopharynx, one of the most important causes of referred otalgia.

Dental causes—caries, dental abscess and impacted lower molars are all common causes of earache. Malocclusion may give rise to dysfunction of the temporo-mandibular joint (Costen's syndrome). These patients often have a history of dental extractions or a badly fitting denture and tenderness will be found over the joint especially on movement, which may be restricted.

Pharynx. Tonsillitis, pharyngitis and even the initial stages of the common cold are all accompanied by earache which may vary from a mild stinging pain to very severe pain. The postoperative period after tonsillectomy is very consistently a time of quite unpleasant earache. This can be relieved by aspirin which has both a general and local action. Other simple pharyngeal causes are a quinsy, impacted foreign bodies or scratches due to trauma from bones and sharp objects that have been swallowed.

The most important group from a diagnostic point of view are malignant lesions of the nasopharynx, pharynx, laryngopharynx and larynx. Earache is found very consistently in these conditions and careful examination is always necessary if there is any doubt about a possible local cause.

Cervical spine. Cervical osteoarthritis or cervical spondylosis causing pain in the C2 and C3 regions may lead to referred pain around the ear in the middle-aged or elderly people who may have a history of trauma, such as 'whiplash injury'.

Neurological causes

A number of conditions come under this heading.

Herpes zoster oticus. Herpes zoster of the geniculate ganglion gives rise to lesions of the meatus, pinna and sometimes the palate and fauces. If facial palsy occurs (Ramsay–Hunt syndrome) this coincides with the vesicles and follows some days of severe otalgia

which may precede all other signs. Sometimes there is tinnitus and vertigo.

Other cranial and upper cervical nerves are also affected by herpes.

Glossopharyngeal neuralgia. Very severe pain radiating from the throat to the tongue and ear is a rare condition sometimes associated with an elongated styloid process. There is often a trigger area in the throat in the same way as a trigger area may initiate trigeminal neuralgia or *tic doloreux* which, though usually involving the face, may also largely affect the ear.

A. G. D. Maran

Enuresis

(*See also* URINE, INCONTINENCE OF)

Enuresis means incontinence of urine in children and can be diurnal, nocturnal or both. Children vary in the age at which they become reliably continent of urine. The majority of children are continent during the day by age two-and-a-half years and by night by three-and-a-half years. The prevalence of wetting diminishes with age and is approximately 20 per cent of 4 year olds, 10 per cent of 5 year olds, 7 per cent of 7 year olds and 1.4 per cent of 14 year olds.

The commonest organic disease to lead to enuresis is urinary tract infection especially in girls; enuretic girls have a four-fold increased likelihood of having a urinary tract infection compared to non-enuretics. Dribbling urinary incontinence may be the presenting sign of an ectopic ureter draining below the sphincter or overflow from an obstructed bladder. Secondary enuresis (having previously been reliably continent) should be considered suspicious of a urinary tract infection especially when associated with other symptoms such as urinary frequency, abdominal pain, dysuria and wetting in the daytime. Secondary enuresis can be caused by neurological problems such as neurogenic bladder (associated with spina bifida or other cord lesions such as tumours). Polyuria often leads to enuresis in children and so diseases such as diabetes mellitus or insipidus, or chronic renal failure must be considered. Emotional problems can lead to enuresis which compounds the psychological difficulties because of parental reaction (similar to encopresis). Secondary enuresis is common following family break-up or bereavement. Child sexual abuse may present in this way.

G. S. Clayden

Epistaxis

It is important to realize that epistaxis is a sign not a disease. The causes of the condition are shown in (*Table* E.2).

Table E.2. Causes of epistaxis

A. Local causes

Trauma to Little's area
Dryness of nasal mucosa, e.g. drugs
Abnormal anatomy, e.g. septal deviations
Ulceration and excoriation
Nasal fracture
Nasal infections
Tumours of the nose and sinuses
Septal granulomas and perforations
Foreign bodies

B. Systemic causes

Coagulopathy—haemophilia, Christmas disease, von
  Willebrand's disease, purpura, leukaemia
Hypertension
Drugs, anticoagulants, aspirin, cytotoxic drugs
Arteriosclerosis
Hereditary haemorrhagic telangiectasis
Vitamin deficiency—vitamin C, vitamin K
Renal dialysis

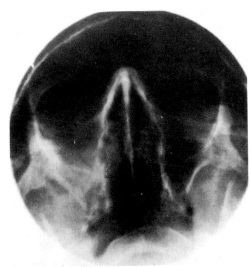

Fig. E.4. Carcinoma of the antrum. Note the opaque antrum and dehiscent orbital floor on the left side. (*Dr Lorna Davison.*)

Epistaxis usually occurs from the anterior part of the nasal septum, an area known as Little's area. The feeding vessels are the greater palatine artery, the facial artery, the anterior ethmoidal artery and the sphenopalatine artery. At the junction of these vessels the area is very vascular and is easily traumatized, since it is at the front of the most prominent feature of the face.

Bleeding higher up the nose usually comes from the sphenopalatine arteries or the anterior ethmoidal arteries. It is important to try to identify the site as accurately as possible because, in the event of persistent epistaxis where packing has failed, a vessel may need to be tied. Different approaches are needed for the anterior ethmoidal artery, a branch of the internal carotid, and the sphenopalatine artery, a branch of the maxillary artery as the terminal branch of the external carotid and so as accurate identification as possible is required.

The management of epistaxis is the management of the cause. If the nose has been traumatized then it is possible that a spicule of ethmoid bone has penetrated the anterior ethmoid artery and an open reduction may be required. Neoplasms of the nose and sinus need to be identified and treated accordingly (*Fig.* E.4). Coagulopathies require the appropriate medical therapy and if the patient is on anticoagulants or aspirin then the effects of these need to be reversed. Many patients are hypertensive and a period of bed-rest and adequate sedation is helpful. Patients with hereditary telangiectasis may require skin grafting of the septum.

The most usual cause in children is bleeding from Little's area. In this instance the blood vessels are easily identified if the nose is packed for a short time with cocaine and adrenalin. Once the vessels are identified

they can be easily cauterized either with electrocautery, silver nitrate or trichloracetic acid.

Bleeding that comes from areas other than Little's area often requires admission to hospital. The first thing to do is to replace the blood volume, put the patient to bed and adequately sedate him. The nose is packed with $\frac{1}{2}$-inch ribbon gauze impregnated with an antiseptic such as BIPP or an antibiotic such as terracortril. It is left in place for 48 hours and then removed. If the epistaxis recurs then the nose is packed again. If there is a further recurrence then either the anterior ethmoidal artery or the maxillary artery is ligated. The access to the maxillary artery is through the maxillary sinus.

A. G. D. Maran

Exophthalmos (or proptosis)

This may be bilateral or unilateral.

Bilateral exophthalmos

The commonest cause of this condition is *Graves' disease*, or primary hyperthyroidism in which the exophthalmos is associated with thyroid gland swelling, with other general symptoms such as tachycardia, fine tremors and general nervousness. The degree of prominence of the eyes is variable, in some cases being so great that there is inadequate lid coverage of the cornea on attempted eye closure. A protrusion causes the upper lid to be unusually raised and the eyes look wide open, giving the patient an expression of alarm or astonishment (Stellwag's sign). When the eyes are lowered, the upper lids lag behind the downward excursion of the eye, leaving a broad portion of the sclera visible above the cornea (von Graefe's sign). The extent of exophthalmos may be asymmetrical with minimal involvement of the fellow eye. The condition sometimes appears to be unilateral. Increasing oedema of the lids along with inflammation of the conjunctiva and dilatation of the vessels over the insertion, particularly of the lateral rectus, are significant findings. The myopathy of Graves' disease most frequently involves the vertically acting muscles with limitation of upward eye movement. Other uncommon causes of bilateral exophthalmos are septic thrombosis of the cavernous sinus, historically associated with skin infection at the inner angle of the eye, or ethmoidal sinus suppuration, bilateral lymphomatous deposits or pseudotumour and in children the craniodysostoses or other rare causes.

Unilateral exophthalmos

Unilateral exophthalmos may be due to:

Orbital cellulitis
Orbital haematoma
Cavernous sinus thrombosis
Pseudotumour
Lymphoma
Cavernous haemangioma
Lacrimal gland tumour
Peripheral nerve tumour
Meningioma
Mucocele
Metastatic and secondary tumours
Carotico-cavernous arterio venous fistula

Orbital cellulitis can begin as a primary inflammatory process in front of the orbital septum, thereafter extending backwards or rising from direct orbital extension of paranasal sinus infection. The dire complication of further progression is septic cavernous sinus thrombosis. The general signs and symptoms of cavernous sinus thrombosis are more grave than in uncomplicated orbital cellulitis. Headache, nausea, vomiting and altered consciousness are early signs. Venous congestion produces gross chemosis and proptosis with a bluish discoloration of the eyelids. There is early onset of pan-ocular motor paresis. Bilateral involvement is virtually diagnostic of cavernous sinus thrombosis. Pseudotumour involvement of the orbit usually first appears above, but may also be found in the inferior retrobulbar tissues. Another involvement is at the apex of the orbit, visual loss may be of early onset. A pseudotumour along the superior orbital fissure causes a painful external ophthalmoplegia (Tolosa-Hunt syndrome).

Capillary haemangioma is the commonest cause of unilateral proptosis in childhood, the adult cavernous haemangioma causes a slowly progressive exophthalmos.

Orbital lymphomas usually occur in the anterior orbit involving the conjunctiva and lids. However posterior orbital involvement may occur and it is important to exclude a primary systemic lymphoma. Lacrimal gland tumours occur characteristically at the upper lateral portion of the orbit, causing painless downward and medial displacement of the globe and irregular enlargement of the lacrimal fossa.

Dermoid cysts specifically appear in childhood at the upper lateral quadrant of the orbit. Superior and medial swellings are more suggestive of mucocoeles of the frontal or ethmoidal sinus. Teratomas may occur congenitally or in very early life. Rhabdomyosarcoma is the commonest intraorbital malignant tumour of childhood presenting within the first decade. Development of proptosis is rapid, occurring within 1–3 weeks. The rapidity of progression is more or less pathognomonic of this tumour.

Optic nerve gliomas usually manifest before the age of 5, resulting in a downwards nasal and forward proptosis. Meningiomas usually occur in older women, but can occur in childhood and their course is much more rapid.

Ultrasound scan, CT, MRI and biopsy are all useful in assessing cases of exophthalmos.

Orbital haemorrhage may arise from trauma or sudden extreme physical effort causing bleeding from orbital varices leading to alarming, progressive orbital swelling. Arteriovenous fistula can occur following fracture of the base of the skull, with rupture of the internal carotid artery as it passes through the cavernous sinus. The carotico cavernous fistula causes a pulsatile proptosis of the eyeball associated with a bruit which is synchronous with the pulse. Gross dilatation of the conjunctival vessels is visible with arterialization of the conjunctival veins. Compression of the ipsilateral internal carotid diminishes the pulsation and audible bruit. Intermittent unilateral exophthalmos in children following coughing or crying is nearly always associated with a deep cavernous haemangioma.

S. T. D. Roxburgh

Eye, blindness of

The World Health Organization defines blindness as a central visual acuity of less than 3/60 (1/20) or a visual field of less than 10 degrees. An alternative functional definition is loss of vision sufficient to prevent one from being self-supporting in an occupation, making the individual dependent on other persons, agencies and devices in order to live.

Colour blindness is a genetically determined disorder which is a minor handicap and is not true blindness.

The causes and prevalence of blindness through the world vary from country to country. It is estimated that 75 per cent of blindness in the world is avoidable.

The leading causes of blindness world wide are trachoma, leprosy, onchocerciasis, xerophthalmia and cataract. In western countries age-related macular degeneration, diabetic retinopathy and glaucoma are the most common problems.

Different categories of the blind have different needs and the agencies for the blind access the individual blind person's requirements and provide a variety of services, including mobility training, visual magnifying aids, talking books, training of Braille, educational assessment, job rehabilitation and psychological counselling.

S. T. D. Roxburgh

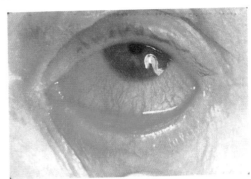

Fig. E.5. Acute conjunctivitis.

Eye, inflammation of (red eye)

Inflammation of the eye may involve the conjunctiva (as a *conjunctivitis*), the cornea (*keratitis* — usually in the form of a *corneal ulcer*), and less commonly the uvea (*uveitis*) and sclera (*scleritis*). Localized patches of *episcleritis* may superficially resemble conjunctivitis, and the dusky circumcorneal congestion in an *acute glaucoma* may stimulate that from an acute anterior uveitis. The character of the inflammation varies with the type of the disease, but certain symptoms, such as *pain, photophobia* and *lacrimation*, are common to all inflammatory conditions, and are by themselves of little value in the differential diagnosis.

Conjunctivitis

In conjunctivitis the conjunctival vessels are dilated; they are freely movable over the subjacent sclera, and the conjunctival injection is most evident at a little distance from the corneal margin; the circumcorneal portion of the conjunctiva, owing to its firmer attachment to the sclera in this region, being relatively less injected. If the condition is purely conjunctival the cornea is clear and bright, the anterior chamber and iris are normal in appearance, the pupil is black with normal reactions. Purulent discharge may occur and there is often a feeling of grittiness as of sand or dust in the eye. Hyperaemia of the conjunctiva may be

secondary to a foreign body on the cornea or on the conjunctiva itself, particularly underneath the upper lid.

Inturning of the eyelid (entropion) allows the eyelashes to rub against the cornea and conjunctiva (trichiasis) producing conjunctival hyperaemia and predisposing to conjunctivitis.

The use of topical drugs may produce an allergic conjunctivitis which is often associated with signs of allergy of the skin of the lids. Strong ultraviolet irradiation damages the conjunctival corneal epithelium, when using a sun-lamp or arc-welder without eye protection, producing conjunctival hyperaemia with considerable irritation or pain.

Conjunctivitis may be associated with a *mucopurulent* ocular discharge (*Fig.* E.5). The lids may be stuck together after sleep, the pain is generally slight, and allayed by closing the eyes. Mucopurulent conjunctivitis is characterized by more profuse discharge and is frequently due to infection by the staphylococcus or streptococcus and haemophilus species.

Some particular forms of conjunctivitis deserve special mention. In *ophthalmia neonatorum* (acute conjunctivitis of the newborn), caused by infection from the birth canal (chlamydia, staphylococcus or gonococcus), there is often profuse mucopurulent discharge; the condition is differentiated from imperfect canalization of the nasolacrimal ducts by the fact that in the latter the discharge is present without the accompanying inflammation. Untreated cases are at grave risk of secondary corneal ulceration and require identification and early antibiotic therapy.

In *trachoma* (*Fig.* E.6), a chlamydial infection, endemic in the Middle East, but rare in the UK, the conjunctiva is studded with enlarged follicles, particularly on the under-surface of the upper lid and in the upper conjunctival fornix causing partial ptosis, with excess lacrimation, and, in the later stages, vascular infiltrate (pannus) of the upper part of the cornea. In the later stages of trachoma the infiltration is followed

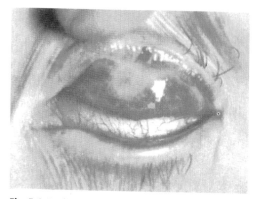

Fig. E.6. Trachomatous scarring of everted upper lid. (*Institute of Ophthalmology.*)

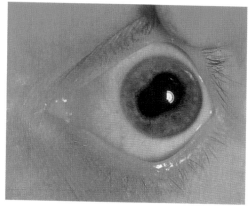

Fig. E.7. Iridocyclitis synechiae. (*Institute of Ophthalmology.*)

by scarring which may buckle the tarsal plate, leading to cicatricial entropion and trichiasis.

Conjunctival *allergies* are characterized particularly by oedema of the conjunctiva (conjunctival chemosis) and of the skin of the lids, epiphora and itch. They include non-specific responses to a wide miscellany of drugs, cosmetics and other irritants, and three specific clinical forms are recognized: (1) *Hayfever*, from exogenous pollens, etc.; (2) *Phlyctenular conjunctivitis* (due to an allergic reaction, e.g. to staphylococcus), featuring marked photophobia and one or more round yellowish raised masses at the corneoscleral junction surrounded by a localized area of vascular conjunctiva. In some cases the phlycten encroach on the corneal surface, being followed by a trail or leash of conjunctival vessels; (3) *Spring catarrh*, exists in a palpebral and a bulbar form, the former showing polygonal flat-topped conjunctival nodules resembling cobblestones, the latter showing focal gelatinous limbal thickening.

Keratitis

Corneal ulcers produce greyish or white opacities of the corneal stroma with loss of the corneal epithelium. In more serious untreated cases infiltrations of the cornea may lead to loss of corneal tissue and progress to perforation of the cornea. In severe cases there may be pus in the anterior chamber—hypopyon. The diagnosis presents no difficulty; the ulcers are obvious if the cornea is examined carefully, and stained with fluorescein.

Iritis

In iritis or 'anterior uveitis' the eye is congested and painful (in contrast to a 'posterior uveitis', or choroiditis, which simply blurs the vision). This vasodila-

tion differs from that in a conjunctivitis in that it is most evident in the circumcorneal region, with the tarsal conjunctiva remaining unaffected and that the colour of the injection is brick-red rather than pink. The cornea retains its clarity, but the aqueous may be turbid due to the presence of cells and protein, and there may be punctate deposits of leucocytes on the posterior surface of the cornea (*keratic precipitates*), or rarely a hypopyon or pus level within the anterior chamber. Owing to the increased vascularity of the iris, and to the exudation into iris substance, its volume is increased and its mobility impaired; hence the pupil becomes small and sluggish. The presence of blood and exudate in the substance of the iris also changes its colour—a blue iris becomes greenish, and the fine detail of the iris structure is blurred and obliterated. Adhesions are apt to occur between the iris and the lens at the point of their immediate contact, the edge of the pupil; in the constricted state of the pupil these may not be seen, but on dilatation with cyclopentolate or atropine these adhesions or *posterior synechiae* prevent the enlargement of the pupil at certain points, and it therefore becomes irregular in shape (*Fig.* E.7). Small masses of iris pigment may also be seen on the anterior surface of the lens where the mydriatic may have broken down some of the weaker adhesions. An exudate into the pupillary aperture may form a fibrinous membrane completely or partially blocking the pupil.

An important form of iritis (or, more properly, of 'uveitis', since the ciliary body and choroid are also involved), may occur in the second eye following a perforating injury in the first—'sympathetic ophthalmitis'. This possibility must always be borne in mind in cases of previous perforation of the globe, as it relentlessly leads to blindness unless suppressed by steroid treatment at an early stage.

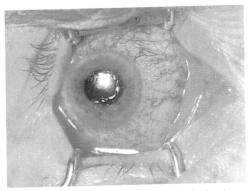

Fig. E.8. Acute glaucoma. (*Institute of Ophthalmology.*)

Glaucoma

Acute angle closure glaucoma is a disease of the later years of life, and of hypermetropes rather than myopes. It is precipitated by any of the factors that may provoke dilatation of the pupil.

At first the chief complaint in subacute attacks is of temporary obscuring of vision and the appearance of haloes or rainbows around light sources; there is often a feeling of tension in the eye and a dull frontal headache in addition to the loss of vision. In acute attacks the pain is severe radiating from the eye to the head, the ears and teeth, and is associated with nausea, a symptom that *may* lead to the mistaken diagnosis of migraine. The lids may be oedematous and the conjunctiva injected (*Fig.* E.8). The cornea is hazy due to oedema, the anterior chamber shallow, the iris discolored, and the pupil mid-dilated and fixed. The eye is hard to the touch and very tender. Vision fails rapidly, even down to bare perception of light, within a few hours.

The distinction between subacute or acute glaucoma, as just described, and chronic simple glaucoma is easily made. Chronic simple glaucoma is an asymptomatic disease, and is usually discovered in the course of routine examination. No pain, blurring of vision, haloes or feeling of tension are complained of; and the visual field loss which characterizes this disease is rarely noticed by the patient in the early stages.

The importance of discriminating between iritis and acute angle closure glaucoma cannot be overemphasized; the use of atropine or some similar mydriatic is a basic treatment of iritis, while in acute glaucoma it is disastrous (*Table* E.3).

Acute inflammation of the eye may be seen in *episcleritis* and *scleritis* (*Fig.* E.9). Episcleritis may be simple or nodular producing localized injection of the episcleral vessels. In either type the condition is normally idiopathic and asymptomatic with the patient merely complaining of redness of the eye. Scleritis is a more serious condition, often associated with the connective-tissue disorders. In contrast to episcleritis, the eye is painful and tender with a deep-seated bluish injection. Recurrent episodes of inflammation of the

---

Table E.3. A summary of the points of distinction between conjunctivitis, iritis and acute glaucoma and keratitis

	Conjunctivitis	Iritis	Acute glaucoma	Keratitis
Conjunctiva	Conjunctival vessels bright red and injected; movable over subjacent sclera; injection most marked away from corneoscleral margin; colour fades on pressure	Ciliary vessels injected, deep-red; most marked at corneoscleral margin; colour does not fade on pressure	Both conjunctival and ciliary vessels injected but dusky in colour	Conjunctival vessels red and injected. Injection most marked near the corneoscleral margin
Cornea	Clear, sensitive	Clear, sensitive	Steamy, hazy, insensitive	Irregular reflex, corneal opacity
Anterior chamber	Clear; normal depth	Aqueous may be turbid	Very shallow	Normal, hypopyon
Iris	Normal	Swollen, adherent to lens and muddy-coloured	Injected	Normal
Pupil	Black, active (normal)	Small and fixed, later festooned after adhesions form to lens	Mid-dilated, fixed, oval	Black active (normal)
Intraocular tension	Normal	Normal	Raised	Normal

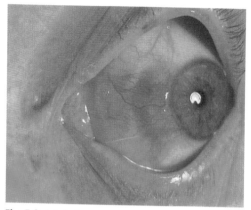

Fig. E.9. Episcleritis.

sclera may produce progressive scleral thinning. Early treatment with systemic anti-inflammatory drugs or corticosteroids is mandatory.

S. T. D. Roxburgh

Eye, pain in

Pain in the eye is not by itself pathognomonic of any particular lesion; but it may occur in a variety of circumstances, grouped as follows:

1. Pain associated with visible inflammatory changes

Due to:

Foreign body
Entropion or ingrowing lashes
Conjunctivitis
Keratitis
Iritis
Acute glaucoma

The differential diagnosis between these is discussed in the section on EYE, INFLAMMATION OF

2. Pain without visible changes in the eyeball, with loss of sight

Loss of vision in retrobulbar neuritis is usually unilateral and progresses during the first week sometimes to perception of light only.

The pain is generally referred to the back (retrobulbar) rather than to the front of the eye, and is exacerbated by ocular movement. The diagnosis is suggested if considerable loss of sight occurs in an eye, which, on examination, proves not to be affected by intraocular haemorrhage, detachment of the retina or any other visible lesion. After days or weeks, the pain may disappear and sight return to normal. On the other hand, in more severe cases, the inflammation in the optic nerve may extend forward to the back of the eyeball and become visible as a papillitis. The cause of the optic neuritis may be difficult to determine. Most commonly it is due to multiple sclerosis; often it remains obscure; sometimes it is traced successfully to some acute viral illness such as influenza.

3. Pain without inflammation and without impaired sight

An indefinite discomfort, sometimes (erroneously) labelled 'eyestrain', with a feeling of fatigue and congestion in the eyes, usually occurs in the evenings after prolonged close work which may be enhanced by difficulty in focusing (inadequate presbyopic correction), or an unclear image from incorrect glasses. If the refractive error is largely to blame, this is usually because of over-correction, as absence of glasses rarely causes eyestrain. Much more commonly the primary troubles are inadequate (or excessive) illumination, infrequent blinking, and especially a mild chronic blepharitis. The sensitivity of patients to such errors of refraction is variable, and is largely conditioned by the neurotic tendencies of the individual, for the errors to which eyestrain is attributed are usually of very small degree. It should be emphasized that myopia does not cause eyestrain, but simply a blurring of distance vision, that presbyopes normally complain of having to hold the book too far away, and that before the general availability of astigmatic lenses, a few decades ago, eyestrain was rarely mentioned—even among close workers, in poor illumination. A further occasional cause of eyestrain is an error of muscle balance, notably convergence insufficiency, which commonly responds to orthoptic exercises.

4. Pain in the eyes due to febrile or other constitutional causes

The most familiar example in this category is *influenza*. The pain is generally referred to the backs of the eyeballs rather than to the eyes themselves, but the complaint is one of pain in the eyes. The trouble occurs both at an early stage of the disease and as a sequel when the fever has subsided. The diagnosis is made from the course of the pyrexia and the general symptoms. There may be coryza as well as pain, for instance in the early stages of measles. In other conditions, such as meningitis, there is photophobia rather than pain in the eyes.

5. Pain in the eyes due to inflammation in ethmoid, sphenoid or frontal air sinuses

Sinusitis is probably the commonest cause of pain referred to the eye. It may be influenced by posture, and is commonest on waking (after prolonged recumbency).

W. M. Haining

Eyelids, disorders of

Apart from those conditions considered under EYE, INFLAMMATION OF, there are various others of which the patient may complain that deserve mention.

Blepharitis, or inflammation of the lid margin, is normally a sequel to seborrhoea with an allergic aggravation; and, if secondary infected with staphylococci, may become ulcerative. The margins are red, scales or crusts are found between the lashes, which are often small, distorted or destroyed. Entropion or trichiasis (ingrowing of the eyelashes) may result. The symptoms can normally be allayed by steroid/antibiotic applications.

External stye is a suppurative inflammation of an eyelash follicle. The condition is common and easily recognized; it is nearly always secondary to blepharitis, and is provoked by impairment of the general health.

A *Meibomian cyst or internal stye* is a similar infection of a Meibomian gland (in the posterior half of the eyelid margin). It may clear spontaneously, or the inflammatory signs and symptoms may recede, leaving a pea-sized swelling (which may also develop without antecedent inflammatory signs) called a 'chalazion'.

Entropion, or rolling inwards of the lid margin, may be *spastic* or *cicatricial*. *Trichiasis*, or rubbing of the lashes on the eye, with consequent discomfort and inflammation, is a frequent result. The opposite condition of *ectropion* may also be *spastic* or *cicatricial*, but it also occurs as a *senile* and *paralytic* phenomenon.

Symblepharon, or adhesion of the conjunctival surface of the lids to the globe, usually results from caustic burns. *Ankyloblepharon* is the term applied to adhesion of the two lids to each other, and may be due to similar causes, or may be congenital.

Xanthelasma is a slightly raised plaque, yellowish in colour, found in the skin at the inner end of either lid, often symmetrical and multiple. It may occur spontaneously or in association with hypercholesterolaemia. It should be removed if sufficiently disfiguring. A small clear cyst situated among the lashes is due to retention of secretion in a *gland of Moll*. Removal of the anterior wall results in its disappearance.

Molluscum contagiosum often occurs on the lids. The nodules are small, white, umbilicated and characterized by the ease with which contact with another portion of skin (not infrequently during removal) may allow the virus to provoke the appearance of further nodules.

Naevi or *moles* may occur on the lid, especially the margin, and involve the conjunctiva as well. They are usually pigmented. *Haemangiomata* may be similarly sited, as may *papillomata*. The commonest malignant tumour of the lid is a *basal cell carcinoma* or *rodent ulcer*. Congenital lesions of the lid already mentioned include ptosis, symblepharon, ankyloblepharon, ectropion, entropion and trichiasis. *Coloboma* occurs as a notch in the lid margin, usually towards the nasal end in the upper lid. A double row of lashes (*distichiasis*) may be found as a congenital malformation, possibly causing trichiasis. A frequent site for a *dermoid cyst* is near the outer canthus; there is often a corresponding bony defect, and the condition needs careful distinction from *meningocele* before exploration. *Epicanthus* is a disfiguring semilunar fold of skin across the inner canthus, usually disappearing as the nose develops. Though not primarily diseases of the lids, inflammatory conditions of the lacrimal gland or sac cause swelling and oedema in this region. *Dacryo-adenitis* is rare; it causes a painful swelling in the outer end of the upper lid; a similarly situated, though painless, swelling is caused by tumours of the lacrimal gland, histologically resembling the mixed parotid tumours. In *Mikulicz's disease* there is enlargement of both lacrimal and salivary glands, probably lymphomatous in nature. *Acute dacryocystitis* causes a painful red swelling at the inner end of the lower lid; it should be treated as an abscess, and no attempt made to relieve the underlying condition surgically (dacryocystrhinostomy) until the inflammation has subsided. The abscess may rupture through the skin, or require incision. It is frequently preceded by chronic dacryocystitis and epiphora.

A disturbing symptom sometimes complained of, especially by elderly people, is 'flickering' of the lid — a periodic clonic spasm of the orbicularis muscle. It may respond to general sedatives, though obstinate cases may call for blockage of the peripheral branches of the facial nerve by injecting botulinum toxin.

It is important to note that swelling and oedema of the lids, and oedema of the conjunctiva (*chemosis*) may be so intense as to suggest a far more serious state of affairs than the local inflammatory lesion which is its usual cause. Chemosis may occur from acute conjunctivitis, ocular inflammations or orbital cellulitis, obstruction to the lymph-flow from an orbital tumour may be the cause; or general disorders, such as anaemia or angioneurotic oedema.

W. M. Haining

Face, abnormalities of appearance and movement

The patient's features, expression and facial movements can in many cases suggest an instant diagnosis. While such 'spot' diagnoses may often be wildly inaccurate, in many cases they prove more telling than many investigative procedures done later to prove or disprove a diagnosis. Experience alone can teach the student to detect all that is to be learned from the patient's facies. The more subtle abnormalities of expression, the play of the emotions and the response of the features to questioning and intellectual and emotional challenge are transient and fleeting and cannot be recorded or reproduced and are sometimes so intangible as to defy any attempt to describe them. The passive vacant aspect of a chronic alcoholic, the tremor of his mouth when he opens it to protest his temperance, are clinical observations which cannot be reproduced visually, except by a television camera. The shifty eyes of the drug addict, the fatuous placidity of the patient with advanced multiple sclerosis, the anxious look of those within a few days of death, the explosive suddenness with which the victim of multiple sclerosis or brain damage bursts into laughter or tears, the vacant stare of the mentally defective child, the unsmiling sad appearance of the melancholic, the distant removed look of the schizoid personality, the excessive vivaciousness of the hypomanic—these are a few of the many familiar and striking lessons of the face which must be seen in real life if they are to be learned and utilized. It is upon the appearance of the face that people most rely for the judgement of general health and well-being, for this is the only part of the body which everybody is habitually accustomed to see—plumpness or wasting, the complexion, the expression, the carriage of the head, the way the eyes, brows, cheeks and mouth move, for example, may all suggest certain disorders. Appearances may be deceptive however (*Fig.* F.1). Pallor is by no means the same thing as anaemia; a ruddy complexion is not necessarily a sign of rude health; it is often far from easy to distinguish the appearance of illness from the expression of unhappiness; it is all too easy to mistake for aggression what is really shyness.

CRETINOID FACIES

Compared with the general stunted growth of the rest of the body the head of the child hypothyroid from birth is relatively large. The expression is dull or

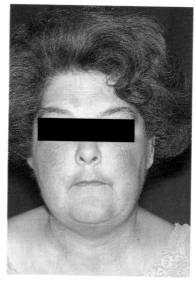

Fig. F.1. Red moon face in an anaemic woman on large doses of corticosteroids. Note the increased hair growth on the upper lip.

stolid. The face is broad, and remarkable for thick eyelids, broad flat nose, thick lips and widely spaced eyes (*Fig.* F.2). The mouth is usually open, the tongue may be more or less constantly protruded, and the chin is poorly developed. The hair is scanty and

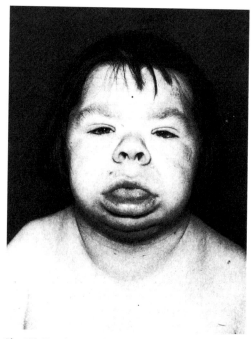

Fig. F.2. Female cretin, showing half closed eyes, thick nose, tongue and lips, fat chin and squat neck. (*Dr R.G. Ollerenshaw, Manchester Royal Infirmary.*)

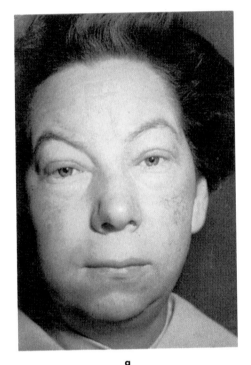

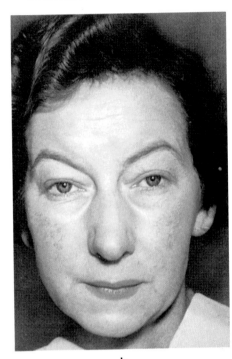

a   b

Fig. F.3. Facies in myxoedema (a) before and (b) after thyroxine treatment. (*Dr P. M. F. Bishop.*)

brittle, the skin coarse, dry or muddy, and often almost yellow.

MYXOEDEMATOUS FACIES

The dulled intelligence of the patient is betrayed by the apathetic physiognomy (*Fig.* F.3). The skin of the myxoedematous face of hypothyroidism is coarse, dry, sallow, pale and waxy, with occasionally a tinted rose-purple flush over each cheek. The puffiness of the eyelids may suggest acute glomerulonephritis, but the subcutaneous tissue everywhere is of firm consistence, and doughy rather than oedematous. The tongue is enlarged. The nose is broadened, the ears are thickened and the lips swollen. The hair is scanty, receding from the forehead, the eyebrows are thin and sparse (although the scantiness of the outer half often regarded as a diagnostic feature occurs too frequently in normal subjects for this to be reliable), the nails brittle and striated. Masses of fatty tissue may be found in the neck and trunk. The slow, husky speech, the expressionless face, and the general attitude of the patient may superficially suggest Parkinsonism, but the diagnosis may be made by paying attention to other clinical features. In hypopituitarism, the eyelids and nose, in contrast to myxoedema, are unaffected, and show no undue thickening. Another point of differ-

entiation is that in pituitary disease complete loss of axillary and pubic hair is common, a feature that does not always occur in myxoedema. In hypopituitarism the face is hairless in males or females (*Fig.* F.4) and

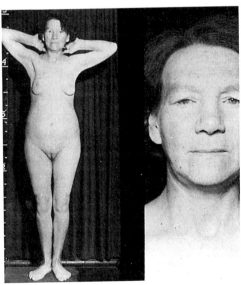

Fig. F.4. Sheehan's syndrome (hypopituitarism following haemorrhage at childbirth) here gives a very different picture from that of primary hypothyroidism (myxoedema).

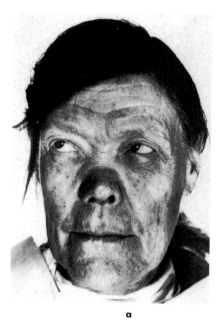
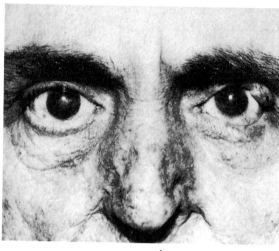

a   b

Fig. F.5. *a*, Congenital syphilis, showing depressed nasal bridge and rhagades. (*Dr J.C. Houston.*) *b*, Interstitial keratitis and nasal scarring in congenital syphilis. (*Mr Rex Lawrie.*)

unduly wrinkled. The features are those of a middle-aged Peter (or Pauline) Pan. In contrast the patient with myxoedema looks like a wax doll who has been left in a sunlit shop window too long. In hypopituitarism the skin is soft and smooth and the hair of soft texture, whilst in myxoedema hairs and skin are of coarser quality. The voice in myxoedema is a husky croak, in hypopituitarism normal.

CONGENITAL SYPHILITIC FACIES

The victims of congenital syphilis, now an extreme rarity, after 10 or 12 years of age, may present a facies which is unmistakable—an overhanging forehead, perhaps frontal bosses, a depressed nasal bridge (*Fig. F.5*), striated scars radiating from the corners and other parts of the lips, with a sallow, earthy complexion. Closer observation of the eyes and teeth may detect the opacities of old keratitis and the changes in the upper incisors which were stated by Jonathan Hutchinson to be pathognomonic (*Fig. F.6*). These teeth are wide-gapped, irregular, and so deficient in enamel over the anterior and median parts of their cutting edges that the resulting crescentic notch imparts a striking appearance.

MYOPATHIC FACIES

Many cases of myopathy show no characteristic facies; in *facioscapulohumeral dystrophy* the face is always

involved, the muscles around the mouth being affected most with a loose pout of the lips at rest and 'transverse' smile (*rire en travers*). These features are due to defective facial musculature, particularly to weakness of the orbicularis oris. Paresis of the orbiculares palpebrarum is only evident when an attempt is made to close the eyes, although it may sometimes lead to prominent and perhaps staring eyeballs. Inability of the patient to whistle or to blow out his cheek demonstrates the weakness of the orbicularis oris which is often rendered obvious by the large amount of labial mucous membrane exposed while the mouth is at rest.

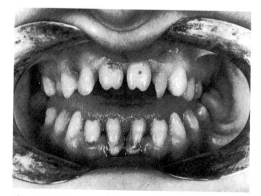

Fig. F.6. Hutchinson's teeth in congenital syphilis. Note the upper central incisors which are peg-shaped and notched. (*Professor W.E. Herbert.*)

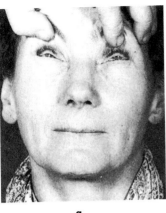
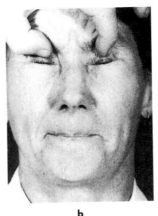
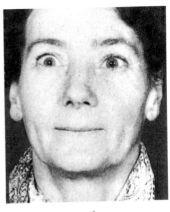

a   b   c

Fig. F.7. Myasthenia gravis showing: *a,* Inability to keep eyes closed against light traction on upper eyelid; *b,* Effective resistance after neostigmine—note the return of power to the orbicularis oris; *c,* Normal facies under the influence of neostigmine. (*Dr R.G. Ollerenshaw, Manchester Royal Infirmary.*)

In *dystrophia myotonica (myotonia atrophica, Steinert's disease)*, ptosis, facial weakness and dysarthria occur. There is a characteristic weakness and diminution in the size of the sternomastoids and the masticatory muscles are poorly developed or waste early, giving a long lean facial appearance. In males, frontal baldness is common. In the rare *ocular myopathy* there is progressive ptosis of the eyelids and immobility of the eyes.

MYASTHENIC FACIES

In patients suffering from myasthenia gravis there are two types of facies. The first is the patient whose lids lag with fatigue (*Fig.* F.7). The second depends on the characteristic myasthenic smile, almost a sneer. This unfortunate and misleading facial expression is the result of deficient action on the part of the zygomatic and risorius muscles and exemplifies the curious way in which in this disease some muscles are affected and others escape, even when they derive their innervation from the same source. In patients with this disorder facial weakness is worsened by repeated movement but responds rapidly but transiently to anticholinesterase drugs such as intravenous edrophonium which acts more rapidly than neostigmine. In ocular myasthenia only the extra-ocular muscles are involved.

HYPERTHYROIDISM

The *facies of hyperthyroidism* depends chiefly upon the 'stare' (*see Fig.* T.7). Surprise or terror is suggested by the prominence of the eyeballs and the retraction of the eyelids. The degree of exophthalmos varies greatly and it may be completely absent; it is sometimes unilateral. The sclera is visible between the edge of the iris and the eyelids; the usual harmony of movement between the eyeball and the eyelid is lacking; normal blinking is much diminished or entirely in abeyance. The surface of the conjunctiva may be abnormally bright and glistening, and the secretion of tears may be excessive. In contrast with the white of the eyeballs, there is often considerable dark pigmentation of the eyelids which may also be the site of some oedema.

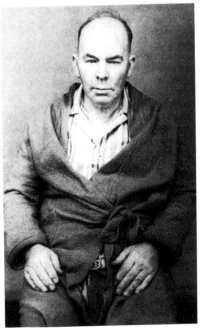

Fig. F.8. Paralysis agitans (Parkinson's disease) showing expressionless gaze and typical rigid immobility. (*Dr R.G. Ollerenshaw, Manchester Royal Infirmary.*)

The size of the pupils varies, undue dilatation occurring only in exceptional cases. The upper eyelid lags as the eye follows the examiner's finger downwards. Eye movements are often diminished in range due to intrinsic muscle weakness and the muscles of the brow are wasted, giving diminished wrinkling on raising the eyebrows (Joffroy's sign). A moist skin and a readiness to flush may often be remarked in the face.

THE FACIES OF PARKINSONISM

In this disease a cardinal symptom is muscular rigidity which affects the skeletal muscles generally as well as those of the face (*Fig. F.8*). The ocular muscles, however, escape and, as a consequence, while the face as a whole is expressionless or 'mask-like', the eyes appear to move with natural or even abnormal rapidity; for instance, they will turn in the direction to which the patient desires to look before the head has assumed a corresponding position. The face has often a staring expression, the eyelids being retracted by the tonic spasm of levator palpebrae. An absence of normal blinking has been ascribed to the same cause. In contrast with the slow development of facial expression, under the influence of emotion there may be marked want of control over the fully developed emotional movement, and the patient protests that the exuberance of his laughter or tears is entirely out of proportion to his feelings of merriment or sorrow. The poverty of facial and general movement may falsely suggest a lack of intelligence and mental activity.

Parkinsonism may occur in patients who are suffering or have suffered from an attack of *encephalitis*. This syndrome, which is now very rare, may often be distinguished from primary Parkinson's disease by the presence of disturbances in pupillary and other reflexes, tics, localized spasms and the so-called 'oculogyric crises' in which the eyes are suddenly deviated upwards, downwards or sideways so that only the white of the eye is visible to the observer. These crises, highly unpleasant for the patient, usually last for several minutes and occasionally for hours. The facies of Parkinsonism may also be caused by certain drugs, which interfere with the action of dopamine within the basal ganglia; these include chlorpromazine, phenothiazines, butyrophenones and reserpine in large doses. In most cases, the abnormalities disappear after stopping the drug except for tardive dyskinesia which may become permanent. This serious variety of drug-induced extrapyramidal disease consists of involuntary 'mouthing' movements of the lips, lip-smacking and protrusion of the tongue. Neuroleptic drugs with the least anticholinergic activity, such as haloperidol, produce the larger number of cases of drug-induced Parkinsonism. Thioridazine has potent anticholinergic activity and does not have this side-effect. Less common causes of Parkinsonism include carbon monoxide and manganese poisoning.

TABETIC FACIES

In a considerable number of the few remaining cases of tabes dorsalis the appearance of the face is sufficiently striking to afford a clue to diagnosis. The small size or the inequality of the pupils reacting to accommodation but not to light (Argyll Robertson pupils) may first attract attention. The drooping of the upper eyelids, combined with some wrinkling of the forehead produced by a compensating effort on the part of the frontalis muscle, imparts a sad expression. This drooping of the eyelid is not due to any paresis of the levator palpebrae superioris, as may be shown by the raising of the lid when the patient is looking upwards, but depends on the fact that this muscle, like most of the muscles of the body, is in a condition of hypotonia so that under the influence of gravity the lid hangs like a half-raised curtain in front of the eyeball. In other respects the face may be normal, but the majority of tabetics have a sallow complexion and very little subcutaneous fat, two conditions which contribute to their generally unhealthy appearance. Many victims of this disease exhibit a deficiency of the emotional reflex movements of the facial muscles; during conversation the play of the features appropriate to the subject of their talk is not so noticeable as in the case of healthy individuals.

FACIES OF ACROMEGALY (*Fig. F.9*)

In acromegaly changes in appearance frequently take place to such a degree that the patient becomes unrecognizable to friends, who have known him or her only before the onset of the disease. These are the result of abnormal growth of the bony and subcutaneous tissues especially in the skull and extremities. The characteristic facies is brought about by osseous hyperplasia of the frontal ridges, the mastoid, zygomatic, malar and nasal processes, while the lower jaw is usually enlarged in all directions. The prominent, arched brows, with retreating and wrinkled forehead, the massive nose, the long, thick upper lip and the heavy chin (*Fig. F.9*) form the most conspicuous features. The lower teeth are unduly wide apart and may project some distance in front of the upper. The tongue may be so enlarged as to keep the mouth open and to display many fissures and indentations as the result of its pressure against the teeth. In some cases the lower jaw is not affected, and the face may be described as abnormally square (*type carreé*).

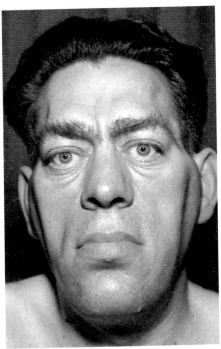

Fig. F.9. A case of acromegaly, exemplifying the heavy enlargement of the front of the lower jaw.

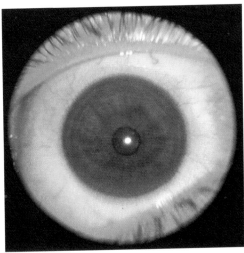

Fig. F.10. Kayser–Fleischer ring in a patient with Wilson's disease, due to deposition of copper-containing pigment in the cornea. (*Courtesy of Dr R. Guiloff.*)

DOWN'S SYNDROME

This facies is so distinctive that the diagnosis may usually be made at a glance. The head is brachyce-phalic; the palpebral fissures slant obliquely inwards and downwards towards a broad flat nose, rendered even broader by the presence of epicanthus; the eyelids show signs of chronic blepharitis; the ears are large and pitcher-shaped; the lips are fissured and often left open to allow a coarse tongue to protrude; the forehead is downy, and the hair of the scalp scanty, wiry and frequently mouse-col-oured; the complexion is florid and mottled. The almond-shaped eyes, the presence of epicanthus, the florid complexion and the absence of fatty masses serve to distinguish Down's syndrome from cretinism.

THE ADENOID FACIES

This used to be described in the child sufferer with wide open mouth resulting in the oral breathing demanded by nasal obstruction, and the overslung lower jaw and dental occlusion with consequent incomplete musculature of the mouth and receding cheeks.

FACIES OF HEPATOLENTICULAR DEGENERATION (WILSON'S DISEASE)

The characteristic facies of this disease is seen only in advanced cases, and may be described as one of 'fixed emotion'. The slightest attempt to engage in conversa-tion may evoke a sustained expression of exaggerated mirth, which is quite unlike that seen in other diseases of the nervous system. There is also a tendency to fall to one side when in the sitting position. The malady is associated with bilateral degenerative changes in the lenticular nuclei together with cirrhosis of the liver, due to the excessive amounts of copper in the tissues. The most remarkable feature of the disease is the Kayser–Fleischer ring, present in about 50 per cent of patients; this is a ring of rusty-brown pigment at the periphery of the cornea (*Fig.* F.10). Radiating brownish spokes of copper carbonate on the anterior or posterior lens capsule less often cause the character-istic 'sunflower' cataract.

FACIES OF MITRAL STENOSIS

It is occasionally possible to suspect mitral stenosis at sight, on account of the remarkable malar hyperaemia and dark-crimson lips contrasting with the yellowish pallor of the forehead, peri-oral and perinasal skin. If one covers the malar regions and the lips the face looks sallow, yet the malar flush and the dark-crimson lips give a look almost of plethora (*Fig.* F.11). When cardiac failure occurs and the liver becomes engorged, an element of icterus may be added.

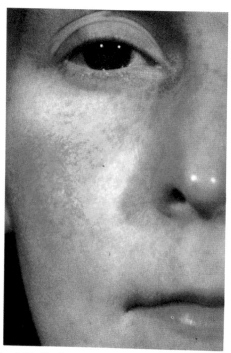

Fig. F.11. The facies in mitral stenosis, showing the malar flush. (Dr R.G. Ollerenshaw, Manchester Royal Infirmary.)

FACIES OF PRIMARY POLYCYTHAEMIA

The coloration of the nose, lips, ears and palpebral conjunctiva is the chief feature of the facies in this malady, presenting an appearance which may be described as a combination of exposure to weather, of plethora and of cyanosis. The diagnosis depends on discovering pronounced polycythaemia, and generally a large, firm spleen. Polycythaemia may also be secondary to other conditions, cardiac, pulmonary or malignant disease (*Fig.* F.12).

FACIES OF CIRRHOSIS OF THE LIVER

There is nothing characteristic in the facies when cirrhosis of the liver is in an early stage. Nor can one diagnose the existence of cirrhosis with certainty even when the facies is that of chronic alcoholism, with its telangiectases over the cheeks, coarsening of the tissues, especially on and around the nose and mouth, with purplish reddening in general. But in the later stages of cirrhosis the sallow, dull, diffusely pigmented facies is often distinctive, though the actual peculiarities are not easily described.

FACIES OF ADDISONIAN PERNICIOUS ANAEMIA

Though today rarely seen, the facies in untreated Addisonian pernicious anaemia may be absolutely characteristic in the later stages. There is no emaciation, but the colour is remarkable. Often described as 'lemon-yellow', it is more often a pale primrose yellow, with a peculiar delicacy in the yellowish tint that is unmistakable when it is fully developed.

FACIES OF ACUTE GLOMERULONEPHRITIS

The generally swollen half-bloated look, the partial closing up of the eyes by oedema, are usually unmistakable, but a somewhat similar appearance may be presented by the effects of insect bites, of angioneurotic oedema, or after the administration of aspirin or

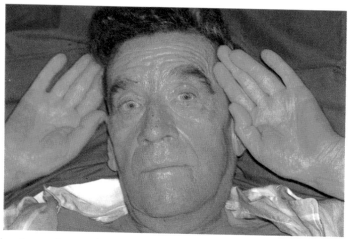

Fig. F.12. Polycythaemia secondary to malignant hepatoma.

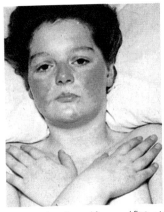 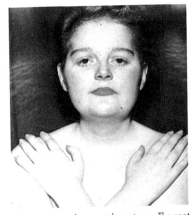

Fig. F.13. Female patient with prolonged fever and flitting joint pains due to systemic lupus erythematosus. The contrast is striking between the red butterfly rash of the disorder and the Cushingoid appearance on full steroid therapy 1 month later.

other drugs to which the patient is allergic. In the nephrotic syndrome, kwashiorkor and many other conditions with extensive oedema this may extend to involve the face but not usually in cardiac or starvation oedema which affects the dependent parts. In leprosy a similar puffy appearance of the face, particularly around the eyes, may be seen; a variety of skin lesions may occur with nodules, plaques and thickening of the skin. The ear lobes may enlarge and the lines of the face may coarsen and become deeper, giving the so-called 'leonine facies'. Patches of depigmentation may occur or bronzed hyperpigmentation. Eyebrows and eyelashes may fall out and lips swell. Nasal blockage may occur and a saddle-nose deformity develop.

FACIES OF ARTHRITIS AND CONNECTIVE TISSUE DISORDERS

In *dermatomyositis* the most characteristic rash consists of a dusky red eruption on the face, over nose and cheeks, periorbital regions, occasionally on the forehead and on the neck, shoulders, front and back of the chest and on the arms. The erythema may be mottled or diffuse and either intensely red or cyanotic or a mixture of both. Sometimes on the upper eyelids a dusky lilac hue is seen, the so-called heliotrope rash said to be typical of dermatomyositis. Telangiectasia may be present as it may in systemic lupus erythematosus and scleroderma.

A common skin lesion of *lupus erythematosus* has a 'butterfly' distribution over the bridge of the nose and the cheeks (*Fig.* F.13). The facial skin lesion of *sarcoidosis* may have the same distribution but the eyelids and ears may be infiltrated with brownish nodules.

In *scleroderma* the parchment-like skin may be so tightly drawn over the underlying muscles that the face becomes completely expressionless (*Fig.* F.14) and the mouth cannot open widely.

In *giant cell (temporal) arteritis*, the inflamed temporal arteries are tender to touch and become thrombosed. Vision may be affected if the retinal arteries become involved. Tophi in the ears (*Fig.* F.15) indicate the presence of *gout*.

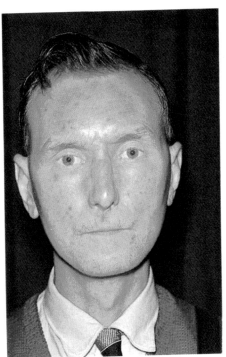

Fig. F.14. Scleroderma, showing the pigmented, mask-like smooth expressionless face.

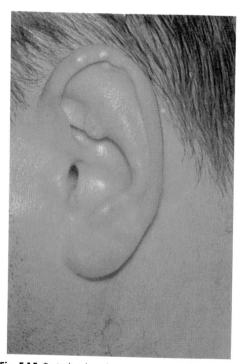

Fig. F.15. Typical tophi in the ear in a patient with gout. They are opaque to transillumination.

associated with a malignant process be differentiated from the disease without this association.

Other colorations of diagnostic significance are those of *haemochromatosis*, where over 90 per cent of patients show bronzing of the skin from melanin deposition, about half having haemosiderin deposition also causing a slate-grey colour. The bluish tinge of the cartilage of the ears and sclerae in *ochronosis* appears usually between the age of 20 and 30. The cartilages of the ears may be slate-blue or grey and are often thickened and irregular. Pigmentation of the sclera is usually localized to a small area half way between the cornea and the inner or outer canthus. The skin over the malar areas and nose is often darker than usual. Other abnormal colours which may be seen in the face include the patchy pigmentation of the chloasma of pregnancy or that of vitiligo or albinism, and that resulting from prolonged administration of arsenic.

FACIES OF ADDISON'S DISEASE

Generalized darkening of the skin of the face may be the first thing to attract attention in a case of Addison's disease, but the distinctive character of the pigmentation is that it occurs in the mucous membranes within the mouth (*Fig.* F.16), where it tends to be grey,

FACIES OF ACANTHOSIS NIGRICANS

The outstanding feature of this disease is the extreme pigmentation which develops in various parts of the body, as in the axillae, groin, nipples and umbilicus, but also in the neck or face; the degree may be described as what would, more or less, result if a collier's hands were stroked over the skin, producing massive darkening, almost blackening, in the areas affected. Although rarely generalized it is usually bilateral and symmetrical, blending into adjacent normal skin. Although the disease usually indicates abdominal carcinoma, especially carcinoma of the stomach, the patient may present himself for treatment on account of the pigmentation only, without any suggestion at the time that there is malignant disease anywhere. It is probably an extreme degree of the liability to diffuse pigmentation of the skin that malignant disease in general tends to produce. It may precede malignant disease or follow it but usually appears at the same time. It may also occur in Cushing's syndrome, acromegaly, the Stein–Leventhal syndrome, suprarenal insufficiency, pituitary or hypothalamic tumours or other lesions at the base of the brain. When associated with a malignant process these tend to be aggressive and rapidly fatal. Neither clinically nor histologically can acanthosis nigricans

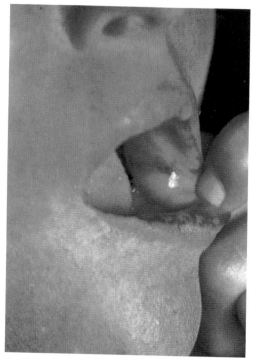

Fig. F.16. Buccal pigmentation in untreated Addison's disease. Under treatment with cortisone all pigmentation disappeared within a few weeks.

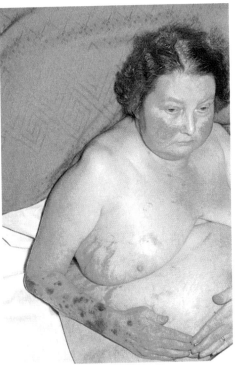

Fig. F.17. The Cushingoid picture of corticosteroid therapy. Note also the striae and subcutaneous haemorrhages.

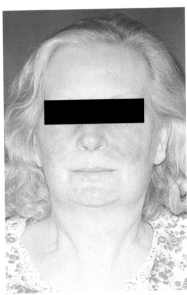

Fig. F.18. Cellulitis involving the cheeks in an elderly woman.

as well as on the skin of the face and other parts of the body, where it is dark brown.

FACIES IN CUSHING'S SYNDROME

The red 'moon face' and hirsutism (q.v.) are characteristic and often seen as the result of corticosteroid therapy (*Fig.* F.17). Although the features look plethoric there is no true polycythaemia. This is one point of differentiation from the features of simple obesity, others being the presence of bruising (ecchymoses), muscle weakness, wide purple red striae (those in simple obesity being more narrow and pink) and hypertension. In Cushing's syndrome the cheeks may become so chubby that seen full-face they obscure the ears.

FACIES OF ARGYRIA

This condition is rare nowadays. It may still be met with amongst workers in silver. The coloration is even and uniform; it has a blue-grey appearance which persists when pressure is applied to the skin, and does not blanch as does a cyanotic skin. It is a subcutaneous rather than a dermal pigmentation.

The features in *pachydermoperiostosis*, a rare familial condition associated with pseudohypertrophic osteoarthropathy (with finger clubbing), are typical with thickening and furrowing of the face, with deep nasolabial folds, greasy skin of face and scalp and often excessive sweating. It appears to be transmitted by an autosomal dominant gene with variable expression.

FACIES OF ACUTE ILLNESS

Erysipelas, measles, scarlatina and mumps often permit an immediate facial diagnosis. Cellulitis, also, is self-evident (*Fig.* F.18). In lobar pneumonia the bright eyes, flushed cheeks, active alae nasi and labial herpes constitute what may fairly be termed a typical picture. Respiratory distress advertises itself by expression of anxiety and fear in pulmonary and cardiac disease, although alterations in colour due to cyanosis contribute to the appearance. Labial herpes (herpes febrilis) may also accompany many other febrile diseases, even a simple coryza, and may be due to sun sensitivity. Herpes zoster may affect the face and the periorbital region (*Fig.* F.19) and, when the nasociliary nerve is involved, lesions appear on the end of the nose and on the cornea.

ALTERATIONS IN CONTOUR

Slight facial asymmetry is very common. Marked asymmetry occurs in patients with lipodystrophy, hemiatrophy or hemihypertrophy, or congenital

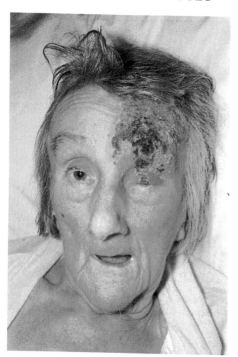 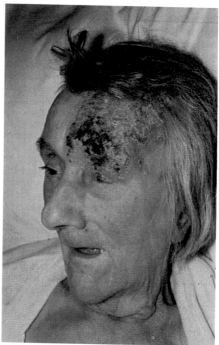

Fig. F.19. Severe herpes zoster affecting the brow and sclera. Not only may scarring interfere with vision subsequently, but at this age post-herpetic neuralgia is common, causing persistent pain in the area subsequently.

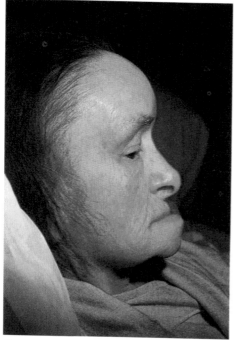 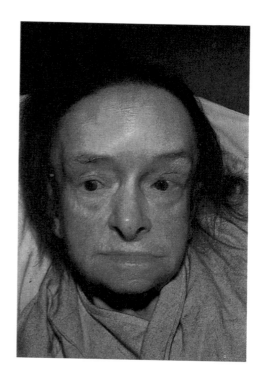

Fig. F.20. Typical Paget's disease.

absence of the condyle of the mandible. Lack of teeth or bad dentures may contribute to asymmetry as may swelling of the parotid or other salivary glands or of the lymph nodes. Some rarer conditions may be mentioned as generally identifiable at sight. In osteitis deformans (Paget's disease) the face has the shape of an inverted triangle and, in consequence of the prominence of the forehead, appears to be toppling forwards (*Fig.* F.20). In leontiasis ossea there is progressive irregular enlargement of the bones of the cranium and face, with consequent asymmetry; the superior maxilla is particularly prominent. The rare condition of oxycephaly ('steeple head') need to be seen only once to be subsequently recognizable.

THE EYES

The eyes alone often provide diagnostic evidence of general as well as local disease. Pigmentation, oedema of the lids and exophthalmos have been mentioned. A squint or ptosis may demand a detailed consideration of the central nervous system, as will spontaneous nystagmus. Icterus of the conjunctiva may be evidence of hepatic disease and the comparatively rare but striking appearance of blue sclerotics points to fragilitas ossium. 'Bags under the eyes' are generally devoid of any baleful significance but may possibly point to lack of sleep or overindulgence in alcohol.

VOLUNTARY MOVEMENTS

Weakness of the facial muscles is discussed in FACE, PARALYSIS OF.

Abnormal movement of the jaw may be due to any painful condition of the temporomandibular joint.

INVOLUNTARY MOVEMENTS

Besides the tremor of the head of old age and Parkinsonism, tremor may be due to alcohol, tobacco or other drugs. There is also a familial tremor of the hands, face and/or head affecting several members of the same family, usually commencing before the age of 25 years. The head-nodding of children may be mentioned in this connection. Other involuntary movements point to chorea, which may be hereditary (Huntington's), rheumatic or, rarely, senile, to habit spasms, or to tics. In aortic regurgitation there may be a constant jerking of the head synchronous with the heart beat (De Musset's sign). Facial paralysis and the peculiar condition of facial hemi-atrophy or hemi-hypertrophy are sometimes obvious, sometimes evident only on careful examination.

EXPRESSION

The patient's expression, at interview, may give an indication of his attitude not only to his illness but also to his physician and what he expects of him or her. Differentiation of the emotional from the physical factors may be very difficult. There may be an expression of melancholy or depression, of anxiety, nervous tension, or querulousness. In some cases depression hangs over the patient like a black cloud, the face being dull, without hope for the future, expressionless, and uninterested in what is going on around.

F. Dudley Hart

Face, paralysis of

Facial paralysis is seen in three clinical forms: (1) upper motor neurone paralysis, in which the lower half of the face is affected, and the upper half spared; (2) lower motor neurone paralysis, in which there is loss of movement in all the muscles on the affected side; (3) myopathy.

Upper motor neurone paralysis

This is due to a lesion of the corticopontine fibres of the pyramidal tract anywhere between the cortex and the middle of the pons. The eye can be closed and the forehead wrinkled, but the teeth cannot be bared on the affected side and there is weakness of the lips and buccinator muscles. In some cases involuntary emotional movements remain normal despite loss of purposive movements. In bilateral pyramidal lesions the upper part of the face is paralysed as well as the lower, and emotional movements are also involved. Rarely, emotional movements are lost and voluntary movements retained; this is occasionally seen in tumours or other lesions of the temporal lobe and premotor cortex.

Upper motor neurone facial paralysis occurs in many conditions—vascular accidents, neoplasms, cerebral contusion, degenerative cerebral disease and so on. It is usually associated with hemiparesis, or with weakness of the upper limb owing to the condensation of fibres which occurs in the pyramidal tract in the internal capsule and below, and in cortical and subcortical lesions it may occur independently.

Lower motor neurone paralysis

This occurs as a result of a lesion of the 7th nucleus or of the nerve itself. The upper and lower halves of the face are affected equally, and there is none of the dissociation of emotional and voluntary movements which may occur in upper motor neurone paralysis. If there is no recovery contractures may occur, the corners of the mouth being drawn to the affected side, thereby giving a false impression of weakness on the normal side. Fasciculation may be seen. Twitching movements are not uncommon in irritative lesions of the 7th nerve.

By far the most common form of peripheral facial palsy is *Bell's palsy*, which appears to be due to an inflammatory lesion in the facial canal of the temporal bone near the stylomastoid foramen. The onset is rapid, the patient often waking up in the morning to find the face paralysed on one side; in other cases the condition takes a day or two to reach its climax. There is often slight pain just below the mastoid process at the onset. The eye cannot be closed and is liable to injury by dust; slight ectropion of the lower lid leads to epiphora. Taste in the anterior two-thirds of the affected side of the tongue may be perverted or lost if the disease has spread up the bony facial canal. At a still higher level, paralysis of the nerve to the stapedius may cause hyperacusis.

Other causes of facial paralysis are less common than Bell's palsy. *Trauma* stands relatively high on the list, whether it be due to stab wounds, gunshot wounds, surgical attacks on the parotid gland and mastoid, or fracture of the petrous portion of the temporal bone. Paralysis usually occurs immediately in the fracture cases, but may appear for the first time a week or more after the injury, in which the event the prognosis for recovery is good.

Among infective causes are *poliomyelitis, infectious mononucleosis, polyneuritis cranialis, polyneuritis of Guillain Barré type, gummatous or other form of meningitis* and *leprosy*. The swelling of the parotid gland which occurs in *uveoparotid polyneuritis*, a form of sarcoidosis, is often associated with a bilateral facial paralysis. *Geniculate herpes*, in which herpes of the tonsil, soft palate, auditory meatus and pinna is associated with facial paralysis, is so named from the belief that it is due to a zoster infection of the geniculate ganglion as suggested by Ramsey Hunt.

Neurofibroma of the 8th cranial nerve stretches the adjacent facial nerve at an advanced stage of its growth and so adds facial palsy to the deafness, vertigo and tinnitus which occur early in the condition. As the tumour grows it encroaches upon the trigeminal nerve above, with loss of the corneal reflex and sensory loss in the face, and causes cerebellar symptoms by posterolateral pressure on the cerebellum. A glioma of the pons may have a somewhat similar symptomatology, but if the nucleus of the facial nerve is involved by the growth the adjacent 6th nucleus is likely to be affected too. Primary and secondary *tumours of the petrous bone* are a rare cause of facial paralysis.

Congenital bilateral facial paralysis is due to absence of the facial nerves. The upper part of the face is sometimes affected alone, or the entire face may be affected. The condition is always bilateral and is then easy to distinguish from facial palsy due to birth injury.

Diseases of muscle

Myopathy may cause facial weakness. This occurs in the heredofamilial dystrophies and myotonic dystrophy, but in these conditions the affection is not limited to the face, the weakness is bilateral, and confusion is unlikely to occur. *Myasthenia gravis*, with its ptosis, diplopia, characteristic aggravation by exercise and ready response to edrophonium chloride (Tensilon), is usually easy to recognize. *Facial hemiatrophy* may, superficially, resemble unilateral facial paralysis, but it is differentiated by the fact that the weakness is associated with an atrophy of all the tissues—skin, muscle, bone, nasal cartilage and even the eye.

Ian Mackenzie

Face, swelling of

In this article are included only swellings of the skin and subcutaneous tissues. Malignant and other diseases of the facial bones, etc., are considered under Jaw, Swelling of; Bone, Swelling of and Salivary Glands, Swelling of. It is necessary therefore to determine the anatomical site of the lesion before considering the pathology. Swelling of the parotid gland will lie below and in front of the ear, or in the anterior prolongation of the gland, lying on the outer surface of the masseter. Swelling of the lingual gland will be seen in the floor of the mouth close to the fraenum, while lateral to this will be felt the submandibular gland, which is also palpable bimanually from outside in the submandibular fossa.

Occasionally a patient may present himself with painless symmetrical *oedema of the face*, commonly of the eyelids where the tissues are loosest. This will almost certainly be of renal origin, cardiac oedema causing oedema primarily in the dependent parts. Another form of oedema which may involve the whole face, but chiefly the eyelids and lips, is angioneurotic oedema. The recurrent attacks, each of sudden onset, the familial history, the associated symptoms of burning and irritation and the presence of similar areas of other parts of the body should clinch the diagnosis.

Swelling of the face and neck is seen in Cushing's syndrome whether primary or secondary to corticosteroid therapy, and when there is obstruction to the venous return to the heart from the head and neck, as is seen with mediastinal and bronchial neoplasms. In trichiniasis oedema of the eyelids is common, though more diffuse oedema of the face may occur.

A well-defined *cystic swelling* on the face is most commonly a *sebaceous cyst*, a structure freely movable on the deeper tissues but attached to skin. *Dermoid cyst* is much rarer and occurs only at lines of suture, the commonest site being above the outer canthus of the eye (*external angular dermoid*). A cyst in this situation is strongly suggestive of dermoid origin, and the diagnosis is confirmed if there is attachment to bone but not to skin, and particularly if depression of the bone has occurred, as it does in long-standing cases, the edge of the depressed area being palpable. *Meningocele* may occur occasionally as a translucent swelling at the root of the nose. It will be present at birth and will exhibit an impulse on coughing or straining. *Haemangiomas* are frequently found on the face and may appear cystic on palpation, but their dusky colour and surrounding dilated vessels will give the clue to their identity; they empty on pressure. Pigmented naevi will be recognized on sight.

Solid tumours of the face are *lipomas* and *fibromas*. The latter are fairly common and include an important variety, the neurofibromas. These tumours vary in size from being quite minute to an inch or more in diameter, and may be hard or soft. Other stigmas of von Recklinghausen's disease such as pigmentation, either diffuse or in multiple café-au-lait spots, or a profusion of soft, fleshy neurofibromas in other parts of the body, chiefly the trunk, help in the diagnosis. The condition sometimes runs in families.

Rodent ulcer (basal-cell carcinoma) is particularly common on the face and eyelids; it is the exception to find it elsewhere. It starts as a small nodule, often with a 'pearly' appearance, but soon breaks down to form the characteristic indurated ulcer with hard rolled edges (*Fig. F.21*). *Epithelioma*, with its raised everted margin and indurated base, and possibly secondary enlargement of regional nodes, is another malignant condition found on the face, particularly the lips (*Fig. F.22*). Confusion may arise in distinguishing epithelioma from the innocent condition *molluscum sebaceum*. However, molluscum runs a short course and the centre sloughs leaving an unsightly scar. Biopsy must be done early in any suspicious lesion.

Various inflammatory swellings are found on the face, of which the following are some of the most important:

Boils and carbuncles are common, particularly around the lips. They have the same character as elsewhere, except that oedema is more marked.

Erysipelas is prone to occur on the face. It is marked by a vivid red oedematous swelling associated

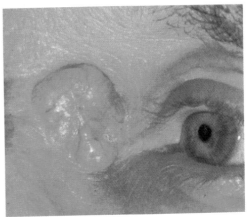

Fig. F.21. Rodent ulcer (basal-cell carcinoma) at the root of the nose.

with fever. The redness tends to spread, the edges being raised and well defined from the healthy skin. The oedema may be continuous, or it may disappear in one place and reappear in another. In very severe cases the fever is high, rigors occur, the cuticle may be raised in blebs, and sloughing may ensue.

Alveolar abscess and *dental caries* are fertile sources of facial swelling, as is abscess in the nasal sinuses. (*See* JAW, SWELLING OF).

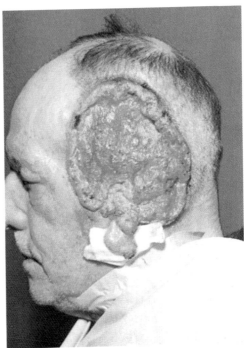

Fig. F.22. Epithelioma of the scalp and pinna. (*Courtesy of the Gordon Museum, Guy's Hospital.*)

Anthrax chiefly affects operatives in wool and horse-hair factories and workers of raw hides. The disease is characterized by the formation of a vesicle, which bursts, forms a scab, and then becomes surrounded by a ring of vesicles around which is an area of oedema. The diagnosis is confirmed by discovering anthrax bacilli in the discharge; a fluid prepared from a drop of fluid from one of the vesicles contains long chains of large, square-ended, Gram-staining bacilli, which have a characteristic growth on culture media.

Vaccinia. An accidental infection about the face may be mistaken for an anthrax pustule. If inquiry into the attendant circumstances is not sufficient to exclude the graver disorder, a bacteriological examination should be made.

Primary syphilitic sore, if found on the face, is generally situated on the upper lip, though it may also occur upon an eyelid, the nose or elsewhere. It is not so indurated as when on the glans penis, but the surrounding oedema is more marked, and the neighbouring lymphatic nodes become enlarged. The condition is often missed because it is not expected. An absolute diagnosis can be made by finding the spirochaetes in the serum discharged from the ulcer, and by serological tests, though the latter may not yet be positive if the facial chancre is of recent date.

Insect bites or stings—from mosquitoes, gnats, bees, etc.—often cause large, lumpy, irritating swellings. The only difficulty in diagnosis is when the original bite or sting has become indistinguishable owing to infection with pyogenic organisms.

Harold Ellis

Face, ulceration of

Most ulcers of the face have a serious cause (*see Table F.1*). If in doubt any persistent ulcer on the face should be subjected to biopsy. The more benign causes include neurotic excoriations of the face—so-called *acne excorieé des jeunes filles*—and ulceration due to accidental thermal or chemical burns. Such traumatic ulceration can, of course, be non-accidental—*dermatitis artefacta* (see *Fig.* F.23). Anaesthetic skin is soon traumatized and often prevented from healing by recurrent excoriation, and this can lead to extensive ulceration, as seen following surgery to the Gasserian trigeminal nerve ganglion for trigeminal neuralgia (*Fig.* F.24). Other causes of facial anaesthesia include posterior inferior cerebellar artery thrombosis and syringobulbia.

Facial ulceration always raises the possibility of malignancy. Perhaps the best-known malignant ulcer on the face is the *rodent ulcer* (basal-cell carcinoma)

Table F.1. Causes of face ulceration

Benign
Excoriation
Trauma
Artefacta (*Fig.* F.23)
Anaesthetic areas (*Fig.* F.24)

Tumours
Basal-cell carcinoma (*Figs* F.21, F.25)
Squamous-cell carcinoma (*Fig.* F.22, *see Fig.* L.17)
Keratoacanthoma (*Fig.* S.12)
Malignant melanoma (*Fig.* S.8)
Lentigo maligna

Infection
Syphilitic chancre
Gumma
Yaws
Leishmaniasis
Lupus vulgaris (*Fig.* F.26)
Swimming pool granuloma
Buruli ulcer

Other
Pyoderma gangrenosum
Cancrum oris (*Fig.* F.27)
Dental sinus (*Fig.* F.28)

(*Figs* F.21, F.25) seen chiefly on exposed white skin. There is usually a background of solar skin damage. The hallmark of a rodent ulcer is its edge, which is raised and rolled with a pearly colour and crossed by multiple

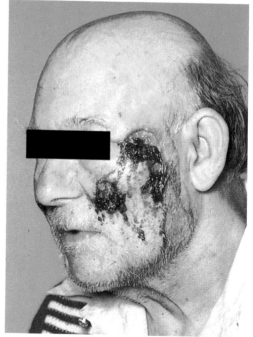

Fig. F.23. Dermatitis artefacta. (*Westminster Hospital.*)

deeply pigmented making the true diagnosis less obvious, with simulation of a banal seborrhoeic wart, or malignant melanoma. *Squamous-cell carcinoma* is also common on sun-damaged skin (*see Fig.* L.17), especially the lower lip, and may ulcerate. Lesions begin as firm fleshy tumours, and grow slowly and asymmetrically. A *keratoacanthoma* is also a fleshy papular tumour on sun-damaged skin, but the lesion is too symmetrical and grows too rapidly to be a malignancy. There is a central keratin plug which may extrude, the whole lesion then having an ulcerated appearance. If not surgically removed, such lesions involute spontaneously within 3 months, leaving depressed scars. Ulcerating *malignant melanoma*, both melanotic and amelanotic, are also seen on the face. *Lentigo maligna* (Hutchinson's freckle) is an indolent black patch on elderly exposed skin. Pigmentation within the patch is variegate and histology shows stage I malignant change of melanocytes. Later fleshy pink nodules and/or ulceration indicate change to a more aggressive and vertical growth phase; despite this, lethal distant spread is unusual.

Infectious causes of facial ulceration are also usually serious. A primary *syphilitic* chancre may occur anywhere on the face, but especially on the lips (usually the upper). It develops rapidly from a small nodule to an indurated, painless ulcer with associated marked lymphadenopathy. Its rapid growth should distinguish it from neoplasms, save keratoacanthoma,

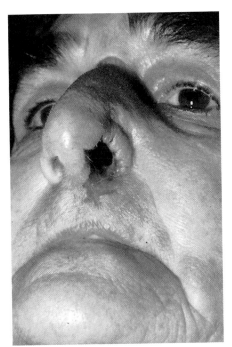

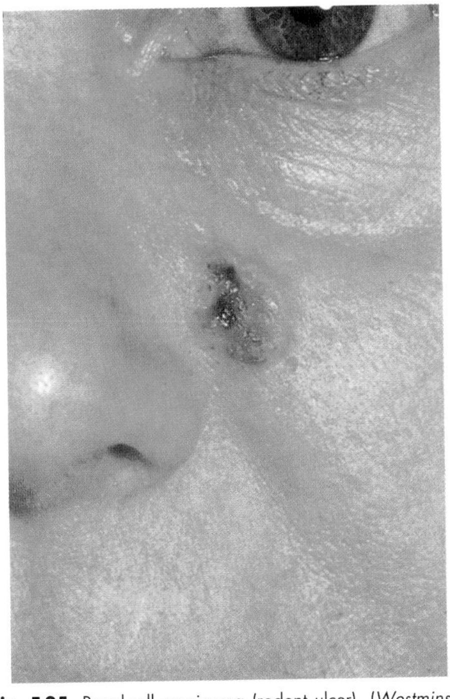

Fig. F.24. Ulceration of anaesthetic skin. (*Dr Paul August.*)

telangiectatic capillaries; usually there is central ulceration but some lesions remain nodular or cystic for many months before ulcerating. Rodent ulcers can be

Fig. F.25. Basal-cell carcinoma (rodent ulcer). (*Westminster Hospital.*)

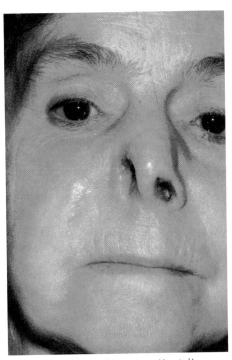

Fig. F.26. Lupus vulgaris. (*Westminster Hospital.*)

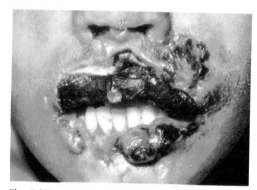

Fig. F.27. Cancrum oris. Herpes simplex in a leukaemic patient. (*Dr Richard Staughton.*)

and *Treponema pallidum* can be found in large numbers on dark field examination of the serous exudate. Serological tests will be positive 10–14 days from the onset of the chancre. A tertiary *syphilitic gumma* tends to ulcerate rapidly, extending at the margins, healing centrally. A primary *yaws* ulcer is rare on the face; in the secondary phase there are exudative nodules around the mouth, but tertiary gummatous ulcers can cause facial ulcers as well as destruction of the nasal septum or palate, as seen in syphilis. Cutaneous *leishmaniasis* may also cause a facial ulcer.

The lesion begins at the site of a sand fly (phlebotomus) bite, usually on a visit to South America or the Mediterranean littoral. Within a few weeks a livid papule develops and grows to 1–2 cm in size before ulcerating. The smear at this stage will be positive for Leishman–Donovan bodies. Untreated most such ulcers heal with scaring in 12–18 months. In *lupus vulgaris*, which is now very rare, the ulceration is chronic. It begins with deep-seated nodules, which after a time break down to form a granulomatous ulcer, covered with crusts. Around the edge the characteristic 'apple-jelly' nodules may be seen. Necrosis of cartilage of the nose and pinna is not uncommon (*Fig. F.26*), but bone is never attacked (in contrast to syphilis and malignancy). Lupus vulgaris usually begins in childhood. Other mycobacteria can produce granulomatous ulcers on the face, e.g. *swimming pool granuloma* and *Buruli ulcer* (e.g. in Uganda, *Mycobacterium ulcerans*). Rare causes of facial ulceration include *pyoderma gangrenosum*, *cancrum oris* (*Fig. F.27*) and *ulcerating dental sinus* (*Fig. F.28*).

Richard Staughton

Faeces, abnormal consistency and shape

Sometimes abnormal consistency and unusual shape of stools may give some indication as to the underlying diagnosis.

Large bulky stools are characteristic of malabsorption and steatorrhoea. Classically the stools are pale brown, yellow or white. Small hard stools may be associated with motility problems secondary to tumours in the colon or irritable bowel syndrome. Narrow ribbon-shaped stools may indicate the presence of anal stenosis. This condition, usually in children, is associated with straining at defaecation and may lead to the development of fulminating enterocolitis.

Watery stools containing large quantities of fluid may be a feature of acute exacerbations of inflammatory bowel disease, especially Crohn's disease, or coeliac disease. They may also be characteristic of cholerheic diarrhoea associated with bile acid malabsorption and increased faecal excretion of bile acids leading to a secretory state with excess amount of water and electrolytes in the faeces. Cholerheic diarrhoea may occur in severe ileo-caecal Crohn's disease or after resection of the terminal ileum for Crohn's disease or caecal tumour. Watery diarrhoea of similar type is also a characteristic of severe infection such as cholera and more common infections such as dysentery.

R. I. Russell

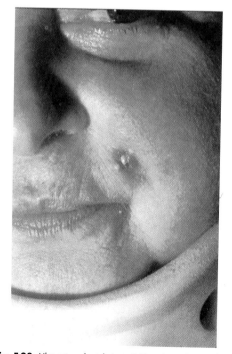

Fig. F.28. Ulcerating dental sinus. (*Westminster Hospital.*)

Faeces, abnormal contents

Abnormal contents of faeces include blood, mucus, pus, bacteria and viruses and worms.

Blood

Red blood in the stools suggests a bleeding lesion at or near the anal margin but the source may be anywhere in the colon. This may be due to ulcerative colitis or, more rarely, Crohn's disease, haemorrhoids, fissures, tumours (benign or malignant), dysenteric infections, diverticular disease of the colon, or angiodysplasia of the colon. Patients with bleeding haemorrhoids usually complain of the passage of blood following defaecation. Bleeding anal fissures are intensely painful. Intussusception is classically associated with red-current stools, comprising blood-stained mucus, due to engorgement and ischaemia of the bowel; pain and abdominal distension are usually also present.

Melaena stools are black in colour, containing altered blood which is due to bleeding from a lesion in the upper gastrointestinal tract proximal to the ileocaecal junction such as gastric or duodenal ulcer or tumour or a small bowel lesion (*see* MELAENA). Rarely a lesion in the low ascending colon may manifest as melaena.

Investigations into the presence of blood in the stools include digital rectal examination, sigmoidoscopy, colonoscopy and radiology (plain X-ray of abdomen and barium enema contrast examination).

Mucus

The presence of mucus in the stool may indicate an inflammatory process and is characteristic of acute exacerbations of ulcerative colitis, sometimes Crohn's disease, or infective lesions. This is particularly so if blood and pus are present. However, mucus may be a normal constituent of the stool without indicating any disease process. Patients occasionally mistake mucus strands for worms. Mucus with or without altered bowel habit may occur in the irritable bowel syndrome.

Bacteria and viruses

Infection with bacteria or viruses generally leads to diarrhoea, often with watery stools. Bacterial infections range widely from common pathogenic organisms, dysentery, pseudomembranous colitis and other infections due to a wide range of viruses associated, particularly in children, with watery diarrhoea. These include rotaviruses, enteroviruses, reoviruses, adenoviruses, Norwalk, astrovirus, coronoviruses and others.

Bacteria can generally be isolated from stool culture but viruses are rarely grown. They may be identified by electron microscopy.

Worms

Occasionally worms may be found in faeces.

TAPEWORMS

A common indication of tapeworm infestation is the passage per rectum of detached segments in either long or short tape-like strips. Close examination reveals the regular segmentation of a tapeworm and examination with a lens reveals the glandular structure of the uterus in tapeworm segments.

Patients may be symptomless or may complain of abdominal discomfort or diarrhoea; anaemia and eosinophilia may be present. The four forms of tapeworm which occur in the human intestine are *Taenia solium* (pork tapeworm), *T. saginata* (beef tapeworm), *Hymenolepis nana* (dwarf tapeworm) and *Diphyllobothrium latum* (fish tapeworm). *T. saginata* is the commonest tapeworm found in Britain. Microscopic examination of the faeces will show the characteristic eggs. Identification of the species is generally possible by the gravid proglottides. Tapeworms may also be seen on a plain X-ray film of the abdomen, or occasionally on barium meal examination.

ROUNDWORMS

The only roundworm which infests man in Britain is *Ascaris lumbricoides*. Symptoms of intestinal colic or biliary obstruction, particularly in children, may occur together with pneumonitis, urticaria and eosinophilia. There may be no symptoms until a worm is found in the stool; typical ova may be discovered in faeces. They are of relatively large size and of oval shape.

THREADWORMS

Oxyuris vermicularis, if present, generally occurs in large numbers. They can be detected by naked eye examination of the faeces. Each parasite is 3–10 mm in length and is colourless. They may be associated with frequency of micturition, pruritus ani, irritability and restlessness.

Other worm infections include hookworm (*Ankylostoma duodenale* and *Necator americanus*). The ova are oval with a clear transparent shell detected on a direct faecal film or a slide mounted in saline or iodine solution, commonly associated with iron deficiency anaemia. *Trichuris trichuria* (whipworm) is very common worldwide and presents with nocturnal pruritus ani. The worm is visible to the naked eye in the stool or perianal area.

Pus

The presence of pus in the stools indicates an infective lesion such as an abscess most commonly at or near the anal margin or in the distal colon. It may also be associated with conditions such as Crohn's disease, ulcerative colitis, tumours, diverticular disease, fistula or appendicular abscess.

The diagnosis may be made by digital rectal examination, sigmoidoscopy, colonoscopy and contrast radiology if indicated. Pus in the stools in large quantities indicates the rupture of an abscess into the gastrointestinal tract. The less the pus is mixed with other intestinal contents, the nearer to the anus is the site of rupture. A complete clinical history is essential and a vaginal examination may be required. Other abscesses leading to pus in the stools include pericolic, pelvic, prostatic, perirectal and pyosalpinx.

Microscopical amounts of pus in the stools may be due to any of the above lesions but is most commonly associated with ulcerative colitis, Crohn's disease, dysenteric infections, cholera, dengue fever, tumours, tuberculosis, typhoidal or venereal ulceration of the bowel.

Pus cells are generally identified under the microscope; digital rectal examination, sigmoidoscopy, barium enema, X-ray and isotope scanning using labelled white cells may be helpful in making the diagnosis.

Undigested food

The presence of undigested foodstuff in the faeces suggests a malabsorption/maldigestion problem such as severe coeliac disease, Crohn's disease or more likely pancreatic insufficiency. Tests of small intestinal and pancreatic function will provide the diagnosis. Another cause is an intestinal fistula between stomach and colon or distal small bowel.

R. I. Russell

Faeces, colour

(*See also* MELAENA p. 258)

Change in colour of the faeces can sometimes be helpful in suggesting a diagnosis. However, severe changes generally require to be present before significant alterations in colour of the faeces are present.

Yellow or white stools

The presence of excess amounts of fat in the faeces characteristically gives yellow or white stools, known as steatorrhoea. It is associated with maldigestion and/or malabsorption states, but is most marked when maldigestion is present. It may be found in chronic pancreatic insufficiency, cystic fibrosis, pancreatic tumours or postgastrectomy conditions; it occurs more rarely in malabsorption states such as coeliac disease, tropical malabsorption, Crohn's disease, intestinal lymphangiectasia, bacterial overgrowth, small bowel ischaemia, chronic liver disease, endocrine abnormalities, lymphoma and Whipple's disease.

The presence of steatorrhoea can be confirmed by collecting stools over 3 or 5 days and measuring the amount of fat present together with the daily weight of stools. Steatorrhoea is defined as a fat content greater than 20 mmol per day. Daily weight of stools should normally not be more than 200 g and is often increased in the presence of steatorrhoea.

The range of causes of maldigestion and malabsorption should be systematically considered in the patient found to have steatorrhoea (*Table F.2*).

Clear-coloured stools

Clear-coloured or pure white stools are a characteristic feature of biliary obstruction or biliary atresia. In the newborn this is generally regarded as an inflammatory process, a progressively sclerosing cholangitis affecting both the extrahepatic and intrahepatic biliary tree. It may be of viral origin in some cases, and the progression from hepatitis to ductal hypoplasia or obliteration being observed. It may also be a congenital abnormality in some infants.

It is associated with liver damage and the clinical features are persistent jaundice, hepatomegaly and clear-coloured faeces. The diagnosis can be suggested by ultrasound or sometimes percutaneous liver biopsy although laparotomy may often be required in infants. Complete obstruction in the adult extrahepatic biliary tree may occur: bile duct or pancreatic cancers, sclerosing cholangitis, gallstones, following surgical trauma or occlusion due to round worms.

Red or reddish-brown or deep brown stools

Red stools may indicate the presence of blood and suggest a bleeding lesion fairly near the anal margin. This may be due to ulcerative colitis, or, more rarely, Crohn's disease (in which there is rectal bleeding, diarrhoea, mucus and abdominal pain), fissure, haemorrhoids, tumours (benign or malignant), dysenteric infections, angiodysplasia of the colon or diverticulitis.

Table F.2. The causes of maldigestion and malabsorption

Gastric
Resection
Gastroenterostomy
Vagotomy
Gastrinoma

Pancreatic
Cancer
Chronic pancreatitis
Resection
Cystic fibrosis
Hypoplasia (Schwachman's syndrome)
Congenital enzyme defects

Hepatic
Cholestatic liver disease
   Drugs
   Primary biliary cirrhosis
   Viral
   Pregnancy
   Alcohol
   Biliary tract obstruction

Small intestinal causes
Infections and infestations
Resection
Bacterial overgrowth
Coeliac disease
Tropical sprue
Crohn's disease
Eosinophilic enteritis
Whipple's disease
Vasculitis
Vascular insufficiency
Lymphoma
Lymphangiectasia
Drugs
Systemic sclerosis
Visceral myopathy
Autonomic neuropathy
Ulcerative ileojejunitis
Immunodeficiency
Graft versus host disease

Investigations include digital rectal examination, stool culture, sigmoidoscopy and radiology if necessary.

Red-current stools are a classical feature of intussusception, commonly in infants. The engorged and ischaemic intussusception bleeds and oozes mucus, the combination of the two resulting in red-current stools; pain and distension are also present. Occasionally the intussusception is palpable per rectum. Plain X-ray of the abdomen or contrast radiology may be helpful in confirming the diagnosis.

Deep-brown stools may also occur due to excess urobilinogen associated with haemolytic jaundice. Urobilinogen can be measured in stools to confirm its presence.

Dark red or reddish-brown faeces may be a feature of porphyria. It may also be associated with deep-red or reddish-brown colour in the urine. The presence of porphyrins and porphobilinogen are tested for by taking a small piece of faeces which is shaken hard in 2 ml of solvent. A red fluorescence under an ultraviolet light confined to the upper (solvent) layer suggests the presence of porphyrins in urine or in faeces chlorophyll. Further extraction of the fluorescing solvent layer from faeces with 1·5 N HCl will remove porphyrins but not chlorophyll. Ingestion of large quantities of beetroot colour the stools red; large amounts of liquorice turn the stools a reddish-black colour.

R. I. Russell

Faeces, incontinence of

The individual affected by the inadvertent voiding of rectal contents per anum exists in a state of social alienation and professional isolation. Contrary to popular belief, of those who seek treatment, the disorder is most frequently seen in women of middle age. The overall estimated community prevalence for women is 1·7 per 1000 aged 15–64 and 13·3 per 1000 aged 65 or more. The latter figures suggest that many elderly patients are failing to attend for treatment, partly because of embarrassment and partly because many medical practitioners mistakenly adopt a defeatist attitude to functional problems in this age group.

Anorectal control is maintained under normal conditions by a combination of several factors the most important of which include: (*a*) the internal anal sphincter; (*b*) the external anal sphincter; (*c*) the puborectalis muscle component of levator ani; and (*d*) anorectal sensation. The role of the internal anal sphincter appears to be largely one of support, providing a 'fine-tuning' mechanism. Weakness of this muscle (e.g. following manual dilation of the anus or sphincterotomy) leads to incontinence of flatus and soiling in the presence of diarrhoea but not to major functional disturbance. The external anal sphincter can contract vigorously for approximately 60 seconds before fatiguing. This is probably a mechanism to prevent soiling (for a short period) should the anal sphincters become 'threatened' by the presence of loose stool in the rectum. A major contribution to anorectal control is provided by the contraction of the puborectalis muscle which creates an angle between the lower rectum and upper anal canal (the anorectal angle). Sharp angulation permits a flap-valve mechanism to operate such that increases in intra-abdominal pressure cause the anterior rectal wall to close over the top of the anal canal, excluding it from rectal contents.

The sensation of a full rectum is probably caused by tension on pressure receptors situated in the pelvic floor rather than within the rectum itself. The discrimination of the nature of rectal contents is achieved by a simple locally mediated reflex whereby rectal distension (from flatus or faeces) initiates internal anal sphincter relaxation. A sample of rectal contents thereby intrudes into the anal canal and makes contact with the sensory rich anoderm at the dentate line where it is perceived.

A complete classification of the causes of faecal incontinence is provided in *Table F.3*. At the outset it is of importance to establish the degree of disability since clearly the management of the patient with partial

Table F.3. Classification of the causes of faecal incontinence

Normal sphincters and pelvic floor
Faecal impaction
Causes of diarrhoea (e.g. infection, inflammatory bowel disease)
Faecal fistula/colostomy

Abnormal sphincters and/or pelvic floor
Minor incontinence
Internal sphincter deficiency
    Previous surgery (e.g. anal dilatation, sphincterotomy)
    Rectal prolapse
    Third degree haemorrhoids
    Idiopathic
    Minor denervation of external sphincter and pelvic floor

Major incontinence
Congenital anomalies of the anorectum
Trauma
    Iatrogenic
    Obstetric
    Fractures of the pelvis
    Impalement
Denervation
    Obstetric
    Rectal prolapse
    Peripheral neuropathy (e.g. diabetes mellitus)
    Cauda equina lesion (tumour or trauma)
    Tabes dorsalis
    Lumbar meningomyelocoele (spina bifida)
Upper motor neurone lesion
    Cerebral
        Multiple strokes
        Metastases and other tumours
        Trauma
        Dementia and other degenerative disorders
    Spinal
        Multiple sclerosis
        Metastases and other tumours
        Degenerative diseases (e.g. B_{12} deficiency)
Rectal carcinoma
Anorectal infection (e.g. lymphogranuloma)
Drug intoxication (particularly in the elderly)

soiling secondary to a prolapsed haemorrhoid will differ from that in a patient with frequent and incapacitating incontinence of formed stool. In all patients a full clinical examination with special reference to the anorectum should be carried out. Digital examination of the anorectum will provide a subjective assessment of anorectal function which ought to be supported, wherever possible: by (*a*) proctography; (*b*) anal canal manometry; and (*c*) electromyography of the external anal sphincter and puborectalis muscles.

Faecal incontinence in the presence of normal anal sphincters and pelvic floor

It is important to stress that the symptom of faecal incontinence need not necessarily imply deficiency of the anal sphincters or pelvic floor. Hence, any patient experiencing severe diarrhoea will frequently develop soiling of varying degree. The commonest cause of faecal incontinence therefore is probably *gastroenteritis*. Patients with severe *inflammatory bowel disease* frequently state that the urgency and frank faecal incontinence is the most distressing aspect of the disease and this, rather than the bleeding, may militate towards a surgical approach to management. Elderly patients and those who have *depressed cortical awareness* of rectal filling (e.g. following CVA or spinal cord section) may develop faecal impaction. Incontinence in these patients probably results from over-activation of a visceral reflex whereby the internal sphincter relaxes in response to rectal distension. A wide open internal sphincter then permits the leakage of stool of looser consistency.

Minor faecal incontinence

This is defined as the inadvertent loss of flatus or liquid stool per anum and is usually the consequence of a weak internal anal sphincter. This situation may arise secondary to some *surgical procedures* (e.g. manual dilatation of the anus) or be caused by a stretch effect in patients with a full thickness *rectal prolapse* or with third degree *haemorrhoids*. In some patients internal sphincter dysfunction is observed *without any underlying cause* apparent; in these patients there may be disease affecting the autonomic supply to this muscle. Finally, minor degrees of incontinence may result from *denervation* and other *injuries* affecting the external anal sphincter and pelvic floor; these are discussed below.

Major faecal incontinence

This is defined as the inadvertent and frequent loss of fully formed stool per anum and, as such, represents the most severe degree of functional impairment of the anorectum. *Congenital abnormalities* of the lower gut may be associated with anorectal incontinence particularly in some forms of rectal atresia where there has been total failure of development of the pelvic floor musculature. *Traumatic damage* may be inflicted on the external sphincter during vaginal delivery in which case the damage sustained is usually confined to the anterior section of the sphincter (third degree perineal tear) or by the surgeon during treatment of anal fistula when perhaps the puborectalis portion of the levator ani muscle or too much external sphincter muscle has been inappropriately divided. The pelvic floor can be damaged by 'shearing' forces when there has been complete disruption of the bony pelvis following compression injury to the pelvis. Rarely, impalement injuries to the anal sphincters and pelvic floor can lead to severe functional loss.

The greatest number of patients presenting for treatment of major faecal incontinence are found to have *denervation of the striated component of the anal sphincter musculature*. The source of nerve damage seems to be local (i.e. pudendal) in the majority and a major factor would appear to be traumatic childbirth where the pudendal nerves (S2, 3, 4) are subjected to undue compression and stretching forces. Damage may also be sustained in patients who strain excessively with defaecation and less commonly in patients with peripheral neuropathies, particularly diabetes mellitus. Finally, very rarely, lower motor neurone lesions can be the consequence of cauda equina tumours. If there is a history of severe perineal pain and the history of incontinence is brief this diagnosis should be considered and a myelogram or spinal MRI obtained.

Upper motor neurone lesions cause faecal incontinence for imprecise reasons. There is little doubt that interruption of suprasegmental control causes incontinence partly as a consequence of a motor deficit and partly because of sensory loss which in turn leads to impaction.

Rarely *rectal carcinoma and infection* (specifically by lymphogranuloma venereum) can give rise to extensive destruction of the pelvic floor such that faecal incontinence might be the presenting symptom.

M. M. Henry

Fingers, dead (white, cold)

Primary Raynaud's phenomenon

The digital arteries of the fingers serve two purposes: (a) to supply blood for nutrition of the finger and (b) by controlling blood flow through the skin of the fingers, they vary the heat loss and assist in regulating the core temperature of the body. Thus, on exposure of the body to cold they normally constrict, reducing blood flow through, and heat loss from, the fingers. In some people this reflex appears to be excessive and the digital arteries close completely so that the finger becomes 'dead' white and numb. With rewarming the arteries open up again and blood flushes vigorously through the fingers, often causing throbbing discomfort ('rewarming pain'). This condition of primary Raynaud's phenomenon probably occurs in about 5 per cent of healthy young females in Britain. It is sometimes seen in males. A family history is common, indicating a constitutional basis for the condition. It virtually always begins between the ages of 10 and 30, and does not progress beyond this stage. The fingers remain healthy and normal in appearance and do not develop ulcers or gangrene.

Secondary Raynaud's phenomenon

Much less common is Raynaud's phenomenon secondary to some underlying disease. In these patients the phenomenon usually appears later in life, often middle age, though it can occur in younger patients and men are affected more often than in primary Raynaud's phenomenon. From the beginning the digital ischaemia tends to be more severe and is often at first asymmetrical. The white colour phase is often followed by a blue colour phase persisting for a long time and, in cold weather, the fingers may be permanently blue and cold. Within a short time, and usually within a year or two, the fingers begin to change in appearance, becoming shrunken with tight skin and loss of subcutaneous tissue. Ulcers commonly appear under the fingernails (*Fig. F.29*) and, when healed, leave puckered scars (*Fig. F.30*). Repeated attacks lead to loss of tissue of the terminal phalanx with resorption of the phalanx and curved overhanging nails (*Fig. F.31*).

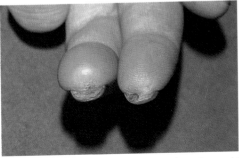

Fig. F.29. Subungal ulcers in secondary Raynauds' phenomenon.

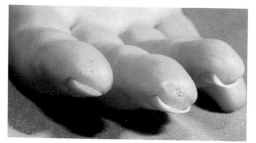

Fig. F.30. Healed ulcers in secondary Raynauds' phenomenon.

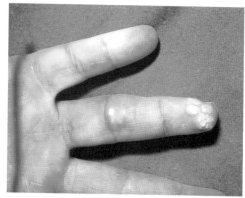

Fig. F.32. Subcutaneous calcification in scleroderma (CRST syndrome).

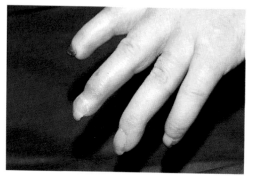

Fig. F.31. Loss of tissue and overhanging nails in secondary Raynauds' phenomenon.

The causes of secondary Raynaud's phenomenon may be listed as follows:

A. THE MORE COMMON CAUSES

Scleroderma (CRST syndrome)
Systemic lupus erythematosus
Rheumatoid arthritis
Vibration injury

B. THE LESS COMMON CAUSES

Beta-blocking drugs
Chronic ergot administration
Thrombo-angiitis obliterans (Buerger's disease)
Cold agglutinins

Scleroderma is the commonest cause of secondary Raynaud's phenomenon. It is usually the variety of scleroderma known as the CRST syndrome (Calcinosis, Raynaud's phenomenon, Sclerodactyly, Telangiectases). At first only one or two of these four components of the syndrome will be present, usually the Raynaud's and the telangiectases. The telangiectases are first seen on the nail bed but later larger ones appear on the fingers and face. Subcutaneous calcification eventually appears, which at first is felt as tender nodules under the skin of the fingers but eventually extrude through the skin (*Fig.* F.32). Although severe involvement of the fingers often leads to loss of digits it does not usually

affect vital organs and does not usually shorten life-expectancy. Progressive systemic sclerosis with widespread skin involvement and involvement of vital organs is a rare cause of Raynaud's phenomenon and ulceration and gangrene of digits is unusual.

Systemic lupus erythematosus (SLE) may cause severe digital arteritis with Raynaud's phenomenon and repeated attacks of digital gangrene causing extensive loss of digits (*Fig.* F.33). *Rheumatoid arthritis* can similarly affect the fingers with digital gangrene.

Vibration injury, e.g. in foundry workers using pneumatic powered hand-held buffers and grinders, caulkers and welders in the shipbuilding industry and forestry workers using hand-held power driven saws, can cause severe Raynaud's phenomenon. The disorder may appear within a few months in foundry workers but takes longer to appear in shipyard and forestry workers. In addition to the white fingers these patients develop numbness and tingling of the fingers.

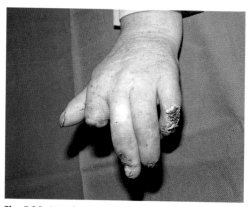

Fig. F.33. Digital gangrene in patient with SLE.

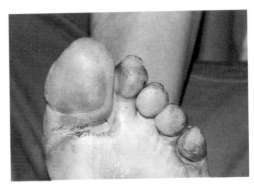

Fig. F.36. Frostbite of toes at 10 days.

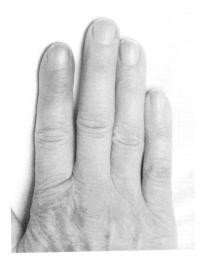

Fig. F.34. Persistent digital ischaemia.

Although the Raynaud's phenomenon can be very severe and a considerable nuisance during cold weather, ulcers and gangrene generally do not occur.

Beta-blocking drugs used in the treatment of angina and hypertension, commonly cause cold hands but do not seem to induce classic Raynaud's phenomenon, i.e. digital vasoconstriction, in patients who would not otherwise have Raynaud's but may make Raynaud's worse in those already suffering from the condition.

Persistent digital ischaemia

Sudden onset of ischaemia of one or more digits persisting for days, weeks or months (persistent digital ischaemia) is not uncommon in the middle aged and elderly. On examination the finger is usually blue and cold (*Fig*. F.34) but capillary circulation is present and the finger usually survives. In younger patients this

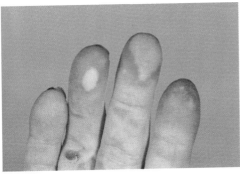

Fig. F.35. Limited early (within 12 hours) frostbite.

condition is usually due to some form of arteritis, e.g. *SLE* or *Rheumatoid disease* but in older patients investigation usually fails to reveal any abnormality except the presence of atheroma and in these patients the ischaemia is due to rupture of an atheromatous plaque higher in the arterial tree with cholesterol debris embolizing the digit.

Frostbite

Prolonged exposure of the fingers to cold, e.g. in hill walkers or outdoor workers in winter, may result in the patient complaining of cold, dead, numb fingers. This is due to freezing of the superficial layers of the skin. In the early stages there are white and dead patches of skin on the fingers (*Fig*. F.35) but later and in more severe cases, gangrene of the skin appears and may envelop the whole digit (*Fig*. F.36). Although it appears alarming at first, the gangrene is limited in most causes to the superficial layers of the skin and the skin will eventually peel off leaving a normal digit beneath.

E. Housley

Flatulence

Excess gas in the abdomen, wind, or flatulence is one of the most common complaints encountered in medical practice and yet it is seldom possible to offer a rational or convincing explanation, and therapy is often unrewarding. While it is widely believed that excessive gas in the gut is a frequent cause of abdominal discomfort there is objective evidence to suggest many of the patients who complain of bloating, pain, and gas are suffering from a disorder of intestinal motility rather than any increased production of intestinal gas.

Nitrogen, oxygen, hydrogen, carbon dioxide and methane make up more than 99 per cent of intestinal gas; the most important quantitatively are carbon dioxide, hydrogen and methane. Hydrogen and methane are not produced by human metabolic processes but are the consequence of the action of bacterial flora in the gastrointestinal tract. Carbon dioxide arises from bacterial metabolism and from the interaction of bicarbonate and hydrogen ion.

There are three ways in which patients with flatulence may present; with excessive belching, intestinal distension or meteorism, and the passage of excess flatus.

Belching

Air that is belched has always been swallowed and intraluminal production plays only a minor role. Because carbon dioxide, hydrogen, methane and swallowed air (nitrogen and oxygen) are odourless, it is normal for eructation not to have any odour. All healthy subjects may produce methane but only when production reaches a threshold does it appear in the breath. Excessive bacterial action in an oesophagus or stomach that is obstructed may produce gas which is unpleasant in odour. This may occur, for example, in pyloric stenosis from a chronic duodenal ulcer or a pyloric carcinoma or following the operation of total vagotomy without an adequate gastric drainage procedure.

Bacterial gases may become detectable when the extrapulmonary route of removal is defective as in fetor hepaticus which results from the failure of the liver to clear volatile bacterial metabolites such as mercaptans from the blood. Patients with excessive gastric air may complain either of excessive or troublesome eructation of gas, or when the gas is unable to be belched, a discomfort in the left upper quadrant, the so-called *gas bloat* syndrome.

Hypersalivation or chewing gum may give rise to flatulence but sucking sweets, smoking or loose dentures are implicated on less secure grounds.

Intestinal distension and excess flatus

It is convenient to consider these two complaints together. Excess gas in the intestine usually arises from fermentation although aerophagy may contribute. The patient complains of distension, bloating, borborygmi which may be audible, discomfort, cramping abdominal pain and the passage of excessive volumes of flatus. Many patients are socially embarrassed and some admit to a fear of cancer. Gas accumulating in the splenic flexure may give rise to pain in the left upper quadrant, a condition which has been called the *splenic flexure*

syndrome and which may possibly be a variant of the irritable bowel syndrome. Most patients who complain of excessive flatus are producing intestinal gas (hydrogen, carbon dioxide and methane) in the colon rather than the swallowing of excessive air (oxygen and nitrogen).

It is a common experience that certain types of food regularly cause flatulence and excessive flatus in normal individuals. The storage carbohydrates of vegetable material are resistant to the digestive enzymes and become available as substrate for bacterial enzymes. Those most commonly implicated include nuts, beans, raisins, onions, cabbage, brussels sprouts, prunes and apples. Patients who have carbohydrate malabsorption such as lactose or starch will produce excessive gas from the breakdown of unabsorbed oligosaccharides. The production of hydrogen following the ingestion of carbohydrates is utilized in the breath hydrogen test which can be used as a test for malabsorption of carbohydrate or bacterial overgrowth in the gut. Methane differs from hydrogen in that about two-thirds of the population produce very little of this gas. Increased quantities of methane are produced in the presence of carcinoma of the colon but this gas is not thought to play any role in the pathogenesis of the malignancy.

There is a group of young or middle-aged women who complain bitterly of abdominal distension prior to the menses or at the time of menopause and for whom no cause can be identified. These patients complain that they cannot fasten or comfortably wear clothing about the abdomen and they often maintain that they feel socially embarrassed although physical examination usually fails to reveal any abdominal swelling. This syndrome is probably a variation of the irritable bowel syndrome and should not be regarded as a syndrome involving excess intestinal gas.

The quantity of flatus which is passed varies between 200 and 2000 ml per day with a mean of about 600 ml daily in normal persons. Flatus varies from being odourless to unpleasantly odiferous. There is little information about the nature of the odiferous gases. Carbon dioxide, hydrogen, methane and swallowed air are odourless. Gases which can be detected by the human nose in concentrations of small amounts include ammonia, hydrogen sulphide, skatol, indole, volatile amines and short fatty acids. The ingestion of certain foods such as French green cheeses may also be a factor in creating foul-smelling flatus.

The flatus frequently contains quantities of hydrogen and methane which are within the explosive range and a dramatic, though rare event, is gas explosion during electrocautery of the colon.

Ian A. D. Bouchier

Flushing

Flushing is a slowly spreading erythema of the skin due to a temporary dilatation of the capillaries and is conventionally differentiated from emotional blushing only by severity, duration and extent. Flushing may be caused by many conditions and is often accompanied by light-headedness, a sense of suffocation, tremors, tinnitus and sometimes nausea and vomiting. The skin of the face, neck and upper anterior chest may be involved. In general flushing is more common in women than in men.

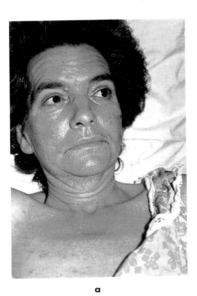

a

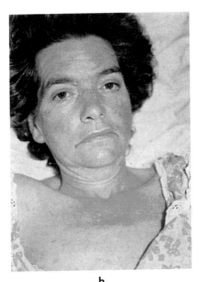

b

Fig. F.37. Before and after carcinoid flush. (*Dr Richard Staughton.*)

Menopausal flushing ('hot flushes') is extremely common at and just after the menopause, but may occur earlier following bilateral oophor-ectomy. The flushes, which can last 15 minutes, may be accompanied by sweating and develop sponta-neously, sometimes even during sleep. The mecha-nism is still unknown though presumably neurohormonal.

Alcohol-induced flushing can be related to quantity or variety of drink consumed. Large amounts of histamine are found in sherry and some red wines though none in distilled spirits. Histamine causes flushing, and certain drugs and food may release enough from mast cells to cause a blush. Some diabetics on chlorpropamide flush with alco-hol as do those taking disulfiram, metronidazole, and after percutaneous absorption of the anti-sca-betic Tetmosol (monosulfiram). Flushing is the com-monest clinical feature of the *carcinoid* syndrome (*Fig. F.37*), also comprising diarrhoea, dyspnoea and right-sided heart lesions. In this condition, as in recurrent flushing of any cause, persistent cheek telangiectasis eventually occurs. In *systemic masto-cytosis* severe flushing attacks, often accompanied by headache, may occur spontaneously or after trauma to skin lesions. Episodes of flushing and diarrhoea may accompany the *Zollinger–Ellison syndrome*, and fainting with flushing can occur with an adrenaline-secreting *phaeochromocytoma*. It may also occur in insulin-dependent *diabetics* with both hypo- and hyperglycaemia. It may be part of an *epileptic* aura.

Postprandial flushing of the face, especially the muzzle area, is a characteristic of *rosacea*. In this disease reddening later becomes permanent with telangiectasia, as well as papules and pustules.

A flushed facial appearance is seen in patients with Cushing's syndrome, polycythemia rubra vera and ACTH secreting bronchogenic tumour.

Richard Staughton

Foot and toes, deformities of

A deformity of the foot and ankle is described as a 'talipes' and this is the generic term commonly used for foot deformities of congenital origin. The primary deformities of the foot are *varus* (the heel is inverted), *valgus* (the heel is everted), *equinus* (the foot is plantar flexed) and *calcaneus* (the foot is dorsiflexed). A *cavus* foot is one with a high arch and a combination of deformities may occur so that a cavo-equino-varus foot may be seen.

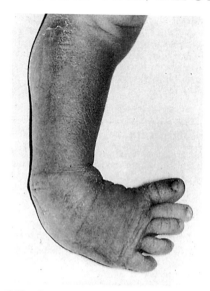

Fig. F.38. Talipes equino-varus.

Talipes equino-varus or club foot

The term 'club foot' is routinely restricted to a talipes equino-varus and it may be congenital or acquired (*Fig. F.38*).

CONGENITAL CLUB FOOT

The incidence is approximately 5 per 1000 live births in the United Kingdom and approximately 2 per 1000 live births are severe. The factors involved are partly genetic and partly environmental with the latter features acting upon the fetus in utero. There is a familial incidence with a greater incidence among the male offspring of a female patient. The male is predominant but there is no recognizable pattern of inheritance. The very moulded baby in utero with an oligohydramnios may present with a club foot. Congenital contractures in arthrogry-

phosis multiplex congenita or in spina bifida may produce a congenital club foot.

The club foot is one in which the foot and ankle are in equinus and the forefoot is moulded into varus. The heel is in marked varus and there may be some minor cavus deformity associated.

CLINICAL FEATURES

There is a great variation in the degrees of talipes equino-varus from a mild deformity to one in which the sole and the toes touch the medial side of the lower leg. In the severe deformity there is an associated incidence of congenital dislocation of the hip, and the spine must be carefully examined for neurological abnormality.

Talipes varus

A minor varus deformity of the foot is frequently seen after intra-uterine moulding. Manual stretching will produce easy correction and spontaneous resolution is expected.

Talipes calcaneo-valgus

This is a common position of the foot of the newborn and is considered due to intra-uterine moulding (*Fig. F.39*). It is a benign condition and simple stretching will rapidly correct this position. The eventual prognosis is one of normality.

Congenital metatarsus varus

Adduction of the forefoot is again a common deformity in the baby and toddler. The constant face-lying of the baby tends to aggravate the position and alteration of the sleeping posture should be encouraged. Spontaneous resolution occurs in the vast majority without

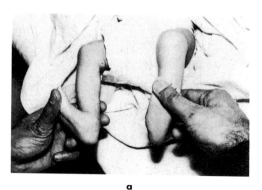

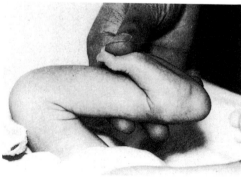

a   b

Fig. F.39. *a.* Calcaneo-valgus feet in the neonate. *b.* The dorsum of the foot easily reaches the anterior shin.

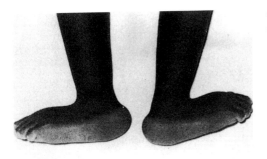

Fig. F.40. Valgus feet in spina bifida paralysis.

treatment and only very rarely is surgical correction required.

Pes valgus (Fig. F.40)

A flat foot is one in which the heel is in some valgus and is common. The structure of the skeleton of this foot is normal and there may be associated ligament laxity. A painless flat foot should be considered normal, but if the foot is in spasm and painful the possibility of an abnormal tarsal coalition should be considered (peroneal spastic flat foot).

Pes cavus

Pes cavus is a fixed deformity of the foot with a very high arch in which there is an equinus deformity of the forefoot on the hindfoot (*Fig.* F.41). There is associated clawing of the toes and the term 'claw foot' is sometimes used to describe this extremity. The cavus deformity of the foot is usually associated with some underlying neurological abnormality. There may be associated muscular dystrophy, Charcot–Marie–Tooth or peroneal muscular atrophy causing the peripheral muscular imbalance. Poliomyelitis and Friedreich's ataxia are also causes. Spastic hemiplegia may also

cause a rigid pes cavus. In those feet in which a neurological deficit cannot be demonstrated, the term 'idiopathic pes cavus' is used.

Acquired talipes: paralytic causes

It is possible for any paralytic condition of neurological or muscular origin to produce deformities of the foot: (*a*) spastic paralysis due to upper motor neurone lesions; (*b*) flaccid paralyses due to lower motor neurone lesions; (*c*) cerebellar ataxias; (*d*) muscular dystrophies.

   a. Lesions of the upper motor neurone (Figs F.42, F.43)

Cerebral palsy is usually due to a birth injury and produces a spastic paresis. Acquired lesions such as meningeal infections or cerebrovascular accidents may cause similar spastic weakness. The cord may be

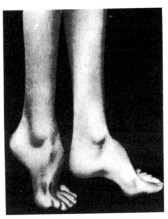

Fig. F.42. Infantile hemiplegia causing extreme talipes equinus of the right foot.

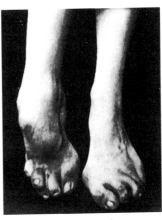

Fig. F.43. Bilateral talipes equinus from congenital spastic paraplegia.

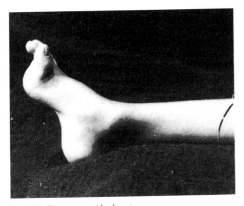

Fig. F.41. Pes cavus with claw toes.

affected by injury, haemorrhage, thrombosis and tumour. Spinal dysraphysm, a malformation arising from abnormal splitting of the notochord, may produce cord lesions and a diastematomyelia or congenital splitting in the upper part of the spine may affect the cord with a bony or fibrous bar obstructing the spinal canal.

b. Lesions of the lower motor neurone

Spina bifida affecting the cauda equina, poliomyelitis, peroneal muscular atrophy (Charcot–Marie–Tooth disease), progressive muscular atrophy and amyotrophic lateral sclerosis may all cause a foot deformity (*Figs F.44, F.45*). The nerves of the cauda equina or lumbar and sacral plexuses may be compressed by tumours, by untreated disc prolapse and by congenital bone abnormalities and in particular the bony abnormality associated with diastematomyelia.

c. Lesions of the cerebellum

Friedreich's ataxia may produce a talipes equino-varus.

d. Primary muscular disease

Pseudo-hypertrophic muscular paralysis (Duchenne disease) produces an equino-varus deformity. The family history, the enlargement of the calves and the way in which the patient raises himself from the supine position is characteristic. Amyotonia congenita is a similar condition with similar effects.

Foot deformities may develop in a variety of other rarer conditions such as Volkmann's ischaemic contracture with peripheral lower limb ischaemic changes analogous to that occurring in the forearm. Acute flat foot may be due to inflammatory softening of the plantar ligaments as is seen in acute arthritis (Reiter's disease). Contracting scars following injuries or burns may cause deformity and the hysteric may produce what appears to be a fixed deformity but which in the early stages may be corrected during sleep or under anaesthesia.

Hallux valgus

The hallux is deviated into valgus at the metatarsophalangeal joint. There is a genetic predisposition and the female is more commonly affected. The commencement of the deformity may occur in adolescence and it may be exacerbated by the use of overtight and pointed shoes.

A bunion develops in associated with hallux valgus. The apex of the angle between the toe and the metatarsal may be pressurized in the patient's shoe. Reactive new bone produces a metatarsal head exo-

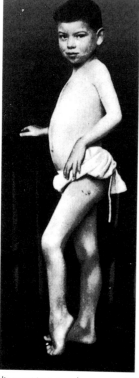

Fig. F.44. Talipes equino-varus due to spina bifida.

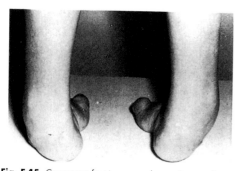

Fig. F.45. Cavo-varus feet in peroneal muscular atrophy.

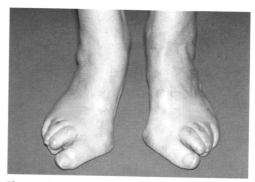

Fig. F.46. Gross bilateral hallux valgus with associated bunions.

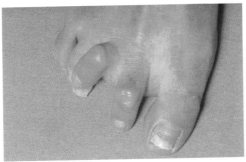

Fig. F.47. Hammer toes affecting the second and third digits.

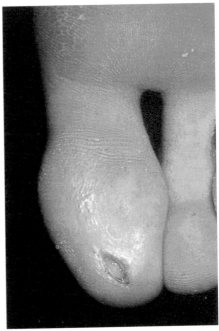

Fig. F.48. Ischaemic ulcer. (*Addenbrooke's Hospital.*)

stosis and the adventitial bursa medial to it becomes enlarged, inflamed and sometimes infected (*Fig.* F.46), the so-called 'bunion'.

Hammer toe

The constant lateral pressure of the hallux against the other digits may produce a hammer toe. The proximal interphalangeal joint flexes and becomes contracted with a painful and tender dorsal callosity (*Fig.* F.47). The distal joint hyperextends. The same hammer deformity may occur if the second digit is extremely long.

Claw toes

Clawing of the toes may occur if there is a neurological imbalance with partial paralysis of the foot intrinsic muscles. This is seen in poliomyelitis and peroneal muscle atrophy. A pes cavus may be found in association (*Fig.* F.41). This deformity is also seen in Volkmann's contracture involving the lower limb, where it may be accompanied by hallux flexus and a plantar flexion deformity at the ankle.

Paul Aichroth

Foot, ulceration of

Perforating ulcers of the foot usually occur under the ball of the great toe, but may affect any pressure area. Ulcers can form under hard *callouses*. Anaesthesia appears to be the most important factor and such lesions are seen in patients with *sensory neuropathy* of any cause, e.g. *diabetes, leprosy, alcoholism*, etc. Diabetes is the commonest cause of a sensory neuropathy in the Western World, while leprosy heads the list in developing countries. Pressure ulcers are also seen

in paraplegics of any cause. Chronic ulceration of the sole can be the presentation of *ischaemia* (*Fig.* F.48), and occurs in those with *arteriosclerosis, heavy smokers* and patients with *familial hyperlipidaemia*. Ulceration of the feet can be the presenting feature of *cryoproteinaemia* (*Fig.* F.49). Deep fungal infections can cause foot ulceration, e.g. *blastomycosis, sporo-*

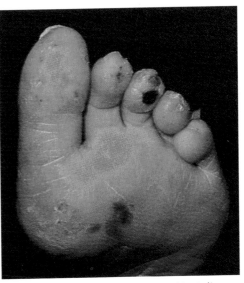

Fig. F.49. Cryoproteinaemia. (*Westminster Hospital.*)

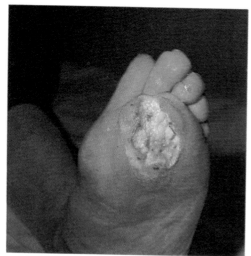

Fig. F.50. Squamous cell carcinoma. (*Dr Richard Staughton.*)

trichosis and *maduromycosis*. Rare causes include *syphilitic gumma* and neoplasms, e.g. *carcinoma cunniculatum*, *malignant melanoma* and *squamous-cell carcinoma* (*Fig.* F.50).

Richard Staughton

Gallbladder, palpable

Physical signs

On rare occasions a grossly distended gallbladder in a thin subject may be visible as a distinct globular swelling in the right upper abdomen. However, palpation is the physical method of examination in detecting enlargement of the gallbladder. One may feel an oval, smooth swelling moving downwards close behind the anterior abdominal wall when the patient inspires, descending either from beneath the right costal margin near the tip of the 9th rib, or attached to the undersurface of a palpable liver in the right nipple line. As it enlarges, the tumour generally extends inwards as well as downwards so that it may ultimately cross the midline below the level of the umbilicus. It may be large enough to be palpable bimanually in a thin patient but it does not fill out the loin in a way that a renal swelling may do. It may or may not be tender,

depending on whether the cause of the enlargement is or is not associated with inflammation. It feels firm and tense rather than hard. An impaired but not quite dull note is obtained on percussion.

Diagnosis from other swellings

It has to be distinguished particularly from four groups of conditions: (1) from *carcinoma* arising in the bile ducts or gallbladder itself; (2) from *tumours* in or attached to the liver in the neighbourhood of the gallbladder—secondary new growth, primary hepatoma or more rarely gumma, abscess or hydatid cyst; (3) from *mobile kidney, hydronephrosis* or *renal tumour*; (4) from *tumours in the neighbouring organs*, such as carcinoma of the pyloric antrum or the right suprarenal.

Clinical features, as described below, will often enable an accurate diagnosis to be made. These may be supplemented by appropriate radiological studies and by ultrasound or computerized tomography imaging—if necessary with fine needle aspiration.

1. CARCINOMA OF THE GALLBLADDER

It is often difficult to decide whether a tumour is merely an enlarged gallbladder or a growth infiltrating and replacing it, since in either case there may be a history extending over years of gallstones, with biliary colic, pyrexia and even jaundice, and primary carcinoma of the gallbladder is often associated with gallstones. The rapidity of the enlargement in the absence of any definite cause will suggest growth, particularly in a person of the cancer age; careful palpation may show that the mass is not smooth as in the case of most simple gallbladder enlargements, but more or less nodulated or covered with bosses or irregularities, which in themselves suggest new growth. In some cases there may be secondary deposits in the liver, ascites, and sometimes the enlargement of the left supraclavicular lymph nodes points to malignant disease with metastasis.

Modern imaging techniques of ultrasonography and CT scanning, if necessary with image-guided percutaneous needle biopsy usually provide an accurate differential diagnosis.

2. TUMOURS ATTACHED TO OR IN THE LIVER

Those most likely to be mistaken for enlargement of the gallbladder are Riedel's lobe, secondary carcinoma of the liver and, much more rarely, hepatoma, gumma, abscess or hydatid cyst. It may, by physical examination, be impossible to distinguish a *Riedel's lobe* from an enlarged gallbladder or from a mobile kidney. Speaking generally, a Riedel's lobe usually descends from the liver farther to the right than does a gallbladder, and it is more apt to simulate an enlarged or a mobile kidney.

Metastatic deposits in the liver nearly always cause considerable and sometimes enormous enlargement and great hardness of the organ, not infrequently associated with jaundice (see pages 181–2). The diagnosis depends, first, upon the discovery of a primary growth, which in the case of carcinoma is likely to be in the stomach, pancreas, colon or rectum, or, in the case of melanoma, the eye, and secondly, on the discovery in the liver of several separate nodules, some of which may be felt to be umbilicated, that is to say depressed in their central part and raised around the edges.

Hepatoma, although rare in Great Britain, occasionally occurs in cirrhotics and may be multifocal. In the Far East and in eastern Africa it is far more common and, in patients from those areas, is an important condition to consider in differential diagnosis.

Gumma of the liver is rarely encountered nowadays, and when it occurs is usually mistaken for new growth unless there is a convincing history of syphilis or the effects of tertiary lesions are visible elsewhere, especially gummatous lesions of the skin or leucoplakia of the tongue. The diagnosis may be confirmed by obtaining a positive serological reaction, or by the beneficial effects of antisyphilitic treatment, though this does not always lead to rapid disappearance of a gumma of the liver. Even when the liver is inspected at laparotomy the diagnosis between gumma and new growth is not always easy.

Abscess of the liver, if it is to simulate an enlargement of the gallbladder, is likely to be a single large one which, if it has not arisen in some pre-existent mass, such as a gumma, new growth or hydatid cyst, is almost certain to have been acquired in a tropical country where the patient has suffered from amoebic dysentery. The diagnosis may not be evident until laparotomy is undertaken or the mass is punctured with an exploring needle.

Hydatid cyst of the liver is seldom situated in such a position as to cause difficulty of diagnosis for gallbladder enlargement; more usually the cyst is embedded in the liver substance, or projects from its upper surface. The diagnosis might be entertained if the patient were known to have hydatid cysts elsewhere or came from an area where this disease is endemic; but in most cases it is suggested by ultrasonography or CT of the liver and sometimes determined only when laparotomy has been performed. It might have been suggested by the discovery of eosinophilia, and also by the specific hydatid serum reaction if the hydatid cyst is alive and active. But latent or calcified hydatid cysts cause no symptoms, do not produce an eosinophilia and are not associated with a positive hydatid blood-serum reaction. Their walls, if calcified, can be seen on radiographs of the region.

3. THE DISTINCTION BETWEEN AN ENLARGED GALLBLADDER AND A MOBILE KIDNEY OR HYDRONEPHROSIS

There may be no jaundice to suggest gallbladder trouble, nor need there be any urinary changes to suggest kidney, so that the diagnosis may have to be made chiefly by palpation. Facts to stress are that a gallbladder is more easily felt anteriorly than posteriorly, whilst the reverse is the case with the kidney; that the kidney is, as a rule, the more freely movable of the two; that it is seldom possible to demarcate the upper pole of an enlarged gallbladder in the way that the top of a movable kidney can sometimes be defined; that with kidney tumour the loin is dull, whilst with gallbladder enlargement it is resonant; and that, on rather firm bimanual palpation, the patient may experience a perculiar sickening sensation which is characteristic of kidney. In cases of doubt, an intravenous pyelogram will demonstrate whether or not the right kidney is normal. (*See also* KIDNEY, PALPABLE.)

4. TUMOURS OF OTHER ORGANS SIMULATING ENLARGEMENT OF THE GALLBLADDER

These may be distinguished to some extent by the fact that new growths of the pylorus, transverse colon or suprarental big enough to simulate an enlargement of the gallbladder seldom have the smooth oval outline that the gallbladder nearly always possesses. In addition, there may have been symptoms attributable to the primary growth, such as dilatation of the stomach, coffee-ground vomit, or evidence of secondary deposits in the liver, in the left supraclavicular lymph nodes, or elsewhere, to indicate the diagnosis.

Modern imaging techniques (ultrasound and CT scan) can usually give anatomical delineation of an enlarged gallbladder and differentiate the other masses enumerated above. Nevertheless in some of these cases it is impossible to exclude enlargement of the gallbladder without resorting to laparotomy.

The causes of enlargement of the gallbladder

Empyema of the gallbladder
Chronic pancreatitis.
Carcinoma of the head of the pancreas.
Cholecystitis from: (1) gallstones; (2) new growth.
Typhoid fever.
Obstruction of the common bile duct by a gallstone.
Obstruction of the cystic duct by a gallstone.
Simple mucocele.

It is noteworthy that *gallstones* comparatively seldom lead to enlargement of the gallbladder. If the associated inflammation does not progress to empyema, the gallbladder usually becomes thick-walled, contracted and embedded in dense adhesions which prevent it from dilating even when the cystic or common bile ducts become obstructed by a stone. Indeed, in a middle-aged patient in whom there has not been any very definite attack of biliary colic, the occurrence of progressive and considerable enlargement of the gall-bladder, associated with a deepening jaundice and without ascites, arouses serious suspicion of a *lesion of the head of the pancreas* which has extended along the pancreatic duct so as gradually to occlude the common bile duct, the commonest cause of these symptoms being either *chronic pancreatitis* or *carcinoma* of the head of the pancreas or of the ampulla of Vater. In obstruction of the common bile duct due to gallstones, the gallbladder is as a rule not palpable; in obstruction due to carcinoma of the head of the pancreas it is usually distended and is palpable in about 50 per cent of patients (Courvoisier's law, which states: 'in the presence of jaundice, a palpable gall bladder is unlikely to be due to stone' *Fig.* G.1). Painless progressive jaundice suggests a carcinoma arising at the ampulla of Vater and, if this ulcerates, the stools may be positive for occult blood. Jaundice preceded by epigastric or upper lumbar pain is more likely to be due to carcinoma or chronic pancreatitis of the body of the pancreas. Sometimes sloughing of part of the tumour allows the pent-up bile to escape into the duodenum with puzzling temporary remission or even disappearance of the jaundice. In cases in which gallstones are the cause of the enlargement there is nearly always tenderness over the gallbladder and pain when it is palpated firmly, associated with a rise of temperature, possibly with rigors, especially if the inflammation has spread to the bile ducts (infective or suppurative cholangitis). Leucocytosis, with a relative increase in the polymorphonuclear cells, would indicate that in addition to gallstones there is *empyema of the gallbladder* demanding urgent surgical treatment.

Another cause of empyema of the gallbladder, albeit rare, is *typhoid fever*. The diagnosis is not difficult as a rule, for in most of the cases there will be

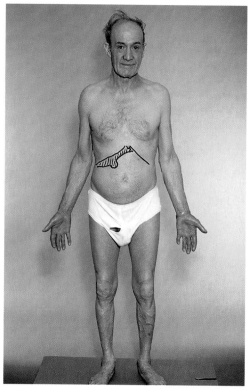

Fig. G.1. Courvoisier's law. Obstructive jaundice due to a carcinoma of the head of the pancreas. The liver is smoothly enlarged due to biliary obstruction. The gallbladder forms a globular palpable mass at its lower border.

no question of new growth or of gallstones and the patient will have been suffering from a prolonged asthenic fever already diagnosed serologically. In some typhoid patients bacillary infection of the gallbladder causes it to enlarge rapidly even to the extent of rupturing spontaneously and causing general peritonitis. In less severe cases, the inflammatory products discharge themselves naturally by the bile passages.

Simple mucocele of the gallbladder is a relatively unusual event which results from impaction of a gallstone at the outlet of the gallbladder when it happens to be empty. The walls of this organ continue to secrete mucus so that it becomes greatly distended with perfectly colourless mucoid liquid, free from bile pigment though sometimes containing crystals of cholesterol. The fluid is sterile. There are usually no symptoms. Such a mucocele may be mistaken for a mobile kidney. Usually the differential diagnosis can be established by radiological examination (cholecystography or intravenous urography) or by ultrasound or computerized tomography. However, the diagnosis of the nature of the mass is sometimes obscure until revealed by operation.

Harold Ellis

Gangrene

Gangrene means death of a part of the body from deprivation of its blood supply with superadded bacterial infection of the dead tissues. Ischaemia without infection results in a sterile infarction. This obstruction to the blood vessels may be mechanical, infective, degenerative, spasmodic or neoplastic.

Common causes of gangrene

TRAUMA

Division of the main artery to a limb, or pressure by splints or plaster-of-Paris. The effect of extreme heat or cold — frostbite, etc.

DISEASES OF THE BLOOD VESSELS

Embolism, thrombosis, Buerger's disease (thrombo-angiitis obliterans), Raynaud's disease, arteriosclerosis, venous gangrene.

INFECTION

Carbuncle, 'gas gangrene', etc. (Both arteriosclerotic and infective gangrene are common in diabetes mellitus.)

Less common causes

TRAUMA

Electric shock, chemical burns.

INFECTION

Septic wounds, erysipelas, anthrax, cancrum oris.

Complicating the following diseases and due to slight trauma

The typhoids, typhus, measles, marasmus, cholera, plague, yellow fever, malaria, poisoning by snake venom, leukaemias.

Neuropathic

Peripheral neuritis, syringomyelia, tabes dorsalis, leprosy, myelitis, meningomyelitis, lesions of the spinal cord.

Circulatory

Rheumatoid arthritis, syphilitic endarteritis, ergotism, erythromelalgia, carbolic dressings, aneurysm, poly-

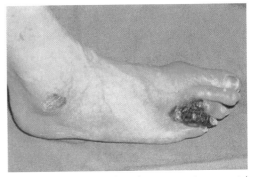

Fig. G.2. Gangrene of the foot, due to arteriosclerotic arterial obliteration.

arteritis nodosa, systemic lupus erythematosus, intra-arterial injection of barbiturates and other drugs, obstruction by new growth, following carbon-monoxide poisoning.

The clinical picture of gangrene is exemplified best in the extremities. Here the failing blood supply is often first manifest by cramps in the muscles on exercise (intermittent claudication), and cyanosis of the toes or fingers, which may be colder than normal. Later, in the case of the legs, there is pain at rest, especially in bed at night when the warm environment raises the metabolic requirements of the part beyond that with which the inadequate circulation is able to cope. Finally some minor trauma, such as friction from a tight shoe or irritation from a protruding nail in the shoe, enables ingress of bacteria and gangrene supervenes. The toes, heel and malleoli are especial sites for trauma and hence for commencement of the gangrenous process.

Adjacent to the dead area there is a zone of inflammatory hyperaemia (*Fig.* G.2) distal to which a definite line of demarcation eventually develops. This classic picture is modified in different sites, and dependent upon the presence and degree of infection, so that it will be necessary now to examine the individual causes of gangrene and see how these may be differentiated according to the clinical picture presented.

It is of paramount importance to confirm or exclude the diagnosis of associated diabetes mellitus in all cases of gangrene (*Fig.* G.3).

Trauma

The diagnosis of the pathology of traumatic gangrene can rarely give rise to any difficulty in that the history will betray the cause. Nevertheless, it may be important to ascertain *where* the vascular obstruction has

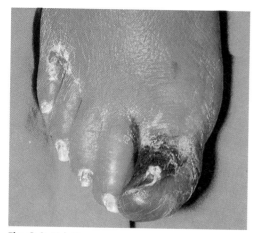

Fig. G.3. Diabetic gangrene.

occurred, and, although there are exceptions, it may be stated that where the distal half of the foot becomes gangrenous the obstruction is probably in the region of the popliteal artery; when the gangrene affects the lower half of the leg, the obstruction is at about the level of the bifurcation of the common femoral artery, observations which hold good whatever may have been the cause of the obstruction.

Diseases of the blood vessels

EMBOLUS

Gangrene due to embolism will be sudden in its inception and rapid in its onset. The embolus is commonly from vegetations on cardiac valves from a thrombus within the left atrium associated with mitral stenosis and atrial fibrillation, and occasionally from thrombi forming on the wall of the left ventricle after a coronary thrombosis, or from atheromatous plaques detached from large-bore vessels proximal to the site of the obstruction. Rarely a *paradoxical embolism* originates from a peripheral vein in a subject with a right to left heart shunt resulting from an atrial or ventricular septal defect.

The condition must be differentiated from acute thrombosis. Both may require urgent surgery, but an embolus is treated by balloon embolectomy whereas acute thrombosis may necessitate urgent endarterectomy or a by-pass procedure.

If, in a case of acute onset, the heart is known to be diseased and the valves known to have vegetations, while the peripheral vascular system is normal, the diagnosis of embolism may be made with confidence and the only problem of diagnosis is to ascertain precisely where the embolus has lodged. If, on the other hand, the patient is known, or can be shown, to have atheromatous disease of the peripheral vessels then the case may be one of embolism or acute thrombosis, and arteriography is necessary to differentiate between the two, the filling defect in an embolism showing a smooth, rounded outline like a cigar butt, that of acute thrombosis being irregular and merging indefinitely with the jagged outline of the locally diseased vessels.

The diagnosis as to *where* the embolism has lodged depends partly on clinical signs and symptoms, but in the last analysis upon arteriography which, if the limb is to be saved, should be performed upon these cases of acute vascular obstruction, in the first place to exclude acute thrombosis, and in the second to localize the obstruction with precision. Nevertheless, the level of the developing gangrene (*see below*) will be of some help, particularly if it be remembered that emboli commonly ride astride a vessel at its point of bifurcation. The site of the initial pain may be misleading and attempts should always be made, by palpating along the course of a vessel, to find at what point the pulse is lost.

THROMBOSIS

Gangrene from this cause is usually of slow onset and always accompanies localized arterial disease, which latter may of itself have already obstructed the blood supply to a considerable extent; in fact the final occlusion, whatever the underlying pathology, is almost invariably due to thrombosis. Cases of acute thrombosis can only be diagnosed from embolism by arteriography (*see above*).

Venous gangrene is rare but is seen occasionally in the foot in severe cases of iliofemoral venous thrombosis (*Fig.* G.4).

BUERGER'S DISEASE (THROMBO-ANGIITIS OBLITERANS)

This disease affects the medium-sized arteries, chiefly of the lower extremity, and usually in men under the age of 45. Heavy smoking is invariable and the condition is more common in Eastern Europeans than in other population groups. The first symptom of vascular insufficiency is generally intermittent claudication and later rest pain at night in bed. There are often minor attacks of superficial thrombophlebitis. Examination of the affected leg may show absence of pulsations in the line of the dorsalis pedis and posterior tibial arteries. In advanced cases the popliteal pulse is also absent, but femoral pulsations usually persist indefinitely. The affected foot and toes are at first blue and cold; later gangrene of one or more toes ensues.

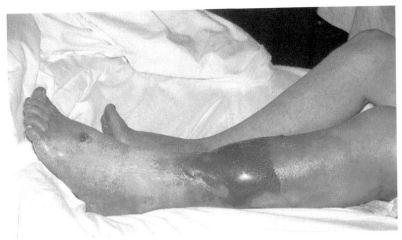

Fig. G.4. Gangrene secondary to iliofemoral venous thrombosis.

Buerger's disease usually affects both legs eventually, although, one being slightly worse than the other, the intermittent claudication in the more advanced leg brings the patient to a halt and masks the symptoms which would otherwise soon develop on the other side. In very advanced cases the upper limbs are also affected and very occasionally the upper limbs may be the first to suffer. Smoking is absolutely forbidden in these cases as nicotine aggravates the condition.

RAYNAUD'S PHENOMENON (SEE ALSO FINGERS, DEAD)

This may be primary Raynaud's disease, almost invariably in young females, or Raynaud's phenomenon, secondary to some other lesion, e.g. scleroderma (see below), polyarteritis nodosa or other collagen diseases; it may occur in patients with cryoglobulinaemia, or it can result in men working with vibrating tools. It is important to exclude other causes of cold, cyanosed hands, for instance pressure on the subclavian artery from a cervical rib or main vessel occlusion from arteriosclerosis or Buerger's disease.

As a result of exposure to cold, the fingers become white and later slate-blue. As they are 'thawed out' they change from a livid purple to deep red, this cycle being readily precipitated by plunging the hands into a basin of cold water. Because the disease affects only the terminal vessels, the radial pulse is normal and, in those cases where the toes are affected, the dorsalis pedis and posterior tibial pulsations are not lost. The disease, as might be expected, is subject to exacerbations in the winter and remissions in the summer, but at least for some years is gradually progressive so that, in a severe case, the tips of the fingers become gangrenous (Fig. G.5). Raynaud's phenomenon is commonly associated with scleroderma, in which the skin over the fingers becomes thickened and stiff so that they are held immobile in a position of semiflexion; and microstomia, a similar condition affecting the skin of the face and causing, as the name implies, a contraction of the mouth with radiating creases at the corners, together with pinching of the nostrils. Disappearance of the distal half of the distal phalanges causes shortening of the fingers and this effect is well demonstrated radiologically. In addition there may be calcinosis, or the deposit of calcium salts in the subcutaneous tissues.

ARTERIOSCLEROSIS (ARTHEROSCLEROSIS)

This term is used here to cover the degenerative process which affect the arteries with age. In a proportion of cases the arterial deprivation is sufficiently severe to produce gangrene (almost invariably in heavy smokers), and in this event it is usually the lower limb which is affected, and the stages of intermittent claudication and rest pain are passed through just as in Buerger's disease. In fact the condition mimics Buerger's disease very closely apart from the age of onset, which is usually over 50, the presence of calcification in the arteries which may be shown-up by radiographs, and other evidences of vascular degeneration as revealed by palpation of the brachial artery or by retinoscopy. Just as in Buerger's disease, too, the peripheral pulsations are lost progressively in the leg, but the femoral pulses are usually retained. Sooner or later an embolus or more often thrombus (see above) may completely occlude the already constricted vessel and gangrene will rapidly ensue. Diagnosis can be confirmed by femoral arteriog-

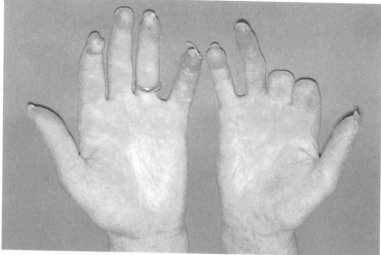

Fig. G.5. Raynaud's disease. Note loss of pulp and parts of fingers.

raphy, which will also enable the surgeon to decide if vascular reconstruction is possible surgically (by endarterectomy, balloon angioplasty or by-pass graft).

Infective gangrene

The inclusion of carbuncle, cancrum oris and 'gasgangrene' together with the causes of gangrene hitherto described is such a well-established convention that no account of this syndrome is held to be complete without mentioning them. Nevertheless, carbuncle, cancrum oris, 'gas-gangrene' and other acute infections with thrombosis of the surrounding vessels are distinct clinical entities and are hardly likely to be confused with other types of gangrene.

Listed above, under the heading 'Less Common Causes' are mostly those conditions in which gangrene is an incidental complication of a clinical picture otherwise coloured by the primary condition; or, on the other hand, local causes, such as carbolic acid dressings and the accidental injection of pentothal sodium into an artery, where the diagnosis is clear cut. Finally, it may be explained that a degree of trauma, which under normal conditions would produce little in the way of tissue damage, may, where the body is wearied by infection or racked by the torments of an unsuitable environment, lead to widespread gangrene. In this connection one may recall the fate of the slight injury to the finger of Evans on Captain Scott's second polar expedition, or the high incidence of *sphacelatio* which complicated the epidemics (? typhoid, ? typhus) ravaging the armies of Rome in their North African campaigns against the Numidians, or later, the similar fate which befell the invading French Armies of 1848,

when the conditions in Algeria so decimated their ranks and gangrene was so common that the whole venture ended in catastrophe.

Ergotism

This now rare cause of gangrene arises from frequent ingestion of rye bread made from infected grain attacked by *Claviceps purpura*. The fingers are affected more frequently than the toes. Nowadays this phenomenon, once called 'St Anthony's fire', is much more likely to be seen following excessive use of ergotamine for migraine.

Harold Ellis

Groin, swellings in

The general surgical clinic would seem incomplete without a number of patients with swellings in the groin whose diagnosis depends almost entirely on history and physical examination. As many of the patients are not urgent they become ideal subjects for both undergraduate and postgraduate examinations, particularly as they demonstrate the need for meticulous clinical assessment and for careful classification of the likely pathologies.

Anatomy

The groin is a region not easily defined anatomically but which may be divided into the inguinal and femoral regions by the inguinal ligament (not the groin crease). Swellings above the medial part of the inguinal

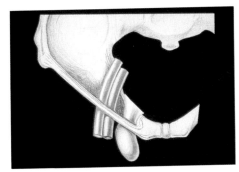

Fig. G.6. Anatomy of the groin.

Table G.1. Classification of groin swellings according to tissues of origin

1. Skin and subcutaneous tissue
Sebaceous cyst
Lipoma
Neurofibroma
Traumatic fat necrosis

2. Lymphadenopathy
Reactive or inflammatory
Metastatic abscess
Metastatic tumour
Lymphoma

3. Body wall
Simple inguinal bulge
Inguinal hernia
Femoral hernia

4. Arteries and veins
Femoral aneurysm
Saphena varix

5. Miscellaneous
Ectopic testis
Psoas abscess
Extension from a pelvic tumour

ligament might be described as *inguinal* with those below the ligament *femoral*. The femoral triangle is more easily described as it is bounded by the inguinal ligament above, the medial border of the sartorius laterally and the medial border of adductor longus medially. These boundaries are not apparent in obese patients but the anterior-superior iliac spine and the pubic tubercle, representing the two ends of the inguinal ligament, allow most groin swellings to be appropriately classified. The mid-point of the inguinal ligament, above which lies the internal inguinal ring, can easily be identified and should not be confused with the *mid-inguinal point* which bisects the line drawn between the anterior superior iliac spine and the pubic symphysis. Deep to this latter point, the external iliac artery passes beneath the inguinal ligament to become the common femoral artery (*Fig. G.6*). These anatomical points should always be used as the groin skin crease may vary considerably, sometimes by as much as 5 cm in obese patients.

Classification

As there are many potential causes, it is logical to classify groin swellings by the structures from which they may arise. Within the various structures the potential pathologies may also be classified as congenital, acquired, traumatic, inflammatory or neoplastic in the usual way (*Table G.1*).

A classification such as this enables a considered and complete assessment of any groin swelling. In practice by far the most common are inguinal or femoral hernias, lymphadenopathy and saphena varices whose features will be described in more detail.

SKIN AND SUBCUTANEOUS TISSUES

Sebaceous cysts are considerably less common in the groin than they are on the scrotum. Benign skin polyps, papillomas and pendunculated lipomas are all frequent in this region and may be easily diagnosed by their typical features. Other skin pathology may occur, as anywhere in the body, but are infrequent. Lipomas represent by far the most frequent swellings arising from the subcutaneous tissue and may also be found in the inguinal canal, although these may merely represent herniating extraperitoneal fat. Occasionally a minor injury may result in fat necrosis where a firm lump of saponified fat may initially be tender with features of inflammation that may be confused with either an inflamed and irreducible hernia or an abscess. This should be resolved by a careful history and examination but where a firm tender lump is related to the inguinal or femoral canal, exploration may be the safer option.

LYMPHATICS

There are three groups of lymph nodes in the groin. The inguinal nodes lie in the subcutaneous tissue just below and occasionally anterior to the inguinal ligament and drain the external genitals, the perineum and anus, the lower abdomen, buttock and upper third of thigh. The femoral nodes are around and below the sapheno-femoral junction and drain the lower two-thirds of the lower limb. The iliac nodes lie above and deep to the inguinal ligament and follow the iliac artery. They drain from the femoral and inguinal nodes but also may become enlarged secondary to intra-abdominal or pelvic pathology.

Table G.2. Common causes of lymphadenopathy

A. Inflammatory
Non-specific (reactive)
Mechanical irritation
Septic foci in the feet, legs, genitalia or perineum
Part of generalized lymphadenopathy (e.g. viral)

Specific
Tuberculosis lymphogranuloma inguinale
Cat scratch fever
Syphilis

B. Neoplasms
Primary non-Hodgkin lymphoma
Low, intermediate or high grade

Hodgkin's lymphoma
Lymphocyte predominant
Nodular sclerosing
Mixed cellular
Lymphocyte depleted

Metastatic carcinoma
Malignant melanoma
Squamous cell carcinoma
  Penis
  Scrotum
  Anal canal
  Lower limb skin

Groin lymphadenopathy is usually multiple but a large single node near the femoral canal ('the gland of Cloquet') may be confused with a femoral hernia. Essentially the causes of lymphadenopathy may be classified as either inflammatory or neoplastic and by custom non-specific inflammatory lymphadenopathy is described as *reactive* (*Table* G.2).

Inflammatory lymphadenopathy

There is usually a history of an inflammatory lesion involving the tissue drained by the relevant lymph nodes. This may appear trivial and the lymphadenopathy may continue for up to 3–4 weeks following resolution of the initial cause. In the early phase the node may feel indurated and tender, following which it becomes firm and softens as it resolves. Reactive lymphadenopathy may be single or multiple but the nodes usually feel discrete. Should resolution fail to occur over 3–4 weeks then biopsy becomes important to identify specific infections or malignancy.

SPECIFIC INFECTIONS

Tuberculous lymphadenopathy is now uncommon in the groin but may be associated with a chronic sore on the foot or leg which had not been recognized as tuberculous. The nodes are indurated but with little signs of inflammation in the overlying skin. They tend to become hard and usually do not suppurate or ulcerate for months. Ultimately chronic discharging sinuses will form.

Syphilitic nodes related to a primary chancre or part of the lymphadenopathy of secondary syphilis are hard and, like lymphogranuloma inguinale and other venereal infections, extremely uncommon in this country. On histology *Spirochaeta pallida* may be identified but serology may occasionally be negative. Frei's serological test is positive in lymphogranuloma inguinale.

Cat scratch fever is due to *Rochalimaea hense-lae*, of the Rickettiae group of small bacilli. Suppuration often occurs in the affected nodes but the pus is sterile on routine culture. If necessary, diagnosis can be confirmed by the positive skin test given to the antigen from human lymph node pus.

GENERALIZED LYMPHADENOPATHY

A range of viral infections will cause generalized lymphadenopathy but when sustained over weeks with ill-health and malaise the Paul Bunnell antibody reaction may be requested where infectious mononucleosis is suspected. The blood film shows leucocytosis with predominance of atypical monocytes. In modern practice toxoplasmosis and other causes of lymphadenopathy related to AIDS should be considered. In these cases the appearance and feel of the lymph nodes are similar to that with other reactive lymphadenopathies, but in AIDS lymphadenopathy is more common in the neck and axillae. Where generalized lymphadenopathy fails to settle within 2–3 weeks and serology is negative for both infectious mononucleosis and AIDS then biopsy may be indicated. Histology is more reliable if a node is taken from the neck or axilla.

Neoplastic lymphadenopathy

Relentlessly progressive lymphadenopathy requires urgent biopsy as neoplastic disease is very much more common than specific infections.

LYMPHOMA

The clinical features of both Hodgkin's and non-Hodgkin's lymphomas are similar but in non-Hodgkin's lymphoma the nodes may be hard and more closely resembling those of metastatic carcinoma. In Hodgkin's lymphoma the nodes often have a typical rubbery feel and may be matted together such that a clinical diagnosis can be quite confident. The diagnosis is confirmed by biopsy which should include an intact node taken, if possible, from a region other than the groin. Once the diagnosis has been confirmed then the extent of the disease should be fully identified (staging) by further investigations which include chest X-ray and CT scanning of chest and abdomen.

Metastatic carcinoma

Firm, hard nodes that grow into a confluent fixed mass as the disease progresses are typical of metastatic carcinoma which may be confirmed by either biopsy or needle aspiration cytology. If the primary has not been identified then a careful search must be performed for primary lesions in the territory drained by the relevant lymphatics. This includes rectal examination with proctoscopy and sigmoidoscopy, careful examination of the perineum and scrotum and a thorough search of the legs, feet and between the toes. Occasionally in melanoma the primary lesion may resolve despite rapidly progressive metastatic melanoma in the regional lymph nodes.

Body wall

Groin hernias are the most frequent type of hernia and may give rise to a number of acute complications. They are distinguished by simple clinical features readily identified on examination.

Inguinal hernia

The inguinal hernia is by far the most common variety of hernia. Approximately 3-5 per cent of the population have some variety of hernia with 70-75 per cent of these being inguinal. Inguinal hernias are very much more common in men and represent over 90 per cent of all hernias in men. In women, inguinal hernias are also nearly twice as common as femoral hernias although there is a misconception that as femoral hernias commonly occur in women they are also more common than inguinal hernias.

Most groin hernias present as a soft lump in the groin that may be associated with local pain or discomfort on standing, lifting or after heavy work. The clinical features of an inguinal hernia are of a lump arising just superior to the lower one third of the inguinal ligament. Most hernias are reducible, in which case there will be an impulse on coughing. In small hernias the sensation of reduction is perhaps the most reliable clinical sign confirming the presence of a hernia. This sensation of reduction helps to distinguish a genuine hernia from the bulge throughout the inguinal canal which is so often seen in thin men (Malgaigne's bulges) and which has little significance.

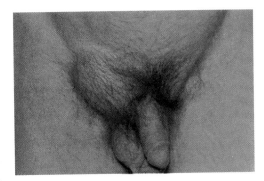

Fig. G.7. Right inguinal hernia.

ANATOMY

The inguinal canal is formed by the descent of the testis from the posterior abdominal wall during early development and passes obliquely through the anterior abdominal wall extending from the internal inguinal ring at the mid-point of the inguinal ligament to the external inguinal ring just above the pubic tubercle. The anterior wall is formed by the external oblique aponeurosis and incorporates the lower-most fibres of the internal oblique at the internal ring. Inferiorly there is the inguinal ligament and posteriorly the transversalis fascia reinforced medially by the fibres of the conjoint tendon. The internal oblique and transversus muscles arch over the canal superiorly. Indirect inguinal herniae arise through the internal ring passing into what is probably a congenital sac consisting of a persistent patent processus vaginalis. Direct inguinal herniae occur as a result of weakness in the posterior wall of the inguinal canal medial to the inferior epigastric artery which passes in the medial border of the internal ring.

CLINICAL FEATURES

The vast majority of patients notice a lump in the groin which may be asymptomatic or cause an aching or dragging sensation (*Fig.* G.7). Occasionally the presenting symptoms are those of small-bowel obstruction when bowel herniates and then becomes stuck in the sac with oedema and obstruction at the hernia ring. A local, irreducible and acutely inflamed lump suggests either inflammation in an irreducible hernia or strangulation of the hernial contents which may be extra-peritoneal fat, omentum or intestine.

Inguinal herniae in infants and children

These are almost invariably indirect with 90 per cent in boys. The lump may be noticed by the mother while bathing the child or when the child is straining, coughing or upset, or may be detected either during the postnatal examination or as the child first starts to walk. It is frequently difficult to demonstrate the hernia in the clinic but a clear history from the mother is sufficient to make a confident diagnosis. As there is a definite risk of obstruction and strangulation the surgeon should not refrain from exploring the affected side where an appropriate and reliable history can be obtained. The differential diagnosis consists of a hydrocele, encysted hydrocele of the cord, undescended testis or torsion of the testis.

Inguinal hernia in adults

Essentially adults may have either indirect or direct inguinal hernias with sliding hernias representing a variety, usually indirect, in which an adjacent partly peritonealized organ herniates as part of the hernia sac wall. This usually involves the caecum, the sigmoid colon or the bladder.

INDIRECT HERNIAS

These arise from the internal ring lateral to the inferior epigastric vessels and pass down the inguinal canal within the cord. Frequently they pass down into the scrotum and may reach substantial size (*Fig.* G.8). This variety of hernia is ten times more frequent in men than women and is more common than the direct variety. It is identified by an impulse passing obliquely from lateral to medial as the hernia is produced on coughing and by the sensation of reduction in the line

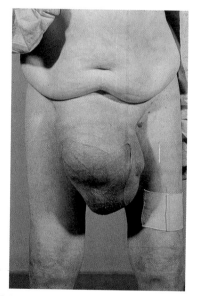

Fig. G.8. A massive indirect right inguinal hernia. Note that the penis has 'disappeared' beneath the scrotal skin.

of the inguinal canal on gentle pressure. Once the hernia is reduced it can be controlled by digital pressure over the internal ring even with the patient standing or coughing. A finger gently introduced from the upper scrotum into the neck of the inguinal canal at the external ring may identify filling from above and laterally rather than from posteriorly.

DIRECT INGUINAL HERNIA

This variety of hernia is extremely rare under the age of 40 and typically presents in the elderly. A bulge is identified over the most medial part of the inguinal ligament which may reach sizeable proportions but rarely descends into the scrotum (*Fig.* G.7). It is uncommon for direct hernias to obstruct and they usually have an obvious and prominent cough impulse which appears to come directly out through the body wall rather than obliquely in the line of the inguinal canal.

The differential diagnosis of inguinal herniae include encysted hydrocele of the cord, herniated extraperitoneal fat or lipoma of the cord, inguinal lymphadenopathy, ectopic testis and femoral hernias. The inguinal hernia is best distinguished from the femoral hernia by carefully identifying the pubic tubercle where the insertion of the inguinal ligament can usually be felt. The inguinal hernia arises above the inguinal ligament, passing over this point towards the medial side. The femoral hernia, which may appear to fold over the inguinal ligament, can be felt to arise in its deeper part from the femoral canal below and lateral to a finger on the pubic tubercle.

Femoral hernia

Although relatively common as a cause of small-bowel obstruction, femoral hernias are less common than inguinal, incisional and paraumbilical hernias, representing only 3–5 per cent of all hernias. They are two to three times more common in women than men, so that femoral hernias do represent over 20 per cent of all hernias in women. They more frequently occur on the right side and over 30 per cent present with a complication such as obstruction or strangulation.

ANATOMY

The femoral hernia descends through the femoral canal bordered medially by the lacunar ligament, posteriorly by the iliopectineal band and anteriorly by the inguinal ligament. As these three rigid walls limit femoral canal expansion, which can only occur by displacing the femoral vein laterally, there is a definite risk that the hernia will become irreducible, obstruc-

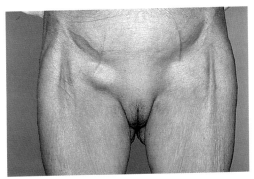

Fig. G.9. Right side femoral hernia.

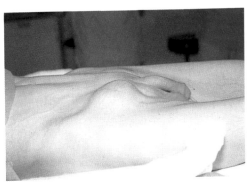

Fig. G.10. Pseudoaneurysm in the right groin 8 years following aorto-bifemoral bypass using a Dacron graft.

ted or strangulate. The sac then descends to the saphena-femoral junction where least resistance turns the hernia forwards and upwards to lie anterior and sometimes even extends above the inguinal ligament (*Fig.* G.9).

CLINICAL FEATURES

Femoral herniation is rare before late adult life. It may present as a firm or even rubbery lump in the groin which often represents no more than herniated extraperitoneal fat together with the tissue accumulated around the sac as it descends through the femoral canal and up through the cribriform fascia. As a result, the hernial sac can almost invariably be palpated in the upper medial femoral triangle even when the contents are reduced. It is unusual to feel a cough impulse in a femoral hernia unless it contains omentum or gut which is freely reducible. An irreducible hernia, particularly in the presence of obstruction or strangulation will be tender, tense, often inflamed and will not have a cough impulse. On careful palpation of the pubic tubercle the neck of the sac may be felt below and lateral as it passes under the inguinal ligament.

Vascular swellings

Vascular swellings in the groin should be easily recognized and yet the saphena varix is often mistaken for a femoral hernia. Aneurysms of the common femoral artery are relatively rare and most frequently seen following previous arterial surgery as a pseudoaneurysm (*Fig.* G.10). Occasionally an inflamed pseudoaneurysm or mycotic aneurysm may present in a drug addict who has used the femoral artery for vascular access. The diagnostic importance of this is that it may be mistaken for an abscess with catastrophic results when drainage is attempted.

Saphena varix

ANATOMY

The saphena varix develops when there is incompetence of the saphena-femoral junction and long saphenous system. The proximal part of the long saphenous becomes dilated where reflux of turbulent blood impinges on the anterior wall of the vein. It lies in the upper femoral triangle just below the usual location for a femoral hernia and just medial to the femoral pulse.

CLINICAL FEATURES

A saphena varix is only visible or palpable when the patient stands and disappears on lying. A cough impulse is pronounced and is usually associated with a fluid thrill which clearly feels different from the impulse in a hernia. On compression the swelling collapses completely and reappears immediately the finger is withdrawn. Almost invariably there are varicose veins in the distribution of the long saphenous vein from which a tap impulse may be transmitted into the saphena varix.

Femoral aneurysm

Aneurysms of the femoral artery are not common but usually involve the common femoral just above its bifurcation. Atherosclerotic aneurysms rarely cause symptoms but occasionally thrombose spontaneously with resulting acute ischaemia or claudication. More worrying are pseudoaneurysms following bypass to the groin using prosthetic grafts such as Dacron which may expand rapidly and rupture. Needle puncture (often iatrogenic during arteriography) may result in pseudoaneurysm formation or, in drug addicts, mycotic aneurysm.

ANATOMY

The common femoral artery lies immediately below and medial to the mid-point of the inguinal ligament. Aneurysms rarely extend into the profunda or superficial femoral artery and resulting bleeding tends to involve the groin tissues, spreading up and down in the line of the inguinal canal promoting swelling and bruising of the scrotum or labia.

CLINICAL FEATURES

In the absence of inflammation the diagnosis is obvious, with easily palpated pulsation. A rapidly expanding pseudoaneurysm or more particularly mycotic aneurysm may be mistaken for an abscess. Gentle palpation through the induration will always reveal substantial and abnormal pulsation. Occasionally there may be swelling of the distal limb due to compression of the vein or lymphatics.

Miscellaneous

ABSCESS

Groin abscesses are not infrequent and may arise primarily from skin or subcutaneous infection, by metastasis to the regional lymph nodes or by extension from the hip, sacroiliac joint or lumbar spine in chronic abscesses.

In achieving a diagnosis a careful search must be made for a primary source of infection either from the toes, foot or leg or from the scrotal or perineal skin including the perianal region.

CHRONIC ABSCESS

Abscesses from the retroperitoneum, either arising from skeletal structures or occasionally from appendicitis or regional enteritis (Crohn's disease) may track down the psoas sheath to point just below the inguinal ligament. An abscess such as this must be distinguished from a femoral hernia as incision into an irreducible or strangulating femoral hernia will almost certainly result in fistula formation. Aspiration may aid in the diagnosis, remembering that occasionally tuberculosis infection of the spine or fallopian tubes may present in this way as may actinomycosis of the appendix, which is now extremely rare.

A number of rarer lumps may develop in the groin including all the usual soft tissue or mesenchymal tumours that may occur in any other part of the body such as a neurofibroma or neurolemmoma. These are rare in the groin and more usually extend from pelvic tumours. An ectopic testis may be felt in the region of the external inguinal ring where it occasionally lies superficial to the inguinal ligament, in the upper femoral triangle or just above and lateral to the scrotum. This diagnosis may be suspected when the testis is absent in the scrotum and is usually obvious as the patient recognizes the sensation on gentle compression.

C. McCollum

Gums, bleeding

Bleeding from the gums is a common complaint and the predominant underlying local cause is infection, both bacterial and viral, as the induced inflammatory response renders the mucosa very susceptible to minor trauma. The coexistence of systemic disease can exacerbate this gingival inflammation or may even initiate it through a reduced resistance to infection or a defect in blood coagulation.

Dental diseases

Periodontal disease is almost endemic within the human race. The most significant factor is poor oral hygiene, leading to the accumulation of food debris and bacteria in the supporting tissues, which subsequently becomes organized into dental plaque and calculus. Bacterial toxins cause destruction of the periodontal ligament supporting the teeth; pockets form, where further bacteria may accumulate. Slow progressive destruction and infection of the supporting tissues follow. The gingival mucosa becomes swollen and hyperaemic, leading to a reluctance to clean the teeth, which aids further infection. Any minor trauma to this swollen and inflamed mucosa, such as mastication or toothbrushing, causes bleeding. There may also be a purulent discharge from the necks of the teeth and the breath smells unpleasant (*Fig.* G.11).

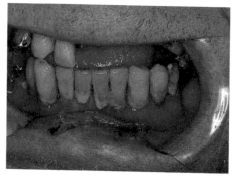

Fig. G.11. Gingival erythema due to chronic periodontal disease.

Dental caries, when present, may be obvious to the naked eye, or, less conspicuously between the teeth or beneath the gingival mucosa. This also allows an accumulation of bacteria leading to localized infection and, again, gingival hyperaemia and haemorrhage.

If both these conditions are left untreated then eventually abscess formation will occur which is discussed in the section JAW, SWELLING OF

Blood dyscrasias

Abnormal or defective bone marrow activity as in aplastic anaemia, or neoplastic infiltration, will cause bleeding of the gums due to a reduced resistance to infection and a reduction in the number of circulating platelets. The gingival mucosa becomes acutely inflamed, swollen and bleeds readily. In acute leukaemia the swelling is also due to the local accumulation of leukaemic cells in the gingival tissues. Thrombocytopenia also occurs as part of marrow disorders, any of which may give rise to purpura in the oral cavity. Purpuric spots may best be seen in the hard and soft palates and haemorrhage from the gums occurs readily. In the mucosal tissues of the cheeks and lips, where the surface epithelium is not so tightly bound down to the underlying supporting connective tissue, large ecchymoses may be found.

The coagulation defect in haemophilia and von Willebrand's disease may cause spontaneous haemorrhage within the oral tissues and may be particularly troublesome after dental extraction unless appropriate measures are taken.

Disorders of blood vessels

Scurvy can be conveniently discussed under this heading, as the main defect is of abnormal collagen production causing capillary fragility. There is also a general lack of tissue resistance which, in the gingival mucosa, may lead to superimposed infection. It is probably this latter aspect which produces the majority of the gingival enlargement characteristic of the disease, as in the presence of good oral hygiene the swelling is far less marked. Whilst scurvy in the developed world is now an uncommon disease, it can still be found amongst old and neglected people with a restricted diet and, in people who for dietary reasons reduce their input of food containing ascorbic acid. It may also be found in alcoholics and patients with peptic ulceration existing on a milk diet.

Hereditary haemorrhagic telangiectasia (Osler–Rendu–Weber syndrome) (*Fig*. G.12) is caused by a capillary abnormality and the head and neck region is a common site. In the mouth these abnormal vessels

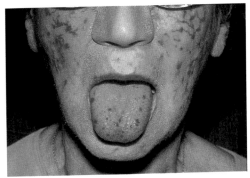

Fig. G.12. Hereditary haemorrhagic telangiectasia.

are visible through the mucous membrane and minor trauma may produce a persistent haemorrhage, which is difficult to control. Von Willebrand's disease and Henoch-Schonlein purpura both may occur in the oral cavity but are not a predominant feature of the disease.

Chemical poisoning

Mercury was previously used in the treatment of syphilis and frequently produced a severe acute stomatitis with profuse salivation, halitosis and painful swellings of the lips, gums, tongue and cheeks. The patient suffered a metallic taste and the regional lymph nodes could be involved. This method of treatment has long been discontinued but poisoning can still occasionally occur from industrial exposure. The gums become hyperaemic and tend to bleed which, as always, is aggravated by poor oral hygiene. Eventually necrosis of the gingival mucosa may occur.

Phosphorus was at one time responsible for severe stomatitis, going on to necrosis of the jaw — 'phossy jaw' — not infrequently ending in death as the result of fatty degeneration of the liver and heart. Since restrictions are now laid upon the use of crude yellow phosphorus in the manufacture of matches it is now almost unknown. Apart from occupation, the patient may, with suicidal intent, have been taking a rat paste or other vermin-killer containing phosphorus.

Arsenic and *lead* are rare causes of gingival bleeding and usually arise from industrial contamination. The gingivae are again inflamed, swollen and bleed easily and, in the case of lead, there is a characteristic blue line at the gingival margin known as the Burtonian line. Other signs of poisoning may be present, particularly pigmentation of the skin, vomiting, diarrhoea, hyperkeratosis of the soles of the feet and the palms of the hands. Generalized peripheral neuritis may be found in the case of arsenic and the symptoms given under anaemia in the case of lead.

Arsenic may be found in excess in the hair, or lead may be detected in the faeces, or in the urine.

Pregnancy

The hormonal changes which take place during pregnancy may have the effect of exacerbating a pre-existing gingivitis. Generalized swelling of the gingival mucosa may occur, or it may be confined to one papilla, giving rise to a pregnancy tumour (*Fig.* G.13). Histologically this tissue consists of immature granulation tissue and is extremely vascular. Haemorrhage readily occurs and, provided the diagnosis is certain, all that is necessary are oral hygiene measures, as once the pregnancy is completed, the vascular tissue will recede. Isolated lesions which, however, remain should be excised.

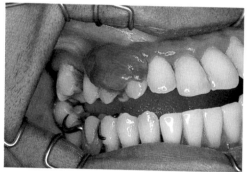

Fig. G.13. 'Pregnancy tumour'.

Malabsorption

Patients with malabsorption may show signs of anaemia in the mouth with a red and swollen tongue and pallor of the mucosa. In addition to this, the gingival mucosa may haemorrhage readily.

Iatrogenic

Overdose with the drug Warfarin may produce spontaneous bleeding of the oral mucosa and will require vitamin K preparations or transfusion of fresh frozen plasma to arrest the haemorrhage. In the mouth with pre-existing gingivitis, the drug phenytoin, used in the control of epilepsy, may produce hypertrophy of the gingival mucosa, predominantly involving the interdental papillae. Regular maintenance of good oral hygiene becomes very difficult and further secondary infection supervenes. At this stage, the gingival mucosa becomes inflamed and is associated with local haemorrhage. Treatment is thorough scaling and polishing of the teeth and the maintenance of good oral hygiene

but, in some cases it may be necessary to withdraw the drug or excise the hyperplastic tissue.

Radiotherapy

Radiation to the oral cavity in the management of malignant tumours induces a severe mucositis of the oral mucosa, which is characterized by erythema, superficial ulceration and pain. Good oral hygiene is difficult to maintain and supra-infection, especially with candida may ensue. Spontaneous haemorrhage of the mucosa during mastication and tooth cleaning is not uncommon.

Chemotherapy

Because of their toxic effect on the bone marrow, cytotoxic agents may produce changes in the oral cavity similar to those which are seen with the blood dyscrasias.

Infection

The oral cavity is commonly involved in bacterial infection due to dental causes. However, generalized infection of the oral mucous membrane due to bacteria is rare, the majority being caused by viruses.

BACTERIAL

The most important example of the former is acute ulcerative gingivitis, which is characterized by a proliferation of Vincent's organisms, *Treponema vincentii* and *Fusiformis fusiformis*. The predominant features are bleeding of the gums, soreness and halitosis. There is a characteristic ulceration and blunting of the interdental papillae and there is considerable debris and slough in the gingival crevice. There may be an associated fever, malaise and regional lymphadenitis.

Infection may be associated with pre-existing poor oral hygiene and stress has also been implicated. It may also be a feature of patients with a reduced resistance to infection as in acute leukaemia, agranulocytosis and those undergoing cytotoxic chemotherapy. In the African continent, the association with measles and the suppression of the immune system by malnutrition leading to cancrum oris is well described. Here, small areas of dark necrosis occur in the cheeks or lips, which rapidly progress to produce widespread necrosis and destruction of the circum-oral and oral structures.

VIRAL

Acute inflammation of the oral cavity occurs with viral infections, the most common being herpes simplex and herpes varicella-zoster. The primary infection with herpes simplex may often be subclinical, but if not then acute herpetic gingivostomatitis is encountered. This is characterized by severe inflammation and vesicle formation, leading to ulceration of the entire oral mucous membrane with constitutional symptoms of fever, malaise and enlargement of the regional lymph nodes.

The gingivae are acutely inflamed, swollen and bleed easily. The disease is usually self-limiting after a few days and only symptomatic relief is required and the maintenance of oral hygiene. Secondary infection of the vesicles may be prevented by chlorhexadine or tetracycline mouthwashes.

The reactivation of the herpes zoster virus (shingles) in the distribution of the trigeminal nerve may cause severe erythema, ulceration and haemorrhage of the oral mucosa in the exact distribution of the branch involved, usually the maxillary branch. The condition is again self-limiting and the intraoral lesions require only symptomatic relief, although one of the new antiviral agents may be valuable in the protracted case.

The Epstein–Barr virus (infectious mononucleosis) may cause a gingivostomatitis where the gingivae are characteristically red, swollen and haemorrhagic, similar to the appearance found in acute leukaemia or scurvy. Acute bacterial ulcerative gingivitis may follow. A high proportion of patients show petechiae in the soft palate, which, because it is so characteristic, is of diagnostic importance.

Autoimmune disease

The oral mucous membrane is frequently involved by autoimmune conditions whereby the mucosa undergoes superficial bullous formation followed by ulceration. This is invariably associated with inflammation, a degree of secondary infection and haemorrhage. The commonest is aphthous ulceration of the minor and major type, but the mouth is also not infrequently involved by systemic lupus erythematosus, pemphigus, mucous membrane pemphygoid, bullous erythema multiforme and epidermolysis bullosa. The autoimmune skin condition lichen planus frequently involves the mouth and the erosive type is associated with widespread ulceration and haemorrhage.

Neoplastic disease

The commonest malignant tumour of the oral cavity is the squamous cell carcinoma, which is liable to undergo central necrosis, producing ulceration and secondary infection. This may produce intermittent haemorrhage, especially if the tumour erodes one of the adjacent blood vessels.

Developmental lesions

The oral cavity may be involved by capillary or cavernous haemangiomas and on occasions lymphangiomas. All these lesions are liable to bleed with trauma and are particularly hazardous following dental extractions, should they involve the bone of the mandible or the maxilla.

Inflammation

The fibrous epulis, denture granuloma, pyogenic granuloma and the giant-cell epulis have a similar clinical and histological appearance. These soft-tissue swellings arise within the oral or gingival mucosa and consist of a fibrous tissue stroma which may be vascular and covered by squamous epithelium. These swellings when subjected to trauma will be a source of haemorrhage within the oral cavity.

P. T. Blenkinsopp

Gums, hypertrophy of

True hypertrophy of the gingival mucosa is relatively rare, accordingly, enlargement can conveniently be classified into that caused by predominantly *fibrous tissue* and that caused by a *cellular infiltration*. It should be remembered that the commonest cause of gingival enlargement is infection associated with the dental structures, and this is discussed in the sections on Bleeding Gums and Jaw, Swelling of.

Fibrous infiltration

Hereditary gingival fibromatosis is a rare autosomal dominant condition in which all the gingival tissues become enlarged to such an extent that the teeth may become almost buried, and in the child will interfere with their eruption. Mucosal inflammation is not always a feature and treatment is by surgical reduction and the maintenance of good oral hygiene. There may, in addition, be hirsutism and thickening of the facial features, associated epilepsy and mental retardation.

A high proportion of patients taking the anticonvulsant drug phenytoin over a long period of time will develop fibrous hyperplasia of the gingival tissues but this predominantly affects the interdental papillae (*Fig.* G.14). Again, the enlargement may be such as partially to obscure the teeth from view and is made worse by the presence of chronic infection. In severe cases, it may be necessary to consider substituting a different drug; local measures consist of improving the oral hygiene and gingivectomy.

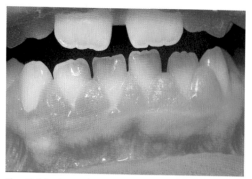

Fig. G.14. Gingival hypertrophy as a result of phenytoin therapy.

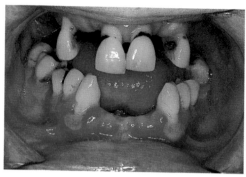

Fig. G.15. Gingival recession due to chronic periodontal disease.

Vascular or inflammatory enlargement

Pregnancy gingivitis, acute leukaemia and scurvy have been discussed under Gums, Bleeding. Wegener's granulomatosis is a disease of focal necrotizing vasculitis affecting the upper and lower respiratory tracts. Occasionally, a proliferative gingivitis may occur which arises interdentally and spreads mainly along the buccal gingivae. Extensive periodontal destruction may occur and the diagnosis can only be obtained by biopsy.

Infiltration of the gingivae by angiomatous tissue occurs as part of a haemangioma (*see* Jaw, Swelling of) and should be distinguished from a localized proliferation of capillaries due to chronic irritation, such as that which is caused by a carious tooth or a retained dental root. The latter will resolve with removal of the irritant stimulus, while the former is usually part of a more extensive proliferation involving adjacent structures.

P. T. Blenkinsopp

Gums, retraction of

Retraction of the gingival mucosa is mostly associated with chronic periodontal disease (*Fig.* G.15). Accumulation of dental plaque causes progressive destruction of the alveolar bone supporting the teeth and the mucous membrane, if not swollen by inflammation, recedes with the bone. So common is this process with age, it is often referred to as 'getting long in the tooth'. Vigorous attention to the periodontal tissues will limit the rate of bone loss but in some patients it is progressive with little evidence of infection.

Retraction of the gingivae may also be associated with intraoral scarring as occurs in epidermolysis bullosa, submucous fibrosis and various connective tissue disorders. Occasionally high muscle attachments will cause localized recession due to recurrent traction during function.

P. T. Blenkinsopp

Gynaecomastia

Gynaecomastia is enlargement of the male breast due to an increase in the duct tissue and in the periductal stroma. If the condition lasts for longer than a year the stroma becomes fibrous and the gynaecomastia tends to persist. The condition should not be confused with fat in the mammary region; in this case no glandular tissue is palpable behind the areola. Other conditions which cause swelling in the breast should be excluded, such as carcinoma, lipoma or neurofibroma.

Gynaecomastia is common in neonates and at puberty. When it occurs in older age-groups a pathological cause is more likely, though in the elderly it may be a physiological accompaniment of declining testicular function.

The pathophysiology of gynaecomastia is poorly understood. In some cases there has been shown to be a decreased ratio of free androgens to free oestrogens. In other cases the cause may be an undue sensitivity of breast tissue to normal circulating hormones; sometimes the enlargement is unilateral. The causes of gynaecomastia are set out in *Table* G.3.

Table G.3. Causes of gynaecomastia

Physiological
Neonatal
Pubertal
Senescent

Familial
Endocrine pathology

Hypogonadism
  Prepubertal testicular failure
    Agenesis
    Bilateral torsion of the testes
    Klinefelter's syndrome
    Reifenstein's syndrome
    Noonan's syndrome
    Cryptorchidism
  Destructive lesions of the testes
    Trauma
    Castration
    Mumps orchitis
    Tuberculous orchitis
    Leprous orchitis
    External radiation
    Defects in testosterone synthesis

Testicular tumours
Leydig-cell tumour
Sertoli-cell tumour
Chorion carcinoma
Teratoma
Seminoma

Other tumours
Bronchogenic carcinoma

Thyroid
Hyperthyroidism
Hypothyroidism

Suprarenal
Adrenocortical carcinoma or adenoma

Pituitary
Acromegaly
Chromophobe adenoma

Hypothalamic lesions
Disorders of sex differentiation
Male pseudohermaphroditism
True hermaphroditism

Liver dysfunction
Hepatitis
Cirrhosis
Haemochromatosis
Hepatic carcinoma

Neurological disorders
Traumatic paraplegia
Dystrophia myotonica
Friedreich's ataxia
Syringomyelia

Respiratory disorders
Carcinoma of the bronchus
Chronic suppurative lung disease

Renal disorders
Chronic renal failure
During maintenance haemodialysis
Renal carcinoma

Gastrointestinal disorders
Chronic ulcerative colitis
Following extensive gut surgery

Polyostotic fibrous dysplasia (McCune–Albright syndrome)

Renutrition following starvation and malnutrition

Drugs

Hormones
Oestrogens
Human chorionic gonadotrophin
Methyl testosterone
Desoxycorticosterone

Androgen antagonists
Spironolactone
Progestogens
Cyproterone
Cannabis
Cimetidine
Griseofulvin
Digitalis glycosides
Flutamide

Other drugs
Amphetamines
Tricyclic antidepressants
Methadone
Amphetamines
Diethylpropion
Isoniazid

Neonatal gynaecomastia

Seventy per cent of male neonates have some breast enlargement. In just over half of these fluid ('witch's milk') can be expressed on squeezing. The breast enlargement is probably due to the effect of placental oestrogens and human chorionic gonadotrophin stimulating the Leydig cells of the baby's testes to produce oestrogen. The witch's milk may possibly be the result of maternal prolactin. Histological examination shows the typical features of a lactating breast.

Pubertal gynaecomastia

The vast majority of boys develop a minor degree of gynaecomastia at the time of puberty (*Fig.* G.16a). Before the gynaecomastia appears there is a rise in plasma oestradiol which anticipates the expected pubertal rise in plasma testosterone. Along with the increased oestradiol there is an increase in prolactin, but the levels fall as the gynaecomastia develops. In boys in whom pubertal gynaecomastia does not occur, this sequence of hormonal events does not take place. In some boys the gynaecomastia is more marked and may even approximate to the normal female breast (*Fig.* G.16b). Often the condition arises in one breast only, or develops on one side some weeks or months before it appears in the other. Occasionally fluid can be expressed. In an appreciable number of cases there is a history of neonatal gynaecomastia, or even a family history, suggesting that there may be a constitutional sensitivity to oestrogen secreted by the Leydig cells of

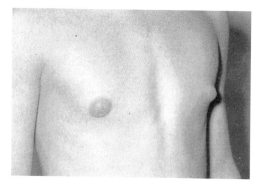

a

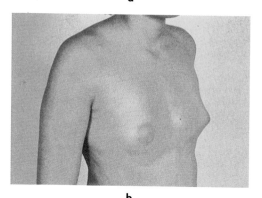

b

Fig. G.16a and b. Gynaecomastia in boys at puberty.

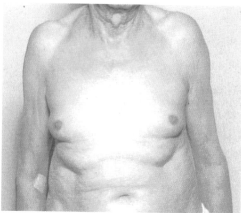

Fig. G.17. Gynaecomastia in elderly man.

the testis. This sensitivity could possibly be mediated by increased numbers of oestrogen receptors in breast tissue.

Mild, early gynaecomastia usually regresses, but moderate to marked degrees of it tend to persist. Although anti-oestrogens such as tamoxifen should theoretically be of value, they seem to have little effect on anything but mild gynaecomastia. The patient is best referred early for plastic surgery. A peri-areolar incision should leave a virtually invisible scar.

It is important to consider other causes of gynaecomastia in a pubertal boy, such as drug ingestion, and to examine the testicles carefully for the presence of a tumour. If one testis appears to be normal and the other one is small, the 'normal' testis may be harbouring a tumour. The oestrogens produced by the tumour may have suppressed pituitary gonadotrophins and caused failure of development of the contralateral testis. Testicular ultrasonography is a useful way of detecting small tumours.

Senescent gynaecomastia

Occasionally patients in the sixth or later decades of life may develop gynaecomastia (*Fig.* G.17). There may be associated loss of libido and occasionally hot flushes. The plasma testosterone is reduced. Plasma oestradiol levels remain normal, but plasma oestrone rises due to increased conversion from androstenedione. Sex hormone binding globulin levels rise with a consequent increase in the binding of testosterone. The result is a further reduction in free testosterone and an imbalance in the ratio of free testosterone to free oestrogens. The serum gonadotrophins are raised. It is important, however, in this age group to consider other causes of gynaecomastia, such as bronchogenic carcinoma, drug ingestion, liver disease, etc.

Testicular disorders

HYPOGONADISM

Gynaecomastia is usually due to testicular agenesis or to Klinefelter's syndrome. In cryptorchidism, while sterility is the rule, Leydig-cell function is usually normal, so gynaecomastia is not a common feature. It should be noted that gynaecomastia is not usually a feature of hypogonadism secondary to pituitary or hypothalamic disease.

Destructive lesions of the testes such as castration, trauma and mumps orchitis are relatively commonly associated with gynaecomastia.

Rare defects in testosterone synthesis due to enzyme deficiency have been associated with gynaecomastia.

TESTICULAR TUMOURS

Testicular tumours such as those of the Leydig cell produce gynaecomastia because of increased oestrogen secretion. Others, e.g. chorion carcinoma, do so because human chorionic gonadotrophin (hCG), produced by the tumour, stimulates testicular tissue to secrete oestrogens. In the early stages chorion carcinoma of the testis may be impalpable, so estimations of serum hCG are important in the investigation of gynaecomastia, particularly since chorion carcinoma is the commonest testicular tumour to cause it.

Leydig-cell tumours are rare before puberty but should be considered as a cause of gynaecomastia in adult males. Seminomas rarely may cause gynaecomastia. The rarest testicular tumour of all, the Sertoli-cell tumour, frequently presents with gynaecomastia and loss of libido.

Thyroid disorders

Five per cent of male thyrotoxics have gynaecomastia. There is an increased conversion of androgen to oestrogen in the liver. Increased oestrogen levels and excess thyroid hormones both lead to a rise in sex hormone binding globulin (SHBG) levels, so that more testosterone is bound and the free testosterone to free oestradiol ratio falls.

Rare patients with hypothyroidism have been noted to have gynaecomastia; the mechanism is uncertain.

Suprarenal tumours

Adrenocortical carcinoma and, more rarely, adenoma may produce oestrogens and lead to the development of gynaecomastia. Plasma or urinary oestrogens may be raised and gonadotrophin levels may be suppressed. Urinary 17-oxo-steroids can be increased or normal. The testes are small and aspermia is present. Testicular biopsy may show hypoplasia of Leydig cells. Localization by computerized tomography should be carried out.

Pituitary tumours

Acidophil or chromophobe tumours of the pituitary causing acromegaly or chromophobe tumours not producing excess growth hormone not infrequently secrete large amounts of prolactin. This occurs particularly when associated with secondary hypogonadism and an alteration in the free testosterone: free oestradiol ratio may lead to gynaecomastia. Some pituitary tumours have caused gynaecomastia because of the secretion of luteinizing hormone.

Hypothalamic disorders

Lesions in the hypothalamus may give rise to precocious puberty and gynaecomastia.

Disorders of sex differentiation

Male pseudohermaphroditism is a term used to describe individuals who have testes and an XY chromosomal constitution but ambiguous external genitalia. There are two main varieties. The first is due to abnormal testicular function, usually deficient testosterone production. This may be caused by certain enzyme deficiencies occurring in congenital adrenal hyperplasia (20, 22-desmolase deficiency, 3-β-hydroxysteroid dehydrogenase deficiency and 17-α-hydroxylase deficiency), to failure of conversion of testosterone to dihydrotestosterone because of 5-α-reductase deficiency or to failure of testosterone production because of 17-β-hydroxysteroid dehydrogenase deficiency. The clinical manifestations vary widely from hypospadias only to grossly abnormal appearances with a small penis exhibiting chordee, a bifid scrotum, a persistent urogenital sinus and a vagina opening into the posterior urethra. A rudimentary uterus and Fallopian tubes may be present. The testes are undescended or present in the labio-scrotal folds. Gynaecomastia may appear at puberty.

In the other variety of male pseudohermaphroditism (*testicular feminization syndrome*) there is end-organ resistance to the action of androgens due to lack of androgen receptors (*Fig.* G.18). The appearance is female, there is absent pubic and axillary hair, the external genitalia look like those of a normal female, but there is a blind vagina. Testes are usually intra-

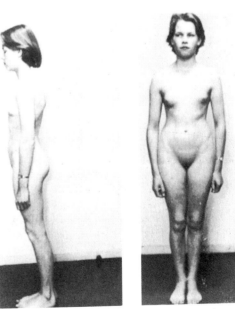

Fig. G.18. Testicular feminization. Normal female configuration. Note absence of pubic hair. (*Courtesy of the Gordon Photographic Museum, Guy's Hospital.*)

abdominal, but may lie in the inguinal canal or in the labia majora. The breasts are those of a normal female except that the nipples and areolae are often small.

Liver dysfunction

In chronic liver disease there is a decline in testosterone production and an increased conversion of androgens to oestrogens. The sex hormone binding globulin goes up and reduces further the level of free testosterone. During recovery from liver diseases such as hepatitis the gynaecomastia may be due to an improvement in nutrition.

Neurological disorders

About 20 per cent of patients with *traumatic paraplegia* develop gynaecomastia. In the cases in which testicular histology has been studied the findings are similar to those found in Klinefelter's syndrome. Traumatic paraplegia is followed by a period of catabolism with marked loss of protein. It is possible that this is responsible for the testicular changes.

Patients with *dystrophia myotonica* very rarely develop gynaecomastia and then it is usually accompanied by extreme physical debility. The same applies to patients with *syringomyelia* and *Friedreich's ataxia*. In all of them the histological appearances in the testis are similar to those of Klinefelter's syndrome.

Respiratory disorders

Carcinoma of the bronchus may secrete human chorionic gonadotrophin (hCG), which by stimulating the testes may lead to increased oestrogen production. In most cases where bronchial carcinoma has caused gynaecomastia there has been associated hypertrophic pulmonary osteoarthropathy. In patients recovering from chronic suppurative lung disease the gynaecomastia is probably due to improved nutrition.

Gynaecomastia may occur in any chronic debilitating disease such as renal failure, neoplasia, congestive cardiac failure, tuberculosis, cirrhosis and diabetes, particularly during a recovery phase. It has been especially noted during maintenance dialysis. The mechanism is probably similar to that noted in starving ex-prisoners of war when re-fed. In them gonadotrophin levels which were depressed during the period of starvation rise following the receipt of food. The testes become stimulated again and the individual goes through what is, in effect, a second puberty. However, in renal failure there are low levels of testosterone and evidence of testicular resistance to gonadotrophin action.

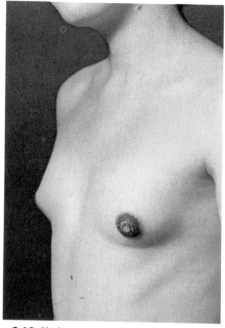

Fig. G.19. Black pigmentation of the nipples and gynaecomastia in a man to whom stilboestrol has been administered. (*Courtesy of the Gordon Photographic Museum, Guy's Hospital.*)

Drugs

Drugs are an important cause of gynaecomastia, especially in adults. Oestrogen therapy invariably produces gynaecomastia and when stilboestrol is used a deep brown pigmentation of the nipple and areola develops (*Fig.* G.19). Gynaecomastia has been described in workers in the pharmaceutical industry who were involved in the manufacture of oestrogens. Human chorionic gonadotrophin administration may cause gynaecomastia when used for the treatment of undescended testicles. Methyl testosterone can occasionally lead to breast enlargement, possibly because of peripheral conversion to oestrogens. Any drug which is an androgen antagonist (*see* Table G.3) may cause gynaecomastia by allowing the unopposed action of oestrogens on breast tissue. However, the major reason for the association of digitalis glycosides with gynaecomastia may be because they are used for the treatment of heart failure and it may be that the improvement in the individual's health and nutrition is the important factor.

A few other drugs have been reported as causing gynaecomastia (*see* Table G.3). It is possible that with isoniazid, used for the treatment of tuberculosis, the most important factor in the causation of gynaecomastia is the recovery from a chronic disease.

Ian D. Ramsay

Haematemesis

Causes of haematemesis

Gastrointestinal haemorrhage commonly presents as vomiting of blood or blood-stained gastric content; this is defined as haematemesis.

1. Swallowed blood

Epistaxis
Haemoptysis
Bleeding from mouth or throat
Spurious

2. Diseases of the oesophagus

Hiatus hernia and reflux oesophagitis
Oesophageal varices
Mallory–Weiss syndrome
Oesophageal ulcer
Mediastinal tumour perforating oesophagus and aorta
Foreign body perforating oesophagus and aorta

3. Diseases of the stomach

Gastric ulcer
Acute gastritis and haemorrhagic erosions
Tumours, carcinoma, haemangioma, leiomyosarcoma
Pseudoxanthoma elasticum
Hereditary haemorrhagic telangiectasia (Osler–Rendu–Weber syndrome)

4. Diseases of the duodenum

Duodenal ulcer
Diverticula
Tumours, primary or invasion from pancreas
Gallstones ulcerating into duodenum

5. Portal obstruction

Hepatic cirrhosis
Portal vein thrombosis

6. Disordered haemostasis

Thrombocytopenia
Polycythaemia
Purpura
Leukaemia and related disorders
Aplastic anaemia
Haemophilia and related disorders
Von Willebrand's disease
Scurvy
Chronic liver disease

7. Drugs

Anticoagulant therapy
Non-steroidal anti-inflammatory drugs (NSAIDs), aspirin, phenylbutazone; indomethacin and many others

8. Miscellaneous

Abdominal aneurysm opening into stomach or duodenum
Uraemia
Abdominal surgery, trauma or burns (Curling's ulcer)
Polyarteritis nodosa, systemic lupus erythematosus
Malignant hypertension
Acute febrile disorders, variola, scarlet fever, measles, malaria, yellow fever, Dengue, infective endocarditis

The commonest causes of profuse haematemesis are acute gastric erosions, gastric ulcer, duodenal ulcer and cirrhosis of the liver. A long history of typical peptic ulcer symptoms may be present in patients bleeding from gastric or duodenal ulcer but this may not always be present. Acute erosions are particularly common in patients taking aspirin or other non-steroidal anti-inflammatory drugs or may follow acute alcohol ingestion. A history of alcoholism may point to cirrhosis of the liver and may be accompanied by jaundice, palmar erythema, spider naevi and ascites; the liver may be enlarged and the spleen may also be palpable. Absence of these features does not exclude the diagnosis. Endoscopic examination of oesophagus, stomach and duodenum is essential in all cases of significant haematemesis.

1. Swallowed blood

EPISTAXIS

Bleeding from the nose may be followed by haematemesis when blood has been swallowed and then vomited; this may occur at night when blood has been swallowed during sleep.

HAEMOPTYSIS

Blood coming from the lungs may be swallowed, especially if haemorrhage occurs during sleep. The patient may cough up blood which is subsequently swallowed.

BLEEDING FROM THE MOUTH AND THROAT

Bleeding may occur from the gums, tongue and fauces, and blood from these sources may be swallowed and subsequently vomited. Bleeding from the gums may occur in scurvy or mercurial stomatitis.

SPURIOUS

Some patients suffering from a variant of the Munchausen syndrome may swallow blood in secret and subsequently vomit this with an intent to deceive.

2. Diseases of the oesophagus

HIATUS HERNIA AND REFLUX OESOPHAGITIS

Hiatus hernia is common but is mostly associated with the symptoms of acid reflux and oesophagitis than with gastrointestinal bleeding. Blood loss in oesophagitis and hiatus hernia is usually chronic, presenting as iron-deficiency anaemia, but occasionally haematemesis does occur. This most commonly occurs from the gastric side of the oesophago-gastric junction and is more common with a paraoesophageal rather than a sliding hiatus hernia. Haematemesis may be associated with Barrett's syndrome, in which ulceration of gastric mucosa may occur in the lower oesophagus.

OESOPHAGEAL VARICES

Varices developing at the lower end of the oesophagus or the upper end of the stomach as a result of portal hypertension are generally associated with cirrhosis of the liver and may be the cause of profuse haematemesis if rupture occurs. Stigmata of chronic liver disease may be present such as jaundice, ascites, palmar erythema or spider naevi. The absence of these features does not exclude the presence of portal hypertension and varices. The distended varices beneath the mucosa of the lower oesophagus and cardiac region of the stomach can be demonstrated on barium swallow but are more certainly visualized by fibre-optic oesophagoscopy.

MALLORY–WEISS SYNDROME

Rupture of the gastric mucosa at the oesophago-gastric junction may result in haematemesis. This may follow vomiting and is particularly common in alcoholics. Such tears are generally linear, at or just below the mucosal junction, and may extend into a submucosal plexus of thin-walled vessels. The characteristic clinical picture of retching and vomiting followed by haemorrhage is not the only way the Mallory–Weiss syndrome presents, as early endoscopy in patients has shown this to be a relatively common cause of haematemesis.

OESOPHAGEAL ULCER

Such ulcers may be benign or malignant and may be associated with hiatus hernia and reflux oesophagitis.

Although a relatively uncommon cause of haematemesis, significant bleeding may occur, the diagnosis being confirmed by endoscopy with biopsy.

MEDIASTINAL TUMOUR PERFORATING OESOPHAGUS AND AORTA

This is an infrequent complication of such tumours but may occur if the tumour erodes into the oesophagus. It may be associated with compression and invasion of large veins leading to oedema of the neck and extremities, cyanosis and dilated superficial veins.

FOREIGN BODY PERFORATING OESOPHAGUS AND AORTA

This rare cause of haematemesis may be induced by a fish bone, pin or dental plate perforating both oesophagus and a large vessel or aorta. A history of a foreign body being swallowed, followed by a feeling of discomfort in the oesophagus, suggests the condition which is generally confirmed by radiology or endoscopy.

3. Diseases of the stomach

GASTRIC ULCER

Haematemesis may occur in acute or chronic gastric ulcer. Gradual loss of blood may allow sufficient time for acid gastric juice to convert haemoglobin into haematin which gives the vomit a dark brown or 'coffee-ground' appearance. Severe bleeding may occur if a medium-sized or large vessel is eroded. Profuse haemorrhage causes a feeling of faintness, restlessness, syncope and a rapid feeble pulse. There may be abdominal pain, nausea, vomiting and associated melaena. The pain is generally epigastric, but many haematemeses from ulcers are associated with no abdominal discomfort.

Endoscopy is the most important investigation in determining gastric ulcer as a cause of haematemesis; the site of the ulcer can be positively identified, the severity of the bleeding assessed and biopsy obtained to determine if the ulcer is benign or malignant. Usually a biopsy is not taken from bleeding ulcers, the endoscopy being repeated in a few days for the purpose of obtaining suitable biopsies.

ACUTE GASTRITIS AND HAEMORRHAGIC EROSIONS

In acute gastritis the mucosa is congested and small haemorrhages and erosions are identified at endoscopy. Generally slight haemorrhage occurs although it may be occasionally profuse. Haemorrhagic erosions are small or minute ulcers, the differences between these and multiple small gastric ulcers being that of degree rather than of kind.

Acute gastritis and haemorrhagic erosions may be associated with the ingestion of irritating foods, alcohol, or corrosive and irritant poisons. There may be a feeling of discomfort and tenderness in the epigastrium, nausea and vomiting.

Non-steroidal anti-inflammatory drugs are now perhaps the commonest cause of bleeding from erosive gastritis.

Other causes of bleeding from such lesions are very severe acute infections such as variola, infective endocarditis, yellow fever, black water fever and Dengue fever.

Gastritis and haematemesis may also be due to corrosive poisons, strong acids or alkalis destroying the surface membranes of mouth, throat, oesophagus or stomach, causing intense pain, dysphagia, retrosternal discomfort, abdominal distension, collapse and haematemesis. In arsenic poisoning the mucous membrane of the stomach is red, inflamed, partly detached and covered with blood-stained mucus. The principal symptoms are nausea, severe sickness, burning epigastric pain and diarrhoea. The vomitus is usually brown, turbid fluid mixed with mucus and streaked with blood in which arsenic may be detected by appropriate tests; severe diarrhoea may come later.

TUMOURS

Severe haematemesis is relatively rare in *carcinoma of the stomach*, accounting for less than 5 per cent of all haematemeses. The patient may have epigastric discomfort, nausea, vomiting, anorexia and weight loss. Pyrexia, anaemia, cachexia and an abdominal mass may also be present. Sometimes no preceding symptoms occur and the patient presents with haematemesis. Pain is variable but when present is generally central, sometimes being referred to the back. If narrowing at the pyloric area has occurred, the patient may have regular vomiting streaked with blood of 'coffee-ground' appearance. If the tumour is at the cardia, regurgitation of food may occur rather than true vomiting, and may occur a few minutes after eating. Troisier's sign—enlargement of the left supraclavicular lymph node—is a rare finding but if present strongly suggests malignant disease.

Gastric tumours are best diagnosed by endoscopy through which adequate biopsies under direct vision can be obtained.

Other tumours of the stomach may rarely occur; these include haemangioma—a benign tumour comprising newly formed blood vessels—and leio-myoma—characterized by large spindle cells of unstriped muscle. These are rare tumours but are likely to ulcerate and bleed.

PSEUDOXANTHOMA ELASTICUM (GRÖNDBLAD–STRANDBERG SYNDROME)

This is a hereditary disease characterized by widespread atrophy of elastic tissue throughout the body. Disintegration of submucosal artery elastica leads to severe haemorrhage from the stomach. Characteristic appearances of the skin of head, neck and body may suggest the diagnosis.

HEREDITARY HAEMORRHAGIC TELANGIECTASIA (OSLER–RENDU–WEBER SYNDROME)

This is caused by dilatation of normal vascular structure following congenital thinning of arterial muscle coat and absent elastin in arteriolar walls. There are multiple telangiectasia which are commonly found on the lips and mucous membranes of the mouth and throughout the gastrointestinal tract. There may also be arteriovenous fistulae in the lungs and liver. The condition is inherited as an autosomal dominant. The most common presentations are gastrointestinal tract bleeding, often haematemesis, sometimes melaena, or epistaxis. Endoscopic examination of the stomach generally identifies such lesions, but milder bleeding distal to the stomach is often difficult to diagnose.

4. Diseases of the duodenum

DUODENAL ULCER

Haematemesis occurs when a duodenal ulcer erodes a blood vessel, some of the blood regurgitating through the pylorus into the stomach to be vomited, the rest passing down the gastrointestinal tract to cause melaena. If bleeding is severe, red blood may be passed per rectum. It is common for duodenal ulcer and haematemesis to have little pain. If pain is present it is central, upper abdominal and possibly radiating to the back. There may be a dyspeptic history with pain occurring some hours after food, often at night, with symptoms showing periodicity. Generally endoscopy can rapidly identify the presence and site of a bleeding duodenal ulcer.

DIVERTICULA

Duodenal diverticula are fairly commonly seen on radiological examination, but are generally asymptomatic. If inflammation occurs within a diverticulum the symptoms may resemble those of duodenal ulcer although there is generally not the classical regular food relationship. A coexisting ulcer may be present. Haematemesis is rare in association with duodenal diverticula.

TUMOURS

Duodenal tumours are rare, mostly arising from the ampulla of Vater, being associated with jaundice and pale or silvery stools. Occasionally, invasion of the duodenum occurs from tumour in the head of the pancreas resulting in haematemesis.

GALLSTONES ULCERATING INTO THE DUODENUM

This is a rare cause of haematemesis and is generally associated with previous attacks of colicky abdominal pain, classically under the right costal margin, and sometimes associated with jaundice. The diagnosis is generally confirmed by plain abdominal X-ray showing air in the biliary tree, ultrasound examination, or the passage of stone in the faeces, or endoscopy.

5. Portal hypertension

CHRONIC LIVER DISEASE

Chronic liver disease may be associated with disordered haemostasis in the form of thrombocytopenia associated with portal hypertension, or coagulation abnormalities. Thus any other cause of bleeding such as peptic ulceration or oesophageal varices may lead to a major haematemesis because of the abnormal haemostatic mechanisms.

PORTAL VEIN OBSTRUCTION

Extrahepatic portal vein thrombosis usually occurs in infants and early childhood. The cause is usually unknown and infection is rare. The patients present with haematemesis from oesophageal varices, or splenomegaly. There is rarely evidence of liver dysfunction clinically or biochemically. The outlook is good. Surgery should be avoided, but if bleeding is a problem some form of portal systemic shunt surgery is required.

In adults, portal vein thrombosis is usually due to thrombosis, trauma or neoplastic invasion.

6. Disordered haemostasis

A large number of conditions may be associated with disordered haemostasis. These may cause gastrointestinal haemorrhage with haematemesis. Often another lesion in the stomach or duodenum, such as a small erosion or ulcer, may start to bleed but the bleeding may become significant in the presence of conditions leading to abnormal haemostasis.

THROMBOCYTOPENIA

A number of conditions may be associated with thrombocytopenia, including hepatic cirrhosis with portal hypertension, side-effects of drugs or reticuloses. Any of these conditions may be associated with bleeding, becoming significant and leading to haematemesis.

POLYCYTHAEMIA

Patients with polycythaemia rubra vera may develop thrombotic episodes leading to ulceration and followed by bleeding from the stomach or duodenum.

PURPURA

Purpuric conditions may be associated with haemorrhage from any mucous membranes, anywhere in the gastrointestinal tract. The underlying cause of the purpura should be investigated.

LEUKAEMIA AND RELATED DISORDERS

Leukaemia and other related conditions such as Hodgkin's disease, lymphomas and other reticuloses may develop haemorrhages from any part of the gastrointestinal tract, leading to haematemesis. Enlargement of the spleen may indicate the underlying condition. The diagnosis is established by blood, lymph node or bone-marrow examination.

APLASTIC ANAEMIA

Aplastic anaemias may be related to a range of conditions including viral infection and the side-effects of drugs. They may rarely be associated with gastrointestinal haemorrhage and haematemesis. The diagnosis is again established by blood or bone-marrow examination.

HAEMOPHILIA AND RELATED DISORDERS

Excessive bleeding from many sites may be associated with haemophilia and other disorders of coagulation. Gastrointestinal bleeding presenting as haematemesis is relatively common in these conditions; the diagnosis has generally been made before such bleeding occurs. Haemorrhage into joints may be present.

VON WILLEBRAND'S DISEASE

Deficiency of Von Willebrand factor leads to ineffective platelet adhesion. Bleeding may result, although the defect is generally mild. Sometimes there may be an associated haematemesis.

SCURVY

Haematemesis may occur in severe cases of scurvy. The patient may also have swollen spongy gums, anaemia, cutaneous haemorrhages and subcutaneous indurations. The patient may give a history of a diet deficient in fresh vegetables or there may be underlying conditions such as Crohn's disease or coeliac disease leading to malabsorption and malnutrition. Measurement of the ascorbic acid level in blood will give the diagnosis.

7. Drugs

A number of drugs may be associated with haematemesis, the cause being suspected by an accurate and detailed drug history from the patient or the presence of a disorder such as arthopathy, suggesting that the patient may be having, or have had, drugs such as non-steroidal anti-inflammatory agents, which may lead to gastrointestinal haemorrhage.

ANTICOAGULANT THERAPY

Anticoagulants may be indicated in various conditions including deep venous thrombosis or pulmonary thromboembolism, and patients on long-term anticoagulant therapy may have significant gastrointestinal haemorrhage from relatively minor lesions in the stomach or duodenum such as small ulcers or erosions. An accurate drug history should provide a guide to the cause.

NON-STEROIDAL ANTI-INFLAMMATORY DRUGS (NSAIDS)

These drugs are widely used in all forms of arthropathy and may lead to the development of haemorrhagic erosions or erosive gastritis in the stomach or duodenum, with haematemesis. They are being more widely used especially in elderly patients. An accurate drug history should provide the clue to the cause but endoscopy will localize the site and assess the severity of the lesion.

8. Miscellaneous

A number of rarer conditions may be associated with gastrointestinal haemorrhage and haematemesis. These include severe bleeding from an abdominal aneurysm opening into the stomach or duodenum, uraemia associated with chronic nephritis (in which the presence of high blood pressure, cardiac hypertrophy, retinopathy, polyuria and urine of low specific gravity with albumin or blood present may point to the diagnosis); abdominal surgery; trauma or burns (Curling's ulcer); auto-immune disorders such as polyarteritis nodosa or systemic lupus erythematosus. Gastrointestinal bleeding may be associated rarely with malignant hypertension and acute febrile disorders.

R. I. Russell

Haematuria

Haematuria means the presence of red blood cells in the urine and, although free haemoglobin may be present in the urine as a result of lysis of cells in the urinary tract, it should not be confused with haemoglobinuria in which the pigment alone is filtered through the glomeruli. In clinical practice there are two main ways in which haematuria may pose a diagnostic problem. Macroscopic haematuria may be a presenting feature, with or without other symptoms, or blood may be found in the urine only by 'dipstick' testing or microscopy. In the former case the remainder of the history and examination together with special investigations will be aimed directly at finding the site and cause of the bleeding. In the latter, the finding of microscopic haematuria will either support a diagnosis already made or suspected or will prompt specific investigations; the only reason for ignoring this finding, temporarily, is when blood is found on routine urine testing in a menstruating woman.

In a patient complaining of frank haematuria, with no other symptoms, enquiry should be directed to the details of the symptom itself. The colour of the blood may be of some slight significance as, if it is bright red, it is more likely to have come from the bladder or urethra. The opposite does not apply as dark-coloured blood is of no diagnostic significance. The time at which the blood appears *during* micturition is rather more helpful. Thus, if the blood appears only during the final expulsive efforts or the terminal urine is more deeply blood-stained than the rest, the bleeding is almost certainly from the bladder; if it is the first urine passed which is most blood-stained, the urethra or prostate are the likely source. Even distribution of the blood throughout micturition suggests either that the source of bleeding is in the kidneys or ureters or that the bleeding is profuse from any site above the urethra. The amount of blood present is also of diagnostic importance; in the absence of trauma, a large quantity of blood is suggestive of a tumour of the urinary tract although profuse bleeding is quite common in several other conditions, for example benign prostatic hypertrophy.

The history should, naturally, include the patient's past and family history together with details of his or her occupation and of any drugs being taken. All other symptoms are relevant until proved otherwise and, specifically, symptoms related to the urinary tract should be enquired about. Thus unilateral lumbar pain, passing forward into the groin, with occasional attacks of colic, would suggest a renal lesion while increased frequency of micturition or penile pain immediately after micturition would suggest vesical disease. Sacral pain would suggest malignant disease in the bladder or prostate. The site of associated symptoms may, however, be misleading. For example, a tumour in the bladder might, by occluding a ureteric orifice, cause unilateral hydronephrosis with lumbar pain and tuberculosis of the kidney and ureter can cause increased frequency of micturition in the absence of vesical infection.

Physical examination must be thorough as there is virtually no abnormal physical sign which may not be associated with one of the numerous causes of haematuria. The kidneys should be palpated to determine their size, if possible, and to elicit any tenderness. Suprapubic palpation will detect a distended bladder and may cause pain in the presence of cystitis but it is by rectal and vaginal examination that the pelvic viscera are most easily palpated. On rectal examination the uniform, elastic and movable prostate affected by benign hypertrophy can be distinguished from the hard, nodular, often immovable gland without a median groove characteristic of carcinoma. Thickening of the lower end of the ureter is suggestive of tuberculosis and infiltration at the base of the bladder may be present with a vesical carcinoma. Lymphatic spread from a carcinoma of the bladder or prostate may be palpable as thickening in the lateral pelvic space. Vaginal examination will also allow palpation of the bladder base and lateral pelvic space as well as of the other pelvic organs; in the fornices the lower end of each ureter can sometimes be felt if it is diseased or contains a calculus. The testes should be examined, particularly for evidence of tuberculosis of the epididymis.

The urine itself should be examined. Macroscopic inspection may reveal clots, which can be studied by floating them in the urine diluted with water in a flat tray. Their shape may suggest the source of bleeding; thus, clots formed in a renal pelvis may be triangular in shape while those formed in a ureter are likely to be thin and 'worm-like'. Microscopy of the urine is more revealing but it must be carried out on a fresh specimen. The presence of red-cell casts is

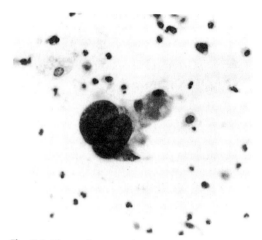

Fig. H.1. Clumps of transitional carcinoma cells in the urine in a case of carcinoma of the bladder. (*Dr J.O.W. Beilby, Middlesex Hospital.*)

pathognomonic of glomerular bleeding. Large numbers of oxalate crystals may indicate a tendency to oxalate stone formation; the much rarer crystals of cystine are diagnostic of cystinuria, with its strong tendency to the formation of calculi. The finding of clumps of transitional epithelial cells (*Fig.* H.1) is suggestive of carcinoma or papilloma of the bladder and is an indication for formal cytological examination of the urine. Rarely fragments of renal papillae may be seen, sometimes with the naked eye, in papillary necrosis associated with chronic interstitial nephritis. The presence of leucocytes is not very helpful as they are likely to be found not only in bacterial infections but also in tuberculosis, tumours and benign prostatic hypertrophy.

Further investigation of haematuria should usually include plain X-rays of the abdomen, ultrasound scanning of the urinary tract and, in many cases, intravenous and retrograde urography; cystoscopy can rarely be omitted unless there is strong evidence of a glomerular lesion causing the bleeding. The latter investigation will reveal not only tumours and other lesions of the bladder but, even if the bladder is normal, may help to locate the site of bleeding if bloodstained urine is seem issuing from one ureteric orifice.

The main causes of haematuria are summarized in *Table* H.1.

Renal causes of haematuria

Haematuria can follow *trauma* of any degree of severity. A history of an accident or a blow or kick to the lumbar region suggests damage to the kidneys. Even slight injury to the loin, of which there may be no

Table H.1. Causes of haematuria

Renal
Trauma
Tumours
Calculus
Glomerulonephritis
Polycystic kidneys
Tuberculosis
Pyelonephritis
Infarction
Polyarteritis nodosa
Chronic interstitial nephritis
Hydronephrosis
Irradiation nephritis
Hydatid disease
Medullary sponge kidney
Relief of bladder tension

Ureteric
Calculus
Tumours

Vesical
Trauma
Tumours
Prostatic enlargement
Tuberculosis
Calculus
Cystitis
Foreign body
Disease of adjacent organs

Urethral
Urethritis
Calculus
Tumours
Foreign body
Caruncle

General
Drugs
Bleeding disorders

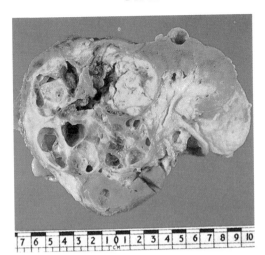

Fig. H.2. Carcinoma of the kidney.

recollection or external sign, can cause haematuria, especially if there is a pre-existing renal lesion. The kidney may be palpable but this must be distinguished from an extravasation of blood in the perinephric tissues. In any case of haematuria following trauma it is essential to distinguish an injury to the kidney from one to the urethra or bladder. With urethral injury the canal may be merely contused or partially or completely ruptured. Blood may be found at the meatus or may be present only in the first portion of urine passed; complete rupture will produce signs of extravasation of urine with an inability to micturate. Evidence of extravasation of urine or of fluid in the peritoneal cavity causing peritoneal irritation may accompany haematuria following injury to the bladder. Evidence, including radiographic, should be sought of fracture of the bony pelvis which may have caused the vesical or urethral injury.

Renal tumours are important causes of haematuria. The commonest presenting symptom in *carcinoma of the kidney* ('hypernephroma') (*Fig.* H.2) is profuse intermittent haematuria. A mass may be felt in the loin and there may be pain in that region resulting from increasing tension or colic from the passage of clots. Occasionally the initial symptom is unexplained fever and polycythaemia or hypercalcaemia may also be found; hypertension is present in about 30 per cent of cases. An intravenous urogram will show deformity of the renal pelvis or calyces but the most useful investigations are CT scanning and renal arteriography; the latter will show a characteristic pattern of vessels in the tumour. In children with *nephroblastoma* (Wilms' tumour) the presenting feature is commonly abdominal distension and a mass is almost always palpable; haematuria occurs later. An *adenoma* of the kidney or an *angioma* at or near the apex of a papilla can cause profuse haematuria. Both are rare and can usually be diagnosed only at surgery or post-mortem, although angiography may sometimes show a tumour 'blush'. *Papilloma* or *papillary carcinoma* of the renal pelvis is uncommon; either may cause profuse haematuria and enlargement of the kidney due to hydronephrosis. Pyelography may show a filling defect in the renal pelvis. Clinically the benign and malignant lesions are indistinguishable although the older the patient the more likely is the tumour to be malignant. *Squamous-cell carcinoma* of the renal pelvis is a very rare cause of slight or moderate haematuria.

Renal calculus seldom causes profuse bleeding but haematuria, and often pyuria, may occur, especially after exercise or the jolting of a journey. An aching pain in the loin is common while the stone remains in the kidney and may be followed by renal

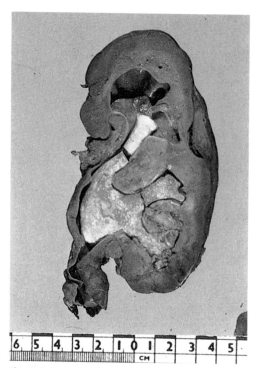

Fig. H.3. Large phosphatic stag-horn calculus of the kidney.

colic if the stone begins to descend down the ureter. This typical very severe pain passes from the loin downwards and forwards to the groin, upper part of the thigh and testicle and is accompanied by a frequent desire to micturate. The previous passage of a small calculus per urethram following an attack of renal colic is an important diagnostic feature. The radiographic diagnosis of ureteric calculus is discussed below (p. 160). A renal calculus may become too large to pass into the ureter and may then cause hydronephrosis·or pyonephrosis with corresponding symptoms including haematuria (*Fig.* H.3).

Glomerular disease is a common and important cause of haematuria, macroscopic or microscopic. *Post-streptococcal glomerulonephritis* is now rare in the Western world but is still common in developing countries where it often follows streptococcal skin infections. The characteristic features are haematuria, producing the typical 'smoky' appearance, and proteinuria, generalized oedema and hypertension. A similar lesion is a common complication of *infective endo-carditis*, in which the glomerular changes are focal and segmental. Careful examination of a fresh specimen of urine will show red cells in a majority of cases of endocarditis and thus is an important diagnostic procedure. In both these conditions the glomerulitis is due to deposition of immune complexes as it is in *shunt*

nephritis associated with infection of shunts used to drain hydrocephalus and in the nephritis occasionally associated with *chronic sepsis. Rapidly progressive glomerulonephritis* is a cause of macroscopic haematuria with loin pain; it causes rapid deterioration and can lead to acute renal failure within a few days. It can occur in Henoch-Schönlein syndrome, cryoglobulinaemia, microscopic polyarteritis, Wegener's granulomatosis and the nephritis associated with the development of antibodies to glomerular basement membrane (*anti-GBM nephritis*). The latter is often associated with pulmonary haemorrhage (*Goodpasture's syndrome*). Another cause of recurrent macroscopic or micro-scopic haematuria is *Berger's nephritis (IgA disease)*. The aetiology is unknown but the episodes of haematuria commonly follow upper respiratory tract infections; the characteristic histological feature is the deposition of IgA in the glomeruli. It predominantly affects children and young adults; when it was first described, the prognosis was thought to be good but it is now known to account for a significant number of cases of chronic renal failure. Nephritis is also a common feature of *Henoch-Schönlein syndrome* which, although occa-sionally severe (*see above*), is more often a relatively benign condition characterized by haematuria with typical purpuric and oedematous skin lesions, arthritis and abdominal pain with intestinal bleeding. A number of hereditary varieties of nephritis can also cause haematuria; of these the most common is *Alport's syndrome* in which a renal lesion, often severe but less so in females, is associated with nerve deafness; the differential diagnosis, which can be made by renal biopsy, includes *familial benign haematuria* in which proteinuria and deafness do not occur and intermittent or persistent microscopic haematuria continues for many years without any deterioration in renal function. Nephritis with haematuria is also a feature of several systemic diseases of which the most important is *systemic lupus erythematosus* (SLE); of the numerous manifestations of this disease, arthritis, cutaneous lesions and hypertension are those most often asso-ciated with nephritis. Haematuria is not one of the typical features of the nephrotic syndrome but some of the causes of the latter, including SLE, produce sufficient glomerular inflammation to cause haemor-rhage. Apart from this, *renal vein thrombosis* which is a recognized complication of the nephrotic syndrome, causes sudden deterioration in renal function together with haematuria, which is often macroscopic. *Postural proteinuria*, i.e. proteinuria occurring *only* in the erect position, is occasionally associated with slight haematu-ria which does not affect the generally good prognosis; also haematuria may occur with the proteinuria associated with *vigorous exercise*—so-called 'jogger's nephritis'.

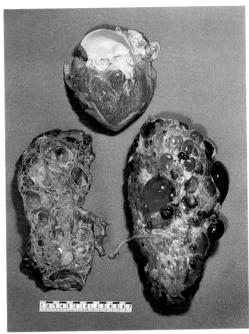

Fig. H.4. Bilateral grossly enlarged polycystic kidneys. Note the associated hypertensive cardiomegaly.

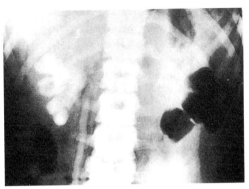

Fig. H.5. Pyelogram of tuberculous right kidney. Note the fine scattered calcification in the upper pole. The calices are dilated and clubbed.

Adult polycystic disease of the kidneys is frequently associated with haematuria, either painless or with clot colic; it can be precipitated by mild trauma. Both kidneys are usually palpable and hypertension is common (*Fig*. H.4). The differential diagnosis includes bilateral hydronephrosis; in the latter haematuria is less common and there will usually be evidence of a lesion of the bladder, prostate or urethra causing obstruction. The pyelographic appearances are quite different; in polycystic disease the calyces are narrow and elongated, quite unlike the dilated pelvis in hydronephrosis.

Haematuria in *renal tuberculosis* is usually slight and is associated with pyuria; occasionally an episode of gross haematuria is the presenting feature. The patients affected are usually young adults who may complain of a dull ache in one loin with occasional exacerbations resembling renal colic. Once the tuberculous focus has ruptured into the renal pelvis the characteristic symptom is increased frequency of micturition both by day and by night even without any involvement of the bladder. The bleeding is rarely increased by exertion, unlike with renal calculus. The thickened lower end of the ureter may be palpable on rectal or vaginal examination and, in males, nodules may be felt in the prostate or seminal vesicles. The cystoscopic appearance of the ureteric orifice may be distinctive. Hydronephrosis may develop in the affec-

ted kidney and intravenous urography will reveal characteristic changes (*Fig*. H.5). The diagnosis can be confirmed by culture of early morning specimens of urine. Other infections of the kidney, such as *acute pyelonephritis*, occasionally cause haematuria.

Vascular lesions of the kidneys can cause haematuria. *Infarction* is usually due to an embolus arising, for example, from a fibrillating left atrium, mural thrombus following myocardial infarction, a large vegetation in infective endocarditis or, very rarely, left atrial myxoma. Infarction can also occur in *macroscopic polyarteritis nodosa*; the diagnosis can be confirmed by arteriography. *Sickle-cell disease* may cause haematuria as a consequence of vascular damage and *aneurysm of the renal artery* and *intrarenal arteriovenous fistula* are also rare causes of haematuria. Accelerated ('malignant') hypertension can cause haematuria, usually microscopic but occasionally macroscopic.

Less common causes of haematuria include *chronic interstitial nephritis* due commonly to the ingestion of analgesics; bleeding may be profuse when there has been recent papillary necrosis. Recurrent bleeding in such a case should, however, prompt a search for transitional-cell carcinoma of the renal pelvis which is a recognized complication of this condition. In *hydronephrosis* likewise haematuria is more likely to be due to an obstructive lesion than to the hydronephrosis itself. *Irradiation nephritis* is a rare cause of haematuria with modern radiotherapeutic techniques as is, in the United Kingdom, *hydatid disease*. *Medullary sponge kidney* is usually symptomless but haematuria and renal colic may occur as a result of calculus formation. *Relief of tension* by the sudden emptying of the bladder in a case of chronic urinary retention may cause bleeding, commonly from the bladder but sometimes from the kidney.

Ureteric causes of haematuria

Ureteric calculus may cause haematuria, either during the descent of the stone or when it becomes arrested without causing complete obstruction to the flow of urine. The diagnosis is usually easy from the history and the character of the pain, accompanied by the increased desire to micturate; but, in some cases, a calculus on the right side may be mistaken for appendicitis. A previous history of the passage of a calculus or of symptoms of renal stone may be elicited. A calculus may become impacted in any part of the ureter, though most commonly in the pelvic portion. Cystoscopy may show swelling and ecchymosis of the ureteric orifice if the stone is near the bladder or occasionally it may be seen projecting from the orifice. Radiographic examination may show an opacity in the line of the ureter, but this should always be confirmed by a stereoscopic radiograph taken with an opaque bougie passed into the ureter or by intravenous urography. Shadows very similar to calculi may be caused by phleboliths or calcified nodes; these are frequently multiple and calcified nodes show variations in density with indistinct outlines but, if single and apparently in the line of the ureter, may cause diagnostic confusion unless investigations are carried out as described above.

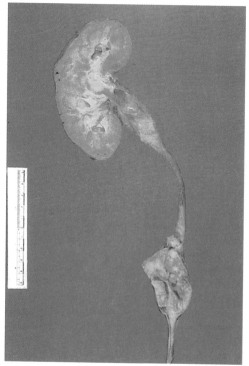

Fig. H.6. Carcinoma of the ureter producing hydronephrosis and treated by nephro-ureterectomy.

Papilloma of the ureter may cause haematuria, even after the removal of the primary disease in the renal pelvis by nephrectomy. For this reason it is usual to carry out complete ureterectomy at the same time as the nephrectomy, if this cause of haematuria is suspected.

Carcinoma of the ureter is rare (*Fig.* H.6); it can be diagnosed by the filling defect in the ureter with dilatation above on ureterography, and by the brisk bleeding which occurs when a ureteric catheter is passed. The differential diagnosis of the negative shadow produced by a tumour in the ureterogram includes a non-opaque calculus and an air bubble.

Vesical causes of haematuria

Intermittent profuse painless haematuria is characteristic of *papilloma* or *papillary carcinoma* of the bladder. Other symptoms which may be present include an urgent desire to micturate or retention of urine due to clot formation in the bladder or, with carcinoma, increased frequency of micturition. Bimanual pelvic examination under general anaesthesia may provide evidence of carcinomatous infiltration of the base of the bladder or of the pelvic lymphatics but an innocent tumour can rarely be felt per rectum. Cystoscopy with biopsy is the essential diagnostic procedure and a malignant tumour will most commonly be seen at the base of the bladder above and lateral to a ureteric orifice. This orifice may be occluded causing hydronephrosis so that a bladder carcinoma may cause renal pain and swelling and, initially, be confused with a renal tumour. A papilloma of the bladder may occur at any age but is rare below the age of 25; a papillary carcinoma is uncommon before the age of 45. Papillomas may be multiple, either from direct implantation or as a result of an inherent tendency of some vesical mucosae to produce multicentric lesions.

Nodular and *ulcerative carcinomas* occur in elderly patients and cause slight but fairly constant haematuria. Other symptoms are commonly present; these include increased frequency of micturition by day and by night and penile pain following micturition. Pyuria is also common. The blood often appears as a few drops at the end of the stream or may be present throughout micturition. Usually the tumour is seen at cystoscopy at the base of the bladder but there is a rare form of adenocarcinoma, derived from the urachus, which occurs at the dome of the bladder.

Sarcoma of the bladder is rare. It occurs in children and, occasionally, in adults and forms a rapidly growing mass, sometimes resembling a bunch of grapes (sarcoma botryoides). *Haemangioma* may occur as a flat lesion or as a solid tumour of considerable size.

Profuse haematuria is common in patients with *prostatic enlargement*, either benign or due to carcinoma. It is, surprisingly, more common with the former. The patient is usually over the age of 50 and there is typically a history of gradually increasing frequency of micturition. The enlarged prostate can be felt on rectal examination and, at cystoscopy, dilated veins ('prostatic varices') can be seen over the surface of the gland.

Vesical tuberculosis occurs most commonly in young adults. Persistent frequency, slight haematuria and pus in a urine sterile on normal culture are very suggestive features although, as indicated above, such symptoms can occur in renal tuberculosis before bladder infection has occurred. Evidence of tuberculosis elsewhere, in the lungs or the genital organs, may be found. Cystoscopy will reveal evidence of vesical infection. Examination of a spun specimen of urine may reveal acid fast bacill, but usually confirmation of the diagnosis depends on culturing the mycobacterium using specific culture technique.

Vesical calculus also causes slight haematuria, usually as a few drops in the terminal urine. In the absence of cystitis, increased frequency of micturition by day but not by night is typical. There may be pain of a pricking character in the glans penis after micturition and sometimes a history of sudden stoppage of the urinary stream. The patients are usually male and there may be a history of previous renal or vesical calculi. Stones are often visible in radiographs, except for urate calculi which contain little calcium and are, therefore, not very radio-opaque. Haematuria is more likely to be associated with the spiky oxalate calculi than with the smooth urate and phosphate calculi.

Acute cystitis is often accompanied by haematuria; the diagnosis will usually be obvious on other grounds. There is, however, a form of haemorrhagic cystitis in which bleeding predominates over other symptoms; a similar form of haemorrhagic cystitis is a complication of treatment with cyclophosphamide.

Simple ulcer of the bladder may occur as a result of severe localized inflammation in acute cystitis.

Chronic interstitial cystitis (Hunner's ulcer) in the female is often associated with painful haematuria and increased frequency of micturition from a small contracted bladder.

Radiation cystitis following pelvic radiotherapy is characterized by multiple telangiectases in the vesical mucosa which may bleed severely. Vesical *schistosomiasis* causes slight haematuria and other symptoms similar to those of vesical tuberculosis. There is likely to be a history of residence in an endemic area such as Iraq and the neighbouring countries, Egypt and much of Africa. The typical ova of schistosoma haematobium may be found in the urine and at cystoscopy so-called 'sandy patches' may be seen; these consist of numerous ova without any inflammatory reaction. *Foreign bodies* may be introduced into the bladder by accident or design and cause bleeding; their presence will be revealed by cystoscopy or radiography.

Haematuria may occur as a result of spread of *disease of neighbouring viscera* to the bladder. Carcinoma of the uterus, vagina, rectum or pelvic colon can all invade the bladder, usually at a late stage of the disease. Of more clinical importance is the haematuria which may result from contact of an acutely inflamed appendix with the bladder wall and consequent localized cystitis; this is obviously a possible source of diagnostic confusion but the other symptoms of acute appendicitis are likely to be present and rectal examination will reveal the inflammatory process in the right side of the pelvis. More rarely, acute salpingitis or pelvic abscess can cause haematuria by a similar mechanism. Haematuria can also be caused by direct spread of inflammation from tuberculous or dysenteric ulceration of the intestines or from diverticulitis of the colon; the latter is particularly likely to lead to a vesico-colic fistula with pneumaturia as well as haematuria.

Urethral causes of haematuria

Lesions of the urethra can cause blood to appear spontaneously at the meatus as well as haematuria. Such conditions include *acute urethritis, calculus*

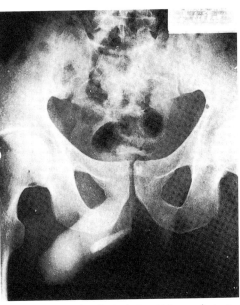

Fig. H.7. Elongated urethral calculus which caused retention of urine visible on a plain X-ray of the pelvis.

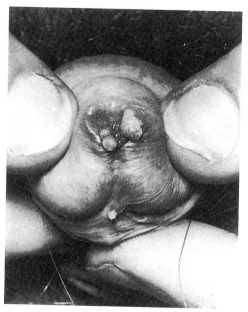

Fig. H.8. Papillomas of the urethra projecting from the external urinary meatus.

(*Fig.* H.7), *papilloma* (*Fig.* H.8) and *carcinoma*. *Angiomas* are rare but can bleed heavily; there may be other similar lesions elsewhere in the body. *Foreign bodies* may be introduced into the urethra as a form of sexual excitement and, in females, a *caruncle* at the urethral orifice may cause haematuria which is inexplicable unless a thorough physical examination is carried out.

General causes of haematuria

Several drugs have been implicated as causes of haematuria but *anticoagulants* are the only ones of practical importance. Haematuria is common if control is poor but it must be remembered that, in such a patient, the fact that he or she is on anticoagulants does not exclude other causes of haematuria; bleeding apparently induced by anticoagulant therapy can be the first sign of renal carcinoma. Finally *thrombocytopenia* and disorders of platelet function can cause haematuria as can *haemophilia*, *Christmas disease* and, occasionally, *scurvy*. In these conditions the diagnosis will usually be clear on other grounds.

Peter R. Fleming

Heartburn

Heartburn is a burning restrosternal discomfort, sometimes amounting to pain, which is usually perceived to originate in the high epigastrium and radiate towards the neck. Many who suffer from it find difficulty in describing the quality of the sensation, for which adjectives such as burning, hot, sharp, rough or acid are not wholly satisfactory but most sufferers will readily identify the discomfort as being felt up and down the midline anterior chest. The location of the discomfort may therefore be of greater value than descriptions of its quality in distinguishing heartburn from other varieties of chest pain.

Heartburn characteristically develops after meals and may be brought on by changes in posture such as stooping or lying down. Relief follows sitting or standing up, and may be derived from antacids and by drinking water, milk, tea or any other non-acid fluid.

The sensation of heartburn originates in the lower oesophagus and is produced by gastro-oesophageal reflux. Sensitivity of the oesophageal mucosa to acid appears to be at the root of the sensation, although the sensory mechanisms are ill-defined. Oesophagitis—inflammation and erosion of the oesophageal mucosa—is often present, but not invariably so and it is important to appreciate that many patients with troublesome heartburn have no detectable abnormality of the oesophageal mucosa on fibreoptic oesophagoscopy.

Gastro-oesophageal reflux occurs to some degree in most healthy individuals. Excessive gastro-oesophageal reflux, which is likely to produce troublesome heartburn, arises most commonly from malfunction of the lower oesophageal sphincter. Loss of the normal anatomical relationships of the gastro-oesophageal junction, as occurs in hiatus hernia, impairs sphincter function to some extent but in most individuals with excessive gastro-oesophageal reflux there is an intrinsic failure of the sphincter to remain tightly closed and relax only in response to swallowing.

The term gastro-oesophageal reflux disease is currently fashionable to embrace all clinical manifestations and pathological consequences of excessive gastro-oesophageal reflux. Heartburn is its principal and classical symptom. It is clear, however, that many healthy individuals suffer occasional heartburn which they can sometimes relate to dietary indiscretions or overindulgence in alcohol or tobacco. Heartburn is also extremely common during pregnancy. Gastro-oesophageal reflux, and thus heartburn, may also occur in association with gastric and duodenal disorders such as peptic ulceration and acute gastritis, and as an element in the 'dyspepsia' provoked by drugs such as non-steroidal anti-inflammatory agents. The possibility of gastric or duodenal disease should be given particular consideration when upper abdominal discomfort and heartburn coexist.

R. C. Heading

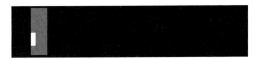

Indigestion

Indigestion is a very common symptom with a prevalence in the community approaching 30 per cent. *Dyspepsia* is synonomous with indigestion which may be defined as upper abdominal discomfort amounting even to pain, nausea, vomiting, heartburn and distension. Severe abdominal pain should not be regarded as either dyspepsia or indigestion. In the past dyspepsia was regarded as indicative of a chronic peptic ulcer. The advent of radiology soon revealed that the majority of patients with indigestion did not have an ulcer and the term 'X-ray negative' dyspepsia was introduced. This term has been superseded since the introduction of fibreoptic endoscopy and a better description for dyspepsia which is not of ulcer origin is 'non-ulcer dyspepsia'. Of all patients with dyspepsia, only 25 per cent have ulcers visible either on endoscopy or radiology. Of those with non-ulcer dyspepsia, about 15 per cent have no identifiable lesion in the gastrointestinal tract. The cause of their dyspepsia is not always apparent and the term 'nervous dyspepsia' has been introduced but this must be used with caution and only in patients in whom a clearly disturbed emotional state can be defined. Indeed, recent work suggests that there is no clear psychological or psychiatric disturbance present in many patients who have no organic cause for their dyspepsia.

Indigestion frequently accompanies the symptoms of nausea and vomiting. The causes of dyspepsia are listed in Table I.1. Under these circumstances the cause for dyspepsia readily becomes apparent. The discussion of indigestion in this section relates to abdominal discomfort which has been present for 1 month or more and is not precipitated by exertion or relieved by rest. The mechanism of dyspepsia is probably varied and can often be accounted for on the basis of a local lesion in the upper gastrointestinal tract, or some more generalized disturbance of gastroduodenal and small intestinal motility. In some circumstances, it is possible that gastric hyperacidity contributes. An attractive concept is that there is a functional disturbance of the upper gastrointestinal tract mediated by gastrointestinal peptide hormones. Although many hormones can be shown to have an influence on gastroduodenal motility, it has not been possible to identify any particular pattern of hormone disturbance which correlates with indigestion. This interesting hypothesis remains to be proven.

Table I.1. Causes of dyspepsia

Common
Duodenal ulcer
Gastric ulcer
Gastritis
  Immune
  H. pylori
Gastric cancer
Hiatus hernia
Oesophageal reflux
Irritable bowel syndrome
Drugs
  Tobacco
  Alcohol
  Non-steroidal anti-inflammatory agents
  Theophylline
  Digoxin
  Iron preparations
  Cytotoxic agents
  Antibiotics
Gallstones
Psychiatric disorder
  Tension/anxiety
  Depression
Food intolerance
Aerophagy
Pregnancy

Less common
Other gastric tumours
  Lymphoma
  Leiomyosarcoma
Other gastric diseases
  Sarcoidosis
  Tuberculosis
  Eosinophilic granuloma
  Syphilis
Adult hypertrophic pyloric stenosis
Hypertrophic gastritis (Ménétriér's disease)
Duodenitis
Other duodenal diseases
  Webs
  Polyps
  Cancer
  Lymphoma
Chronic pancreatitis
Pancreatic cancer
Crohn's disease
Colonic cancer
Metabolic diseases
  Diabetes mellitus
  Uraemia
  Suprarenal insufficiency
  Hyperthyroidism
  Hypothyroidism
  Hypercalcaemia
Coeliac disease
Tropical sprue
Chronic hepatitis
Pulmonary tuberculosis
Congestive cardiac failure
Autonomic neuropathy
Gastric and small intestinal motility disorders
Giardiasis
Strongyloidiasis

Peptic ulcer dyspepsia

Both *duodenal* and *gastric ulcers* may present primarily with indigestion. The classical symptomatology of a *duodenal ulcer* includes intermittent pain felt in the epigastrium or to the left or right of the midline which is located precisely by the patient, and which is worse before meals and relieved by either taking food or antacids. Patients with a *gastric ulcer* tend to be older, and have relatively more pain; this occurs sooner after meals than in a duodenal ulcer and is less likely to be relieved by food or antacids. A characteristic feature of peptic ulcer disease is the periodicity with long periods when the patient is free of pain. Other features include flatulence, nausea and vomiting. One of the more reliable features of distinguishing a duodenal ulcer is the presence of pain which wakes the patient at night. Unfortunately, these characteristic features of gastric and duodenal ulcers are encountered in less than 50 per cent of patients. Not only are the symptoms of peptic ulcer disease non-specific and non-sensitive for the diagnosis of peptic ulcer as opposed to non-ulcer dyspepsia, but in addition it is not possible to distinguish reliably on history between a gastric and a duodenal ulcer. Furthermore, the physical examination is unreliable and there is much evidence to indicate that the physical sign of epigastric tenderness on light or deep palpation is insensitive, not specific, and has a low predictive value for peptic ulcer disease or indeed any other form of gastroduodenal disease. The only certain way of diagnosing either a gastric or duodenal ulcer is either by endoscopy or less reliably by a barium meal.

Non-ulcer dyspepsia

There are many causes for dyspepsia or indigestion which are not due to peptic ulcer disease. These include *gastritis* and *duodenitis, gastric carcinoma, drug dyspepsias, disease* of the *biliary tract, pancreatic disease* and a variety of other less common causes.

Gastritis can present in an identical way to peptic ulcer with indigestion, epigastric discomfort, flatulence, nausea and vomiting. There may or may not be epigastric tenderness. Two types of gastritis are recognized; fundal gastritis, which is commonly associated with pernicious anaemia, and antral gastritis. The latter form of gastritis appears in children and adults and there is a strong association with the organism *Helicobacter pylori*. Although a medical history is a poor discriminator between peptic ulcer and non-ulcer dyspepsia, upper abdominal pain which is not severe, is aggravated by food or milk, and in the absence of night pain, vomiting or weight loss is suggestive of gastritis.

Gastric cancer has become less common in the western world in the past decade. A short history of indigestion in a patient over the age of 55 which is accompanied by marked weight loss and persistent pain with no periodicity should raise the suspicion of a gastric cancer. All patients with indigestion which persists without remit for over a month should be investigated by gastroscopy or by a barium meal.

Indigestion is a poor guide to *cholelithiasis* and *cholecystitis*. The classic features of gallbladder disease include moderate to severe pain felt below the right costal margin or the epigastrium, passing round to the back on the right and occasionally felt in the right scapular area. The pain is of variable intensity. If the stone impacts in the cystic duct the pain will be of a colicky nature. A stone impacted in the common bile duct gives rise to more persistent unremitting pain and will usually be accompanied by the presence of jaundice, dark urine and pale stools. A syndrome of intermittent jaundice, dark urine and pale stools with episodic fever and pain is a feature of stone in the common bile duct associated with infection. There is no characteristic gallbladder dyspepsia. Fatty food dyspepsia is a common symptom in clinical practice but has no relationship to gallbladder disease. Indeed, the mechanism of fatty food dyspepsia remains unclear.

Chronic pancreatitis is usually associated with more severe pain rather than indigestion. However, some patients do have a mild, continual discomfort in the upper abdomen which is accompanied by a bloated feeling and quite often pain which is felt radiating through to the back in the upper lumbar area. *Carcinoma of the pancreas* may present in a similar way with a much shorter history and the appearance of such symptomatology together with the onset of diabetes mellitus in an elderly person should raise the suspicion of a pancreatic cancer. One of the confusing ways in which *cancer of the colon* may present is with the symptomatology suggestive of an upper gastrointestinal disease and it must be borne in mind that should a patient who has presented with indigestion be shown to have no obvious upper gastrointestinal tract disease, a barium enema may well prove to be a fruitful investigation for revealing the cause of the illness.

Drug-induced dyspepsia is not uncommon, particularly with the widespread use of non-steroidal anti-inflammatory agents which is a well-recognized cause of indigestion and upper gastrointestinal discomfort. Other causes include antibiotic therapy, other analgesic agents, prednisolone, digitalis, and theophylline preparations.

Alcoholic gastritis is a well-recognized condition which usually presents with early morning nausea and vomiting but may be accompanied by epigastric discomfort or the latter may be the only feature of this illness. *Smoking* too is a cause of indigestion and may contribute to the dyspepsia of patients with alcohol abuse.

Indigestion is a well-known presenting feature of *pulmonary tuberculosis*. Although this is a less common disease in developed countries, it still occurs with sufficient frequency for a chest X-ray to be necessary in all patients who have dyspepsia which cannot be explained by obvious upper gastrointestinal disease. Two infections in the upper gastrointestinal tract are important causes of indigestion, *giardiasis* and *strongyloidiasis*. Giardiasis is a particularly important condition because it may present with upper abdominal discomfort, nausea and loss of appetite in the absence of diarrhoea or obvious malabsorption. The symptomatology may be quite irregular and misleading unless a specific search is made for giardia in the stool or in duodenal aspirates.

Patients with the *irritable bowel syndrome* frequently have a dyspeptic feature to their illness. Thus, although it is characteristic to have lower abdominal pain associated with a feeling of incomplete evacuation and flatulence with discomfort relieved by the passage of stools, indigestion and upper abdominal discomfort are now recognized with increasing frequency as a feature of this, as yet, unexplained syndrome.

Poor dentition or loss of teeth has been ascribed as the cause for indigestion; but the evidence is poor and it is likely that these are only uncommon causes of upper gastrointestinal discomfort. Similarly it remains controversial to what extent *stress* and other personal factors are responsible for indigestion. A number of well conducted studies suggest that stress is not a major factor in the genesis of dyspepsia and 'functional' dyspepsia is not a condition which can be diagnosed with any ease or certainty. Similarly, it is difficult to demonstrate convincingly a relationship between food and indigestion. Many patients will claim that certain *foods* cause indigestion but such studies that have been undertaken of these patients suggest that only a small number have verifiable specific food intolerance. It is also difficult to know whether the excessive consumption of tea or particularly coffee has a role in the genesis of indigestion. Dyspepsia, nausea and vomiting may be prominent in the early months of *pregnancy.*

Less common causes of dyspepsia include *Crohn's disease, tuberculosis* or *sarcoidosis* of the stomach, *adult hypertrophic pyloric stenosis, hypertrophic gastritis* (Ménétrier's disease). Duodenal lesions which are rare but which may present with indigestion include an *annular pancreas, duodenal polyps* or *webs* and *cancer in the duodenum.*

Indigestion is a common and important symptom in clinical medicine. With careful history and a judicious use of investigations, it is possible to find a cause for many of the patients. However in an appreciable number of patients no clear cause can be identified. It is important that these people should not be falsely diagnosed as either having some psychiatric illness or food intolerance. Usually the dyspepsia subsides over a period of months or years with supportive therapy from the physicians and a judicious use of drugs acting on the upper gastrointestinal tract.

Ian A. D. Bouchier

Infertility

Involuntary infertility may be defined as a failure to conceive when regular intercourse has taken place over a reasonable length of time. After one year 80 per cent of women have managed to conceive and a further 5–10 per cent of pregnancies will have occurred at the end of the second year. The remainder 10–15 per cent of all marriages can be considered as barren requiring infertility investigations.

A precise diagnosis of the cause for infertility is often difficult, and although there are many well-defined conditions which give rise to it, there are a number of cases in which no definite cause can be found. In many patients the failure is due to a number of minor 'infertility factors' unimportant in themselves, but which in aggregate may result in inability to conceive.

In 20 per cent of patients a single cause for the infertile marriage will not be found; factors in the male or female alone may account for a further 30 per cent in each and in the rest both partners may have factors producing infertility. If the examination of a fresh ejaculate of semen shows it to be within normal limits with regard to volume >2 ml and number of spermatozoa (above 20 million per ml), 50 per cent showing motility, and in addition there are not more than 20 per cent of abnormal forms, the husband should not be regarded as subfertile. Repeated checks are not necessary if a fertile specimen has been produced, although the male counts vary much according to the stage of health. Any systemic illness of which fever is a feature depresses spermatogenesis. The effect appears over the weeks after the start of fever and attains its maximum within 6 weeks. Spermatogenesis may not return to normal for several months. If live spermatozoa can be found in the cervical mucus after coitus about the time of ovulation the male can be excluded as the cause of the infertile marriage. Four active progressing spermatozoa to the high-power field is the average. Providing there are some spermatozoa in the ejaculate it is not possible to say that a man is infertile no matter how low the semen count. Pregnancies seem to occur in the face of very low counts.

The causes of male infertility are as follows:

1. Male factors

Impotence, oligospermia, necrospermia, aspermia, varicocele, premature ejaculation and failure to ejaculate during coitus.

Constitutional diseases associated with infertility are: tuberculosis, diabetes mellitus, anaemia, syphilis, alcoholism and dietetic deficiences. *Over-work* of a mental nature can affect sperm production. *Endocrine factors* such as hypothyroidism or hyperthyroidism. Hypopituitarism suggested by underdevelopment of the penis, and obesity. Drugs less commonly cause infertility but they include anti depressants and sulphasalazine.

Men suffering from the chromosomal anomaly, Klinefelter's syndrome (XXY), have undeveloped genitalia with small soft testes and are infertile. Between 3 and 5 per cent of men are infertile because of autoimmunization with circulating antibodies to their own spermatozoa.

The commonest cause of complete sterility in the male is blockage of the epididymis due to gonorrhoea or other infection. Atrophy of the testes following orchitis as a complication of mumps (about 10 per cent of males contracting mumps develop orchitis) may be responsible. The male with both testes undescended is almost certainly sterile.

Failure of the male to ejaculate during coitus is a not infrequent cause when both partners are found to be normally fertile.

2. Female factors

LOCAL

a. *Gross pelvic lesions*
Absence of uterus, vagina, Fallopian tubes or ovaries
Closure of hymen, vagina or cervix
Fibroids, polyps, carcinoma
Tuberculosis of the endometrium
Endometriosis
b. *Cervical lesions*
Cervicitis
Abnormalities of cervical secretion
Stenosis of cervix
c. *Tubal lesions*
Inflammatory lesions
Tuberculosis
Rudimentary tubes
d. *Vaginal and vulval lesions*
Dyspareunia
Vaginismus

e. *Endocrine lesions*
Gross disorders:
Fröhlich's syndrome, myxoedema
Simmonds' disease
Adrenocortical tumours
Menstrual disorders:
Polysystic disease of the ovaries
Amenorrhoea, hypomenorrhoea
Metropathia
Anovular menstruation
Ovarian failure (primary or secondary)
f. *Chromosomal anomalies*
Turner's syndrome (XO)
Super-female (XXX)

GENERAL

Anxiety
Old age
Obesity
Anaemia
Nutritional: vitamin A, B deficiency
Occupational

3. Combined Male and Female factors present together

a. Subnormal sperm count with abnormal cervical secretion in the female
b. Incomplete penetration
c. Lack of seminal plasma
d. Defective germ plasma

The above lists shows that some causes of infertility are primary, others secondary. Thus absence of the uterus or infantile uterus means primary sterility, while failure to ovulate, salpingitis, etc. may occur in women who have had children, and only secondarily because sterile on account of these lesions.

Congenital lesions

Some of the congenital lesions are diagnosed easily, such as *imperforate hymen, absence of the vagina,* or *stenosis of the cervix,* while absence of the essential organs often requires an anaesthetic in order that a bimanual examination may be made satisfactorily or for a laparoscopic examination to be undertaken.

Patients with gonadal agenesis suffer from too short stature, sexual infantilism and primary amenorrhoea. Two-thirds have an XO chromosome complement and other features of Turner's syndrome. Laparoscopy reveals small elongated ovarian streaks of fibrous tissue in place of ovaries. Male pseudo-hermaphrodites with testicular feminization and a 46XY chromosome karyotype have the appearance of a female of normal height and often well-developed breasts. They have absent or scanty axillary and pubic hair, a short, blind vagina, absent uterus and tubes and suffer from primary amenorrhoea. Bilateral testes may be in the abdomen or in the inguinal canal. The cause is end-organ resistance to testosterone or androgen insensitivity. Other members of the family are liable to have the condition.

Acquired lesions

The differential diagnosis of acquired lesions can only be made by complete examination of the patient. This includes a clinical examination of the vulva, vagina, cervix and pelvic organs by inspection and bimanual vaginal examination; an assessment of the Fallopian tubes or salpingography or by injecting dye into the uterus and seeing if it spills out of the fimbrial ends into the pelvis; detection of ovulation by basal body temperatures or blood progesterone levels in the second half of the cycle or the finding of a secretory endometrium on biopsy; a study of the cervical mucus at ovulation time with special regard to the presence or absence of actively progressing sperms in it after intercourse.

Blockage of the Fallopian tubes

This occurs as the result of past salpingo-oophoritis. It can be demonstrated by insufflation of the tubes via the uterus with carbon dioxide (Rubin's test). It can also be demonstrated by injecting into the uterus and tubes a water-soluble substance that is radio-opaque. Radiographs are taken under a fluorescent screen and image intensifier. The tubes may appear to be blocked as the result of spasm (*Fig.* I.1). An alternative investigation and the method of choice is pelvic laparoscopy. This affords an opportunity to study the condition of all the pelvic organs, to see adhesions if they are present and to note if methylene blue dye injected into the uterus comes out freely from the fimbrial ends of the tubes and spills into the pelvis.

When the man's sperm count is adequate and the woman's Fallopian tubes are patent, attention should be paid to the Simms–Hühner *post-coital test*. Mucus is aspirated from the cervical canal at the time of ovulation following intercourse the night before or the morning of the test. The mucus is placed on a slide, covered with a coverslip and examined under the high power of the microscope. There should be at least two, and normally five or more, motile sperms progressing in straight lines across the high power field. A negative postcoital test may be due to abnormal sperm production, inadequate intercourse, failure to ejaculate or hostile cervical mucus.

Endocrine causes of infertility

Endocrine causes are common. Pregnancy is not possible during periods of amenorrhoea because of failure to ovulate. Women who suffer from oligomenorrhoea have their fertility reduced. It is rare for women who menstruate regularly at monthly intervals not to ovulate although some of them do have a defective corpus luteum and a poor or short luteal phase of the menstrual cycle. If an early menopause is suspected serum FSH will be more than 25 u/l and LH more than 25 u/l. The occurrence and timing of ovulation can be verified by taking the temperature by mouth first thing on waking before moving or getting out of bed. The basal temperature in the first half of the cycle is slightly lower than it is in the second half. A characteristic drop followed by a rise at mid-cycle indicates ovulation which, in most women, takes place about 14 days

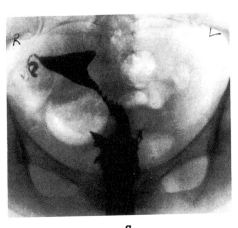
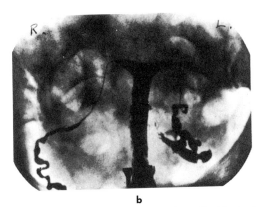

a   b

Fig. I.1. *a*. Radiograph of the uterus and Fallopian tubes after intrauterine injection of radio-opaque solution. The left tube is closed at the uterine end. The right tube is stenosed: *b*. Radiograph of the uterus and Fallopian tubes after intrauterine injection of radio-opaque solution. The left tube is patent. The right tube is closed at its outer end.

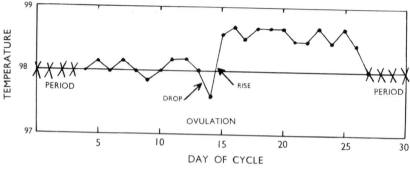

Fig. I.2. A typical basal temperature chart.

before the onset of the next period (*Fig.* I.2). Ovulation is followed by the formation of a corpus luteum and this can be diagnosed by a raised serum level of progesterone (between 2.8 and 64 nmol/l) usually carried out on the 21st day of a normal cycle. Following ovulation the uterine endometrium undergoes the histological changes of the secretory (or progestational) phase which become more and more marked up to the time of the onset of menstruation. The stromal cells enlarge and the glands become tortuous with deep serrations in their walls and secretion in their lumina. A biopsy of the endometrium toward the end of the cycle will show these changes if ovulation has taken place. The finding in the cervix of the typical clear elastic mucus in mid-cycle is further proof that ovulation has taken place. Mid-cycle cervical mucus can be drawn into threads up to 10 cm in length. This is known as *spinnbarkeit* and is an indication of high oestrogen secretion by the ovary. 'Ferning' is another effect of high mid-cycle oestrogen. The mid-cycle cervical mucus is spread thickly on a glass slide, rinsed in distilled water and allowed to dry. A characteristic pattern resembling a fern leaf forms on the slide. Later in the cycle absence of spinnbarkeit and ferning indicate a progesterone effect and functioning corpus luteum.

Although serum levels of hormones are accurate measures of ovarian function, smears of vaginal cells in the hands of the expert cytologist also reflect the hormonal changes. The length and character of the luteal phase can be assessed by doing serial smears. A short luteal phase may prevent a fertilized ovum from embedding in the endometrium.

Other causes of infertility

Generalized endocrine disorders such as hypo- or hyperthyroidism, adrenocortical hypo- or hyperfunction and uncontrolled diabetes may result in infertility. Polycystic ovarian disease (Stein–Leventhal syndrome)

is characterized by bilaterally enlarged polycystic ovaries, secondary amenorrhoea or oligomenorrhoea and infertility. About half the patients are hirsute and many are obese. Infertility is due to failure of ovulation. The enlarged ovaries can be felt on bimanual vaginal examination but are best diagnosed on ultrasonography or laparoscopy. Blood levels of LH are raised and there may be an increased excretion in urine of androstenedione or dehydroepiandrosterone.

N. Patel

Jaundice

Types

Jaundice may be caused by a raised conjugated or unconjugated bilirubin. Unconjugated hyperbilirubinaemia may be due to excessive production of bilirubin (haemolysis), reduced uptake of bilirubin or a failure of conjugation by the liver. Conjugated hyperbilirubinaemia results from hepatocellular damage or obstruction of the bile ducts, either within the liver (intrahepatic cholestasis) or of a major bile duct (extrahepatic obstruction jaundice). Jaundice is also often classified into pre-hepatic (haemolytic), hepatic and extrahepatic types. Clues as to the cause of jaundice may be obtained from the history and physical examination (*Tables* J.1, J.2).

Investigations of jaundice

The simplest investigations are liver function tests and urine examinations; typical abnormalities are shown in (*Table* J.3). The liver enzymes, aspartate (AST) and

Table J.1.   History of jaundice

Haemolytic (Pre-hepatic)	Hepatic		Obstructive (Post-hepatic)
Family history Racial origin Drug history Symptoms of anaemia	Flu symptoms Rashes Joint pains Contact with jaundice Blood transfusions Infections Drug history Alcoholic intake Previous jaundice	Viral	Abdominal pain Pale stools Dark urine Itching

Table J.2.   Physical signs associated with jaundice

Haemolytic (Pre-hepatic)	Hepatic		Obstructive (Post-hepatic)
Splenomegaly, reduced stature	Dupuytren's contractures Parotid enlargement	Alcohol	Scratch marks Mass in abdomen
	Spider naevi Gynaecomastia Testicular atrophy Loss of hair Red hands	Endocrine	Gallbladder In a patient with obstructive jaundice if the gallbladder is palpable the cause is unlikely to be gallstones—Courvoisier's law
	White nails Ascites and oedema	Hypoproteinaemia	
	Bruising	Prothrombin time prolonged	
	Splenomegaly Veins around umbilicus	Portal hypertension	

Table J.3.   Liver function tests and urinalysis in jaundice

	Unconjugated bilirubinaemia (haemolytic)		Hepatocellular jaundice	Obstructive jaundice
Liver function tests	Direct bilirubin↑ AST ALT ALK—P	normal	Indirect bilirubin↑ AST↑↑ ALT↑↑ ALK—P↑	Indirect bilirubin↑↑ AST↑ ALT↑ ALK—P↑↑↑
Urine tests	Bilirubin 0 Urobilinogen normally not raised		Bilirubin + Urobilinogen ++	Bilirubin +++ Urobilinogen 0

alanine transaminase (ALT), are normally contained within the liver cells, and are released during hepatocellular necrosis whereas alkaline phosphatase is excreted into the biliary system and rises in obstructive jaundice.

There is no bilirubin present in the urine of patients with pre-hepatic (haemolytic) jaundice because unconjugated bilirubin is tightly bound to albumin and is not filtered at the glomerulus. On the other hand, conjugated bilirubin is water-soluble and stains the urine dark in hepatocellular and obstructive jaundice. Urobilinogen is produced by bacteria in the gut and is normally partially reabsorbed into the portal vein, taken up by hepatocytes and re-excreted in bile. When the liver is damaged hepatic extraction is less efficient and the concentration of urobilinogen in plasma, and hence in the urine, rises. The presence of urobilinogen in the urine is thus a test of liver function and one of the earliest signs of recovery from hepatocellular jaundice is the disappearance of urobilinogen from the urine as it is again removed by the liver. In complete obstructive jaundice, urobilinogen is absent from the urine as there is no bilirubin in the gut.

All patients presenting with cholestatic jaundice should undergo ultrasound examination of the liver (*Figs* J.1–J.3). This examination is cheap, without complication and in experienced hands accurate at determining whether or not there is obstruction to the biliary tree. If equivocal the ultrasound should be repeated as jaundice deepens and it may then be obvious that there is indeed an obstructive cause. In

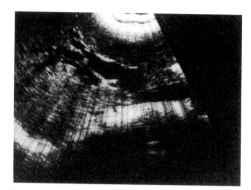

Fig. J.3. Longitudinal ultrasound in obstructive jaundice due to stone in common bile duct.

addition to demonstrating dilated ducts, expert ultrasonographers can often show the cause of obstruction but this is unreliable and definitive cholangiography should be performed in all circumstances. The radiologist may also show dilatation of the gallbladder, cholelithiasis and secondary deposits within the liver. Furthermore the pancreas, portal and hepatic veins and the spleen can be visualized. Once the diagnosis of extra hepatic biliary obstruction has been made the bile ducts should be outlined by cholangiography. This is best done by endoscopic retrograde cholangiopancreatography (ERCP) in which a side-viewing endoscope is passed into the second part of the duodenum (*Fig.* J.4). The ampulla of Vater is first seen and ampullary tumours can be identified and biopsied. The bile duct and pancreas are cannulated and opacified using radiological contrast material. The procedure is successful in approximately 90 per cent of patients in expert hands and, as well as defining the cause of the obstruction, the endoscopist has the capacity to

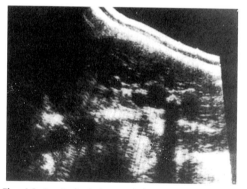

Fig. J.1. Longitudinal ultrasound showing dilated common bile duct and intrahepatic ducts.

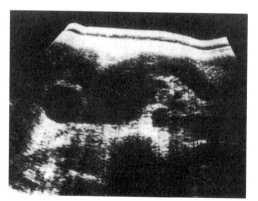

Fig. J.2. Longitudinal ultrasound showing a carcinoma of the head of the pancreas as a cause of obstructive jaundice.

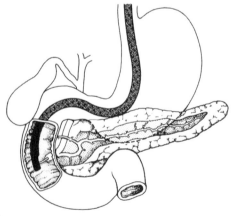

Fig. J.4. Cannulation of the ampulla of Vater via the fibreoptic endoscope.

relieve obstruction by extracting calculi or placing stents within strictures. When the endoscopist fails to achieve a diagnosis the alternative approach to ERCP is to perform a percutaneous transhepatic cholangiogram (PTC) using a 'skinny' needle (*Fig.* J.5). This is a technically easier procedure in patients with a dilated biliary tract but is also successful in approximately 60 per cent of patients with non-dilated bile ducts.

A rational approach to the investigation of jaundice is illustrated in *Fig.* J.6. Liver biopsy confirms the presence of hepatocellular damage, but the differentiation of large duct obstruction from intrahepatic cholestasis may be difficult (*see later*) (*Fig.* J.7).

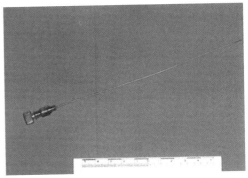

Fig. J.5. Percutaneous transhepatic cholangiography needle.

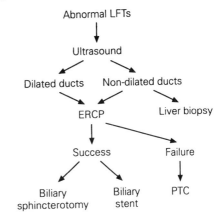

Fig. J.6. Investigation of cholestatic jaundice.

Unconjugated hyperbilirubinaemia

1.   Increased production of bilirubin:
a. Inefficient marrow production
b. Increased breakdown (haemolysis)
     Haemoglobinopathies
     Antibody-mediated
     Drug-induced
2.   Decreased uptake of bilirubin into the liver:
     Gilbert's disease
3.   Decreased conjugation of bilirubin in the liver:
     Crigler–Najjar syndrome
     Neonatal jaundice
     Drugs
     Lucey–Driscoll syndrome

Increased production of bilirubin without haemolysis (shunt hyperbilirubinaemia)

Very rarely inefficient marrow production of haemoglobin results in increased amounts of unconjugated bilirubin being released into the circulation ('early label' bilirubin). The red cells manufactured, however, have a normal life span. This is a rare primary condition and also occurs in a number of other causes of inefficient erythropoiesis, for example anaemia.

Increased production of bilirubin due to haemolysis

Most commonly, unconjugated hyperbilirubinaemia results from haemolysis, either caused by an *intrinsic* abnormality of the red cells or due to the development of an abnormal mechanism of destruction (*extrinsic*). The general investigation of patients with a haemolytic anaemia is summarized below.

a. Evidence of intravascular haemolysis:
     Haptoglobins
     Haemoglobinaemia
     Haemoglobinuria
     Haemosiderinuria
     Methaemalbuminaemia

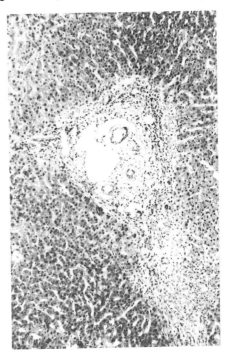

Fig. J.7. Liver histology of large duct obstruction showing expansion of portal tracts and proliferation of bile ducts.

b. Evidence of increased marrow production:
   Reticulocytosis
   Skeletal changes
   Marrow hyperplasia
c. Evidence of red cell damage:
   Fragmented forms
d. Evidence of shortened red cell life:
   Radioactive labelling of red cells

A. EVIDENCE OF INTRAVASCULAR HAEMOLYSIS

Haemoglobin released during intravascular haemolysis is normally attached to haptoglobin, the levels of which are usually reduced in chronic haemolytic states. However, levels may also be reduced by chronic liver disease and increased non-specifically in a number of connective tissue disorders. Haemoglobinaemia associated sometimes with methaemalbuminaemia, haemoglobinuria and haemosiderinuria, provide incontrovertible evidence of intravascular haemolysis, but are frequently absent in chronic haemolytic anaemias.

B. EVIDENCE OF INCREASED MARROW PRODUCTION

In a compensated anaemia, reticulocytosis with a raised mean corpuscular volume (MCV) is common. Increased marrow activity results in skeletal changes which are frequent in thalassaemia and sickle-cell disease but rare in other conditions. The skull of such patients demonstrates a thickened vault and the diploe are widened. Bony trabeculae arising at right angles to the diploe may produce a 'hair-on-end' appearance (*Fig.* J.8). The bones of the limbs have a widened narrow cavity with a coarse trabecular pattern.

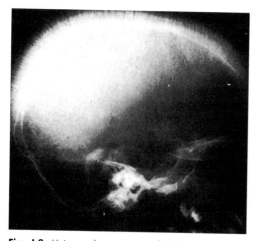

Fig. J.8. Hair-on-end appearance of skull in patient with thalassaemia.

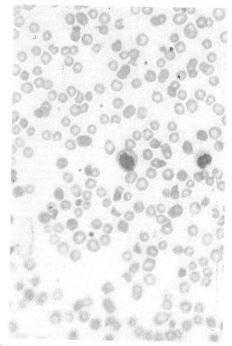

Fig. J.9. Fragmented red cells seen in intravascular haemolysis.

C. EVIDENCE OF RED CELL DAMAGE

Fragmented forms may provide evidence of increased red cell destruction (*Fig.* J.9).

D. EVIDENCE OF SHORT RED CELL LIFE SPAN

The standard clinical test to detect shortened red cell survival is to tag the patient's cells with a radioactive chromium and measure the decline in plasma radioactivity.

Intrinsic defects of the red cells leading to increased haemolysis

a. Spherocytosis
b. Elliptocytosis
c. Enzyme defects
d. Haemoglobinopathies
   i. Sickle-cell disease
   ii. HbSC disease
   iii. Thalassaemia
e. Paroxysmal nocturnal haemoglobinuria

A. CONGENITAL SPHEROCYTOSIS

This is a dominantly inherited defect which probably affects the red cell membrane, rendering it more permeable to sodium. The red cells are spherical rather than the usual biconcave shape and are more readily haemolysed in hypotonic saline (red cell fragility test). The patient usually presents in late childhood, even though jaundice may have been noticed in early childhood; often jaundice is first identified in the teens. Splenomegaly is common; bile pigment stones are frequently formed and patients occasionally present with obstructive jaundice. The disease is characterized by crises of worsening anaemia and jaundice caused by increased haemolysis due to infection. The diagnosis is usually straightforward with splenomegaly, a family history and a typical blood film, but it must be remembered that spherocytes may be a feature of a number of different types of haemolytic anaemia, and that occasional mild cases of congenital spherocytosis do not present until adulthood. Splenectomy is usually followed by long-term remission of symptoms.

B.   CONGENITAL ELLIPTOCYTOSIS

This is another Mendelian dominant disorder and it is usually asymptomatic, without haemolysis. Occasionally a compensated haemolytic anaemia occurs but anaemia sufficient to produce jaundice is extremely rare.

C.   ENZYME DEFECTS

A wide variety of enzyme defects in the red cells have been described which produce a haemolytic anaemia and jaundice. These are usually recessively inherited. Suspicion of this type of disorder is always aroused if haemoglobin electrophoresis and osmotic fragility are normal in a patient with haemolytic anaemia. Splenectomy in these patients is not beneficial. The commonest of these disorders is pyruvate kinase deficiency whose clinical features are more variable in severity, but similar to congenital spherocytosis.

D.   HAEMOGLOBINOPATHIES

The primary structure of haemoglobin is four polypeptide chains attached to a haem molecule. Normal adult haemoglobin has two identical alpha and two identical beta polypeptide chains attached to the haem. In the fetus the haemoglobin has two gamma chains replacing the beta chain (fetal haemoglobin) and a small proportion of adult haemoglobin has two delta chains instead of two beta chains (A2 haemoglobin).

A2 and fetal haemoglobins will increase in disease affecting the beta chains. There are two basic types of haemoglobinopathies. One involves qualitative defects affecting one of the polypeptide chains (usually a single amino acid substitution). The other is a quantitative defect affecting the production of the whole of one long chain.

Qualitative defects of haemoglobin

Single amino acid substitution in the polypeptide chain of haemoglobin commonly produces no disease. Occasionally an amino acid substitution produces a haemolytic anaemia and *sickle-cell anaemia* provides the model for such an illness. Patients who inherit one abnormal gene only (heterozygous or sickle-cell trait) are usually only mildly affected and do not become jaundiced. Patients who inherit two sickle-cell genes have sickle-cell disease. An amino acid substitution in the beta chain produces an unstable haemoglobin molecule which polymerizes into the reduced state into long chains which distort the red cells into a sickle shape. Sickle-cell disease affects blacks predominantly and is characterized by jaundice, anaemia and skeletal changes. Although the clinical manifestations are variable, life for the patient is frequently punctuated by crises of spontaneous sickling in the circulation which produces severe abdominal and bone pain and a high fever. Although splenomegaly is common in children, repeated infarcts of the spleen usually lead to atrophy in adulthood. Gallstones are again common, which may produce obstructive jaundice. The prognosis is serious with many patients still dying either as children or in young adult life.

The diagnosis is made by haemoglobin electrophoresis which will show increased amounts of fetal and A2 haemoglobin, and by demonstrating *in vitro* sickling of cells by addition of a reducing agent to the blood (sickle-cell test).

Sickle-cell HbC disease

Although heterozygous sickle-cell disease is usually asymptomatic, if another abnormal haemoglobin (e.g. HbC) is inherited from the other parent haemolysis and jaundice may result, although the disease is usually milder than homozygous sickle-cell disease. Similar clinical symptoms may occur with the inheritance of one thalassaemia gene and one sickle-cell gene.

Qualitative defects of haemoglobin leading to increased haemolysis (thalassaemia)

The homozygous inheritance of defective production of alpha chains of haemoglobin is not compatible with life. The heterozygous inheritance of defective production of alpha or beta chains (alpha or beta thalassaemia minor) produces a mild abnormality rarely giving rise to jaundice. β-Thalassaemia major is the only homozygous thalassaemia syndrome which may occasionally result in jaundice. This condition is found most commonly in patients originating from the Mediterranean littoral, and anaemia dominates the clinical picture. Hepatosplenomegaly and marked skeletal changes may also occur. The blood picture is similar to that of iron deficiency anaemia and the diagnosis is made by an increased amount of circulating fetal haemoglobin on haemoglobin electrophoresis. For reasons that are unknown, A2 haemoglobin is not usually increased. There is often an *increased* resistance to haemolysis in hypotonic saline (osmotic fragility test).

E.   PAROXYSMAL NOCTURNAL HAEMOGLOBINURIA

Episodes of haemolysis may be accompanied by slight jaundice in this rare condition. Diagnosis can be made by the characteristic history of red urine, which contains haemoglobin, following sleeping. The abnormal haemolysis of the red cells can be demonstrated if the plasma is acidified (Ham's test).

Extrinsic factors leading to increased haemolysis

Autoimmune haemolytic anaemia
Cold haemoglobinuria
Drugs and chemicals
Glucose-6-phosphate dehydrogenase deficiency
Miscellaneous

A.   WARM ANTIBODY AUTOIMMUNE HAEMOLYTIC ANAEMIA

In this condition antibody coats the patient's red cells at 37°C resulting in increased extravascular destruction. The antibody is usually of the IgG class and incomplete (i.e. does not directly cause agglutination or haemolysis). This antibody can be detected by the direct Coombs' test where the addition of antibody to IgG in *in vitro* causes the red cells to agglutinate. Spherocytes are often present in the blood film, the white count may be raised and occasionally the platelets are low, producing purpura. In acute acquired haemolytic anaemia the patient is usually a child with a palpable spleen, jaundice, anaemia and the constitutional symptoms of fever, vomiting and prostration. In the chronic form the onset is insidious, usually in adults but again the patient is usually jaundiced (in 75 per cent of cases) and has a palpable spleen. In half the patients with acquired haemolytic anaemia no cause for the antibody formation is found, but in the rest it is secondary to a number of diseases, most importantly disseminated lupus erythematosus, but also recticulo-

endothelial malignancy, leukaemia and sarcoidosis. Resolution of the symptoms usually occurs following treatment with corticosteroids or, occasionally, splenectomy.

B.   COLD ANTIBODY AUTOIMMUNE ANAEMIA

Occasionally antibody is produced which reacts with the patient's red cells at low temperatures. Depending on the thermal range of the antibody a continuous mild haemolytic anaemia may occur punctuated by paroxysms of intravenous haemolysis with abdominal pain, rigors, transient jaundice and splenomegaly, which may be provoked by exposure to the cold. Cold antibody haemolytic anaemia is frequently secondary to viral infections and malignancy.

C.   DRUG AND CHEMICAL-INDUCED HAEMOLYSIS

Some chemicals (e.g. arsenic and naphthalene in moth balls) produce haemolysis and jaundice which is directly dose related. Haemolysis may occur with other drugs; this is unrelated to the dose and occurs in a few susceptible individuals only (*Table J.4*). The two important mechanisms for producing haemolysis in this situation are an associated deficiency of glucose-6-phosphate dehydrogenase in the red cell, or the production of auto-antibodies, often directed against the drug attached to the red cell membrane, which acts as a hapten. In this type of haemolysis the blood film often shows spherocytes and red cell inclusions (Heinz bodies).

Glucose-6-phosphate dehydrogenase deficiency is common in black people and inhabitants of the Mediterranean littoral. This enzyme helps to maintain

Table J.4.   Drugs occasionally causing haemolysis

a.   In glucose-6-phosphate dehydrogenase deficient subjects

Antimalarials, e.g.	primaquine
	mepacrine
Antibacterials	chloramphenicol
	sulphonamides
Nitrofurans	nitrofurantoin
Quinines	quinidine

b.   Auto-immune

Penicillin
Sulphonamides
Quinine and quinidine
Methyldopa
Mefenamic acid
Sulphasalazine
Para-aminosalicylic acid

the cell concentration of reduced glutathione which is turn stabilizes the haemoglobin molecule.

Favism is a disorder characterized by intravascular haemolysis and jaundice occurring when a glucose-6-phosphate dehydrogenase deficient patient, usually a child from the Mediterranean region, ingests fava beans or inhales the pollen.

Similar episodes occur when the patient is exposed to certain drugs (*see Table* J.4). Haemolysis ceases when the older population of red cells containing less of the enzyme is destroyed.

Autoimmune drug-induced haemolysis is particularly common with methyldopa where the direct Coombs' test is positive in 20 per cent of patients taking the drug, but haemolysis occurs in less than 1 per cent.

D. OTHER CONDITIONS CAUSING HAEMOLYSIS

Acute haemolysis with jaundice may occur with various infections, e.g. malaria and gangrene, and more mildly with viral pneumonia (usually due to cold agglutinins). It may also follow a mismatched blood transfusion or occur in a severely burned patient.

Excessive exercise, particularly on hard roads, may also lead to episodes of intravascular haemolysis (*march haemoglobinuria*).

Microangiopathic haemolytic anaemia is the name given to a group of conditions characterized by haemolysis in association with fragmentation of red cells as they pass through blood vessels damaged by clots. Evidence of disseminated intravascular coagulation is common. Such haemolytic anaemias are present in thrombotic thrombocytopaenic purpura, malignant hypertension, disseminated neoplasia and in association with uraemia in children (the haemolytic uraemic syndrome).

Unconjugated hyperbilirubinaemia caused by impaired uptake of bilirubin into the liver

GILBERT'S DISEASE

There is some debate as to whether this condition exists or whether it represents the upper range of a normal population distribution of unconjugated bilirubin. However, most would accept that it is a common familial condition in which there is a mild degree of unconjugated hyperbilirubinaemia. It is probably inherited as a Mendelian dominant with variable penetrance. The degree of jaundice varies and often increases following an infection or a period of fasting. Episodes of deepening jaundice may be associated with recurrent,

vague abdominal pains. Mild decreases in red cell life span and the liver's ability to conjugate bilirubin are associated with a failure of transport of unconjugated bilirubin into the liver cell. The diagnosis is made by excluding liver disease. It may be confirmed by fasting the patient or by giving an intravenous injection of nicotinic acid. Both of these manoeuvres result in an increase in serum bilirubin concentrations. They are rarely necessary since the diagnosis is usually obvious.

Unconjugated hyperbilirubinaemia caused by impaired conjugation in the liver

1.   CRIGLER–NAJJAR SYNDROME

In this familial condition there is a deficiency of the liver enzyme glucuronyl transferase, which conjugates bilirubin. In severely affected patients (Type 1) death occurs in the neonatal period. A partial enzyme defect with some conjugated bilirubin in the bile and a better prognosis (Type 2) also occurs.

2.   NEONATAL JAUNDICE

Glucuronyl transferase matures shortly before birth and newborn babies, particularly if premature, will become mildly jaundiced. This may be severe in conditions increasing the bilirubin load (e.g. haemolysis) and kernicterus may result. Occasionally prolonged neonatal jaundice is thought to occur in breast-fed babies due to the presence of pregnandiol in the milk.

3.   LUCEY–DRISCOLL SYNDROME

Unconjugated bilirubin has rarely been described in pregnancy due to hormonal inhibition of bilirubin conjugation.

Conjugated hyperbilirubinaemia

HEPATIC CAUSES

The hepatic causes of conjugated bilirubinaemia may be divided into acute hepatocellular damage, associated with considerable increases in hepatic enzymes and a short clinical course, and chronic damage where the course is protracted and there are lesser rises in liver enzymes.

a.   *Acute liver damage*
   i.   Viral hepatitis
   ii.   Non-viral infections
   iii.   Drug induced
   iv.   Poisons
   v.   Fatty liver of pregnancy

b. *Chronic liver damage*
   i.   Cirrhosis
   ii.   Tumours
      a.   Primary
      b.   Secondary
c. *Infiltrations*
   i.   Reticuloendothelial tumours
   ii.   Amyloidosis

Acute hepatic damage

Causes of acute hepatic damage may produce a mild clinical illness or a severe disease (fulminant hepatic failure) with encephalopathy and a high mortality, when cerebral oedema, renal failure and a bleeding diathesis are frequent causes of death.

VIRAL HEPATITIS

Although a large number of viruses occasionally cause hepatitis (including rubella, Coxsackie B, herpes simplex, yellow fever virus and cytomegalovirus) the four common ones are virus A, virus B, virus C and infectious mononucleosis. The recognition of serological markers for hepatitis A and B have revolutionized our understanding of viral hepatitis and it is now realized that many patients with these infections do not become jaundiced.

Virus A (infectious hepatitis)

This is an endemic infection with a short incubation period (15–20 days) causes by a 27 nm RNA virus. Outbreaks usually occur in conditions of poor hygiene or overcrowding. The usual transmission is faeco-oral. Patients present with malaise, anorexia, fever and a rapid onset of jaundice. There is often a vague ache in the right upper quadrant and the liver is enlarged and tender. The spleen may also be palpable. Complete recovery is usually within a few weeks, although relapses may occur. Occasionally patients develop deep jaundice due to intrahepatic cholestasis during the convalescent period. The diagnosis is confirmed by the demonstration of IgM antibody to the virus.

Virus B (serum hepatitis)

This infection has a longer incubation period and arthralgias and rashes may occur in the prodromal period. It is caused by a DNA virus which has an outer coat derived from the host cells and an inner core. Originally only blood transmission was recognized, e.g. blood transfusions, transfusions of blood products (haemophilic globulin), or by needles contaminated with blood in drug addicts and in tattooing. Outbreaks in renal dialysis units produced by blood contamination have caused great concern in the past. The disease is also venereally transmitted as the virus is present in semen. Hepatitis B is common in homosexuals, 10 per cent of whom have serological markers of past infection. Asymptomatic carriers of hepatitis B infection are very frequent in certain parts of the world, e.g. Africa, China and parts of the Mediterranean. These patients may transmit the infection vertically from mother to offspring. The diagnosis of virus B hepatitis is made by the detection of the presence of surface antigen (HbsAg) in the bloodstream. For the patient to be infectious whole virus (Dane) particles must be present in the bloodstream' and the presence of e antigen is a marker for this.

The majority of patients develop an acute viral hepatitis and this is associated with formation of antibodies and clearance of the virus from the liver. Other individuals failed to clear the virus, become carriers and some of these develop chronic liver disease. Patients with persistent hepatitis B virus infection are at risk of developing primary hepatocellular carcinoma.

Patients with known chronic hepatitis B infection may suffer an acute exacerbation of hepatitis due to a coincident infection with the delta virus which secondarily infects only patients with chronic HB hepatitis.

Virus C (non-A non-B hepatitis)

Patients may present with a typical history of viral hepatitis but without evidence of infection with the usual hepatotrophic viruses. At least two types of non-A non-B are recognized. One has a short incubation period and is contracted by transfusion with blood or its products, Virus C. The other is sporadic, has a longer incubation period and is probably contracted by the orofaecal route, Virus E. It has a particularly bad prognosis in pregnant women.

Hepatitis C is characteristically a milder illness than HBV but leads to chronic liver disease in a high proportion of individuals.

Infectious mononucleosis

Up to 15 per cent of patients with glandular fever develop jaundice. The clinical picture is characteristic with malaise, sore throat, skin rashes, lymphadenopathy and splenomegaly. Atypical mononuclear cells are found in the peripheral blood and the test for heterophile antibody (Paul–Bunnell) is usually positive.

Yellow fever

This is a zoonosis and is transmitted to man from a primate pool by the mosquito in tropical Africa, the

Caribbean and South America. The incubation period is short (3-4 days) with a sudden onset of rigors, jaundice and abdominal pain. Its course may be fulminant with renal failure and a bleeding diathesis.

NON-VIRAL INFECTIONS

Relapsing fever

This condition is caused by a spirochaete of the Borrelia group of bacteria and is characterized by jaundice and a fever of up to 40 °C which normally lasts for 4-5 days and then remits. The epidemic form of the disease is usually caused by lice and is common during periods of famine. An epidemic infection is usually transmitted by the tick and is common in the Far East, Africa and America.

Leptospirosis

The spirochaete *L. icterohaemorrhagica* infects a variety of small animals and man contracts the disease by bathing in water contaminated with infected urine. The disease is biphasic with an initial illness a few days after exposure, with a temperature, meningism and prominent myalgias and conjunctivitis. Recovery may occur, or after a week the patient may develop widespread bruising, jaundice and occasionally renal failure. *Leptospira icterohaemorrhagiae* is transmitted by rats' urine, mainly to agricultural and sewage workers, and produces a severe form of the disease where jaundice and renal failure are particularly likely to occur.

Other bacterial infections

Jaundice may complicate any septicaemic illness. Occasionally an infected thrombus in the portal vein may occur (portal pyaemia) following an acute infection in the area drained by the portal system, e.g. appendicitis. The signs of a portal pyaemia are severe prostration, a swinging pyrexia and jaundice.

DRUG-INDUCED ACUTE HEPATIC DAMAGE

Drugs either produce predictable dose-related hepatic necrosis, e.g. paracetamol, or more commonly, damage is produced unpredictably in only a few of the patients exposed to this drug and unrelated to its dosage. There are two basic patterns of liver damage, either acute hepatic cellular necrosis with features identical to viral hepatitis, or intrahepatic cholestasis. It is not possible to give an exhaustive list of drugs producing hepatocellular damage (*Table* J.5) and a high index of suspicion should exist in any jaundiced patient who is taking drugs.

Table J.5.   Drug-induced hepatic damage
Those drugs in italics are the commonest causes of liver damage

	Acute hepatic necrosis	Cholestasis
Paracetamol	+	
Dextropropoxyphene	+	+
Halothane	+	
Tetracycline	+ (in pregnancy)	
Erythromycin estolate		+
Penicillin	+	
Sulphasalazine		+
Nitrofurantoin	+	
Pheniramine maleate	+	
Piperazine	+	
Isoniazid	+	
Rifampicin	+	
Para-aminosalicylic acid	+	+
Chlorpromazine		+
Monoamine-oxidase inhibitors	+	
Methyldopa	+ (? cirrhosis)	
Quinidine	+	
Perhexiline	+ (? cirrhosis)	
Chlorpropamide		+
Phenytoin	+	
Propylthiouracil	+	+
Oral contraceptives		+
Anabolic steroids		+

Paracetamol

Paracetamol overdose is the commonest cause of fulminant hepatic failure in Britain. Hepatic damage is dose-related but death has been reported with amounts as low as 7.5 g. Following ingestion paracetamol is metabolized to a toxic intermediate which is scavenged by glutathione. When glutathione stores are exhausted the metabolite binds covalently to the membrane of hepatocytes causing cell death. Chronic alcoholics whose microsomal enzymes are reduced and whose glutathione stores tend to be depressed are at increased risk following the overdose. Nausea, vomiting and abdominal pain develop within 12–36 hours and jaundice develops 2–3 days later. In severe cases this leads to liver failure with coagulopathy and encephalopathy. A very characteristic feature of paracetamol poisoning is the development of renal failure.

Halothane

Halothane is a very safe anaesthetic but there is an undoubted small incidence (0.003 per cent) of serious acute hepatic necrosis following the use of the drug, which may lead to fever, jaundice and death. Inadvertent repeated use in patients who were previously jaundiced following exposure to halothane results in recurrence of the patient's jaundice. Halothane hepatitis is more common after repeated exposures, particularly in obese patients. Jaundice associated with pyrexia usually occurs 2 weeks after initial exposure but only 10 days after subsequent administration. Halothane should not be reused in patients who have suffered a febrile illness and abnormal liver function tests after a previous anaesthetic with this agent.

Oral contraceptives

The older oral contraceptives containing a relatively high concentration of oestrogen occasionally led to a mild cholestatic jaundice. These individuals are particularly prone to develop cholestasis in pregnancy. In addition the older contraceptives also had a tendency to cause the Budd–Chiari syndrome and a variety of tumours within the liver, in particular benign adenomas. The newer contraceptives, which contain much lower concentrations of oestrogens, are much safer and rarely cause these complications.

Anabolic steroids

The C17-alpha-alkalated-substituted testosterones, e.g. norethisterone and norethanandrolone, produce a dose-related cholestasis by a similar mechanism to the oral contraceptive.

Chlorpromazine

An unpredictable cholestatic jaundice may occur in 1 per cent of patients within a month of starting treatment with this drug. Eosinophilia and mitochondrial antibodies are frequently found in the bloodstream. The patient itches, has pale stools and dark urine. Three-quarters of patients recover on withdrawal of the drug but a few develop prolonged cholestasis resembling primary biliary cirrhosis (see later).

Cytotoxic drugs

A variety of such drugs cause jaundice and liver damage, e.g. methotrexate. However, the primary conditions for which these drugs are administered are often a cause for jaundice.

INDUSTRIAL TOXINS

These are only rarely a cause of jaundice in man. Most seem to act by inhibiting protein synthesis. *Carbon tetrachloride* and less commonly other volatile hydrocarbons produce acute hepatocellular necrosis and jaundice within 1–2 days of exposure. Renal failure, pancreatitis, pulmonary oedema and death may also occur. Dicophane (DDT) and trinitrotoluene (TNT) also occasionally produce hepatic necrosis.

A cholestatic jaundice has been described following accidental ingestion of flour contaminated by diaminodiphenyl methane (so-called 'Epping jaundice', after the place where the outbreak occurred).

Amanita

Ingestion of as little as three wild mushrooms of the Amanita species may be fatal. Abdominal pain and diarrhoea occur within 18 hours of ingestion followed 3 days later by the development of fulminant hepatic failure and jaundice.

ACUTE FATTY LIVER OF PREGNANCY

This condition occurs shortly before or after delivery and is frequently fatal. The cause is unknown but histology shows microvesicular fatty droplets in the liver cells.

Chronic liver damage—cirrhosis

Cirrhosis is defined as diffuse fibrosis with nodular regeneration of the liver which destroys the normal spatial relationship of the lobules. It is classified as micronodular, macronodular or mixed, depending on the size of the nodules. The condition may be suspected in cases of jaundice where the liver is firm and palpable, although sometimes it is shrunken and impalpable. The stigmata of chronic liver disease (*Table* J.2) are often present and the spleen may be enlarged because of portal hypertension. Oedema and ascites are caused by a combination of portal hypertension, sodium retention and hypoalbuminaemia. Hepatic encephalopathy may occur, with a sweet musty odour to the breath (caused by mercaptans originating from gut breakdown of methionine), a flapping tremor (asterixis), disorders of the sleep rhythm and then frank unconsciousness. A chronic form of encephalopathy with slowness and psychiatric changes may also occur. Jaundice is a relatively late complication of cirrhosis and many patients with compensated cirrhosis have relatively normal liver function tests.

Causes of cirrhosis

1. ALCOHOLIC LIVER DISEASE

2. INFECTIONS
  a. Viral (HBV, HCV)
  b. Bacterial (syphilis)
  c. Protozoan (schistosomiasis)

3. CHRONIC ACTIVE HEPATITIS
  a. Lupoid
  b. HBV
  c. Drugs

4. GENETIC DEFECTS
  a. Haemochromatosis
  b. Wilson's disease
  c. Galactosaemia
  d. Glycogen storage diseases
  e. Alpha-1 antitrypsin deficiency

5. BILIARY DISEASE
  a. Long-standing extrahepatic biliary obstruction
  b. Primary biliary cirrhosis
  c. Sclerosing cholangitis
  d. Congenital hepatic fibrosis

6. VENOUS CONGESTION
  a. Cardiac failure
  b. Constrictive pericarditis
  c. Budd-Chiari syndrome

7. JEJUNO-ILEAL BYPASS

1. ALCOHOLIC LIVER DISEASE

There is a strong relationship between the national figures for consumption of alcohol and death from cirrhosis. Women are more susceptible to the effects of alcohol than men, and drinking more than 20 g a day is associated with an increased risk of cirrhosis. In men, over 80 g a day is associated with an increased risk which rises to 25× normal if more than 100 g a day is consumed. Probably steady alcohol consumption for about 10 years is required rather than bouts of drinking. Individual susceptibility is also important as some patients never develop cirrhosis however much they drink. Three types of liver disease are associated with alcohol.

Fatty infiltration does not cause jaundice and does not lead to cirrhosis. *Alcoholic hepatitis* is a clinical syndrome which occurs after a bout of heavy drinking with fever, jaundice and multiple spider naevi. The aspartate transaminase is only mildly elevated but the patient may be deeply jaundiced. The white count is often markedly increased and the prothrombin time may be very prolonged. Such patients have a significant mortality and may later develop cirrhosis, even if they stop drinking completely. Histological changes consist of an acute inflammatory reaction at the portal tract and necrosis of liver cells, often with multiple protein inclusions (Mallory's alcoholic hyaline). These histological changes are seen quite frequently in patients who drink excessive alcohol and are not always associated with the full clinical syndrome of alcoholic hepatitis. In *Zieve's syndrome* alcoholic hepatitis is associated with haemolytic anaemia and hyperlipidaemia in addition to jaundice.

Cirrhosis. Alcohol produces a micronodular cirrhosis and the prognosis is undoubtedly worse if the patient continues to drink. It has been suggested that autoimmune mechanisms, particularly in alcoholic hepatitis, may be important. A combination of alcohol abuse and hepatitis B infection is particularly likely to lead to the development of cirrhosis and strongly predisposes to primary hepatic carcinoma.

2. INFECTIONS

The discovery of markers for hepatitis B and C has demonstrated that these are both important causes of cirrhosis.

Congenital syphilis may produce a pericellular fibrosis but true cirrhosis is uncommon as regeneration nodules do not usually develop.

Schistosomiasis classically produces periportal fibrosis (pipesteam fibrosis) leading to portal hypertension, but cirrhosis may also develop and is thought to be due to associated conditions, e.g. hepatitis B infection which is also very common in these patients.

3. CHRONIC ACTIVE HEPATITIS

Chronic active hepatitis is a consequence of a variety of diseases. The commonest cause worldwide is chronic infection with the hepatitis B virus. A history of drug abuse, homosexuality or exposure to blood products is often elucidated in patients presenting with hepatitis B in the Western hemisphere. Autoimmune chronic active hepatitis (lupoid hepatitis) is an auto-immune disease of women characterized by the presence of circulating smooth muscle antibodies, antinuclear factor and high titres of immunoglobulins (IgG). Chronic active hepatitis may also be due to ingestion of drugs including oxyphenacitin, methyldopa, antituberculous agents or anticonvulsants. Very similar appearances may also be seen in patients presenting with Wilson's disease and the appearances may be indistinguishable from conditions as apparently distinct as primary sclerosing cholangitis.

Chronic active hepatitis presents with malaise, jaundice and eventually with hepatic decompensation. The spleen is frequently enlarged and patients with the autoimmune type commonly have associated arthralgia.

The diagnosis is made by demonstrating abnormal liver function tests, particularly hypertransaminasaemia, which must persist for at least 6 months. There may be evidence of chronic hepatitis B infection, circulating smooth muscle antibodies or antinuclear factor. Liver biopsy reveals an inflammatory infiltrate radiating from the portal tracts and broaching the limiting plates. Fibrosis is almost invariable and may encircle groups of hepatocytes resulting in the formation of rosettes. Frank cirrhosis may be present at the time of diagnosis.

4. GENETIC DEFECTS

a. Haemochromatosis

This is an autosomal recessive disease characterized by increased intestinal iron absorption. The disease is rare in premenopausal women and most patients also abuse alcohol which further increases iron intake. Slate-grey pigmentation develops because of melanin and iron deposition in the skin. Cirrhosis occurs; the liver is invariably enlarged and there is evidence of portal hypertension and hepatic decomposition. Iron deposition in the pancreas causes diabetes mellitus ('bronze diabetes'). Accumulation in other endocrine glands leads to testicular atrophy, gynaecomastia and loss of body hair; hypopituitarism can occur. The diagnosis is

suggested by a high serum ferritin concentration and confirmed by liver biopsy. Primary hepatocellular carcinoma is a relatively common complication and cause of death.

b. Wilson's disease

Wilson's disease is a recessively inherited disease of impaired copper metabolism. Copper accumulates in the liver causing cirrhosis and in the basal ganglia of the brain causing an extrapyramidal neurological syndrome. Patients usually present between the age of 5 and 25 years with either or both liver and neurological disease. The hepatic presentation may be insidious with jaundice and ascites. The liver is usually small and fibrosed. The presentation may alternatively be acute with fulminant hepatic failure and severe haemolytic anaemia.

The diagnosis is made by slit-lamp examination of the eyes when Kayser–Fleischer rings can be demonstrated (*Fig.* J.10). Urinary 24 hour copper excretion is increased and this increases further with penicillamine therapy. In addition serum copper concentrations are increased and caeruloplasmin levels are low. Liver biopsy shows cirrhosis. Copper stains are positive.

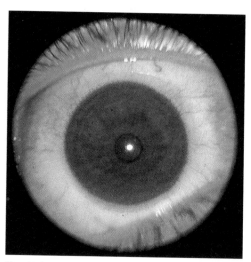

Fig. J.10. Kayser–Fleischer ring in a patient with Wilson's disease, due to deposition of copper-containing pigment in the cornea. (*Courtesy of Dr R. Guiloff.*)

c. Other metabolic errors

All the other metabolic errors leading to cirrhosis and jaundice mentioned above are exceedingly rare. Of the glycogen storage disease, only type IV leads to cirrhosis and jaundice.

d. Alpha-1 antitrypsin deficiency

This autosomally recessively inherited disease may present as a severe neonatal hepatitis or as established cirrhosis in patients below the age of 20 years. There may be associated lung disease characteristically presenting as emphysema, pulmonary fibrosis and respiratory failure. Liver biopsy shows PAS-positive inclusion bodies within hepatocytes.

5. BILIARY DISEASE

Disease affecting the extrahepatic biliary tract, intrahepatic ductules or canaliculi can lead to cirrhosis. Extrahepatic biliary obstruction following trauma to the bile ducts can occasionally cause a secondary biliary cirrhosis; extrahepatic biliary obstruction is considered later. The most important causes of intrahepatic cholestasis are drugs and primary biliary cirrhosis.

Primary biliary cirrhosis predominantly affects middle-aged females and is due to destruction of bile ductules by a cell-mediated auto-immune process. The disease progresses extremely slowly in the majority of patients and usually presents with a cholestatic syndrome comprising itching, pale stools and dark urine. Hypercholesterolaemia is common and may lead to the development of xanthelasmas. The disease is associated with other auto-immune diseases including hypothyroidism, Addison's disease, systemic sclerosis, diabetes and renal tubular acidosis. Other patients present with bleeding oesophageal varices or ascites without a previous history of itching. Physical examination may reveal stigmata of chronic liver disease, jaundice, pigmentation and xanthelasmas. The liver is enlarged and firm; the spleen may be palpable and ascites develop because of portal hypertension.

Primary biliary cirrhosis should be considered in women presenting with cholestatic liver function tests. The mitochondrial antibody is positive in more than 98 per cent of patients. Serum IGM concentrations are increased. A liver biopsy shows chronic inflammatory infiltrate in the portal tract with destruction and paucity of bile ductules. Granulomas may be seen within portal tracts.

Sclerosing cholangitis

Secondary sclerosing cholangitis is a condition in which progressive fibrosis and narrowing of the intrahepatic and extrahepatic biliary tree occurs as a consequence of biliary sepsis. It follows bile duct injury. Primary sclerosing cholangitis is a disease strongly associated with ulcerative colitis. Many individuals are asymptomatic and merely have cholestatic liver function tests. Others present with fluctuating jaundice and in advanced disease this leads to secondary biliary cirrhosis. It is likely that the condition predisposes to the development of cholangiocarcinoma.

6. HEPATIC CONGESTION

True cirrhosis due to heart failure is very uncommon although jaundice may occur in association with heart failure

The Budd–Chiari syndrome

This syndrome is a rare condition in which the main hepatic veins are occluded. It is discussed in the chapter LIVER, ENLARGEMENT OF. The liver scan often shows a central area of uptake which is due to the enlargement of the caudate lobe of the liver whose veins drain separately into the inferior vena cava.

Chronic liver damage—infiltrations

AMYLOIDOSIS

The liver may be involved by infiltration with amyloid, both in the primary disease and where it is secondary to chronic suppuration, myelomatosis or rheumatoid arthritis. Amyloid is an antigen/antibody complex which stains metachromatically with crystal violet and shows birefringence with Congo red staining. The liver is enlarged and rubbery and the patient may show other features of amyloidosis such as nephrotic syndrome, cardiac failure and malabsorption. Hepatocellular failure, and hence jaundice, is rare in this condition, and the diagnosis may be made by liver or rectal biopsy.

Chronic liver damage—tumours

The liver may be affected both by benign and malignant tumours but only the latter will produce jaundice. Secondary deposits are 25 times more common than a primary malignant growth.

PRIMARY HEPATOCELLULAR CARCINOMA

Primary tumours of the liver are a frequent accompaniment of cirrhosis and are said to be found in between 50 and 60 per cent of postmortems in cirrhotic patients. Hepatocellular cancer is particularly common in certain parts of the world especially Africa and China where hepatitis B is the important aetiological agent. Aflatoxin, which is produced by a fungus growing on grain stored in humid conditions, and the now obsolete radiocontrast material Thorotrast (thorium dioxide), are often associated with the development of the tumour.

Primary hepatocellular carcinoma tumours may occur at any age, are five times more common in males than females and should be suspected in any patient with cirrhosis who deteriorates or who develops a lump in the liver. A friction sound is occasionally heard over the tumour and arterial murmurs may be present. The diagnosis is made by finding elevated alpha-feto protein concentrations in the blood, and by liver biopsy.

Primary sarcoma of the liver and malignant haemangiosarcoma

These are extremely rare tumours which may cause jaundice in their terminal stages. Malignant haemangio-sarcoma is associated with exposure to Thorotrast and vinyl chloride.

SECONDARY TUMOURS

The liver is the most frequent site of blood-borne metastatic tumours, whether drained by systemic or portal veins. It is involved in about a third of all terminal cancers, including half of those in the stomach, large bowel, breast and lung. The liver may be normal in size or grossly enlarged with palpable hard deposits. Jaundice may be absent and is usually mild. The serum alkaline phosphatase is often markedly raised.

Reticuloendothelial diseases in the liver

The reticuloendothelial cells of the liver may be involved by any malignant process involving this system. Jaundice is usually mild, and may occasionally be due to haemolysis.

Intrahepatic cholestasis

Drugs
Viral hepatitis
Cirrhosis (occasionally)
Dubin-Johnson syndrome
Pregnancy
Sclerosing cholangitis
Biliary atresia
Recurrent idiopathic cholestasis

In this group of conditions the patient presents with an obstructive jaundice, usually with pale stools, dark urine and itching, but investigations reveal no obstruction of the extrahepatic bile ducts.

DUBIN–JOHNSON AND ROTOR SYNDROMES

These are rare familial benign intermittent conditions producing jaundice with conjugated hyperbilirubin-aemia. In the Dubin-Johnson type the liver is greenish black and contains brown pigment. Jaundice is rarely deep and the alkaline phosphatase remains normal. The diagnosis may be made by a bromsulphthalein retention test in which, after an initial fall, the serum level of BSP rises after 2 hours and remains detectable for 48 hours. The condition is thought to be due to poor transport of conjugated bilirubin into the biliary canaliculi. The Rotor syndrome resembles Dubin-Johnson clinically and biochemically, the main difference being the absence of brown pigment in the liver.

PREGNANCY

Some women develop intrahepatic cholestasis in the last trimester of pregnancy associated with itching, pale stools or dark urine. The mechanism seems similar to that of oral contraceptive-induced cholestasis (see later).

Extrahepatic biliary obstruction

Extrahepatic biliary obstruction can be classified as being due to diseases within the lumen of the bile ducts, those affecting the wall of the ducts or diseases compressing the duct from outside (Table J.6).

Obstruction is usually followed by dilatation of the common bile duct although this may take some time to develop. The architecture of the liver is usually

Table J.6. Causes of obstruction to the bile ducts

Causes within the lumen of the bile ducts
Gallstones
Parasites

Causes affecting the wall of the ducts
Accidental division
Acute pancreatitis
Chronic pancreatitis
Carcinoma of the bile duct
Congenital obliteration of the bile duct

Causes compressing the bile duct or invading it from the outside
Tumours of the pancreas
Peritoneal adhesions
Enlarged portal lymph nodes
Aneurysm of the hepatic artery
Hydatid cysts
Retroperitoneal cysts
Duodenal diverticulum

normal although biopsies show pigmentation, bile plugs and infarcts. Cirrhosis can rarely develop in extremely long-standing obstruction. The patient is clinically jaundiced and the degree of jaundice may be very deep, resulting in a greenish tinge. The urine is dark because of an excess of bilirubin. The stools are pale, clay coloured and bulky because of increased fat content. Biochemical investigations reveal a raised serum alkaline phosphatase concentration, prolonged prothrombin time because of vitamin K malabsorption, hypocalcaemia because of vitamin D malabsorption. The serum albumin concentration is usually maintained until late stages.

The investigation of obstructive jaundice has already been alluded to. The steps involved are ultrasound followed by either endoscopic/or percutaneous cholangiography or liver biopsy.

Causes due to obstruction of the bile duct lumen

A. GALLSTONES

This is the commonest cause of extrahepatic biliary obstruction in the UK. The gallstones are mixed and usually originate from the gallbladder although it is likely that primary bile duct stones may also occur.

The patient presenting with choledocholithiasis and obstructive jaundice may or may not have had a previous cholecystectomy. Severe right upper quadrant pain radiating through to the back usually occurs. Fever associated with rigors is common. The jaundice fluctuates and may disappear completely, presumably because the calculus either passes into the duodenum, or disimpacts from the ampulla, and returns into the lumen of the duct. Another important consequence is gallstone pancreatitis. Occasional patients (usually elderly) present with painless progressive jaundice simulating a carcinoma of the pancreas. Some patients with bile duct calculi have no symptoms and present incidentally with abnormal liver function tests. Examination usually reveals mild jaundice. There may be tenderness of the liver and pyrexia. The gallbladder is usually impalpable.

Investigations reveal cholestatic liver function tests and leucocytosis. Calcified gallstones may be seen on plain abdominal X-ray in 20 per cent of patients with cholelithiasis (*Fig.* J.11). An ultrasound examination may or may not reveal a dilated biliary tree. Stones may be seen within the bile duct although they are often overlooked. Calculi may be identified within the gallbladder although this is uncommon in patients whose jaundice is not caused by choledocholithiasis. Percutaneous transhepatic cholangiography (*Fig.* J.12) and ERCP reveal filling defects within the common bile duct. Gallstones may also be demonstrated by CT scan (*Fig.* J.13).

B. PARASITES

The most important of these is the worm *Ascaris lumbricoides* which is released from an ovum in the duodenum and migrates into the intestinal wall and hence the portal circulation. Worms enter the liver, heart and lungs, migrate in the pharynx and are swallowed. Patients present with haemoptysis, bronchitis and pneumonia; occasionally a worm blocks the bile duct to cause jaundice or act as a nidus for the development of a calculus. Roundworm jaundice is a common cause of icterus in African children.

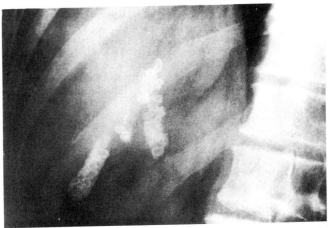

Fig. J.11. Multiple gallstones situated in the gallbladder and common bile duct seen on plain abdominal X-ray. Patient presented with painless obstructive jaundice without any preceding history.

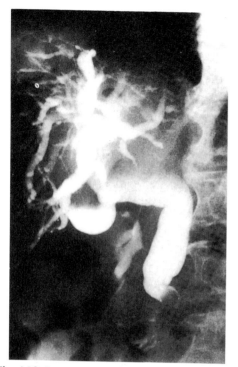

Fig. J.12. Percutaneous transhepatic cholangiogram (PTC) The bile ducts are dilated and the filling defect caused by a stone can be seen at the lower end of the common bile duct.

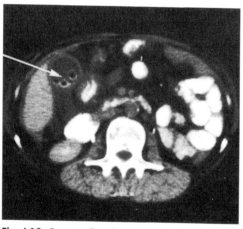

Fig. J.13. Occasionally gallstones may be demonstrated in the course of investigations for other conditions, as in this patient whose CT scan clearly shows the presence of three gallstones situated within the gallbladder (arrowed).

Causes affecting the wall of the bile duct

A.   BILE DUCT TRAUMA

This is usually a consequence of division at operation and is more likely to occur if the surgeon is inexperi-enced, in patients who have had previous biliary operations or who have an inflammatory mass around the bile duct.

B.   CHOLANGIOCARCINOMA

These are epithelial tumours of the bile duct and arise at any point within the biliary tree. Patients present with painless obstructive jaundice and it may be impossible to differentiate the lesion either clinically or by investigation from tumours of the pancreas. One important variant is a tumour arising at the bifurcation of the main left and right hepatic duct (Klatskin tumour). This is an extremely hard, fibrous, but slowly growing tumour and carries a better prognosis than tumours arising elsewhere in the biliary tree.

C.   CARCINOMA OF THE AMPULLA

Tumours arising from the ampulla are uncommon and present with painless obstructive jaundice. They are more slowly growing than carcinoma of the pancreas and should be considered for Whipple's operation.

D.   BILIARY ATRESIA

This presents as deepening obstructive jaundice within 2–3 days of birth. Liver failure develops by the age of 3–6 months. The diagnosis is made by HIDA scanning followed by cholangiography.

E.   SCLEROSING CHOLANGITIS
(*see above*)

Causes compressing the bile duct from outside

A.   CARCINOMA OF THE PANCREAS

The most important cause is carcinoma of the pancreas which invades the common bile duct as it passes through the head of the gland. The patient presents with painless obstructive jaundice although others complain of progressive and continuous pain in the back due to invasion of the coeliac plexus and other retroperitoneal structures. Jaundice is progressive and associated with weight loss. Rigors are unusual.

Examination reveals cachexia, deep jaundice, hepatomegaly and a palpable gallbladder (Courvoi-sier's sign) (*Fig.* J.14). There may be evidence of metastatic spread; in particular there may be supracla-vicular lymphadenopathy or tumour nodules in the umbilicus (Sister Joseph's nodule).

Most tumours arise from ductular epithelium and carry a very poor prognosis. It is important however to remember that some tumours are more amenable to

Malignant obstruction of the extrahepatic bile duct may also be due to enlarged lymph nodes in the region of the porta hepatis and this is usually encountered in patients with breast carcinoma or secondary carcinoma from gastrointestinal origin. Occasionally true secondary deposits occur within the bile duct, usually from melanoma or carcinoma of the breast.

B.   MIRIZZI'S SYNDROME

This is a rare entity in which a stone impacts in Hartmann's pouch. The distended and inflamed gallbladder causes compression and obstruction of the common hepatic duct.

C.   ANEURYSM OF THE HEPATIC ARTERY

This is a rare cause of obstructive jaundice diagnosed by arteriography.

D.   CYSTS

Hydatid cyst is a rare cause of obstruction jaundice; far more commonly these are found incidentally by plain X-ray. Simple cysts or choledochal cysts may also cause obstructive jaundice.

K. R. Palmer

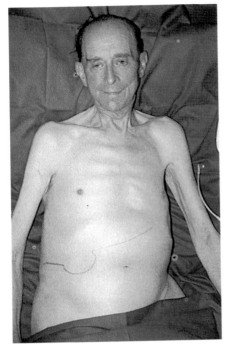

Fig. J.14. Jaundiced patient with enlarged gallbladder. Jaundice due to carcinoma of the pancreas (Courvoisier's sign).

therapy; these include cystadenocarcinoma, a tumour of relatively young women, and apudomas.

Ultrasonography reveals dilated intrahepatic and extrahepatic bile ducts. It may also show a mass within the pancreatic head, which may also be shown on a CT scan. Endoscopy may demonstrate invasion of the duodenum by tumour and the diagnosis can then be confirmed by biopsy. ERCP reveals a stricture within the lead of the pancreas corresponding to a low bile duct malignant stenosis (*Fig.* J.15).

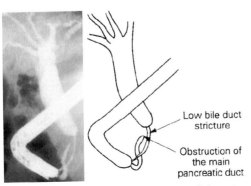

Low bile duct
stricture

Obstruction of
the main
pancreatic duct

Fig. J.15. ERCP showing typical appearances of obstructive jaundice due to pancreatic carcinoma. A stricture in the head of the pancreas is associated with a corresponding stricture in the lower common bile duct.

Jaw, deformity of

The jaws may become deformed by congenital or acquired disease and many of the latter are discussed under the heading JAW, SWELLING OF. The reader should refer to this section for details of pathological conditions causing jaw deformity. Trauma to the jaws may cause deformity due to displacement and this will be maintained if inadequate treatment results in non-union or malunion of the fracture. The majority of conditions, however, to be considered here are of a developmental nature occurring before birth or during the growth period.

CONGENITAL

Cleft palate
Pierre Robin's syndrome
First arch syndrome
Treacher–Collins syndrome

ACQUIRED

Premature synostoses
Achondroplasia
Diseases of the temporomandibular joint
Acromegaly

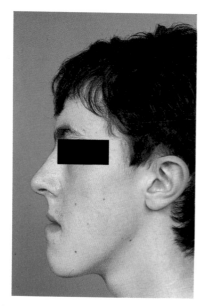

Fig. J.16. Patient exhibiting growth imbalance of the maxilla and mandible.

The mandible forms *in utero* around a rod of cartilage known as Meckel's cartilage, which is replaced by the bone of the mandible, leaving only the condylar cartilage at the temporomandibular joint. Subsequent elongation of the mandible occurs by the growth of this cartilage with secondary ossification and development is completed by surface deposition and resorption.

There is an inherent genetic potential for growth of the facial skeleton, but this is aided by the eruption of the dentition and by the muscular forces placed upon it by the muscles of mastication. A defect in one or more of these mechanisms of growth will produce jaw deformity. However, the majority of cases of jaw deformity arise from a simple imbalance between the growth of the maxilla and the mandible to produce a dental malocclusion (*Fig.* J.16).

Growth of the facial skeleton takes place by sutural growth, surface deposition and remodelling, and cartilagenous growth with secondary ossification. the main stimulus for growth of the maxilla is the growth of the brain, causing an increase in size of the cranial vault and the cranial base to which the maxilla is joined. the cranial base also increases in length by cartilagenous growth at the spheno-occipital synchrondrosis. Growth within the maxilla is stimulated by the development of the nasal capsule and the eyes.

Congenital jaw deformity

CLEFT PALATE

Cleft palate occurs in approximately one in every two thousand live births and is due to a failure of growth and fusion of the palatal shelves in the embryo. Females are affected more than males and there may be an associated cleft of the lip (*Fig.* J.17). There is a genetic disposition to this deformity, but other exogenous factors have been implicated, such as drugs, e.g. phenytoin, or folic acid deficiency. Five per cent of cases of cleft lip and palate are associated with other congenital abnormalities.

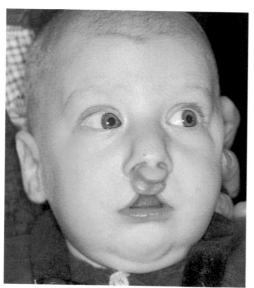

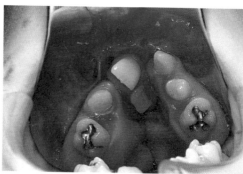

Fig. J.17. *a, b,* Bilateral cleft lip and palate with rotation of the premaxilla.

PIERRE ROBIN'S SYNDROME

This syndrome is thought to be caused by hypoplasia of the mandible, preventing the normal descent of the tongue and thus preventing the fusion of the embryonic palatal shelves. The syndrome is, therefore, characterized by a small mandible, cleft palate and protruding tongue. The baby may present with feeding and respiratory problems, which can be corrected by the construction of a small dental plate and nursing in the supine position.

FIRST ARCH SYNDROME

This syndrome characteristically exhibits a deformed or absent ear, macrostomia and an underdevelopment of the mandibular ramus and condyle. The masticatory muscles on that side are also deficient and there is hypoplasia of the orbit and zygoma on the ipsilateral side (*Fig.* J.18). Other associated abnormalities may be present, particularly of the vertebrae. According to Poswillo, haemorrhage of the stapedial artery in the region of the otic ganglion during uterine development is proposed as the cause.

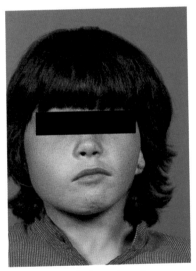

Fig. J.18. Patient with the first arch syndrome.

TREACHER–COLLINS SYNDROME

This is an inherited autosomal dominant condition affecting the facial skeleton in a similar way to the first arch syndrome, but the abnormalities are bilateral and symmetrical. Due to the poor development of the zygomatic arches, prominent nose and small jaw, many of the patients have a fish-like appearance.

Acquired jaw deformity

PREMATURE SYNOSTOSIS

Premature fusion of the cranial sutures are a feature of Cruzon's and Apert's syndrome, producing deformities of the cranial vault. Because of an associated lack of growth of the cranial base, patients also exhibit extreme underdevelopment of the mid-third of the face.

ACHONDROPLASIA

This rare condition usually represents a sporadic mutation; less than 20 per cent will be of a familial nature. The aetiology is not completely understood, but there is a defect of endochondral ossification. Failure of growth at the spheno-occipital synchondrosis and lack of growth in the maxilla produces the characteristic underdevelopment of the mid-third of the face. Curiously, growth of the mandible is unaffected, leading to relative mandibular prognathism.

DISORDERS OF THE TEMPOROMANDIBULAR JOINT

The mandibular condyle may be affected by trauma, infection from the middle ear or juvenile arthritis, all of which will damage the condylar growth centre. The result is under-development of one side of the mandible with compensatory growth on the contralateral side. This produces a facial asymmetry and under-development of the ipsilateral side of the face in the vertical plane. Fractures of the temporomandibular

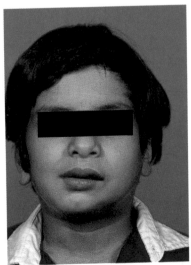

Fig. J.19. Facial deformity due to ankylosis of the right temporomandibular joint.

joint may, on occasions, be followed by ankylosis and this, too, will prevent normal development of the affected side of the face (*Fig.* J.19). Treatment of all these conditions is by surgical correction.

In some patients there may be excessive growth of the condyle known as condylar hyperplasia, resulting in asymmetry of the facial skeleton with, overgrowth of the affected site. Asymmetry may also be caused by hemifacial hypertrophy or hemifacial atrophy. In the latter case there is slow progressive atrophy of the soft tissues of one side of the face with secondary deformity of the facial skeleton. Patients may also exhibit contralateral Jacksonian epilepsy and trigeminal neuralgia. This condition is thought to be due to an abnormality of the sympathetic system and is often associated with scleroderma.

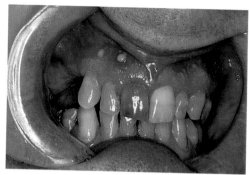

Fig. J.20. Upper right central incisor with gangrene of the dental pulp and pus discharging through the alveolar bone.

ACROMEGALY

Acromegaly follows autonomous hypersecretion of growth hormone caused by hyperplasia or an adenoma of the pituitary acidophil cells. The face is invariably affected by this condition with overgrowth of the mandible to produce prognathism with malocclusion, enlargement of the tongue and deposition of bone at the supraorbital ridges and zygomas (*see Fig.* F.9).

The facial skin also becomes thickened, as does the subcutaneous tissue, producing an accentuation of the normal skin folds. The nose becomes enlarged, especially at the tip, as do the lips. Treatment should be of the underlying pituitary problem and corrective jaw surgery should only be undertaken following stabilization of the condition. Many of these patients have cardiomyopathy and there may be serious complications during anaesthesia.

P.T. Blenkinsopp

Jaw, pain in

Pain in the jaw mostly arises from the dental structures and their supporting bone, the temporomandibular joint and the associated muscles of mastication. In the upper jaw, infections of the nose and paranasal sinuses may additionally cause pain in the maxilla. Disorders of the trigeminal nerve are a relatively rare cause of facial pain, but atypical facial pain which is part of a psychological illness (usually depression) is quite common.

Dental pain

Inflammation in the pulp chamber of a tooth caused by dental caries, inadequately insulated restorations or occlusal trauma characteristically causes pain with thermal stimulation or pressure. This then progresses to an ache which lasts for increasing periods of time or may be worse at night when the patient lies down.

As the inflammation progresses, the pain becomes very severe and constant until such time as remedial therapy is carried out, or gangrene of the pulp occurs. At this stage, the pain diminishes but is replaced by an ache within the alveolar bone should a dental alveolar abscess develop (*Fig.* J.20).

With increasing infection, the visible signs of inflammation become apparent and a swelling develops in the mucous membrane or associated soft tissues (*see* JAW, SWELLING OF). At any stage this pain may be worsened by occlusal trauma to the tooth during mastication or when the teeth are percussed. The pain associated with a periodontal abscess or pericoronal infection is similar to the pain associated with an alveolar abscess; that is, the pain is moderate to severe and throbbing in nature.

Any of the conditions developing within the jaw, e.g. dental cysts, ameloblastoma, etc. (*see* JAW, SWELLING OF) may become infected and again the pain is similar to abscess formation of dental origin. The diagnosis is usually readily apparent following a careful recording of the history followed by clinical and radiographical examination. Should the abscess formation involve the masticatory muscles, then trismus will also be present as well as signs of acute infection.

Acute post-extraction osteitis

This pain commences 2–3 days after the extraction of a tooth and is due to bacterial infection of the bone lining the tooth socket, should the normal healing blood clot break down. The pain is severe, dull, throbbing or gnawing in character. It is usually associated with a bad taste in the mouth and examination will demonstrate an empty tooth socket (dry socket) in which food has collected. Treatment is by local cleansing of the socket and installation of local antiseptic agents. Antibiotics are not normally required.

Acute maxillary sinusitis

Pain arising in the acutely infected maxillary sinus may be confused with pain of dental origin as the tooth roots of the upper teeth have a very close relationship to this structure. Maxillary sinusitis normally follows an upper respiratory tract infection, especially if the normal drainage of the antrum through the ostium is reduced, for example, by a deviated nasal septum. However, maxillary sinusitis can arise from dental infection should the abscess present in the maxillary antrum rather than in the oral cavity. Infection of the maxillary sinus may also follow the creation of an oro-antral fistula after dental extraction.

In maxillary sinusitis, the patient suffers from a throbbing pain in the cheek with radiation towards the eye, but there is never any swelling of the face. The teeth may be tender to percussion and the pain is aggravated by bending forward or lying down. Intranasal examina-tion may demonstrate a mucopurulent discharge through the normal ostium. A reduction in translucency of one maxillary sinus compared with the other suggests that it contains fluid and this will be easily confirmed on an occipitomental X-ray (*Fig.* J.21).

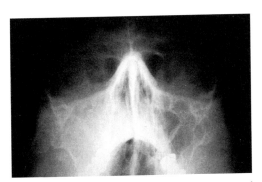

Fig. J.21. Acute right maxillary sinusitis. Note the opacity of the sinus compared to the air-filled left side.

A neoplastic process of the maxillary antrum should be considered if the pain does not respond to normal measures or if there is swelling of the face or oral cavity associated with bone destruction and displacement of the teeth. A tumour of the maxillary antrum may also cause epistaxis and sensory loss in the maxillary division of the trigeminal nerve. If this is suspected, the extent of the tumour can be assessed on a CT scan then a biopsy should be obtained either by antral puncture through the nose or via a Caldwell–Luc approach.

Temporomandibular joint

The temporomandibular joint may be affected by any of the conditions which afflict the other joints, e.g. rheumatoid arthritis, osteoarthritis and septic arthritis; in which case pain and swelling are exhibited in the preauricular region, in the acute phase, with limitation of jaw movements. An acute effusion, as a result of a blow to the jaw or a fracture involving the joint, may arise in the temporomandibular joint, also causing pain and swelling anterior to the ear.

However, the most common form of pain arising in the temporomandibular joint is associated with the temporomandibular joint pain dysfunction syndrome. This is an extremely common and much written about subject without there being a clear cut understanding of the mechanisms involved. The symptomatology is, however, well recorded and consists of pain arising in the region of the temporomandibular joint or ear which may be associated with a 'clicking' noise, and, is aggravated by wide opening of the mouth, as with yawning and chewing hard foods.

When masticatory muscle spasm is also present, which is common in this condition, the patient may have some limitation of jaw opening and complain of facial pain. This radiates across the face from the ear to the region of the eye, or down into the lower jaw on both lateral and medial aspects. Curiously, many patients also state that the face becomes swollen, which is probably a reflection of the shortening of the masseter muscle due to spasm. The alleged mecha-nisms are many, with minor trauma and associated stretching of the ligaments and displacement of the articular cartilage being currently accepted. However, severe dental malocclusion may be a factor and, without doubt, stress is a very important aetiological cause in many people. Patients under stress would appear to clench their teeth, bite their nails or, grind their teeth at night, all of which induces masticatory muscle spasm, ischaemia, and hence pain.

Primary neuralgias

Primary neuralgias may be defined as the disturbed function of a nerve without there being any recognized aetiological factor or pathological process acting at some point along the nerve pathway or its central connections. In the jaws the trigeminal nerve is affected and very occasionally the glossopharyngeal nerve. There is no associated signs and the diagnosis is made from the history.

The pain characteristically affects almost always only one branch of the trigeminal nerve initially, although later on in the disease it may spread to affect two or occasionally three divisions. The disease most commonly affects patients over 50 years old, and the incidence is twice as common in women as in men.

The pain is very severe. It is described as sharp, or similar to an electric shock. It is paroxysmal in nature, lasting only a few seconds with intervals of a few minutes or a few hours. The pain may be felt spontaneously or in response to stimulation within a trigger area on the face. This trigger area may be activated by a cold wind, shaving, washing, eating or cleaning the teeth. Natural remission is fairly common.

The main differential diagnosis is between causes of dental pain and these should be excluded before a diagnosis of trigeminal neuralgia is made. Treatment is with the specific drug carbamazepine but, as it occasionally causes agranulocytosis, regular monitoring of the white blood cell count is essential. Should medical treatment fail then a surgical approach should be considered. In every case, careful examination of the central nervous system should be made to exclude a neoplasm or, in the younger age group, the onset of multiple sclerosis, which can mimic trigeminal neuralgia in the early stages of the disease.

Secondary neuralgias

Here an identifiable pathological process is acting at some point along the trigeminal nerve or its central connections, producing pain at the periphery. The symptoms may be similar to trigeminal neuralgia or may be a duller more continuous pain. Neoplasms are the most significant cause, other examples being aneurysms or compression of the nerve in the bony canal in Paget's disease.

Exact testing of the function of the cranial nerves is essential followed by a full clinical and radiographical examination, including CT scans to establish the diagnosis.

Post-herpetic neuralgia

Involvement of one of the branches of the trigeminal nerve with the virus of herpes zoster will produce pain and vesiculation in the anatomical distribution of that nerve. Once this attack has resolved, scarring of the involved nerve may leave the patient with post-herpetic neuralgia and possibly sensory disturbance. This pain can be severe and very resistent to treatment.

Migraine

Migraine and migrainous neuralgia may occasionally involve the maxilla, although the predominant features are manifested as headache. The diagnosis is normally made from the history, when an intense pain is associated with visual disturbance, nausea and constitutional symptoms. In migrainous neuralgia, the pain is predominantly behind the eye and patients may also experience pain in the maxilla and temple regions. There may be watering of the eye and flushing of the facial skin.

Referred pain

The only important example of referred pain to the jaws is that of coronary artery insufficiency which may produce pain in the left side of the mandible.

Atypical facial pain

Large numbers of patients present with atypical facial pain which is symptomatic of a psychological illness. The pain is described as being very severe, but it does not produce any restriction upon the normal function of the jaws and oral cavity. It does not have an anatomical distribution, commonly involves both sides of the face and jaws and moves from one part of the facial skeleton to another. It does not respond to analgesics and usually there are many other associated symptoms such as a dry mouth, burning tongue, and other complaints throughout the body.

There can be some overlap between this condition, and temporomandibular joint dysfunction caused by stress but, in every case, it is essential to exclude pain due to any one of the other causes just described. Therefore, atypical facial pain is often a diagnosis of exclusion and once made, any underlying depression should be treated by medication or referral for psychiatric help.

P. T. Blenkinsopp

Jaw, swelling of

Swellings of the jaw, once they have reached a certain size, will be obvious as a facial swelling or swelling in the submandibular region. The true nature will, however, only be ascertained by an intraoral examination and in many cases the taking of radiographs will also be required. Smaller swellings may only be visible on examination of the oral cavity or will have been discovered by the patient during normal oral function. Testing of the trigeminal cranial nerve should always be carried out as a change in sensation may have very significant consequences. Swellings of the jaws can, to the inexperienced clinician, be incorrectly diagnosed as swellings of the submandibular salivary gland, submandibular lymph nodes or swellings of the parotid gland.

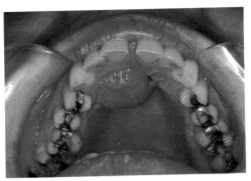

Fig. J.22. Intraoral dental abscess in the palate.

Infection associated with the dental structures

Bacterial infection associated with the dental structures is by far the most common cause of swellings of the jaw. An alveolar abscess arises when gangrene of the dental pulp occurs following dental caries, extensive dental restorations or trauma (*Fig. J.22*). This infection then spreads to the alveolar bone to cause a localized osteitis but remarkably, in the majority of cases, does not cause osteomyelitis. Instead, the abscess as it enlarges becomes localized and perforates either the lateral or medial plate of the outer compact alveolar bone. It is at this stage that it presents as a swelling of the jaw which is tender and covered by inflamed mucosa. Occasionally an alveolar abscess is associated with sensory loss of the mandibular branch of the trigeminal nerve.

A periodontal abscess arises from bacterial infection within the periodontal membrane of the tooth, which is usually associated with previous chronic periodontal disease. A pericoronal abscess arises in the mucous membrane surrounding the crown of an erupting or impacted tooth; the majority being associated with wisdom teeth.

At this stage the swelling is largely confined to the region of the jaws and may discharge intraorally. However, should the bacteria gain access to the adjacent soft-tissue compartments, then facial cellulitis or soft-tissue abscess formation will follow. Depending upon the anatomical position of the infection, the submandibular area may become swollen, or the cheek (buccal space) or more posteriorly the submasseteric space, which may be misdiagnosed as a parotid swelling (*Fig. J.23*).

On the medial aspect of the jaw, swelling in the sublingual space may occur or more posteriorly in the pterygoid, lateral pharyngeal or peritonsillar space. Diagnosis of these latter space infections may be difficult and, if beneath a muscle compartment, are associated with severe trismus.

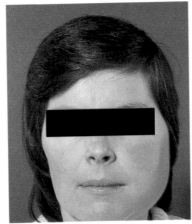

Fig. J.23. Facial swelling due to infection from an impacted wisdom tooth.

These medial swellings are potentially very serious as respiratory obstruction may follow unless the neck is decompressed in severe cases. Ludwig's angina is an acute emergency in which both the sublingual and submandibular spaces are involved in acute infection. Again urgent surgical decompression of the neck is required to prevent respiratory obstruction.

Persistent recurrent infection causing chronic swelling and discharge may be due to an opportunistic infection with actinomycosis.

Osteomyelitis

True osteomyelitis of the jaws is now relatively rare following the improvement in general dental health and the use of antibiotics. However, when established, severe pain with loosening of the adjacent teeth is encountered and usually there is sensory loss of the mandibular branch of the trigeminal nerve. The overlying mucosa becomes swollen and hyperaemic and, indeed, sinuses may develop through which there is a discharge of pus and bony sequestra. In the acute phase, it is invariably associated with significant soft-tissue swelling. The radiographic changes take some time to develop, but show diffuse rarefaction and sequestrum formation. Subperiosteal woven bone may also be a feature and the infected bone may be subjected to a pathological fracture.

Management of all these infections is by antibiotics and drainage in the acute phase and then appropriate treatment of the causative dental structure, which may require extraction.

Trauma

Fractures of the mandible are relatively common and are associated with swelling caused by haematoma formation from the bleeding marrow space and periosteum. The swelling may be made worse by a protruding bone fragment or the presence of a foreign body. The injury may not be sufficient to cause a fracture but may nevertheless produce a haematoma in the soft tissue. This normally resolves without treatment but, occasionally, requires aspiration. The diagnosis of a fracture is normally easy to make from the history, the abnormal mobility of the fragments and the irregularity of the dental arches. In many fractures, a laceration of the oral mucosa is also present. The diagnosis is confirmed by radiographic examination.

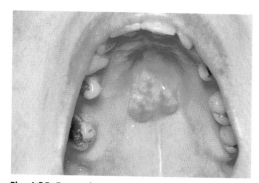

Fig. J.25. Torus palatinus.

Swellings associated with benign dental pathology

Unerupted teeth are a frequent cause of jaw swelling which, commonly, are the canine and premolar teeth in the palate and the premolars in the lower jaw. In the elderly, when the molar teeth have been lost, an erupting wisdom tooth may produce a swelling in the posterior area of the alveolus.

The follicle of unerupted teeth may undergo dentigerous cyst formation, which is an epithelial-lined sac embracing the crown of the tooth (*Fig.* J.24). This slowly enlarges and may cause displacement of the involved tooth or the adjacent teeth. As the expansion continues the alveolus enlarges and, just before perforation, exhibits the phenomenon of 'eggshell crackling'. Once perforated, the swelling is naturally fluctuant. The cyst may slowly enlarge or, should it become infected, acute swelling with inflammation occurs. Other cysts which have a similar clinical presentation are dental cysts, residual dental cysts and keratocysts. Keratocysts, however, tend to be multilocular and have a distinct tendency to recur after removal.

Odontomes, which are developmental abnormalities of the dental lamina, may give rise to a swelling of the jaw and the diagnosis is confirmed by X-ray. Osteomas of the jaw present as hard, round, bony

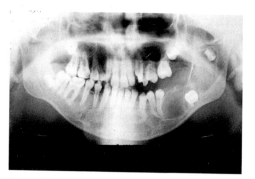

Fig. J.24. Extensive dentigerous cyst formation, left mandible.

swellings which may be endosteal (central) or subperiosteal (peripheral). Multiple osteomas of the facial bones are found in Gardner's syndrome, the other main feature being polyps of the large intestine which have a tendency to become malignant. Radiologically osteomas may be composed of dense radio-opaque bone or may have a high cancellous component, in which case they are relatively radiolucent. Torus palatinus is a developmental abnormality of the midline of the hard palate characterized by a cylindrical enlargement in the region of the midline palatal suture (*Fig.* J.25). Torus mandibularis is a similar slowly enlarging developmental abnormality but it arises on the lingual aspect of the mandible in the premolar region. All these osteomas are simply removed if they prove troublesome as a result of trauma to the overlying mucosa.

Fibrous dysplasia

This condition of bone of unknown origin is characterized by replacement with fibrous tissue and enlargement in all three dimensions. At this stage the abnormal bone is very vascular but subsequently ossification occurs to produce an amorphous radio-opaque appearance on the radiograph. The process tends to cease at skeletal maturity. The jaws are frequently affected in monostotic fibrous dysplasia and may also be involved in polyostotic fibrous dysplasia and Albright's syndrome.

Ossifying fibroma

This is a benign fibro-osseous lesion which causes a well-circumscribed mass of fibrous tissue showing areas of speckled calcification. It normally arises within the substance of the bone and slowly expands in all directions to produce a sclerotic margin. With time, the lesion becomes more calcified and can cause loosening of the adjacent teeth. Treatment is by surgical excision.

Cementifying fibroma

This condition is similar in some ways to ossifying fibroma in that an area of bone is replaced by fibrous tissue, but subsequent calcification resembles dental cementum. Periapical cemental dysplasia is similar to cementifying fibroma but produces multiple sites of ossification with cementum. The diagnosis is usually easy to make from the radiographic appearances but may, in some patients, produce a bony hard irregularity of the dental alveolus.

Cherubism (familial fibrous dysplasia)

Symmetrical enlargement of the facial skeleton occurs in this inherited condition, which is usually apparent in early life and then arrests at puberty. Radiographs show symmetrical multilocular radiolucent areas of the jaws and, histologically, the bone is replaced by fibrous tissue with multinucleated giant cells as a predominant feature. The giant cells, in some cases, make the differential diagnosis difficult from giant-cell granuloma or hyperparathyroidism; the blood chemistry is, however, usually normal.

Paget's disease

This disease of bone of unknown aetiology found in patients in middle to late life may affect the mandible but, more commonly, the maxilla. According to some studies, approximately 15 per cent of cases show involvement of the facial skeleton. Enlargement of the facial bones may produce the characteristic 'leonine facies' and, intraorally, expansion of the dental alveolus occurs with displacement of the teeth. Pain may occur due to entrapment of the trigeminal nerve and the radiograph shows the typical areas of patchy sclerosis. Extraction of the teeth can be difficult due to hypercementosis and postextraction bleeding may be severe. In the active phase of the disease, the serum alkaline phosphatase is raised, which will aid the diagnosis of the condition. Sarcomatous change in longstanding Paget's disease occurs but is relatively rare.

Epulis

This term denotes a swelling arising from the gum of which the majority are either pyogenic granulomas, fibroepithelial polyps or peripheral giant-cell granulomas. They may be sessile or pedunculated in shape and covered by pink or red mucosa (*Fig.* J.26). Histologically they exhibit a core of granulation or fibrous tissue covered by epithelium.

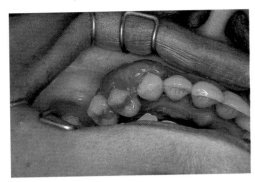

Fig. J.26. Epulis of the gum (pyogenic granuloma).

The pyogenic granuloma and fibroepithelial polyp represent an exaggerated soft-tissue response to minor trauma and are treated by simple excision and curettage. Pyogenic granulomas are common in pregnancy (*see* GUMS, BLEEDING).

Denture granulomas are histologically similar to the fibroepithelial polyp but arise from low-grade persistent denture trauma. Pseudofolds of mucous membrane with a fibrous tissue stroma are formed in the region of a traumatic denture flange. Treatment is again by excision, with attention to the prosthesis.

Papilloma

This benign tumour of epithelium is uncommon in the mouth and, when present, is usually found towards the back of the mouth in the soft palate or on the pillar of fauces. It is predunculated with an irregular surface of pale filiform projections. The lesion should be excised with its base.

Giant-cell granuloma

The aetiology of this lesion is again unknown. It arises in the young age group and is confined to the tooth-bearing areas of the jaws, with the mandible as the most frequent location. Radiographs show a radiolucent area, and histologically, the tissue is vascular fibrous tissue with multinucleated giant cells. The lesion can grow rapidly. The central giant-cell granuloma develops within the jaw, later perforating the alveolar bone to present in the mouth as a spherical purple swelling. Confusion can arise with the brown tumour of hyperparathyroidism but here the occurrence in the older age group with raised serum calcium and parathormone levels would indicate the diagnosis. Additionally, radiographs in hyperparathyroidism show multiple osteolytic lesions, osteitis fibrosa cystica, on skeletal survey. The peripheral giant-cell granuloma is similar in every respect to the central, except that it arises from the gingival margin as a localized fleshy mass which bleeds easily. The treatment of both types is by surgical excision.

Ameloblastoma

Ameloblastoma is a tumour peculiar to the jaws and is a locally invasive neoplasm of odontogenic epithelium. Unless infection supervenes the tumour is quite painless as it slowly enlarges. In underdeveloped countries they may reach enormous proportions before assistance is sought. Radiographs usually show a multilocular radiolucency but, occasionally, unilocular variants may present. Spacing of the teeth may occur but sensory disturbance of the trigeminal nerve is not usually a feature. Treatment is by resection with a margin of healthy bone.

Eosinophilic granuloma

The solitary eosinophilic granuloma produces an area of bone loss in the jaw and there is an associated soft-tissue swelling with gingival ulceration. The condition may first come to be noticed because of loosening of the teeth, the failure of a tooth extraction site to heal or a pathological fracture. The jaws may also be affected by multifocal eosinophilic granuloma where, with loosening of the teeth, there is also generalized inflammation of the oral cavity and gingival enlargement.

Myxoma

Another benign tumour to affect the jaws and cause expansion is the myxoma, which is a rare benign neoplasm arising from odontogenic mesenchyme. It produces a multilocular radiolucent appearance with multiple criss-crossing septi in the defect.

Haemangioma

The endosteal haemangioma is more common in the mandible than the maxilla and, if truly endosteal, presents as a hard, non-tender, painless swelling. Haemorrhage may occur around the necks of the teeth, which may become loosened and severe haemorrhage follows dental extraction.

Minor salivary glands

The minor salivary glands are distributed widely throughout the oral mucosa but are found in abundance at the junction of the hard and soft palate. The important benign causes of enlargement are mucous extravasation cyst and pleomorphic adenoma (*Fig.* J.27).

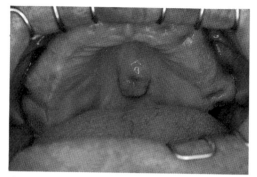

Fig. J.27. Pleomorphic adenoma arising from a minor salivary gland in the palate.

Malignant tumours

Sarcomas of the jaw are rare, with the mandible being affected more often than the maxilla. The tumour presents as a rapidly enlarging swelling with drifting and loosening of the teeth and sensory disturbance of the involved trigeminal nerve. Radiographs demonstrate irregular destruction of the jaw but in the osteogenic sarcoma there are, in addition, radiating trabeculae of new bone formation to give the characteristic 'sun ray' appearance. Treatment is by wide resection and blood borne metastases do not normally occur as rapidly as in osteosarcomas found elsewhere in the skeleton. More rarely a chondrosarcoma may involve the jaws with similar clinical signs to the osteosarcoma. Treatment is again by wide resection.

Intrabony squamous-cell carcinoma is rare but when present it causes a destructive lesion within the mandible on X-ray, sensory disturbance of the trigeminal nerve and expansion of the bone with loosening of the teeth. The more common squamous-cell carcinoma arising in the oral mucous membrane produces swelling of the soft tissue overlying the jaw, usually with central ulceration and underlying bone destruction (*Fig.* J.28).

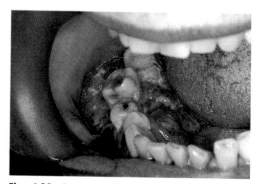

Fig. J.28. Squamous-cell carcinoma of the mandibular alveolus.

Carcinoma of the maxillary antrum and malignant tumours of the minor salivary glands contained within the mucosa of the palate, will eventually cause intraoral swelling of the upper jaw, leading to ulceration. A malignant lesion should be suspected if growth is rapid and is associated with bone destruction, loosening of the teeth, haemorrhage, and sensory disturbance of the trigeminal nerve. In all these malignant tumours, a CT scan provides valuable information on the extent and spread of the growth. The diagnosis is confirmed by biopsy. The important malignant tumours affecting the upper jaw in addition to carcinoma of the antrum are adenocystic carcinoma, adenocarcinoma, malignant pleomorphic adenoma and lymphoma.

Metastatic tumours of the jaws

Secondary deposits of tumours rarely affect the jaws, with the mandible as the commoner site. Tumours of the bronchus, breast, kidney and thyroid produce osteolytic lesions while carcinoma of the prostate tends to form an osteosclerotic deposit. The clinical signs are similar to other intrabony malignant tumours with swelling, pain, loosening of the teeth and sensory disturbance. Eventually pathological facture occurs.

Secondary deposits may also develop in the overlying soft tissue of the jaws, especially at the gingival margin, and may be confused with a benign epulis. Rapid growth usually occurs to produce a fleshy mass, which may be friable and haemorrhagic. These lesions should be excised and all submitted for histological examination lest the diagnosis should be missed.

P. T. Blenkinsopp

Joints, affections of

Joint affections may be acute, as in rheumatic fever, gout or traumatic hydrarthrosis; acute relapsing becoming chronic, as in rheumatoid arthritis or Reiter's disease; chronic with acute onset, as in some cases of generalized osteoarthritis; or insidious and chronic as in most cases of osteoarthritis. The affection may be of one joint, a monarthritis, as may be seen in tuberculous arthritis; or it may be the start of a polyarthritis, as is seen not infrequently in psoriatic arthropathy, in which a number of joints are eventually affected. The pattern of joint involvement may be important: rheumatoid arthritis affects initially and chiefly peripheral joints; ankylosing spondylitis affects the sacroiliacs and spine; polymyalgia rheumatica affects the girdle joints, pelvis and shoulders. The terminal interphalangeal joints are affected commonly

in osteoarthritis (Heberden's nodes) and psoriatic arthropathy, occasionally in adolescent rheumatoid arthritis, but rarely in adult rheumatoid arthritis. Interphalangeal involvement of the toes is rare in rheumatoid arthritis but more common in the arthritis associated with ulcerative colitis or Reiter's disease. Joint involvement may be in the form of a flitting and transient polyarthritis, as in rheumatic fever, some cases of systemic lupus erythematosus and in a number of other conditions or in a recurring or palindromic pattern subsiding completely between episodes, as in some cases of rheumatoid arthritis.

Joints may be swollen because of:

1. Bony enlargement, as in osteoarthritis or Charcot's joints in tabes dorsalis or syringomyelia.
2. New periosteal bone deposition as in hypertrophic pulmonary osteoarthropathy or thyroid acropachy.
3. Synovial effusion. The joint fluid may be:
   clear and acellular in association with, e.g. serious injury; inflammatory and cellular as in rheumatoid arthritis; blood-stained as in traumatic haemarthrosis and bleeding disorders; purulent as in pyogenic infection or acute crystal synovitis; milky as in chylous arthritis associated with filiariasis.
4. Synovial proliferation as in rheumatoid arthritis.
5. Rarely because of malignant changes, as in sarcoma and secondary carcinoma.

Not infrequently joints are swollen from a combination of two or more of these factors. Swelling of synovial tendon sheaths or bursae alongside joints may also contribute greatly to the clinical picture, symmetrical involvement of extensor sheaths on the dorsum of the wrists being very typical of rheumatoid arthritis. Subacromial and semimembranosus bursal involvement may contribute much swelling when shoulders or knees are affected by an inflammatory arthritis. If there is doubt regarding the presence of infecting organisms aspiration should be performed. This will often contribute useful information in non-infective conditions such as gout, chondrocalcinosis, or haemarthrosis if diagnosis is in doubt.

Joints affected by any disease process may show a variable blend of five factors: swelling, pain, stiffness, tenderness and weakness. These five factors in variable combinations cause the dysfunction typical of the particular arthritic disease in question. In progressive systemic sclerosis (scleroderma) stiffness is the dominant component; in gout swelling, tenderness and pain. The joints in rheumatoid arthritis vary and differ depending on activity and stage of the disease process; stiffness in early rheumatoid disease is largely due to joint swelling, in advanced disease to irreversible change, even in some patients, to the point of bony or fibrous ankylosis. In many instances chronic joint swelling produces excessive joint laxity allowing reversible deformity or subluxation. In other cases destruction of joint tissue in rheumatoid arthritis causes gross hypermobility, the so-called 'lorgnette' or 'telescopic fingers' being extreme examples of this.

Two of the cardinal signs of inflammation, heat and redness, are often absent in inflammatory arthritis, while in acute pyarthrosis the joint is hot and in gout hot and red. In most patients with rheumatoid arthritis the joints tend to be cold and moist without erythema, though swollen, painful and tender. Palmar erythema is common in rheumatoid arthritis and in systemic lupus erythematosus, the palms and fingertips being often a bright pink. Inflammatory arthropathies usually cause most discomfort in the early morning, the tissues becoming 'gelled' with disuse in the night. This early morning increase in pain and stiffness of fingers, wrists and shoulders in particular is characteristic of rheumatoid and similar arthropathies; in ankylosing spondylitis a similar increase in stiffness and pain occurs in spine, hips and shoulders. Painful morning stiffness is also seen characteristically in polymyalgia rheumatica in shoulders and hips.

There are very many possible causes of joint involvement in systemic disease; these are listed below. Not all can be discussed and described; the following account deals only with the more common and distinctive.

A list of the arthropathies

1.   CONGENITAL

Achondroplasia and pseudoachondroplasia
Angiokeratoma corporis diffusum (Fabry's disease)
Arthrogryphosis multiplex congenita
Camptodactyly
Chondrodysplasia punctata (Conradi's syndrome)
Congenital indifference to pain
Down's syndrome
Dysplasia epiphysalis multiplex
Ehlers–Danlos syndrome
Familial dysautonomia (Riley–Day syndrome)
Hereditary progressive arthro-ophthalmopathy
Hypermobility syndrome
Marfan's syndrome
Morquio–Brailsford syndrome
Osteodysplasty
Osteogenesis imperfecta
Spondyloepiphysial dysplasia

2.   DEGENERATIVE, TRAUMATIC AND OCCUPATIONAL

Ankylosing vertebral hyperostosis (Forrestier's disease, diffuse interstitial spinal hyperostosis (DISH))
Occupational syndromes, e.g. porter's neck, wicket-keeper's fingers
Osteoarthritis
Traumatic syndromes, e.g. traumatic haemarthrosis

3.   DIETETIC

Fluorosis
Kashin–Beck disease
Rickets
Scurvy

4.   ENDOCRINE

Acromegaly
Cretinous and myxoedematous arthropathy
Diabetic cheiroarthropathy
Hyperparathyroidism
Hypoparathyroidism
Thyroid acropachy

5.   GUT-ASSOCIATED

Acute gastrointestinal bacterial infection
Antibiotic-induced (pseudomembranous) colitis
Crohn's disease
Jejuno-ileal bypass arthritis-dermatitis syndrome
Ulcerative colitis
Whipple's disease

6.   IDIOPATHIC INFLAMMATORY

Acne fulminans arthritis
Behçet's syndrome
Erythema multiforme
Dermatomyositis and polymyositis
Dressler's syndrome
Erythema nodosum
Familial Mediterranean fever
Henoch–Schönlein syndrome (anaphylactoid purpura)
Intermittent hydrarthrosis
Juvenile chronic arthritis (Pauciarticular, Polyarticular, Systemic)
Mixed connective tissue disease
Palindromic rheumatism
Pigmented villonodular synovitis
Progressive systemic sclerosis (scleroderma)
Relapsing polychondritis
Rheumatoid arthritis, including Felty's syndrome, Caplan's syndrome
Sarcoidosis
Spondyloarthropathy, e.g. ankylosing spondylitis, Psoriatic arthritis, reactive arthritis, Reiter's syndrome, Enteropathic arthritis (Crohn's disease, ulcerative arthritis)
SAPHO syndrome
Sjögren's syndrome
Systemic lupus erythematosus

7.   IDIOPATHIC NON-INFLAMMATORY

Osteochondritis dissecans
Osteochondrosis

8.   HAEMATOLOGICAL

Agammaglobulinaemia
Haemophilia and allied disorders
Leukaemia
Sickle-cell disease
Thalassaemia

9.   INFECTIVE

infections due to bacteria, spirochaetes and mycoplasma

Anthrax
Brucella abortus and *melitensis* arthritis
Cat-scratch fever
Clutton's joints
Diphtheria
Erysipelas
Glanders
Haverhill fever
Infective endocarditis
Jaccoud's arthropathy
Leprosy
Lyme arthritis
Lymphogranuloma venereum
Meningococcal fever
Mycoplasma pneumoniae
Poncet's disease
Pseudomonas pseudomallei (Melioidosis)
Pyogenic (staphylococcal, psittacosis, gonococcal, pneumo-coccal, etc.)
Rat-bite fever
Rheumatic fever
Secondary syphilis
Streptococcal reactive arthritis
Tuberculosis
Typhoid and paratyphoid fever
Weil's disease (*Leptospirosis icterohaemorrhagica*)
Yaws

Infections due to viruses

Chikungunya
Dengue
Echo virus infection
Glandular fever (infectious mononucleosis)
Influenza
Measles
Mumps
O'Nyong–Nyong fever
Parvovirus (human)
Poliomyelitis
Ross River virus arthritis
Rubella
Viral hepatitis (mainly 'B')

Infections due to fungi

Actinomycosis
Aspergillosis
Blastomycosis
Coccidioidomycosis
Cryptococcosis (torulosis)
Histoplasmosis
Madura foot (mycetoma pedis)
Sporotrichosis

Infections due to protozoa

Amoebiasis
Giardiasis

Infections due to worms

Chylous arthritis
Dracunculosis (Guinea-worm arthritis)
Filariasis
Trichiniasis
Schistosomiasis
Strongyloidiasis

10.   METABOLIC

Amyloidosis
Biliary and alcoholic cirrhosis
Calcinosis circumscripta (pyrophosphate arthropathy)
Calcinosis uraemica
Chondrocalcinosis
Disseminated lipogranulomatosis (Farber's disease)
Familial hypercholesterolaemia
Familial lipochrome pigmentary arthritis
Gaucher's disease
Gout
Haemochromatosis
Hunter's syndrome
Hurler's syndrome (gargoylism)
Multicentric reticulohistiocytosis (lipoid dermato-arthritis)
Myositis ossificans
Ochronosis
Renal transplant and haemodialysis syndrome
Wilson's disease

11.   VASCULAR

Avascular necrosis (fat emboli, caisson, etc.)
Polyarteritis nodosa
Polymyalgia arteritica (giant-cell arteritis and polymyalgia-jy rheumatica)
Takayasu's (pulseless) disease
Wegener's granulomatosis

12.   NEOPLASTIC

Chondrosarcoma
Haemangioma
Hypertrophic pulmonary osteoarthropathy
Left atrial myxoma
Lymphoma
Metastatic malignant disease
Multiple myeloma
Osteoid osteoma
Paget's sarcoma
Hypertrophic pulmonary osteoarthropathy
Synovioma

13.   NEUROPATHIC

Algodystrophy (shoulder–hand syndrome, transient osteo-porosis, Sudek's atrophy)
Charcot's joints, tabetic or syringomyelic
Diabetic arthropathy (neuropathic and infective)
Paraplegia syndrome
Ulcero-osteolytic neuropathy

14. DRUG-INDUCED

Anticoagulants
Barbiturates
Corticosteroid arthropathy
Hydralazine syndrome (procaine amide, oral contraceptives, etc.)
Isoniazid shoulder–hand syndrome
Quinidine
Serum sickness

15. MISCELLANEOUS

Acro-osteolysis syndrome
Dupuytren's contracture
Knuckle pads (Hale–White) (Garrod)
Paget's disease of bone
Periostitis deformans (Soriano)
Thorn synovitis
Septic focus syndrome
Subacute pancreatitis
Xiphoid syndrome

1. Congenital arthropathies

In classical *achondroplasia* bony growth is abnormal but epiphysial development is normal; premature osteoarthritis is not usual and spinal stenosis may occur. In *pseudoachondroplasia* and the various *spondyloepiphysial dysplasias* epiphyses are involved, rendering these subjects particularly prone to severe premature osteoarthritis in adult life. In *Conradi's syndrome* a widespread patchy calcification in articular and other cartilages is seen in infancy with shortening and asymmetry of the limbs; premature osteoarthritis follows in adult life as it does in *hereditary progressive arthro-ophthalmopathy* where progressive myopia is associated with multiple epiphysial dysplasia.

Arthrogryposis multiplex congenita is a rare congenital condition characterized by joint contractures, usually symmetrical and multiple, affecting lower limbs rather than upper and distal joints more than proximal ones. The subcutaneous tissues may be thick, doughy or gelatinous. While usually apparent at birth and readily recognized, if the patient is not seen until adult life the condition may be confused with advanced rheumatoid arthritis with joint contractures of fingers, knees, elbows and wrists. It is usually, but not always, painless, though secondary degenerative changes may occur later and cause considerable discomfort, particularly in the hips which may become dislocated. Other congenital abnormalities may be present, such as small or absent patellae, high palate, hypospadias and micrognathia. Clubbing of fingers and toes is common, mental deficiency rare.

Camptodactyly is an innocent congenital condition where the little fingers are flexed with thickening of the proximal interphalangeal joints. It is a relatively common condition and important only in that it may be confused with osteoarthritis. Other fingers are less often affected.

In *congenital indifference to pain* the patient traumatizes the joints and other tissues repeatedly and may develop secondary traumatic osteoarthritis or even neuropathic joints. Such patients are usually mentally and neurologically normal otherwise but are constantly suffering the effects of injury, fractures, bruises, dislocations, cuts and scratches, as they do not experience pain as do normal subjects. It is a rare condition.

Dysplasia epiphysalis multiplex is inherited as an autosomal dominant trait. The epiphyses of the long bones become deformed, the hips most commonly. Any or all of the epiphyses of the long bones may be affected, with resultant osteoarthritis, particularly of hips and knees, beginning in early life. The sufferers are often of short stature with short, squat digits. Such children presenting with pain, usually in the hip, are often misdiagnosed as cases of Perthe's disease.

The *Ehlers–Danlos syndrome* is a rare genetically determined disorder of connective tissue, characterized by hypermobile joints and hyperextensible skin which tends to split if mildly injured, with resulting gaping scars. There are probably seven entities included in this title; in one, in particular, the ecchymotic type IV, sudden death may occur from spontaneous arterial rupture or gastrointestinal perforation, though abnormalities in collagen biosynthesis occur also in three other types. Joint subluxations and dislocations occur if the joints are hypermobile and effusions into knees are common. Dislocations of clavicles, patellae, shoulders, radii and hips may occur and recur several times. Other developmental abnormalities are common, such as kyphoscoliosis, anterior wedging of vertebrae, spina bifida occulta, club-foot and genu recurvatum. Bleeding may occur in superficial tissues, or from vagina, rectum or mouth and haemarthrosis may occur. Children may be backward in walking and develop a tabetic-like gait. In the sixth to ninth months of pregnancy joints may become more lax and subluxable than previously. Premature osteoarthritis may occur in a few patients.

Familial dysautonomia (Riley–Day syndrome) is a congenital disorder almost completely confined to Ashkenazic Jews, transmitted as an autosomal recessive trait. Among many manifestations relative insensitivity to pain may lead to neuropathic joints in knee or shoulder in early adolescence.

Maldevelopment of axial and peripheral joints are features of the *mucopolysaccharidoses*. Features of these inherited disorders are due to accumulation of mucopolysaccharides (or glycosaminoglycans) in the tissues as a result of deficiency of lysosomal enzymes necessary for their degradation. In the commonest of these rare disorders, Hurler's syndrome (gargoylism), the onset is from 6 months to 2 years of age but the typical picture of gargoylism does not appear until 4 or 5 years later. The child develops coarse features with thick lips, large bulging head and flattened nose; the cervical spine is short with kyphosis of the lower dorsal and upper lumbar regions. Acetabula are shallow, epiphyses flattened, irregular and retarded in development. Limitation of joint movement is common, particularly abduction of shoulders and hips and extension of fingers, and contractures of hips and elbows may occur, the hands becoming clawed. The children are often intellectually impaired and rarely live beyond 20 years of age. Similar features are found in other mucopolysaccharidoses, the Hunter syndrome, the Sanfilippo syndrome, the Scheie syndrome and the Maroteaux–Lamy syndrome.

In the type IV *Morquio-Brailsford* mucopolysaccharidosis the children appear normal until 1–2 years of age when kyphosis is seen with protrusion of the sternum and prominence of the chin appearing a year later. Growth usually ceases at 10 years, the child showing a short trunk with kyphosis, knock knees, flat feet, waddling gait, muscle weakness and increased laxity of joints, which is in sharp contrast with the contractures seen in the other mucopolysaccharidoses. In a severe case almost every joint may be affected, the spine, hips and knees most often, and cord compression may occur. Aortic regurgitation is common. Keratan sulphate excretion in the urine is increased and, though not invariably present, may be diagnostic. Mentally the children are normal.

Ganglioside storage diseases also result from inherited enzyme deficiencies. *Farber's disease* results from deposition of lipid with a vigorous granulomatous reaction (disseminated lipo-granulomatosis). Arthritis is an early feature with red swollen joints and periarticular pigmented swelling appearing in the first few months of life. It is a very rare condition. Death from respiratory infection is usual before the age of 2.

In the *hypermobility syndrome* generalized joint laxity occurs as an isolated finding, giving rise to recurrent joint pains and effusions, particularly after vigorous exercise. Symptoms, more common in females than in males, usually start from the age of 15. The knees are most commonly affected. Degenerative changes may begin early in the fourth decade. These children, who often consider themselves to be 'double-jointed', often suffer quite severe cramp-like pains in the legs after sporting activities. About 10 per cent of otherwise normal subjects have such hypermobility.

Symptoms are related to the degree of hypermobility but often decrease with advancing age and crippling osteoarthritis is uncommon.

The picture of *Marfan's syndrome* is of a tall, thin loose-jointed youth or girl with long extremities, especially the fingers (arachnodactyly), dislocated lenses, tremulous irides and cardiovascular abnormalities, particularly dilatation of the ascending aorta and aortic regurgitation. Fifty per cent of these patients present with backache, pains in joints and/or effusions. Joints may dislocate readily, hips or shoulders most commonly, but early development of osteoarthritis is unusual. Many other abnormalities may be present, pigeon chest or pectus excavatum particularly. The sexes are affected equally. The distance from pubis to sole exceeds that of pubis to vertex and arm span is greater than height. Distal bones are longer than proximal and subcutaneous fat is sparse.

Osteodysplasty (Melnick and Needles syndrome) is another inherited skeletal dysplasia, probably a congenital disorder of skeletal growth which leads to early degenerative changes in the large weight-bearing joints, including the spine. Radiographs show curvature of the long bones of the limbs with irregular cortex and widening and thinning of the metaphyses. These changes may roughly resemble those of rickets but ribs, clavicles and scapulae are also deformed.

The outstanding abnormality in *osteogenesis imperfecta* is the ease with which bones may be fractured. In addition joints are unduly mobile, thinness of the sclerae gives the eyes the typical pale blue appearance and there is atrophy of the skin with a tendency to subcutaneous haemorrhage. Joints dislocate readily and growth may be arrested by multiple small fractures in epiphyses. Spine and chest deformities may occur and deafness is not unusual. Ligaments are weakened and tendon ruptures may occur.

This list of congenital non-infective arthropathies is not complete and the different causes are not yet clear enough to classify them all accurately. Undue laxity, with recurrent subluxations or increased friability or fragility of tissues, leads to premature degenerative changes in the joints affected. Other coexistent congenital abnormalities are common.

2. Degenerative arthropathies

By *osteoarthritis* is meant the various painful syndromes arising primarily from degenerative changes in the joints (*Figs* J.29, J.33, J.34). Age brings degenerative changes, but the pains experienced vary greatly depending on personality, degree of change and joints affected. Such changes are more likely to occur in any joint previously injured by fracture or dislocation or even mild subluxation or in any joint which is

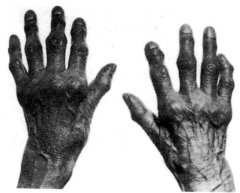

Fig. J.29. Typical osteoarthritic 'Granny's' hands. The enlargement and distortion are essentially bony secondary to degenerative changes in the cartilages.

congenitally abnormal or, because of mechanical factors, working abnormally in the face of abnormal stresses. Repeated 'microtrauma' may also predispose to degenerative changes. Endocrine factors may play a part in some cases as in the so-called *generalized osteoarthritis* which usually affects women 1–5 years or more before or after the menopause. The most commonly affected joints are the terminal interphalangeal joints of the fingers (Heberden's nodes), the thumb bases (carpometacarpal and metacarpophalangeal joints of the thumbs). cervical and lumbar spine, knees and hips and acromioclavicular joints. Less commonly affected are proximal interphalangeal and metacarpophalangeal joints of the fingers. Although essentially degenerative, Heberden's nodes may, in some cases, be tender, red and inflamed in the early stages; inflammation also occurs in osteoarthritis in other joints but does not dominate the scene as it does in rheumatoid arthritis. The hand in osteoarthritis

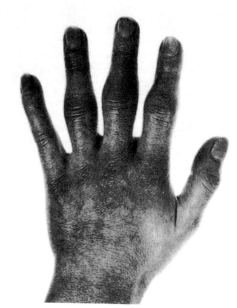

Fig. J.30. Typical spindling of proximal interphalangeal joints in rheumatoid arthritis. The swelling is due to inflammatory changes and increased fluid in these joints.

differs from that in rheumatoid arthritis as shown in *Table* J.7.

In the knee, effusions may occur as a result of trauma and there may also be considerable synovial proliferation. It is not always easy to distinguish an osteoarthritic joint from a rheumatoid one but the pattern of the disease elsewhere in the body and the absence of systemic features in osteoarthritis usually suffice to distinguish the two. In any joint, the absence of inflammatory swelling, nodules and of enlarged lymph nodes favours osteoarthritis rather than inflam-

Table J.7. Differential diagnosis of osteoarthritic and rheumatoid joints

Osteoarthritis	*Rheumatoid arthritis*
Bony joint swelling	Spindle soft-tissue swellings of joints
Terminal interphalangeal joint involvement common (Heberden's nodes)	Terminal interphalangeal joint less commonly involved
Metacarpophalangeal and proximal interphalangeal joints less commonly involved	Metacarpophalangeal and proximal interphalangeal joints commonly involved
Wrists rarely affected	Wrists commonly affected
Tendon sheaths not involved	Swelling of tendon sheaths common
Affected joints not usually very tender	Affected joints usually tender
Gross deformity rare	
Joint effusions rare	Joint effusion common
Radiographs show:	
Juxta-articular bony sclerosis	Juxta-articular osteoporosis
Diffuse joint space loss	Bony erosions
Juxta-articular pseudocysts	Subluxation or deformity
Osteophytes	

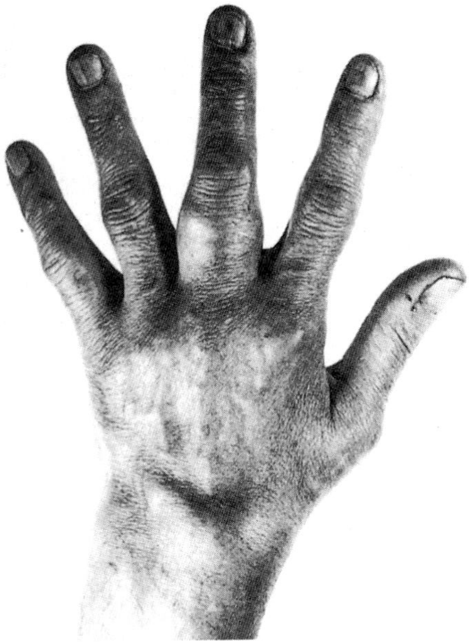

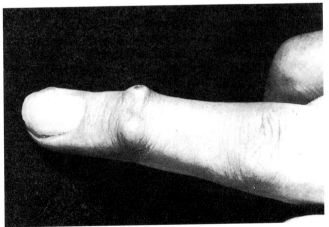

Fig. J.31. Swelling in a rheumatoid hand due to inflammatory changes in extensor tendon sheaths.

matory arthritis. Sedimentation rates are rarely elevated above 30 mm in the first hour (Westergren) in osteoarthritis and are usually normal as are haemoglobin and plasma proteins. Tests for rheumatoid factors are negative. In the cervical spine degenerative changes centre essentially around the lower 5th, 6th and 7th intervertebral discs, the pain often fanning up into the occiput, over the head and into the shoulders; neck movements are restricted and painful. In rheumatoid disease, particularly in childhood, involvement is more diffuse throughout the cervical spine though

pain may be referred in a similar manner. Subluxation of the first on the second vertebra, which occurs in rheumatoid arthritis and ankylosing spondylitis, is not seen in osteoarthritis. A lateral radiograph of the cervical spine will readily distinguish the rough irregularity of disc degeneration from the straight, even intervertebral bridging of ankylosing spondylitis. The condition known as 'ankylosing hyperostosis' of the spine (Forrestier's disease) is a degenerative one occurring not infrequently in diabetics (*see* Back Pain in), usually in the lower dorsal area.

3. Dietetic arthropathies

Kashin-Beck disease is a condition apparently resulting from fusarial infection of flour. In the valleys in eastern Siberia, northern China and North Korea, where it occurred, degenerative changes in joints and spine appeared in relatively young people as a result of cartilage destruction. It is now disappearing with the elimination of infected grain. *Rickets* (*see* Fig. B.14) is much less common than it was and for this reason may be more easily missed. Presenting symptoms may be pains and tenderness over bones, particularly the back, hips, thighs and legs generally. The pains are usually aggravated by rising from resting positions and by exercise. The dangers of missing the diagnosis lie in permanent bony deformities in the pelvis and lower extremities and in the thorax. Pelvic deformities, most serious in females, usually occur in the first year of life. In *scurvy* the child is listless and apathetic with poor appetite. Bones may be painful and tender from subperiosteal haemorrhages and tender swellings may be palpated. The disease is seldom seen in adults; when it occurs dietetic deficiencies are usually due to neglect, alcoholism or obsessional food fads, sometimes medically induced.

Fig. J.32. Rheumatoid nodules masquerading as Heberden's nodes. Note the necrotic (arteritic) centre in the upper one.

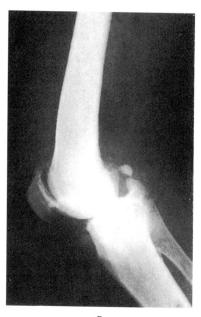
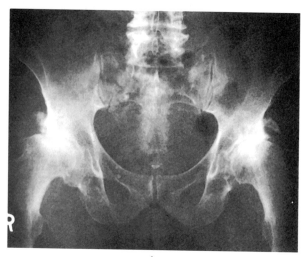

a b

Fig. J.33. *a,* Osteoarthritis of the knee joint. *b,* Osteoarthritis of the hip joints. (*Dr T. A. Hills.*)

4. Endocrine arthropathies

In *acromegaly* recurrent pains in spine and limb joints may be mistaken for those occurring in rheumatoid or osteoarthritis. Effusions may occur in the knees and the carpal tunnel syndrome is not uncommon. The joints may be hypermobile in the early stages due to enlargement of the cartilages, and subluxations and traumatic effusions may occur as in the other hyper-mobility syndromes. Later bony overgrowth restricts movement, so that the picture resembles more that of osteoarthritis, or, because of the fixed bent spine, that of advanced ankylosing spondylitis.

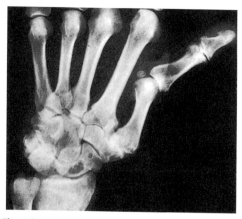

Fig. J.34. Severe osteoarthritis of the carpometacarpal joint of the thumb. (*Dr Keith Jefferson.*)

Diabetic cheiroarthropathy affects the hands of some patients with diabetes mellitus; the fingers may become stiff and partially flexed with thickening of the skin of the palms.

In the original description of *myxoedema*, in 1873 by Sir William Gull, muscular stiffness, joint swelling and broad spade-like hands were noted. In the early stages of the disease, before the classical features of myxoedema appear, the hands may be mistaken for those of early rheumatoid arthritis (*Fig.* J.35). The carpal tunnel syndrome occurs not infrequently and arthralgia is a common complaint. Signs of inflammation are absent but synovial thickening and, occasionally, effusions may occur, the knees and hands being most commonly affected. Traumatic lesions are not uncommon and hip pain may be due to a slipped femoral epiphysis.

In *hyperparathyroidism*, as in some cases of osteomalacia, crush lesions may occur in juxta-articu-lar bone with a traumatic type of synovitis, with effusions and impaired function of the affected joints. Calcification is not uncommon in synovial membrane and cartilage in these cases but it is rare in rheumatoid arthritis, a point of distinction between the two conditions. Not only may 'pseudorheumatoid arthritis' occur but also 'pseudo-gout' due to deposition of crystals of calcium pyrophosphate dihydrate. In idio-pathic *hypoparathyroidism* back pain and stiffness may cause a clinical picture similar to that of ankylos-ing spondylitis but, though ligamentous calcification is present, the sacro-iliac joints are normal. It is asso-

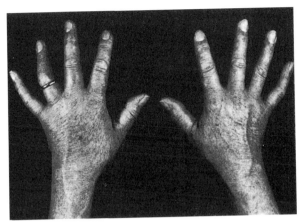

Fig. J.35. Typical swelling of hands in myxoedema.

ciated with hypocalcaemia, cataracts, fits, tetany and rashes. In *thyroid acropachy* subperiosteal thickening is seen in metacarpal and phalangeal bones of the hands in patients with hyperthyroidism who have in many cases been treated and rendered euthyroid. Exophthalmos is common and so-called 'pretibial myxoedema' may be present. The somewhat thickened hand resembles that seen in hypertrophic pulmonary osteoarthropathy, but the condition is milder and less extensive, being usually confined to the hands.

5. Gut-associated arthropathies

The more characteristic of these are considered in the next section under the spondyloarthropathies.

6. Idiopathic inflammatory arthropathies

In *dermatomyositis* and *polymyositis* minimal or moderate transitory arthralgia or arthritis occurs in about one-third of cases. Effusions are less common.

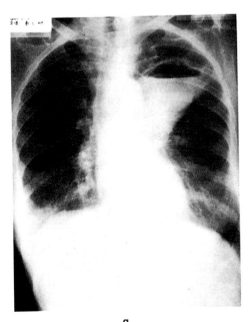

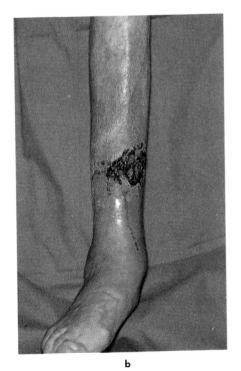

a   b

Fig. J.36. *a,* Lung abscess in neutropenic Felty's syndrome. *b,* Leg ulcer in Felty's syndrome.

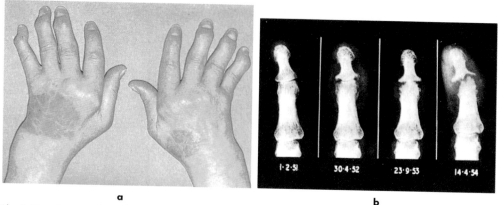

Fig. J.37. *a,* Psoriatic arthropathy, showing involvement of terminal interphalangeal joints. *b,* Advanced radiological destructive changes in psoriatic arthropathy.

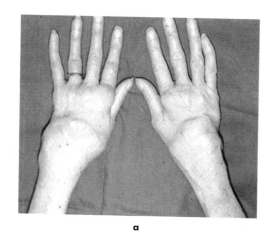

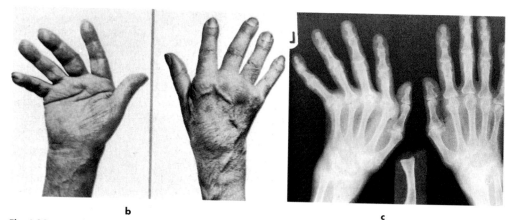

Fig. J.38. *a,* Hands in rheumatoid arthritis. In addition to arthritic changes extensor tendon sheaths are involved. *b,* Rheumatoid arthritis with ulnar deviation and palmar contraction (pseudo-Dupuytren). *c,* Unusual unilateral ulnar deviation with gross bilateral carpal rheumatoid changes. Changes in metacarpophalangeal joints are more marked in the left than the right hand.

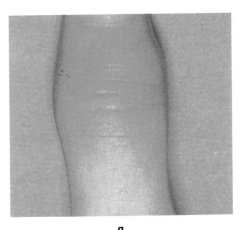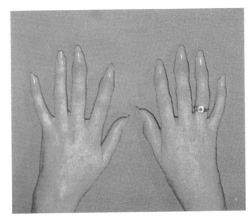

a   **b**

Fig. J.39. *a, b,* Involvement of terminal interphalangeal joints in juvenile chronic polyarthritis.

Fingers and knees are most commonly affected. The skin and muscle manifestations point to the true diagnosis, muscles of the pelvic girdle and thighs and shoulder girdle becoming weak. The association of dermatomyositis with malignant disease in adult cases should be kept in mind.

Dressler's syndrome following myocardial infarction or cardiac injury or surgery occurs around 2–4 weeks or more after the acute episode, with pericarditis, arthralgia and, rarely, arthritis.

The diagnosis *erythema multiforme* probably covers several different entities, some mild, some severe, the so-called 'Stevens–Johnson syndrome' being a severe variant. Arthritis or arthralgia may occur along with other inflammatory reactions in skin, eye, mouth and elsewhere.

Familial Mediterranean fever is an ill-understood disorder characterized by recurrent and sometimes periodic attacks of arthralgia or arthritis. It occurs predominantly in people of Mediterranean origin, Armenians, Arabs and Sephardic Jews. Onset is in childhood or adolescence, episodes of fever recurring with polyserositis, abdominal pain, urticaria and other rashes, arthralgia and arthritis and, later, amyloidosis. Joint manifestations occur in one-third to one-half of the cases, usually arthralgia but sometimes mono- or oligoarthritis. The acute episodes last only a few days, rarely weeks, most cases showing no permanent sequelae. Sacroiliac changes may occur late in the disease.

Henoch–Schönlein syndrome ('anaphylactoid purpura') is commonest in children under 12 years of age. The outstanding feature is a maculo-petechial and sometimes papular rash on the buttocks and extensor surfaces of the lower limbs particularly. Urticaria and purpura may occur. Pain, swelling and stiffness of joints, most commonly ankles and knees, is usually transient and lasts only a few days. Alimentary haemorrhage and haematuria are not uncommon and about 10 per cent of cases develop renal failure.

Intermittent hydrarthrosis, usually in the knees, may resolve without sequelae but approximately 50 per cent of patients eventually develop rheumatoid arthritis or ankylosing spondylitis. Hydrarthrosis may, however, be a manifestation of infective systemic disease such as syphilis or brucellosis. There is usually complete or almost complete remission between attacks. It may also occur after trauma, in osteoarthritis and osteochondritis dissecans; in other words it is a physical sign and not a diagnosis. Some patients recover without showing signs of any other disorder.

Palindromic rheumatism is a name given to recurring episodes of arthritis due to many causes, the most common probably being the early phase of rheumatoid arthritis.

Pigmented villonodular synovitis presents as a persistent but usually relatively painless synovial proliferation with blood-stained joint fluid. Brown nodular masses, possibly due to haemangiomas, form in the synovia; these become traumatized, inflamed and hyperplastic, the hyperplastic synovial cells containing haemosiderin. The condition is usually monarticular, commonly of the knee, and occurs in young adults, males rather than females. The joint may lock repeatedly. The aspirated joint fluid is characteristically blood-stained or dark brown in colour.

In *progressive systemic sclerosis* (scleroderma) the skin is stretched tight over the underlying tissues (*Fig.* J.40), the joints being intact though initially showing changes resembling those of rheumatoid arthritis.

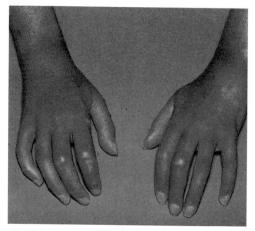

Fig. J.40. Scleroderma (progressive systemic sclerosis). Note the tight shiny skin over the flexed knuckles.

Relapsing (or atrophic) polychondritis is a rare disorder in which the cartilages of joints, ears, nose and trachea soften and collapse; this leads to arthritis, facial changes, dyspnoea or stridor and, occasionally, death.

Rheumatoid arthritis (Figs J.30–32, 38) is sufficiently well known as to need no description. It is as well to remember that tendons and tendon sheaths and bursae are commonly involved by the inflammatory process and these add to the clinical picture. *Juvenile arthritis* is, in only a small minority of cases, an early form of rheumatoid arthritis. In a few cases, particularly in boys, it may be an early form of ankylosing spondylitis but it is usually a sero-negative chronic arthritis. It differs from adult polyarthritis in that splenomegaly and lymphadenopathy are more common, tests for rheumatoid factor usually negative, involvement of terminal interphalangeal joints of fingers and cervical spine more common (*Fig.* J.39), and skin rashes of maculopapular type more common. In the eye, iritis with band opacity in the cornea occurs, sometimes with secondary cataract formation; these are not seen in rheumatoid arthritis in adults. Growth in general may be arrested if the disease is severe and premature fusion may occur in epiphyses adjacent to involved joints. Pericarditis is more common in juvenile arthritis than in adult rheumatoid arthritis.

In *Felty's syndrome* splenomegaly, enlargement of lymph nodes, neutropenia and sometimes pigmentation of the skin are superimposed on the usual picture of rheumatoid arthritis. The only reason for maintaining the title in what is merely a variant of rheumatoid arthritis is to emphasize the importance of the neutropenia, for intercurrent infections are the rule

and splenectomy may be necessary. Leg ulcers are relatively common, the usual site being the lower shin anteriorly (*Fig.* J.36).

The arthropathy associated with *sarcoidosis* is often accompanied by erythema nodosum; a weak or negative tuberculin reaction is usual and the Kveim test may be positive. The arthropathy may be no more than a migratory arthralgia or it may be a true polyarthritis with pain, fever, systemic upset and swelling of several joints, usually the larger ones. In the majority of cases polyarthritis subsides in a few weeks. Hilar node enlargement is common in chest radiographs, and lymph nodes may be palpable in the neck and axilla in some cases. Splenomegaly may be present. Histoplasmosis may also present with hilar lymphadenopathy and joint pains ('pseudosarcoidosis').

The term *spondyloarthropathy* is applied to a family of conditions whose key features are: involvement of the spine and sacroiliac joints; oligo-articular lower limb arthritis; an association with iritis, psoriasis and inflammatory bowel disease; a high prevalence of the HLA B27 antigen.

The principal members of this group are: ankylosing spondylitis; reactive arthritis; Reiter's disease; psoriatic arthropathy; enteropathic arthritis associated with ulcerative colitis and Crohn's disease.

Behçet's syndrome and the Stevens–Johnson syndrome share some features with this family though their inclusion within the group is contentious.

The classical picture of *ankylosing spondylitis* is that of a young male adult with stiff back and chest and often stiff neck and hips also (*see Fig.* B.7). The sedimentation rate is elevated, anterior uveitis is present in 25 per cent of cases at some stage in the disease course, and radiographs show typical changes in sacroiliac joints and usually in the dorsolumbar spine.

Peripheral joint involvement may occur but is usually, though not always, transient. Knee effusions are not uncommon. The pattern of the disorder is essentially central, spine and girdle joints being predominantly affected, peripheral small joints rarely and transiently; this contrasts with rheumatoid arthritis. Nodules do not occur and rheumatoid factor is not present in the serum. The histocompatibility antigen HLA-B27 is found in over 90 per cent of patients.

Reiter's disease comprises arthritis associated with genital-tract inflammation or recent gastrointestinal infection. The syndrome may be caused by either sexually transmitted infection or acute gastrointestinal infection and in either case urethritis or cervicitis may be present. Recognized causal pathogens include *Chlamydia trachomatis*, *Salmonella enteritidis* and *typhimurium*, *Shigella flexneri*, *Yersinia enterocoli-*

tica and *pseudotuberculosis* and *Campylobacter jejuni*. Traditionally arthritis, urethritis and conjunctivitis comprise the classical triad; conjunctivitis is often transient or mild and genital tract symptoms may be mild, overlooked or denied. Diagnosis therefore requires a careful history and a genitourinary examination including microscopic examination of urethral and/or cervical smears. A variety of terms are used to describe this condition; commonly the relationship between infection in the genitourinary or gastrointestinal tract with aseptic arthritis is described by the term 'reactive arthritis'. Arthritic symptoms appear a few days or up to 3 weeks after the initial symptoms of the causative infection. The distribution of affected joints, ankles, heels and knees being principally affected, is characteristic and lesions of buccal mucosa, of the glans penis or prepuce (balanitis circinata), or of skin (keratoderma blenorrhagica) suggest the correct diagnosis. Later, sacroiliac changes may occur and sometimes a clinical picture similar to that seen in ankylosing spondylitis develops. Caucasian patients with Reiter's disease usually have the tissue antigen HLA-B27, those with the picture of ankylosing spondylitis almost 100 per cent. Rheumatoid factor is absent from the blood; nodules do not occur. When skin manifestations are present the condition may closely resemble that of psoriatic arthropathy. The interphalangeal joints of the toes, rarely involved in rheumatoid arthritis, may be affected in Reiter's disease. Iridocyclitis and iritis, rare in rheumatoid arthritis, are not uncommon in Reiter's disease.

In *psoriatic arthropathy* (*Fig.* J.37) the arthritis usually but not invariably follows the skin disorder by several years. The sero-negative, non-nodular polyarthritis tends to be more patchy and less evenly symmetrical than rheumatoid arthritis, and the terminal interphalangeal joints of the fingers are frequently affected, particularly if the nails are affected by the pitting, ridging and separation of psoriasis. When all the joints of a finger are affected by inflammatory arthritis the digit resembles a hot sausage, as was noted many years ago by French rheumatologists. In some cases the sacroiliac joints or the spine are affected, the clinical picture being that of ankylosing spondylitis.

In *Crohn's disease* and *ulcerative colitis* and, less commonly, in *Whipple's disease* (intestinal lipodystrophy) arthralgia or arthritis may occur in the spine or peripheral joints. In all of these, rheumatoid factor is absent from the blood and rheumatoid nodules are not seen. In the arthropathy of ulcerative colitis, the best documented of these three disorders, onset is usually between the ages of 15 and 45 years. It is usually symmetrical and often monarticular with short exacerbations and usually complete recovery, joint erosions being rare and minor in character. It affects both sexes

equally and usually begins acutely, affecting one knee or ankle primarily, subsequent attacks being of similar pattern. The arthritis usually commences long after the onset of the colitis and may coincide with an exacerbation of the disease. In all three conditions, ulcerative colitis, Crohn's disease and Whipple's disease, a picture similar to that of ankylosing spondylitis may eventually appear after some years.

In *systemic lupus erythematosus* any or all systems of the body may be involved in addition to the joints, which are not invariably involved, though arthralgia is usually present at some stage in the course of the disease. The patient, usually a female, is more ill than arthritic in most cases, though joint involvement is present in about two-thirds of patients. The finding of numerous antibodies, including antinuclear antibody, in high titre, and DNA antibody in the blood is strong confirmatory diagnostic evidence. The joint involvement may be flitting, resembling rheumatic fever, or more constant, resembling rheumatoid arthritis. The coexistence of skin lesions and visceral manifestations suggests the correct diagnosis, the typical lupus butterfly rash over nose and cheeks being particularly characteristic (*see Fig.* F.13). Neutropenia and anaemia are common, thrombocytopenia not uncommon. Asthma, proteinuria, neurological signs, splenomegaly, retinal exudates and a number of other coexistent findings in any arthritic should make one think of this disorder or a related connective tissue disease. Epileptiform fits occur in about 10 per cent of cases. Patients with neurological and renal involvement fare worst. Patients having a combination of clinical features of systemic lupus erythematosus, progressive systemic sclerosis and polymyositis with high titres of a circulating antinuclear antibody with specificity for a nuclear ribonucleoprotein are said to have *mixed connective tissue disease*.

7. Idiopathic non-inflammatory arthropathies

In *osteochondritis dissecans* flakes of articular cartilage, sometimes with a portion of the underlying bone, become detached without evident trauma, the condition manifesting itself as recurring attacks of arthritis. The commonest site (85 per cent) is the knee; the radial head is the next most common, hip and ankles being rarely involved. The condition may be bilateral and X-rays are usually diagnostic.

In *osteochondrosis* the diagnosis is also essentially a radiological one. It is essentially a disturbance of epiphysial ossification seen in childhood and early adult life, possibly ischaemic in origin. Early radiographs show dense fragments in the epiphysis and a broadening of the epiphysial line with, later, areas of rarefaction and condensation so that a core of dense bone is seen in a porotic matrix. The epiphyses are affected during the periods of their greatest activity, for instance the femoral head from 4–12 years (Legg–Calve–Perthes disease), the tibial tubercle from 10–16 years (Osgood–Schlatter disease).

8. Haematological arthropathies

It is wise to perform a full blood count, sedimentation rate and examination of plasma proteins in obscure cases of arthritis. Approximately 25 per cent of patients with *agammaglobulinaemia*, congenital or acquired, develop a non-suppurative arthritis not unlike rheumatoid arthritis, the joints showing effusions, pain, tenderness and stiffness. The condition is usually asymmetrical, is unaccompanied by radiological changes, and may be transient, subsiding in a few weeks without sequelae, or may persist for years but with little residual change. Biopsy of synovial tissue does not distinguish between the two conditions. The sedimentation rate is usually normal and tests for rheumatoid factor are negative. In some cases arthritis has been attributed to mycoplasma infection but recurrent infection with the usual pyogenic organisms is also common.

Haemarthrosis may occur in *haemophilia* (factor VIII deficiency) and allied disorders, such as *Christmas disease* (factor IX deficiency), and in patients on anticoagulant therapy but is rare in von Willebrand's disease. In *leukaemia* haemorrhages are common and flitting pains resembling rheumatic fever are not uncommon in acute leukaemia and this, taken in conjunction with a systolic cardiac murmur, may cause diagnostic confusion particularly in acute aleukaemic leukaemia. Pains in bones and joints occur not infrequently in acute leukaemia in childhood and in chronic leukaemia in adults, both myeloid and lymphatic. In children juvenile arthritis is often diagnosed in error.

In *sickle-cell anaemia* painful crises occur which are characteristic of the disorder, and these may occur not only in the abdomen but in bones and joints in children or adults. Although the most common symptoms are those of anaemia, some patients have no complaints except during crises. Aseptic necrosis of bone may occur, particularly in the head of the humerus or femur, radiographs showing subsequently areas of increased density and areas of necrosis. The course of the disease is that of a chronic haemolytic process punctuated by periodic painful crises. Chronic ulceration of the lower legs is relatively common and scars are commonly to be seen around the malleoli. Another striking complication of sickle-cell disease, particularly in children, is salmonella osteomyelitis,

often multifocal. In β-thalassaemia major pains and swelling in ankles and feet may occur.

9. Infective arthropathies

In the infective arthropathies the infecting organism is present in locomotor tissues; in gonococcal arthritis, for instance, gonococci can be isolated from the infected joints or joint; the condition responds to appropriate antibiotics. Any of the infections due to bacteria, spirochaetes or mycoplasma may, if there is destruction of tissue, lead to chronic changes in bones and joints, but if the correct treatment is given early there may be little or no residual disability. In these days of extensive and rapid worldwide travel, conditions previously unknown in residents of one country can occur with resulting arthralgia or arthritis.

Viral arthropathies are common throughout the world but are usually mild and transient. Arbovirus infections including Chikungunya and O'Nyong-Nyong are common in some parts of Africa and South America. To a lesser extent arbovirus infections also occur in Scandinavia (Ockelbo, Pogosta) and Australia (Ross River virus arthritis). In Europe and the USA parvovirus arthritis is the commonest viral joint disease, also associated with a transient rash, upper respiratory infection and malaise (erythema infectiosum, fifth disease). Arthritis following natural rubella is uncommon because of widespread vaccination but may follow vaccination itself. If viral arthritis is suspected hepatitis B infection must also be excluded. Usually joint involvement is polyarticular and symmetrical and carpal tunnel syndrome may develop. Symptoms generally subside within 3 weeks. Postvaccination arthritis may affect a single joint only and persist or recur. Lyme arthritis, named after the part of East Connecticut in which it was first identified, comprises a variable multisystem disease combined with transient asymmetrical oligarthritis. The causative agent is a spirochaete *Borrelia burgdorferi* which is transmitted by tick bites. The disease is only acquired therefore in areas where ticks of the genus *Ixodes* are endemic. The disease responds to antibiotic treatment.

Rheumatic fever is seen much less often today than previously. It is as well to remember that many other arthropathies may present in similar form, joints being successively affected and remitting rapidly, the so-called 'flitting pains' rippling round the locomotor system. Not only may rheumatoid arthritis present in this way, but also systemic lupus erythematosus, ankylosing spondylitis, Hodgkin's lymphoma, leukaemia, brucellosis and a number of other disorders. The heart is rarely seriously involved if rheumatic fever first occurs over the age of 17 years.

Jaccoud's arthritis is an extremely rare disorder following repeated attacks of rheumatic fever, characterized by ulnar deviation of the fingers and hyperextension of the proximal interphalangeal joints without bone destruction.

The arthropathy occurring after *prostatectomy*, and sometimes after gynaecological operations, affects hips particularly, the patient lying in great pain with hips partly flexed. On rising from his bed he may have to walk backwards as forward progression is too painful. The disorder is usually rapidly relieved by draining a pocket of fluid or infective material from behind the symphysis pubis; occasionally true osteitis pubis is present.

10. Metabolic arthropathies

The commonest of these is *gout*. This disorder is characterized by the sudden agonizing nature of the acute attack which is often so severe as to make the patient, almost always an adult male, feel he must have broken a bone in his foot, but for the fact that the disorder frequently starts in bed in the early morning about 5–6 a.m. There are usually clear signs of inflammation, the skin being tense, shiny, hot and red over the big toe metatarsophalangeal joint, ankle or hand, the first named being the commonest. Acute attacks may also occur in the knee (*Figs* J.41–J.43). Although hyperuricaemia is usually present it is not invariably so, and an elevated plasma urate concentration occurs in many other disorders and is not in itself diagnostic. The presence of tophi in ears or elsewhere suggests the diagnosis although the symptoms and signs are usually diagnostic. The only absolute proof is the identification of urate crystals from the affected joint under the polarizing microscope.

In some cases, suggestive of gout, intra-articular crystals turn out to be not urate but calcium pyrophosphate, the condition being *chondrocalcinosis articularis* or 'pseudogout'. This condition affects knees most commonly but other joints are also affected, often in symmetrical fashion, with the appearance of calcification in the joint cartilages. Acute inflammatory episodes occur also in chronic *renal failure* with deposition of calcium salts in the soft tissues alongside, rather than in, joints. This may also be seen in patients following *renal transplantation* from cadavers or living donors other than identical twins. Polyarthritis with effusions, often in the knees, may occur in these patients who may have rheumatoid factor in the blood.

In *calcinosis circumscripta*, calcium salts (carbonate and phosphate) may be deposited under the skin but they are again para-articular rather than in the joint tissues, which appear normal.

Amyloidosis may be secondary to rheumatoid arthritis, ankylosing spondylitis and (more rarely) Reiter's disease, but it may also occur in primary form associated with pains and swellings in joints and, when associated with multiple myeloma, may cause the carpal tunnel syndrome.

Joint symptoms and backache in particular occur in *ochronosis*. Here the diagnosis is made by examination of the urine for homogentisic acid and the cartilage of the ears for pigmentation. Radiographs of the spine are typical, heavy calcification occurring in the intervertebral cartilages (*see Figs* B.1 and B.2).

Multicentric reticulohistiocytosis (lipoid dermato-arthritis) may be mistaken for rheumatoid arthritis in adults as changes in fingers and tenosynovitis occur, but the presence of yellow nodules on ears, forehead, neck, forearms and elsewhere, with groups of purple papules, suggests the true diagnosis which can be confirmed by biopsy. In advanced cases erosion of phalanges leads to shortening of the fingers.

In *Wilson's disease*, characterized by accumulation of copper in the tissues, arthritic changes, commonest in hands, wrists and knees, may start about

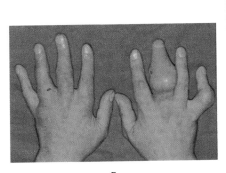 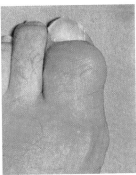 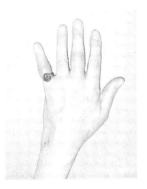

a   b   c

Fig. J.41. *a*, Severe tophaceous gout. *b*, Acute gout in big toe. *c*, Acute gout in middle and little fingers.

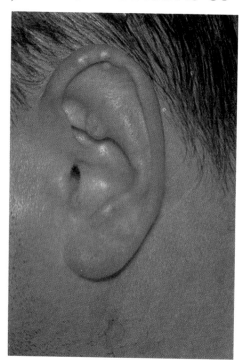

Fig. J.42. Typical tophi of gout in ear. They are opaque on transillumination.

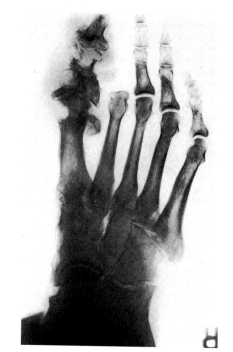

Fig. J.43. Severe destructive tophaceous gout. The second toe was even more severely affected and was removed.

the age of 30. Associated features are hepatic cirrhosis, psychiatric disease, and the Kayser–Fleischer green-brown ring around the cornea is diagnostic (*see Fig. J.10*).

11. Vascular arthropathies

Avascular necrosis occurs in caisson disease (nitrogen or air embolism), from fat embolism, and occasionally in chronic alcoholism. The hips are often bilaterally involved with destruction of parts of the heads of the femurs but shoulders and one or both knees may also be affected.

Giant-cell arteritis and *polymyalgia rheumatica* are probably two facets of the same condition occurring in the elderly as, on existing evidence, both conditions are due to an arteritis of those vessels having an internal elastic lamina. Renal and cerebral vessels are therefore usually spared. The patients, usually over the age of 60, are of either sex, have marked morning stiffness, sedimentation rates up to 100 mm in the first hour (Westergren) and pains and stiffness of shoulder and hip girdles. When the temporal vessels are involved a splitting headache is often present, and the main danger is to vision if branches of the ophthalmic artery become affected.

Pulses may disappear and murmurs be heard at the points of arterial narrowing. The sternoclavicular joints may be affected, but the disorder, as far as the girdle joints in general are concerned, is one of pain and stiffness in hips and shoulders without progressive clinical or radiological change and eventually with full recovery. Diagnosis can be confirmed by temporal artery biopsy.

In *polyarteritis nodosa* arthralgia is much more common than actual arthritis, but any joint may be affected in any pattern, local or general, severe or mild, flitting or constant. The appearance of nodules clinches the diagnosis but these occur in only a minority of cases and many biopsies may have to be done before the diagnosis is confirmed. Eosinophilia occurs in about 15 per cent of cases. Bronchial spasm is among the more common manifestations elsewhere but it is the multisystem distribution of symptoms which may suggest the diagnosis. When asthma, allergic rhinitis and eosinophilia are present the term 'Churg–Strauss vasculitis' is used.

12. Neoplastic arthropathies

Metastatic malignant disease or *multiple myeloma* usually cause bony rather than joint changes. The

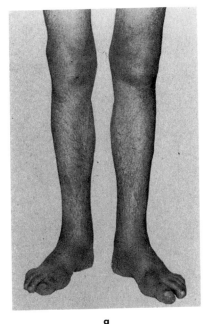

a

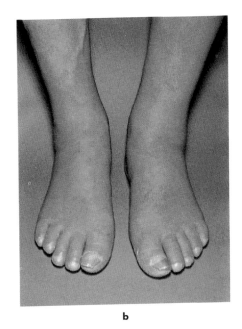

b

c

Fig. J.44. *a*, Hydrarthrosis of knees and swelling of ankles and feet due to bronchial carcinoma, causing pseudohypertrophic pulmonary osteoarthropathy. *b*, Swollen painful ankles in pseudohypertrophic pulmonary osteoarthropathy with *c*, wasting and loss of weight due to right basal bronchial carcinoma.

serum alkaline phosphatase, often elevated in the former, is usually normal in the latter as there is no osteoblastic activity in myelomatosis. Joint changes occur, however, in *hypertrophic pulmonary osteoarthropathy* (Figs J.44, J.45), a condition mostly associated with a bronchial carcinoma, usually a peripheral one. Removal of the primary lesion leads to rapid resolution of the effusions and arthritic changes in the more commonly affected joints, the knees and ankles. Fingers and toes are clubbed and the extremities show a thickening based on new subperiosteal bone deposition which can be seen in radiographs (*Fig.* J.46). Not

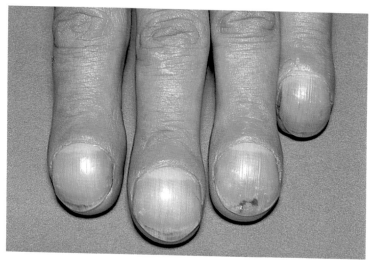

Fig. J.45. Pseudohypertrophic pulmonary osteoarthropathy, showing clubbed fingers.

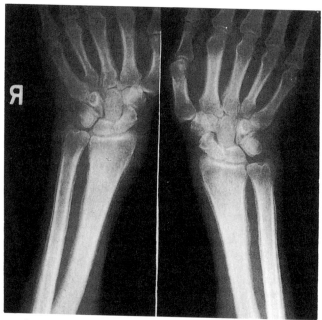

Fig. J.46. Pseudohypertrophic osteoarthropathy of the radius and ulna showing new periosteal bone deposition. (Dr T. H. Hills.)

all cases of hypertrophic osteoarthropathy are secondary to malignancy, however, some being due to cyanotic congenital heart disease, colonic and other conditions. In a familial primary form symptoms of *pachydermoperiostosis* start usually in adolescence, more commonly in males, the hands and feet enlarging with marked clubbing and cylindrical thickening of forearms and legs; recurrent joint effusions may occur. The patient's features thicken, giving a leonine appearance.

Osteoid osteoma is a benign disorder and, although not a disease of joints, it should be mentioned

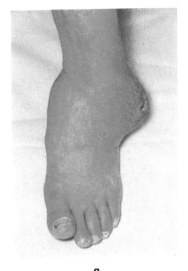
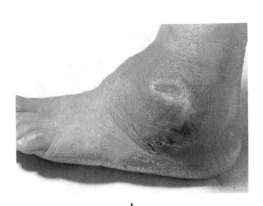

a   **b**

Fig. J.47. Charcot's disease of ankle showing disorganization of the joint (a) and gummatous ulcer (b). (Mr R. G. Beard.)

because of the pain it causes and the difficulties in differential diagnosis. The pain is initially intermittent but becomes more persistent and severe and is often aggravated by movement. There are no physical signs. It affects adolescents and young adults and, although any bone except the skull may be affected, the commonest to be involved are femur and tibia, which account for half the cases. Radiographs show a characteristic central opacity surrounded by a translucent zone, surrounded in turn by a zone of sclerosis. It may affect the bones of the spine, where it is often very difficult to diagnose and is usually not suspected. The pains are sometimes worse at night than during the day.

13. Neuropathic arthropathies

Although the *carpal tunnel syndrome* is not strictly a joint affection, it is so often a manifestation of rheumatoid arthritis that is should be mentioned. It is

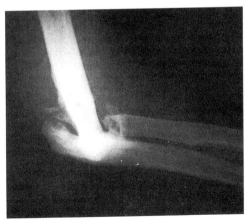

Fig. J.48. Charcot's disease of the knee joints in a patient with neurosyphilis showing the extraordinary mobility arising from joint destruction. The absence of pain is evident from the facies. (Dr Ralph Kauntze.)

Fig. J.49. Charcot's disease of the elbow joint in a patient with syringomyelia producing pathological dislocation. (Dr T. H. Hills.)

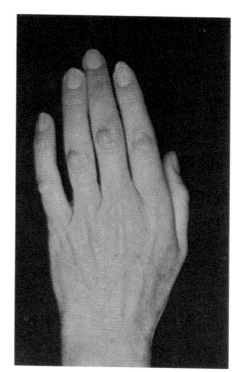

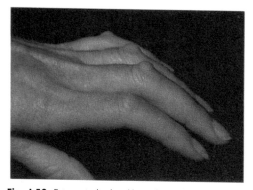

Fig. J.50. Extra-articular knuckle pads (Knobbly Knuckles, K.K. syndrome, Garrod's fatty or Hale White's nodes). They are fibrous, are not painful, and are only important in differential diagnosis from rheumatoid and osteoarthritic nodes.

not infrequently the first sign of this disorder. Other causes are pregnancy, acromegaly, myxoedema, multiple myeloma and amyloidosis. There is also an idiopathic variety with no apparent cause. Characteristic symptoms are tingling and hot and cold electrical sensations up the arms, interfering with sleep.

Neuropathic joints (*Figs* J.47–J.49) in the form of Charcot's joints in tabes dorsalis are characterized by their gross deformity, painlessness and florid X-ray appearances, where numbers of bone islands surround a grossly deformed or disorganized joint. Syringomyelia affects chiefly shoulder and elbow; knee, ankle, hip and spine are more commonly affected in tabes. Diabetic arthropathy is different in that clinical and radiological signs of infection are often present along with poor vascularization and signs of peripheral neuropathy; the condition is usually confined to the feet and toes.

Osborne's syndrome is due to ulnar nerve compression beneath the arcuate ligament just below the elbow.

In the *shoulder–hand syndrome*, a reflex dystrophy, trophic changes follow soon after injury to the shoulder or weeks or months after myocardial infarction; a similar syndrome has been reported in patients on antituberculous therapy and in other pathological conditions. The shoulder is stiff and painful, the skin of the hand shiny and smooth and sometimes hyperaesthetic, the muscles atrophic. There is no joint swelling, though initially there may be considerable swelling of the whole hand and fingers. X-rays show initially osteoporosis of humeral head and wrist, later a more diffuse 'ground-glass' appearance. In many cases there is no apparent cause for the condition.

14. Drug-induced arthropathy

Alcoholics are especially likely to sustain injuries to bones and joints; they are also more prone to septic arthritis and avascular necrosis of bone. Prolonged *corticosteroid therapy* may also be associated with septic arthritis, osteoporosis, and fractures. Crush fractures of lumbar or dorsal vertebrae are not uncommon. A condition very similar to systemic lupus erythematosus with LE cells present in the blood can be due to a large range of drugs, the commonest being procaine amide; this is the so-called *hydralazine syndrome*. Symptoms disappear on stopping the drug. It has also been reported with oral contraceptives, though such cases are very rare.

15. Miscellaneous arthropathies

The *knuckle pads* (Garrod's pads), seen not infrequently on the dorsal aspects of the proximal interphalangeal joints of the fingers (*Fig.* J.50), are usually not accompanied by any symptoms and are best disregarded. They are due to fibrous thickenings the size of small orange pips and are not part of the clinical picture of osteoarthritis or any other form of arthritis. They are not associated with any bony changes, though in some cases they occur with *Dupuytren's contracture* which, in turn, is occasionally associated with Peyronie's disease (induratio penis plastica). The palmar contractures occurring in rheumatoid arthritis may, on occasion, resemble Dupuytren's contracture (*see Fig.* J.38b). *Thorn synovitis* is an inflammatory condition due to a thorn or splinter of wood or a foreign body being knelt on by a child, who is hardly aware of it at the time. The *septic focus syndrome* is a rare disorder where diffuse aches and pains in and around joints are rapidly relieved by removal of a septic focus or drainage of an abscess. No residual changes are left in the tissues. Lastly, the *xiphoid syndrome* refers to pains which stem from a displaced or mobile xiphisternum, often the result of trauma. This simple condition is only noteworthy in that it may be mistaken for more serious disorders of stomach, duodenum, gall bladder or heart.

Joint disease in young children

The following conditions should be considered when children under 5 years of age present with joint symptoms.

Septic arthritis: due to staphylococci, haemolytic streptococci, *H. influenzae*, tuberculosis).

Associated with or *following* infection: adenovirus, rubella, mumps, chickenpox, *Mycoplasma pneumoniae*, cytomegalovirus, rickettsia, Lyme arthritis, Kawasaki's syndrome.

Idiopathic: chronic juvenile arthritis (Still's disease), familial Mediterranean fever.

Vascular and haematological: Henoch– Schönlein syndrome, sickle-cell disease, leukaemia, haemophilia, haemangioma, hypogammaglobulina- emia.

Dietetic: rickets.

Miscellaneous: Farber's disease, the mucopolysaccharidoses (e.g. Hurler–Scheie syndrome), injuries (the battered child syndrome), neuroblastoma, thorn synovitis.

INFECTIVE (SEPTIC CONDITIONS)
Infection in infancy

Staphylococcal infection is common, but many organisms may be responsible. The infant is ill, often rejecting food, vomiting or convulsing, but sometimes only mildly ill with slight fever. The hip is the most common joint to be affected and is held flexed and adducted, oedema appearing around the adductors.

Haemophilus influenzae infection is common in Great Britain. If several joints are affected suspect hypogammaglobulinaemia or some other immune abnormality. Staphylococcal, haemolytic streptococcal and, more rarely, tuberculous infection should be considered.

INFECTIONS

Other infections with adenoviruses often start with pharyngitis followed a few days later by fever, macular erythematous rash and a symmetrical arthritis which lasts up to 6 weeks. A similar transient arthropathy may occur with rubella, mumps and chickenpox. Infection with cytomegalovirus is often associated with abnormal tests of liver function and infection with *Mycoplasma pneumoniae* with erythema multiforme. Other infections not seen in the UK unless imported are rickettsial infections such as Rocky Mountain Spotted Fever or Lyme arthritis where a small red macule or papule enlarges to form a large erythematous ring followed by fever and arthritis, usually of only a few joints. In Japan and the East, Kawasaki's syndrome should be considered a possibility.

NON-INFECTIVE INFLAMMATORY CONDITIONS

Juvenile chronic arthritis often presents under 5 years of age (*see* p. 206). If of inflammatory onset it has to be distinguished from the infective conditions above.

Andrew Keat

Keloid

A keloid is a benign but uncontrolled fibrous overgrowth of the dermis in response to wounding. The tendency to form keloids is a personal trait, more common in blacks, young adults and in the stretched skin of neck and chest. Usually the antecedent damage is obvious, e.g. surgical incisions, pierced ear lobes (*Fig.* K.1), burns and chickenpox. Keloids may follow acne and folliculitis, chiefly on the chest (*Fig.* K.2) and

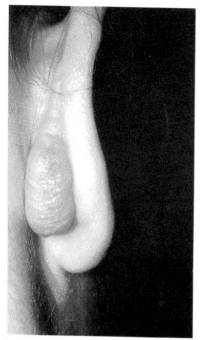

Fig. K.1. Keloid following ear piercing. (*Westminster Hospital.*)

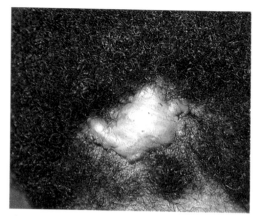

Fig. K.3. Keloid folliculitis on back of neck. (*Dr Richard Staughton.*)

at the back of the neck (*Fig.* K.3), where ingrowing hairs may be a perpetuating factor. Keloids commonly recur following an excision unless intralesional steroids are injected at the time of operation or radiotherapy is administered during the postoperative period.

A keloid can be differentiated from simple hypertrophy in a scar by the observations that the overgrowth extends beyond the limits of the wound itself and continues to enlarge; a hypertrophied scar is confined to the wound limits and tends to regress with time.

Richard Staughton

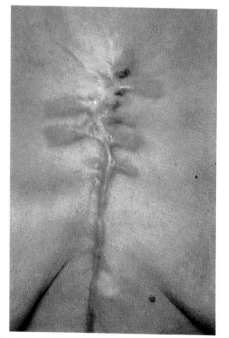

Fig. K.2. Keloid following cardiac surgery. Note the extension of scar tissue beyond the limits of the median sternotomy incision. (*Westminster Hospital.*)

Kidney, palpable

A renal swelling may be so slight that it is only found upon careful clinical examination, or it may be large enough to attract the patient's attention. Hydronephrosis, pyonephrosis, renal tuberculosis or abscess, new growth or cysts (single or multiple) in the kidney have to be diagnosed not only from one another but also from other tumours simulating a renal swelling. The characteristic points of a renal tumour are:

1. The *intestine is in front of the tumour*. When either kidney is merely slightly enlarged, both large and small intestines will be in front of it; but when the organ is so enlarged as to reach the anterior abdominal wall the coils of small intestine are pushed aside. The anatomical relation of the large intestine to the kidney, and the absence of a mesentery, do not allow of the same mobility of the colon, which usually retains its position in front of the kidney, although it is sometimes pushed downwards by a tumour projecting forwards from the lower pole. Hence an area of resonance can usually be obtained in front of a renal swelling; if the

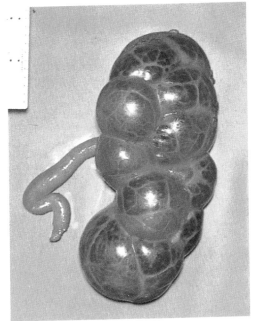

Fig. K.4. Enormous hydronephrosis due to small stone impacted in the distal ureter. The kidney was so large that it could readily be felt on rectal as well as abdominal examination, yet it has retained its reniform shape.

colon is empty it can sometimes be felt in a thin subject and rolled by the fingers on the surface of the tumour. Bowel is almost never placed in front of a splenic tumour, and only rarely in front of a hepatic tumour.

2. The *area of dullness to percussion* is continuous from the lateral aspect of the swelling to the midline posteriorly — that is, there is no area of resonance between the mass and the vertebral spines, as with a splenic or ovarian tumour.

3. A renal tumour usually *retains the shape of the kidney*; it is rounded at its borders and poles, and does not possess any edge or sharp margin, as do splenic or hepatic swellings (*Fig.* K.4). The surface of the tumour may present rounded, smooth, raised bosses in cases of renal growths or in polycystic disease.

4. A *renal tumour* in the process of enlargement *projects forwards and downwards*. It may fill up the natural hollow of the loin, but seldom causes any prominence posteriorly. A perinephric abscess, which often simulates a renal swelling, may cause a distinct prominence in the loin.

5. A renal tumour may be movable downwards or inwards, unless it is fixed in the loin by preceding inflammation, or by the spread of carcinoma into the perirenal tissues; an enlarged kidney may be felt bimanually, and if grasped between the two hands *can*

be pushed into the loin. A renal tumour rarely descends into the iliac fossa but it may be present there in congenital ectopia or in cases of excessive mobility.

6. When a renal tumour is large enough to reach the anterior abdominal wall it commonly comes in contact with it at the level of the umbilicus, at the same time bulging out the iliocostal space. There is usually a line of resonance between the upper margin of the tumour and the hepatic dullness.

7. A *varicocele* may be developed on the same side as the renal tumour due to obstruction of the testicular vein as this drains into the renal vein on the left or the inferior vena cava on the right. This is especially significant on the right side, although it is a rare finding, and I have personally never seen a renal tumour associated with a rapidly developing varicocele due to involvement of the testicular vein.

8. With a renal tumour there may be *changes in the urine* pointing to renal disease; but on the other hand, the urine at any one time may be normal, free from blood or pus, from the fact that the ureter of the diseased side is blocked, or that the disease does not involve the renal pelvis.

9. In exceptional cases, a tumour of the right kidney may extend upwards towards the dome of the diaphragm, rotating the liver so that the anterior margin of the latter descends below the costal margin, and prevents satisfactory palpation of the renal areas.

Although, from the above physical characters, it would seem that a renal tumour should present little difficulty in diagnosis, yet it is by no means infrequent to find that a tumour possessing several of these characters may give rise to considerable doubt in the determination of the organ from which it arises. The following points will assist in the diagnosis of renal swellings from other tumours with which they are likely to be confused.

1. Enlargements of the gallbladder

These are placed immediately below the costal margin, so that no interval exists between the tumour and the lower margin of the liver. They are usually oval in outline, with the long axis in the line between the 9th right costal cartilage and the umbilicus, are freely movable with the respiratory movements, and movable from side to side about an axis at the costal margin. There is dullness on percussion over them, and they cannot be felt in the loin or be grasped bimanually. With an enlarged gallbladder there may be attacks of colic, with or without jaundice. A good radiograph may show the outline of a distended gallbladder distinct from the shadow of the kidney, and gallstones may sometimes be seen, while a cholecystographic examination will show that no contrast medium enters the gallbladder. Ultrasonography is a particularly valuable non-invasive method of demonstrating the distended gallbladder and will also show up gallstones, which are highly echogenic.

2. Enlargements of the liver

These pass downwards from beneath the costal margin so that there is no line or resonance, or area in which the hand can be depressed, between the tumour and the costal margin. Hepatic tumours do not impair the normal resonance in the loin in the same manner as a renal tumour does. A tongue-shaped lobe of the liver (Riedel's lobe) may cause difficulty in diagnosis; but here the lower margin is seldom so rounded as is that of a renal tumour, nor will the mass be felt in the loin on bimanual examination. A tumour or cyst in the concave aspect, or of the left lobe, of the liver is especially liable to cause error in diagnosis, whereas, on the other hand, a tumour of the right kidney which projects upwards behind the liver may so rotate the latter that its anterior margin descends below the costal margin and completely obscures the kidney. In a case of a large carcinoma of the right kidney, the liver may in this way be so depressed as to render palpation of the kidney impossible. A pyelographic examination may reveal a normal renal picture or on the other hand may indicate a hydronephrosis or renal growth. Ultrasonography will readily differentiate between a hepatic and a renal swelling.

3. Enlargements of the spleen

These descend from beneath the left costal margin, and have no bowel in front of them, they are therefore dull to percussion. The edge of a splenic tumour is usually well defined and often notched and there is resonance between the posterior aspect of the tumour and the spinal column. A splenic tumour is more movable than is a left renal tumour. A blood count may help in deciding in favour of a splenic enlargement, and a pyelogram may show a normal kidney. Abdominal ultrasonography will enable accurate delineation of the spleen.

4. Perinephric effusions

Whether of blood, pus or urine, these may form a tumour in the loin which upon physical examination may be mistaken for a renal swelling. A perinephric effusion may arise from some suppurative condition of the kidney, so that the previous history and examination of the urine will not assist in differential; or it may be due to conditions entirely distinct from renal

disease. An effusion of blood around the kidney is, in nearly all cases, caused by an injury to the loin, and will be accompanied by other signs of injury. It may, however, occur from the spontaneous growth and rupture of a renal neoplasm. A perinephric abscess forms a less well-defined tumour than that caused by a renal swelling, is more acute in its general symptoms, such as pain and temperature, and fills up the iliocostal space. The skin over it may be thickened or oedematous, and fluctuation may be felt to be more superficial than in a renal swelling. A perinephric abscess may result from suppuration about a carcinoma or diverticulum of the large bowel, from appendiceal inflammation, or from suppuration in a perinephric haematoma due to injury; it may be a sequel to a specific blow, or be due to a haematogenous infection. Bilateral palpation and comparison of the loins may detect a perinephric swelling by the way the loin is filled out and becomes even convex on the affected side. This is best seen by laying the patient prone and carefully inspecting both sides. A high leucocyte count in the blood with increased percentage of polymorphonuclear cells would be in favour of perinephric inflammation.

5. Tumours arising from the pelvic organs

Tumours arising from the pelvic organs, from the ovary or uterus, may in some cases simulate renal tumours. An ovarian cyst with a long pedicle occupying the loin may be mistaken for an enlarged or movable kidney, and any sudden attacks of pain occurring from torsion of the pedicle may be looked upon as due to renal colic. The usual ovarian cyst or uterine fibroid will seldom be confused with a renal swelling, for it is placed in the midline of the body, can be felt to come up from the pelvis, and can be felt on bimanual vaginal examination to be attached to the uterus or its appendages. These tumours give rise to dullness anteriorly, and do not alter the normal resonance in the loin. In cases of malignant ovarian tumours associated with ascites the lumbar resonance may be lost, but on turning the patient over on one side the previously dull note becomes replaced by resonance in the uppermost loin. In the case of an ovarian cyst with a long pedicle, or of a uterine fibroid of pedunculated, subserous form, the position in the loin may sometimes suggest a renal tumour; it will be found, however, to occupy a more anterior position in the abdomen than a renal tumour, and to possess a much greater range of movement, and it does not slip back into the loin under the costal margin in the same manner as an enlarged kidney does; there is resonance posteriorly, the kidney may be actually palpated as well as the abdominal tumour, while a distinct connection with the pelvic organs can sometimes be traced from the tumour when the latter is drawn up.

In contradistinction to the above a very large cystic renal swelling may be mistaken for an ovarian cyst. It may occupy the greater part of the abdomen, and even be felt per vaginam to be encroaching upon the pelvis; but on careful examination of a renal tumour of this form there will be no line of resonance between the mass and the vertebral column posteriorly, the natural hollow of the loin will be filled up, and there is frequently a distinct bulging in the lower thoracic wall, together with an increased length of the iliocostal space on the affected side. Some assistance may be obtained from the history; a hydronephrosis may have been first noticed as a tumour starting under the costal margin and gradually increasing downwards towards the iliac fossa and inwards across the median line, whereas an ovarian tumour may have been noticed to increase upwards from the pelvis. With an ovarian or pelvic tumour, a pyelogram will show a normal renal pelvis. Ultrasonography usually enables accurate anatomical diagnosis of the pelvic mass.

Laparoscopic examination is a valuable, if interventional, method of direct visualization of suspected pelvic masses.

6. Suprarenal tumours

Suprarenal tumours may occasionally be of sufficient size to form an abdominal tumour, presenting a rounded, movable swelling in the hypochondrium. It is sometimes possible to distinguish them from renal tumours by radiography after presacral insufflation of oxygen into the retroperitoneal tissue, or, more certainly and with far less disturbance to the patient, by computerized tomography.

7. Faecal accumulation in the colon, caecum or sigmoid flexure

These may give rise to a tumour and pain of a colicky nature in the loin; the tumour can sometimes be indented by the examining fingers. They will be distinguished from renal swellings by the general intestinal symptoms, flatulence and the changes in form consequent on the administration of large enemas. A patient with a collection of faeces in the colon may not complain of constipation, but may in fact have a small daily evacuation from the overloaded bowel. A plain X-ray of the abdomen will usually demonstrate the faecal masses.

8. Appendicular inflammatory mass

This will be diagnosed from renal tumours by the situation of the pain and by the swelling being in the iliac fossa rather than in the loin. In some cases, however, the pain may be referred to the lumbar region, or an appendiceal inflammatory mass may spread upwards. This is especially so when the appendix is retrocaecal in position. The onset of the trouble, the acute symptoms, and the febrile disturbance will usually distinguish these cases from renal lesions. There is nearly always a polymorph leucocytosis. Ultrasonography will demonstrate the mass and confirm its distinction from the normal right kidney.

9. Malignant growth of the large intestine

Malignant growth of the large intestine, especially of the ascending or descending colon, may form a tumour in the loin which closely resembles a renal swelling. The mass formed by the growth may be grasped bimanually, is movable in the same directions as a renal tumour, and comes forward under the costal margin. The percussion note over the front of the lump is resonant, and there is usually an aching pain in the loin. If the growth has infiltrated through the wall of the bowel uncovered by peritoneum, the perirenal tissues may be thickened, or proteinuria may be produced by direct invasion of the kidney, when the case will even more resemble a renal lesion. Carcinoma of the large intestine should be suspected if there is any irregularity in the action of the bowels, mucus or blood in the motions, or any symptom of incipient obstruction in the intestine. The tumour may be irregular and nodular, whereas a renal tumour presents rounded margins. The occurrence of a tumour in either side, associated with discomfort or palpable distension of the caecum from the accumulation of faeces, would render a growth in the colon the more suspicious.

The diagnosis of a large bowel tumour can usually be established by a barium enema X-ray examination. Confirmation can be made by direct colonoscopic examination, at which, usually, biopsy material can be obtained for histological examination.

10. Tumours of the omentum, mesentery or pancreas

These tumours, either cystic or malignant, are more median in position, do not project into the loin and seldom resemble a renal tumour. Retroperitoneal and perirenal tumours may closely simulate renal tumours but can be distinguished on pyelography; they displace the ureter medially or laterally.

In many cases in which difficulty arises in the diagnosis of a swelling in the loin, great help may be obtained by excretion urography (p. 227) or by retrograde pyelography by the injection into the renal pelvis and calices of a medium opaque to X-rays, through a ureteric catheter. By these means the renal pelvis and calices may be outlined clearly in their normal position, and any change in position or shape may indicate that the swelling is of renal origin. The detailed anatomy of these masses can usually be demonstrated by CT scan.

THE DIFFERENTIAL DIAGNOSIS OF RADIOGRAPHIC SHADOWS IN THE ABDOMEN AND THE PELVIS

It is necessary for the true interpretation of radiographs that a clear conception should be held of the various conditions which may cast a shadow on an X-ray negative. In the diagnosis of cases of urinary disease much information may be gained by the use of X-rays, and not merely in the confirmation of the presence of calculi in some part of the urinary tract; in a good film the outline and the size of the kidney can be seen, while, by means of excretion urography or by the direct injection of the ureter and the pelvis of the kidney with a radio-opaque solution, the size, position and shape of either may be outlined accurately and

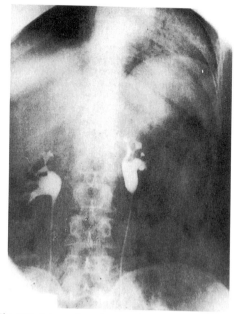

Fig. K.6. Retrograde pyelogram. The right kidney is normal. On the left the calices are clubbed and the pelvis dilated from the presence of a calculus, which is hidden by the contrast medium.

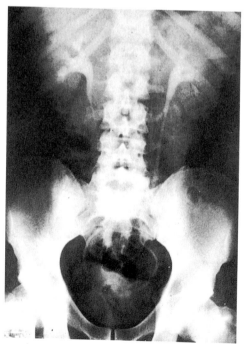

Fig. K.5. Normal excretion pyelogram, 30-minute film after removal of compression. The calices are cupped, the left ureter is filled completely and the right partially.

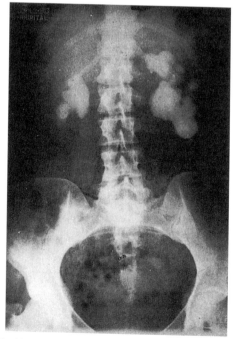

Fig. K.7. Radiograph showing bilateral renal calculi. On the left the dendritic stone forms a cast of the renal pelvis and calices.

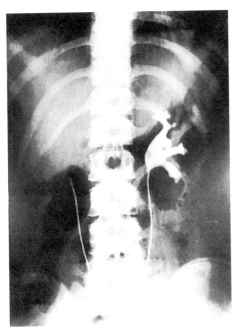

Fig. K.8. Pyelogram outlining a pure uric acid stone in the left kidney. It gave no shadow on the plain film.

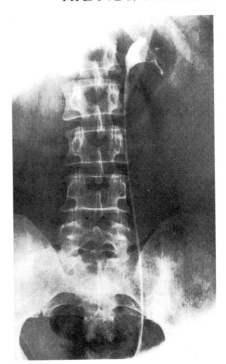

Fig. K.9. Retrograde pyelogram showing a benign tumour as a filling defect in the left renal pelvis.

compared with the normal (*Figs* K.5, K.6). In a good film after efficient alimentary preparation the outline of a normal kidney should be visible, lying opposite the bodies of the 1st, 2nd and 3rd lumbar vertebrae (*Fig.* K.5), and having an excursion of from 4 to 5 cm in forced inspiration and expiration. A *renal calculus* (*Figs* K.6, K.7) in a radiograph casts a shadow superimposed upon the renal shadow. If it is of triangular or branched outline, it is almost certainly a renal calculus; but others may give a shadow of even, uniform density, of sharp outline, yet clearly renal as shown by the manner in which the opacity moves equally with the renal shadow in respiratory movements. In a film taken laterally through the transverse axis of the patient, a renal calculus should make a shadow superimposed upon the bodies of the upper lumbar vertebrae, usually the 2nd, unless the kidney is enlarged, when the shadow of a calculus may be displaced in front of the vertebral bodies. A stone composed of pure uric acid may give no shadow on a radiograph; one of calcium oxalate gives the most dense shadow; next in order of density is the phosphatic; those of urates, cystine and xanthine give a less definite shadow. A radiolucent stone may, however, be shown as a negative shadow in an excretion or retrograde pyelogram; it must be distinguished from a tumour of the renal pelvis, an air bubble or blood clot.

In the case of a stone the contrast medium is more likely to surround the shadow completely (*Fig.* K.8) whilst a tumour will be attached at some point (*Fig.* K.9). Blood clot is irregular and an air bubble can be displaced in a second radiograph.

The shape of a shadow in the renal area will often indicate its position in the kidney and an excretion pyelogram will confirm it (*Fig.* K.10). There are, however, several other conditions which may cast a shadow in the renal area, and it is necessary to differentiate these from the shadow of a renal calculus. The following are the most frequent:

1. Intestinal contents
2. Calcification of mesenteric lymph nodes
3. Gallstones, on the right side
4. Calcification of the costal cartilages
5. Caseous masses in a tuberculous kidney
6. Areas of calcification in a renal growth
7. Foreign bodies

1. INTESTINAL CONTENTS may cast a shadow in the renal area owing to inefficient preparation of the patient or to the fact that he has recently taken as medicine bismuth, magnesium salts, etc. Faecal masses in a loaded colon are often visualized. If any doubt exists a second examination should be made after further purgation. There may be some residue in the intestine from a recent barium meal examination.

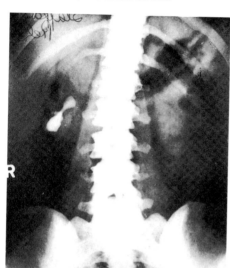
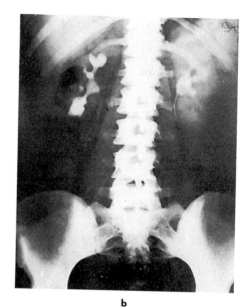

a   b

Fig. K.10. *a.* Radiograph showing a dumb-bell shadow in the right renal area. *b.* The excretion pyelogram shows that the shadow is a stone occupying the lowest calix and pelvis of the right kidney.

2. CALCIFICATION OF THE ABDOMINAL OR MESENTERIC LYMPH NODES may cause a shadow in any part of the abdominal cavity. Though they are most frequently seen near the lower lumbar vertebrae or about the sacroiliac joint, and therefore external to the renal shadow, they may be superimposed upon the latter and cause difficulty in diagnosis. The shadow of a calcified node is usually mottled in appearance, small areas in the shadow showing increased density owing to the irregular deposition of lime salts; calcareous nodes are frequently multiple, but their chief characteristic is their range of mobility. Thus if more than one negative is taken with varying degrees of compression the shadows of calcareous nodes may show a varying position with regard to the renal shadow, whilst in a lateral view a lymph node shadow is usually in front of the bodies of the vertebrae and not superimposed upon them. A calcified node may be placed immediately in front of the kidney and move equally with it, causing great difficulty in diagnosis; or there may be a calculus in one kidney and calcareous nodes imitating calculi on the other side.

A pyelogram will show the relation of a calculus to the renal pelvis (*Fig.* K.10).

3. GALLSTONES may give a shadow in the renal area on the right side. They are frequently multiple, and may be seen to be faceted in a fusiform collection presenting the shape of the distended gallbladder (*Fig.* K.11). A single gallstone superimposed on the renal shadow may cause difficulty; the shadow of a gallstone is less dense than is that of a renal stone, and is

frequently more dense in the central than in the peripheral part. In a lateral view a stone in the gallbladder will occupy an anterior position in the abdomen, though one impacted in the common bile

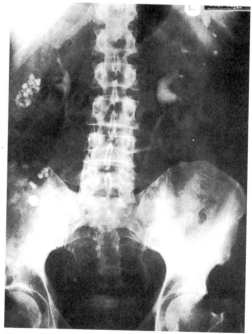

Fig. K.11. Intravenous pyelogram showing a normal renal tract but also a collection of faceted stones in the gallbladder, calcified mesenteric glands in the right iliac fossa and phleboliths in the pelvis.

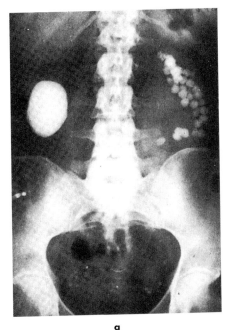
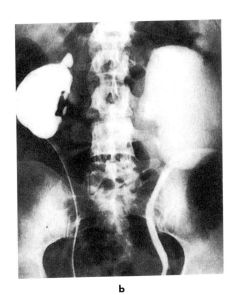

a   b

Fig. K.12. *a.* Large single dense shadow on the right and multiple small ones on the left. *b.* Pyelography shows that the shadows are enclosed in the dilated pelves of a horseshoe kidney. Note the inwardly pointing calices and the flower-vase pattern of the ureters.

duct may be seen opposite the body of the 1st or 2nd lumbar vertebra; in this case there will probably be jaundice. In a cholecystographic examination a gall-stone may cause a filling defect (negative shadow) in the area of the gallbladder occupied by the dye. The distribution of stones in a horseshoe kidney may cause confusion until a pyelogram is done (*Fig. K.*12).

4. CALCIFICATION OF THE COSTAL CARTILAGES may give a shadow in the renal area in an anteroposterior negative. The shadows are not dense, are hazy in outline, and tend to assume a horizontal or oblique axis. In a lateral view they will be placed immediately under the anterior abdominal wall.

5. CASEOUS MASSES IN A TUBERCULOUS KIDNEY. The shadow in this condition is rarely so defined as is that of a calculus, is of moderate density with blurred and indistinct margins, appearing as one or more blotches in the renal area; but occasionally, from the deposition of calcium salts, it may be very like the radiograph of a calculus (*see Fig. H.*5).

6. CALCAREOUS AREAS IN A RENAL CARCINOMA. Rarely faint ill-defined areas may be present in a renal carcinoma. There will, however, be symptoms of a growth, such as haematuria and renal tumour, whilst a pyelographic examination will show a deformity of the pelvis and renal calices.

7. A FOREIGN BODY, such as a shrapnel bullet, lying in front of or behind the kidney may mimic a calculus.

The line of the *normal ureter* lies anatomically along or just internal to the tips of the transverse processes of the 2nd to the 5th lumbar vertebrae, passes with a slight curve outwards in front of the sacro-iliac articulation, and then with a marked curve forwards and inwards to the base of the bladder. A shadow in this line may be due to a calculus in the ureter, but it must be differentiated carefully from other conditions. A calculus is usually small, rounded or oval, with a long axis in the line of the ureter. It may be found in any part of the course of the ureter, but it is seen most frequently in the lower end just before it enters the bladder. The conditions which may give a shadow that is likely to be mistaken for a ureteric calculus are:

1. Calcified lymph node
2. A concretion in the appendix or the intestinal contents
3. Phleboliths in the pelvis
4. A foreign body

1. CALCIFIED LYMPH NODES in the line of the ureter are placed most frequently in the angle between the last lumbar vertebra and the ala of the sacrum. They are usually multiple, forming a group in this situation in triangular form rather than in the longitudinal axis of the ureter; they are mottled in appearance, of irregular density, and are so movable that their position varies in successive radiographs. Should difficulty arise, the examination should be repeated after a radio-opaque catheter has been passed into the ureter by means of a

cystoscope. In many cases a stereoscopic examination of the area with a catheter in the ureter or a radiograph by the 'double-shift' technique in which two exposures are made on the same film, the tube being moved laterally before the second exposure is made, will show that the suspicious shadow is some distance from the ureter. A catheter may often be passed up the ureter alongside and pass a calculus in the duct, but a stereoscopic examination will show that the two are actually in contact with each other.

2. A CONCRETION IN THE APPENDIX may occasionally give rise to a shadow in the line of the right ureter, suggesting a calculus with very similar clinical symptoms. Further examination with a radio-opaque catheter in the ureter will show that the shadow is extra-ureteric.

3. PHLEBOLITHS IN THE PELVIS are liable to be mistaken for ureteric calculi, but they often have a characteristic ring-like appearance, which is quite diagnostic. They are usually multiple and are placed towards the peripheral areas of the pelvis, often about the level of the ischial spine. A stereoscopic examination with an opaque catheter in the ureter will differentiate them from calculi, though it may not be possible to distinguish them from calcified lymph nodes. It must not be forgotten that a calculus may be present in the ureter in addition to phleboliths, but the distinction can be made by excretion pyelography or radiography after the passage of a ureteric catheter. *Fig.* K.13 shows that the shadow of the ureter does not impinge on any of the numerous phleboliths present in the pelvis.

4. FOREIGN BODIES, especially after periods of war, may occasionally lie near the line of the ureter. They are usually more dense than calculi.

A shadow may be present in a pelvic radiograph which must be differentiated from that of a vesical calculus. The latter is usually rounded or oval, occupies a fairly central position in the pelvis, and may show rings of varying density owing to the deposition of layers of urinary salts of different composition. Occasionally one or more vesical calculi may form a shadow in a more lateral position in successive negatives, when a suspicion of their presence in a diverticulum in the bladder will arise. The diagnosis of this condition is discussed below. The following conditions may give rise to radiographic shadows in the pelvis.

1. Prostatic calculi
2. Calcification of a uterine fibroid
3. Opaque masses in a dermoid cyst of the ovary
4. Phosphatic encrustation upon a vesical growth
5. Foreign bodies in the bladder
6. Urethral calculi

1. PROSTATIC CALCULI may be single or multiple, but in the radiograph they occupy a position very low in

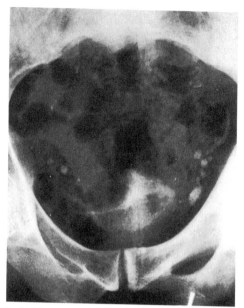

Fig. K.13. Excretion pyelogram showing numerous phleboliths in the pelvis; the left ureter is seen passing between them. Note the 'bite' defect in the bladder caused by a solid carcinoma.

the pelvis, often behind the shadow of the pubis (*Fig.* K.14). They would not be seen by a cystoscope, but might be felt during the passage of any instrument through the prostatic urethra. They are palpable in the gland per rectum, either as a hard, inelastic nodule embedded in the prostate, or by the grating of multiple calculi on each other on pressure.

2. CALCIFICATION OF A FIBROID TUMOUR OF THE UTERUS gives a large, irregular shadow of varying degree of density. Bimanual palpation of a tumour moving with the uterus would point to the diagnosis.

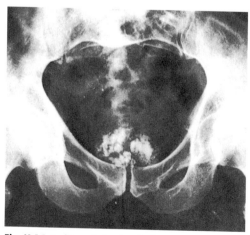

Fig. K.14. Radiograph showing shadows in the pelvis due to multiple prostatic calculi.

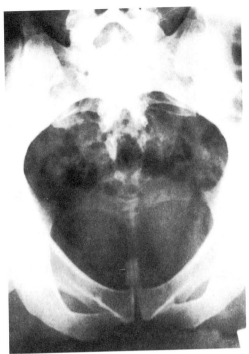

Fig. K.15. Radiograph showing a shadow due to a cystine calculus in the prostatic urethra.

3. OVARIAN DERMOIDS may give rise to irregular shadows in the pelvis due to the formation of bone or teeth in the cyst. They may be present in young adult life, and a tumour would be palpated on abdominal or pelvic examination.

4. PHOSPHATIC ENCRUSTATION UPON A VESICAL TUMOUR may occur in a case of growth in the presence of cystitis and give rise to faint ill-defined shadows in the pelvic radiograph. A cystoscopic examination will reveal the true nature of the lesion.

5. FOREIGN BODIES in the bladder may become so encrusted with urinary salts that a shadow like that of a calculus may be present. A variety of foreign bodies have been found in the bladder, either introduced by intent or by the accidental breaking off of a piece of catheter or the like. In some cases the shadow will show a central area of different density or even a metallic nucleus.

6. URETHRAL CALCULI may be retained in the canal behind a stricture and enlarge *in situ*. They form a shadow in a radiograph above or below the pubic arch (*Fig.* K.15).

Imaging techniques

Much assistance in the diagnosis of urinary disease apart from the presence of calculi may be afforded by means of imaging techniques (radiology, ultrasonog-

raphy and computerized tomography), supplemented by methods used by the urologist; cytoscopy, urethroscopy and, if necessary, the passage of a retrograde ureteric catheter. A good plain film taken in a thin subject may show the outline and size of the kidneys so plainly that one of them may be demonstrated to be enlarged, or the irregularity of outline may give rise to a suspicion of malignant growth. Methods have been devised by which more information may be gained — for example, by the injection of gas into the presacral tissues or by direct introduction into the renal pelvis, calices and ureter of radio-opaque solutions, or by the injection into the circulation of radio-opaque dye which is excreted by the kidneys, or by the injection of such substances into the aorta.

Presacral gas insufflation consists of distending the fatty tissue around the kidney with oxygen, CO_2 or air; by this method a more distinct outline of the kidney is obtained. The injection is made into the retroperitoneal tissues in the presacral hollow. The outline of the kidneys can usually be clearly demonstrated and sometimes that of the liver and spleen. The method is harmless and usually painless. Nowadays this technique has been almost entirely replaced by ultrasound scanning or CT scanning, which, in turn, may be superseded by MRI scanning as these machines come in to more universal use.

The injection of radio-opaque solutions into the renal pelvis and ureter, combined with radiography (*retrograde pyelography* and *ureterography*), has a

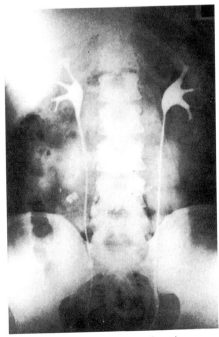

Fig. K.16. A normal bilateral retrograde pyelogram.

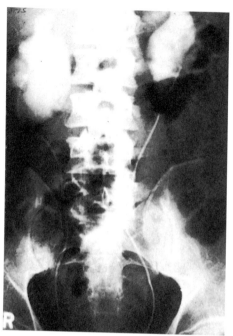

Fig. K.17. Retrograde pyelogram in a case of bilateral hydronephrosis associated with pelvi–ureteric obstruction.

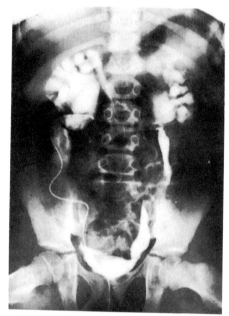

Fig. K.19. Retrograde pyelogram showing bilateral congenital hydro-ureter and hydronephrosis in a girl.

wide application and renders more precise information than can be obtained by the perirenal insufflation method; the two investigations can be successfully combined. A dilute solution of 25 per cent sodium

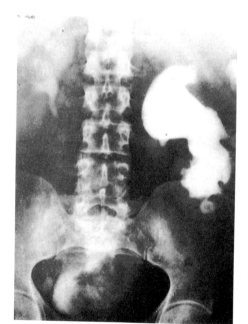

Fig. K.18. An excretion pyelogram showing a giant calculus in the left kidney. Note the filling defect in the bladder caused by a large papillary tumour.

diatrizoate ('Hypaque') or 35 per cent meglumine iothalamate, the drug used for excretion urography, is used. For this method of pyelography (the 'ascending pyelogram') a ureteric catheter is passed by means of the cystoscope through the ureteric orifice; the solution is injected very slowly by means of a small syringe or allowed to run in by gravitation until the patient begins to feel discomfort in the loin, an accurate measure of the amount of fluid injected being recorded. The pelvis of the normal kidney will hold an average of 6 ml before pain is produced. A radiograph is taken immediately, when an exact outline of the renal pelvis and calices is displaced as a dense shadow (*Figs* K.6, K.16). In cases of renal distension a much larger amount can be injected before pain is produced (*Figs* K.17–K.19).

The determination of a normal renal pelvis by radiography has also aided the diagnosis in many cases of doubtful abdominal tumours in which the clinical data have raised a suspicion of renal disease. There may be doubt as to whether a tumour palpable in the abdomen and causing pain in the loin is a renal tumour or whether it originates in the colon, gallbladder, pancreas or suprarenal gland. Examination by pyelography may demonstrate a normal renal pelvis which would in many cases exclude any disease of the kidney.

To obtain a radiograph of the ureter it is advisable to pass a ureteric catheter with an acorn tip only a short distance into the ureter before making the injection; in this way any dilatation or deviation from the normal line of the ureter is demonstrated, whereas the passage of the catheter along the whole length of the canal might straighten out the latter. In some cases the passage of the catheter may be obstructed in the ureter; in these the injection should be made with the catheter in situ, when the fluid may find its way past the obstruction and radiography may show a dilated or tortuous ureter (*Fig*. K.19) with dilatation of the pelvis of the kidney.

Occasionally a radiographic picture of the bladder is required to determine the size of a diverticulum, the vesical opening of which has been found on cystoscopy. For this purpose the same type and concentration of dye is used as in retrograde pyelography. Radiographs are then taken in both the anteroposterior and the oblique planes; it is also of advantage to repeat the exposures after the patient has voluntarily voided the vesical contents, when the diverticulum may be seen to remain filled with the solution.

Excretion urography is a method of pyelography consisting of the *intravenous injection* of non-toxic fluids of high iodine content and depends upon the excretion of the radio-opaque solution by the kidney. For this purpose 40-60 ml of 45 per cent sodium diatrizoate ('Hypaque') or meglumine iothalamate 60 per cent is injected into a vein after the patient has abstained from drinking any liquid for at least 6 hours. Radiographs are then taken at intervals of 1, 5, 15 and 30 minutes after the injection. In cases in which the kidneys are of normal efficiency, a distinct shadow should be obtained of the renal pelvis and calices of each side in the first picture, increasing in definition in the second (*Fig*. K.5). The outlines of the ureters may be seen and in the later pictures the bladder is outlined in the pelvis. This test differs from the ascending method in being dependent upon the functional efficiency of the kidney; if this is impaired the test may fail to show any shadow owing to lack of excretion of the fluid, and therefore it may be used as a test of function as well as a radiographic test. The simplicity of the method has much to recommend it, but it must be said that the outlines of the renal pelvis and calices may be indistinct, and insufficient to rely upon for accurate diagnosis, in which case it has to be sometimes supplemented by the ascending method. In cases in which there is obstruction to the ureter, dilatation of the latter and of the renal pelvis may be distinctly seen. In cases of vesical tumour a distinct filling defect may be seen in the bladder in the later negatives (*Fig*. K.13). Compression of the lower ends of the ureters by a pneumatic belt and pads suitably placed after the first pictures have been taken improves the definition and filling even more.

Aortography is done by the translumbar route or by catheterization of the femoral artery (Seldinger's method). In the translumbar method 20-30 ml of 60 per cent meglumine iothalamate are injected directly into the upper part of the abdominal aorta in order to outline the renal vascular system. It is carried out under general or local anaesthesia with the patient in the prone position; a long needle, up to 10 in (25 cm) in length, is introduced from the left side of the body of the 1st lumbar vertebra below the last rib and passed forwards, inwards and upwards to enter the aorta above the origin of the renal arteries; 30 ml of solution are injected quickly and films are taken as soon as the injection starts and as rapidly as possible whilst it continues. The early ones show the arterial system and the later ones show the nephrographic phase when the whole of the renal substance is opacified; they may also show the veins and sometimes some filling of the pelvis (*Fig*. K.20).

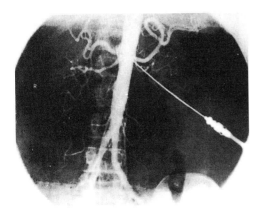

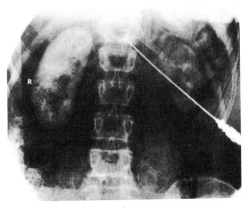

a   b

Fig. K.20. *a*. Aortogram done by the translumbar method: arterial phase. The right renal artery, seen below the hepatic, is of normal size. The left, seen below the splenic, is small. *b*. Nephrographic phase in the same case. The left kidney is small and less densely opacified than the right, it contained a papillary carcinoma in the upper calix.

In the femoral approach by the Seldinger technique (now by far the more commonly used) a fine catheter is passed into the femoral artery and up the aorta as far as the renal vessels where the contrast medium is injected. A method of selective renal angiography has been developed in which the tip of the catheter can be turned to enter one or other renal artery; this gives the best demonstration of the renal vessels but it requires the use of an image-intensifier with a television monitor.

The investigation is of value in demonstrating new growths of the kidney, where pooling of the contrast occurs in the growth, and in detecting congenital abnormalities. It has been of use in verifying the existence of a solitary kidney. It can also differentiate tumours from cysts, which may also be aspirated under radiological control.

Nephrotomography. In this investigation 45 per cent sodium diatrizoate or 60 per cent meglumine iothalamate is injected rapidly into an antecubital vein, and a series of tomograms is taken at 1-cm levels through the whole thickness of the kidney. This investigation has its greatest value in distinguishing a renal tumour from a cyst; the tumour is irregularly and densely opacified; the cyst contains no vessels and remains radiolucent (*Fig.* K.21).

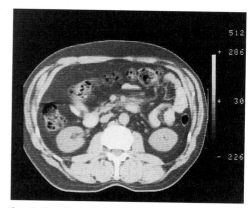

Fig. K.22. CT scan showing normal kidneys. (*Professor Adrian Dixon.*)

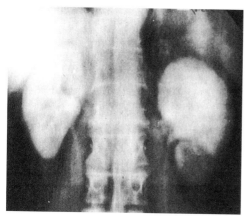

Fig. K.21. Nephrotomogram showing a solid tumour (carcinoma) in the upper pole of the left kidney. (*Reproduced by courtesy of Dr John L. Emmett.*)

Ultrasonography enables the skilled operator to differentiate between a solid and a cystic renal mass and also to detect a hydronephrosis. The simplicity and non-invasiveness of this technique are especially advantageous.

Computerized tomography (CT scan) readily differentiates, again, between solid and cystic enlargements of the kidney and enables clear delineation of other masses in the region which may mimic a renal swelling.

CT enables the extent and local spread of a tumour of the kidney to be delineated and also allow lymph node and hepatic metastatic spread to be defined. Invasion of the vena cava by tumour can be shown if contrast is injected intravenously (*Figs K.22–K.24*).

A kidney may be enlarged and yet not palpable from the fact that it is either wholly above the costal margin or obscured by the liver or the thick abdominal walls of the patient. On the other hand a kidney may be so diseased as to be functionless and shrunken, when it cannot be felt; but the remaining organ may be enlarged in a compensatory degree and may be distinctly palpable. One must remember the danger of regarding an enlarged kidney as the diseased organ when it may in reality be the only functioning one. The kidney of normal size and position is not palpable from the abdomen, or on bimanual examination with one hand on the loin; but, in a thin subject, the lower pole of the right kidney may sometimes be felt to descend between the hands on the patient's taking a full inspiration; if, therefore, a kidney can be felt easily on bimanual examination, it is either unduly mobile, unduly low or enlarged. It is often difficult to say if a kidney that is movable is also enlarged to a slight degree; and a kidney which was thought clinically to be enlarged has often been found to be of normal size when exposed; this is in part due to the thick coverings of the abdominal wall, or to the amount of fatty tissue surrounding the organ.

Causes of kidney enlargement

If the kidney is definitely enlarged, it remains to determine the nature of the enlargement; in this one is guided, not only by the physical characters of the

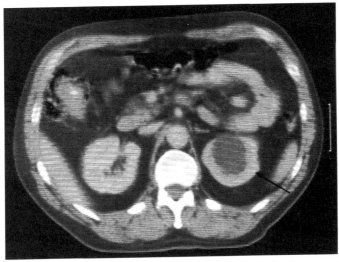

Fig. K.23. CT scan demonstrating a large left renal cyst (arrowed). (*Professor Adrian Dixon.*)

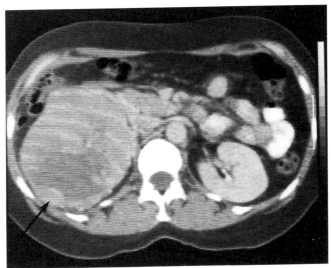

Fig. K.24. CT scan showing a massive clear cell carcinoma of the right kidney (arrowed). (*Professor Adrian Dixon.*)

tumour present, but also by other symptoms that are associated with it, more especially, perhaps, by the altered characters of the urine. The kidney may be enlarged only slightly, as in tuberculosis, pyelonephritis, incipient hydronephrosis or carcinoma; or may be enlarged to a considerable degree in polycystic disease, hydro- or pyonephrosis, and in some forms of malignant growth. From the physical examination of the enlarged organ it is often possible to say that the swelling is fluid or solid in nature, but it is seldom that a true diagnosis of the lesion can be made from palpation of the kidney alone. In the following

diseases, in which renal enlargement is usually present, the diagnosis must be arrived at by the consideration of associated symptoms.

In *renal tuberculosis* the disease occurs in a miliary or in a caseous form. Miliary tuberculosis occurs as part of a general tuberculosis, usually in children, is bilateral and causes no tumour. It is now rarely seen in the Western World. The caseous variety occurs most frequently in young adults who have had tuberculosis elsewhere in the body, as a disease in one kidney, in which one or several foci may be present. These enlarge and soften to form a tuberculous abscess, which invades the medullary tissues, to open eventually and discharge its contents into the renal pelvis. The kidney is slightly enlarged and tender, and there is persistent pyuria and haematuria in small amounts. The epithelial lining of the ureter is quickly invaded by the tuberculous process, becoming thickened and infiltrated, and at the same time shortened, so that cystoscopically the ureteric orifice is seen to be drawn upwards. An early symptom of renal tuberculosis is increased frequency of micturition, even before the bladder has become infected in the downward progress of the disease. The ureter may be felt to be thickened per rectum or per vaginam, or other tuberculous foci may be found in the prostate, vesiculae seminales or epididymes in the male. A thorough search should be made for tubercle bacilli in the urine by microscopy and specific culture. In cases in which caseous areas are present in the kidney, a radiograph may show blurred, indistinct shadows in the renal area, and a pyelographic examination will show a lack of definition of one or more renal calices and occasionally cavitation of the kidney. Intravenous pyelography may fail to show a shadow on the affected side owing to inefficient function of the kidney in the excretion of the contrast.

In *pyelonephritis* the kidney may be slightly enlarged, together with renal pain, pyuria and general malaise. Pyelonephritis is usually bilateral, and due to some infective or obstructive lesion in the lower urinary tract, symptoms of which are usually obvious (*see* Pyuria). Bacteriological examination by culture of a specimen of urine is essential to the diagnosis.

Malignant tumours of the kidney give rise either to an irregular nodular enlargement of the kidney, or to a general, uniform, solid tumour. There is usually aching pain in the loin, with intermittent attacks of profuse haematuria that occur when the growth has infiltrated the renal pelvis or sometimes sooner. The bleeding may be so profuse that clots are formed in the renal calices, pyramidal in shape, which in their passage down the ureter give rise to typical colic. Long worm-shaped clots from formation in the ureter may also be present. The common type of renal tumour in the parenchyma of the kidney, the adenocarcinoma, arises in the renal tubular epithelium. It was formerly supposed to arise in small aberrant areas of suprarenal tissue which may be found in this situation and was known as a hypernephroma (Grawitz tumour). The malignant tumours arise in any part of the kidney, are often fairly well defined from the renal tissues, and are seen on macroscopical section to contain areas of yellow colour and areas of organizing blood clot from former interstitial haemorrhage. Microscopically, they show large polyhedral cells, with clear cytoplasm (clear cell carcinoma), arranged in an alveolar, tubular

or papillary formation somewhat resembling the suprarenal cortical tissue; in some specimens granular cells predominate. They are now classified under the term 'adenocarcinoma'. Their rate of growth varies enormously, but the main symptoms are fairly constant. There is aching in the loin, and enlargement of the kidney may be found on examination (*Fig.* K.24), but at first the symptoms are slight. Haematuria occurs without any apparent exciting cause, and there may be renal colic from the passage of clots down the ureter; the tumour may be of fair size before any haematuria is noticed. Metastases to lungs, brain, liver and bones (skull, vertebrae, pelvis, ribs, upper humerus and upper femur) are common and, indeed, these manifestations may be the first evidence of the presence of the renal primary. A papillary carcinoma of the renal pelvis, ranging from a cell-differentiated 'papilloma' to an anaplastic tumour, is relatively uncommon. It may produce enlargement of the kidney by obstruction of the pelvi–ureteric junction with resultant hydronephrosis. A squamous cell carcinoma of the renal pelvix, associated with squamous metaplasia due to a calculus, is uncommon.

Another form of malignant tumour that occurs in the kidney is that which arises from embryonic tissues, and to which the name 'nephroblastoma' (Wilms' tumour) has been applied. These tumours are formed of mixed tissues, such as striated and non-striated muscle, cartilage or bone, and epithelial structures in tubular or glandular form. They grow in the renal tissues, expanding these to form a spurious capsule. They occur most frequently in children, and haematuria is infrequent. These tumours are of rapid growth, are exceedingly malignant, and the existence of a large tumour in the loin may be the earliest symptom.

Thus, the occurrence of a renal tumour, accompanied by intermittent attacks of haematuria, especially if profuse, should always give suspicion of renal growth in an adult. Renal tuberculosis and calculus may give rise to renal enlargement, but the haematuria is seldom profuse; with calculus, the haematuria is often brought on or increased by exertion, whereas with growth it may come on at any time, even during rest. At the same time it should be remembered that both profuse haematuria and renal enlargement may arise from a vesical tumour which obstructs the normal flow of urine from the ureteric orifice. In all cases, therefore, a full urological examination should be made before any operative measure is carried out. The rapid development of a *varicocele*, especially on the right side, is very rare but it is a point significant of renal growth. The pyelographic picture of a renal growth is usually distinctive. There is displacement or destruction of one or more calices and deformity of the renal pelvis, with frequently a filling defect in the latter (*Fig.*

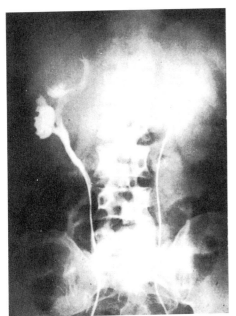

Fig. K.25. Pyelogram in a case of carcinoma of the right kidney. The crescentic filling defect of the upper calix is characteristic of a space-occupying lesion.

size. The tumour is oval or rounded, smooth, and gives a sense of tenseness or elasticity, while occasionally distinct fluctuation may be obtained. Pyelography assists the diagnosis very materially (pp. 225 et seq. and *Fig.* K.25). A hydronephrosis occurs when there is a partial ureteric obstruction, or in cases of repeated attacks of temporarily complete obstruction to the ureter. Bilateral hydronephrosis may also arise from the back-pressure due to any obstruction of the normal passage of urine from the bladder. Hydronephrosis is often accompanied by renal pain, sometimes by renal colic, and occasionally by haematuria. The tumour may show marked changes in size, from the varying character of the lesion producing the obstruction; thus, if the ureter is wholly blocked, the tumour will increase in size and become more tense, whilst if the obstruction is partially relieved the tumour will diminish, synchronously with the passage of a larger quantity of urine of low specific gravity. The presence of any obstruction to the normal flow of urine from the kidney predisposes to the onset of infection of the kidney by microorganisms, so that a hydronephrosis may become converted into a pyonephrosis, or the latter may arise from the obstruction of the ureter of a kidney already the seat of pyelitis. The physical examination of a kidney distended with urine or with pus shows practically no difference between them, but

K.25). A filling defect in the pelvis alone, perhaps with dilatation of the calices, is more suggestive of a pelvic new growth of the papillary type.

Hydronephrosis and *pyonephrosis* form definite enlargements of the kidney, which may attain a large

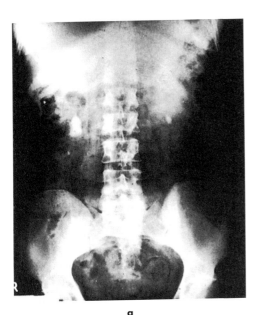

a

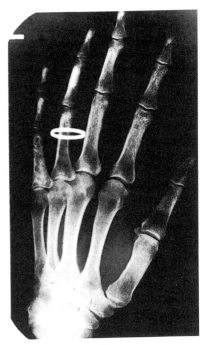

b

Fig. K.26. *a.* Recurrent bilateral calculi of the kidneys in a woman with a parathyroid adenoma. (Plain radiograph of abdomen.) *b.* The left hand of the same patient showing cystic changes in the 5th proximal phalanx.

with pyonephrosis other indications are usually present to assist the diagnosis. Examination of the urine will reveal the presence of pus at some time, although, if the ureter is wholly obstructed at the time of examination, pus may be absent if the other kidney and the bladder are normal. If, however, the ureter is blocked only partially, pus will be found in the urine; in the intermittent form, pus may be present in large quantities at intervals coinciding with the decrease in the size of the renal tumour. With pyonephrosis, also, there will be the general evidence of suppuration, namely, raised temperature, sweating, pallor and often diarrhoea. The most frequent causation of pyonephrosis is renal calculus, so that a careful inquiry into the history of the case for symptoms of calculus may give important indications, and X-ray examination, etc., will be of service (pp. 225 et seq.) unless the stone has been passed. Very occasionally palpation of a kidney enlarged from calculus disease will give rise to distinct crepitation from the friction of one stone upon another. (*Fig.* K.26) illustrates recurrent bilateral calculi of the kidneys in a woman with raised serum calcium and lowered serum phosphate. After removal of the parathyroid tumour and pyelolithotomy there has been no more stone formation and the case also demonstrates the relationship between urinary calculi and the parathyroid glands, because of the influence of the latter upon the calcium metabolism of the body.

Cysts of the kidney

Hydatid cyst of the kidney may give rise to a tumour in the loin exactly resembling a hydronephrosis, and would usually be diagnosed as such. The discovery of hooklets or hydatid elements in the urine, or in the fluid aspirated from a renal cyst, will point to the nature of the disease.

Polycystic disease of the kidney may occur in children or in adults, and forms a tumour which is commonly bilateral, though that of one side may be larger than the other. In adults the disease causes practically no trouble, except the presence of the tumour, in the early stages, but later, symptoms of renal insufficiency develop, with thirst, drowsiness and vomiting. The tumour gives the usual physical signs of a renal enlargement, and may attain a great size on both sides. In thin subjects rounded prominences may be felt on the surface of the tumour. There may be aching pain in the loins and, occasionally, marked haematuria. The urine is of low specific gravity, is increased in amount, and in the absence of blood often contains a small amount of protein. The disease is usually accompanied by arteriosclerosis and raised blood pressure. Indeed, death may result from hypertensive cardiac failure or a cerebrovascular accident. The character of the urine and the bilateral renal tumours are usually sufficient data upon which to form a diagnosis, but with a unilateral tumour, such as occasionally occurs, the diagnosis is very difficult. A hydronephrotic or pyonephrotic kidney may give evidence of fluctuation which will not be obtained with a polycystic kidney. The pyelographic picture of polycystic disease shows the calices to be considerably

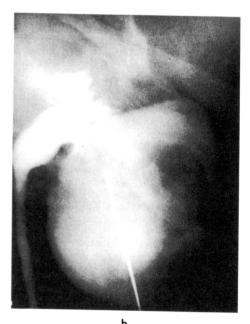

a   b

Fig. K.27. Arteriogram demonstrating a renal cyst. *a*. The avascular filling defect (anterior view). *b*. The cyst after aspiration and confirmation of the diagnosis by injection of contrast medium (posterior view).

lengthened and drawn out by the disease, but shows no cavitation and rarely any pelvic dilatation as in a hydronephrosis.

A large *solitary cyst* of the kidney may produce a renal tumour and may cause aching in one loin. A pyelographic examination shows the calices to be displaced by the enlarging cyst, and in spite of the absence of haematuria, a diagnosis of renal growth is usually made and the true cause of the disease revealed by ultrasound or CT scanning and confirmed, if necessary, by aortography; the renal cyst is avascular in contrast to the marked tumour circulation seen in a renal carcinoma. The cyst can then be both confirmed and treated by aspiration under X-ray or ultrasound control (*Fig.* K.27).

Harold Ellis

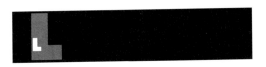

Leg, oedema of

In the great majority of patients with generalized oedema, the legs, particularly the ankles, are likely to be affected (*see* Oedema, Generalized). In most of these cases both legs will be involved but, occasionally and perhaps due to the patient's position in bed, the oedema may be somewhat asymmetrical. In most of the conditions discussed in this section, the oedema is strictly unilateral and there will, therefore, be little difficulty in distinguishing them from the causes of generalized oedema. The causes of oedema of the legs can be classified under the headings of *trauma, inflammation, venous obstruction* and *lymphatic obstruction*.

Trauma

The cause of the swelling associated with sprains and fractures, bites and stings, and burns and frostbite is likely to be obvious. There is, however, a late complication of trauma, of which oedema is a feature, which may present a diagnostic problem. This is *algodystrophy* or *Sudek's atrophy*. This rather rare condition usually follows trauma to a limb, which may be very mild, and, in the leg, most commonly affects the ankle. It is characterized by pain, which may be very severe, and the ankle is warm, red and oedematous, suggesting local inflammation; there is, however, no systemic evidence of inflammation. These changes subside after a few weeks and the skin around the joint becomes

cold, cyanosed and, ultimately, atrophic. X-rays show local osteoporosis. Full recovery is usual but may not occur for many months. The aetiology is unknown but it has been suggested that abnormal autonomic reflexes may be responsible.

Inflammation

Oedema is one of the cardinal signs of inflammation. Local lesions, such as *boils* and *carbuncles*, are easily identified but more widespread inflammatory lesions may initially cause diagnostic confusion. The bright red areas with palpable raised margins of *erysipelas* are characteristic but oedema due to obstruction of cutaneous lymphatics may persist after the acute inflammation has subsided. *Cellulitis* causes more diffuse oedema as does *acute osteomyelitis*; lymphangitis and lymphadenitis are commoner in the former while, in the latter, the constitutional disturbance is greater. *Chronic osteomyelitis* can cause puzzling oedema but imaging will settle the diagnostic issue. *Acute arthritis* of any type is associated with local oedema. In most cases the swelling of the joint itself will make the diagnosis clear but *acute gout* can cause a swelling widespread enough to simulate cellulitis. *Acute rheumatoid arthritis* is less likely to cause confusion but it is worth remembering that, in this condition, more generalized oedema can occur; this is probably due to a combination of hypoalbuminaemia, stasis in an immobile patient and, perhaps, increased capillary permeability. The painful swelling of the calf with ankle oedema caused by a *ruptured Baker's cyst* is easily confused with deep venous thrombosis; a history of prior swelling of the joint, decreasing with the onset of the calf pain, is an important diagnostic feature.

Venous obstruction

Deep venous thrombosis in the calf muscles is an important cause of oedema of the ankle; the swelling will extend further up the leg if thrombus is also present in the femoral and iliac veins (*Fig.* L.1). Venous thrombosis is a common complication of major surgery and of prolonged recumbency for any reason; it can also often occur without any obvious cause. Long coach journeys by the elderly and, in women, the use of oestrogen-containing oral contraceptive agents increase the risk of deep venous thrombosis. In addition to the ankle oedema the calf is typically swollen and tender on pressure from behind and from side to side. Homan's sign (pain in the calf on dorsiflexion at the ankle) may be positive but is of no diagnostic value as it can be positive with any painful lesion of the calf. Very often, none of these signs are

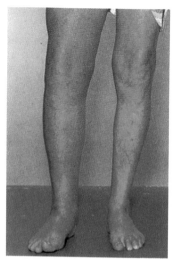

Fig. L.1. Iliofemoral venous thrombosis of the right leg with gross oedema.

present; the first evidence of deep venous thrombosis may be a fatal pulmonary embolism.

Thrombus may spread upwards beyond the iliac veins to involve the *inferior vena cava* and, in that case, the other leg will become oedematous. With such a sequence of events, the diagnosis of inferior vena caval occlusion is clear. Primary occlusion of this vessel, however, will present with bilateral ankle and leg oedema, in which case the differential diagnosis includes all the causes of generalized oedema. Diagnostic assistance may be provided by investigations such as Doppler flow studies but the definitive diagnosis of venous occlusion can be made only by venography or CT scanning. In any patient in whom venous thrombosis has occurred without obvious cause, a thorough general examination, including rectal and vaginal examination, is essential to detect pelvic or abdominal tumours causing pressure on veins.

Varicose veins, with or without previous thrombosis, commonly cause ankle oedema, usually quite mild. Although, in the great majority of cases, it is the veins themselves which are the seat of the trouble, it is wise, at first presentation, to examine the patient with the possibility of external pressure on the large veins in mind, as in patients with acute venous occlusion.

Lymphatic obstruction

The oedema fluid in lymphatic obstruction contains much more protein than the fluid in other conditions causing oedema. Consequently, although, initially, the swelling 'pits' on pressure and disappears overnight, it later becomes firm and non-pitting ('brawny') and is

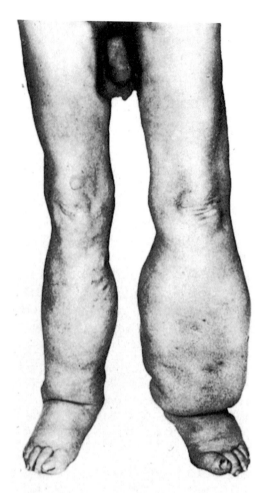

Fig. L.2. Milroy's disease in a man of 74. He had never been abroad. In this condition the lymphoedema may be symmetrical, may affect only one limb or, as in this case, may affect one limb more than the other.

present all the time. Later the skin becomes grossly thickened and, sometimes, ulcerated. The common causes of lymphatic obstruction in Western countries include *neoplastic infiltration* of the lymphatics and lymph nodes, and scarring from *trauma*, surgical or otherwise, and from *irradiation*; recurrent *streptococcal infection* can cause similar damage. In tropical countries, *filariasis* is a common cause of lymphatic obstruction and chronic oedema of the legs known as elephantiasis. The commonest form of filariasis is that due to *Wuchereria bancrofti*; this is widespread in the tropics and causes elephantiasis of the whole leg and also of the genitalia, especially in males. Another filaria, *Brugia malayi*, is found in the Far East, especially South-East Asia; the inguinal lymph nodes are affected, as in Bancroftian filariasis but, curiously, the oedema and elephantiasis are confined to the lower parts of the legs. There is also a *non-filarial elephantiasis* seen in parts of Africa and Central and South America; this is due to chronic lymphangitis apparently caused by microscopic particles of silica absorbed through the skin of the feet; it usually affects the feet and lower parts of the legs. *Lymphatic hypoplasia* is a rare cause of oedema. This occurs in two forms: a congenital variety presenting with oedema in early infancy and a familial form, sometimes known as Milroy's disease. In the latter there is an abrupt demarcation between the swollen and the normal tissue at the level of a joint — ankle, knee or hip (*Fig.* L.2). There is sometimes a history of attacks of pyrexia in association with the spread of the oedema which is typically episodic. Thus, the swelling, having been present at the ankle only for several years, may, rather suddenly, spread to reach the knee and, later, in a similar fashion, the hip.

Peter R. Fleming

Leg, pain in

This section deals specifically with the causes of pain referred into the limb or arising from local lesions rather than generalized diseases. The subdivision of the section is largely anatomical but nerve root compression (sciatica), ischaemia (intermittent claudication) and spinal stenosis (spinal claudication), which are responsible for a very large proportion of pain in the buttock and leg, are considered separately first.

Sciatica may affect the buttock, anterior or posterior thigh, calf or foot or the entire leg. Pain is affected by posture and is aggravated by sciatic and femoral nerve stretch tests; altered cutaneous sensation and motor weakness may or may not be present. Claudication pain occurs only during exercise, though the differentiation between arterial causes and spinal stenosis may be difficult. Most cases of sciatica in the elderly are due to spinal stenosis secondary to osteoarthritis of the apophyseal joints.

Sciatica

CAUSES

Intrathecal

Neurofibroma or other tumour
Irritation of the meninges by haemorrhage
Infection
Intrathecal injections
Hydatid cyst
Postherpetic neuralgia

Extradural

Prolapsed intervertebral disc
Spinal stenosis
Spinal abscess — tuberculous, brucella/osteomyelitis
Vertebral tumour — primary, secondary, myeloma
Fracture-dislocation
Spondylolisthesis

Extraspinal

Cysts and tumours of pelvic viscera
Fetal head during labour
Pelvic inflammatory disease
Neurofibroma of sciatic nerve
Penetrating injuries

Pain radiating from a lumbosacral nerve root into the leg is sciatica. In spite of the multitude of possible causes, in the vast majority of instances sciatica is due to a prolapsed intervertebral disc, apophyseal joint osteoarthritis (spondylosis) or spinal stenosis (especially in the elderly). These lesions do not always cause pain: central disc protrusions may induce cauda equina compression with urinary retention without any other symptoms.

Nerve root compression is characterized by complaints of well-localized pain with or without paraesthesiae, numbness, wasting and weakness. Paraesthesiae including numbness indicate direct involvement of sensory pathways and are not necessarily associated with referred pain. Nerve root pain may be aggravated by coughing and sneezing, straight-leg raising (Lasègue's sign) and by neck flexion. Aggravation of the pain or paraesthesiae by flexion of the hip (which stretches the cauda equina) is a reliable indicator of a root lesion. However, extraneural lesions may be associated with pain on coughing and Lasègue's sign; flexion of the neck may produce a surge of paraesthesiae down the trunk into the limbs (l'Hermitte's sign) in multiple sclerosis, subacute combined degeneration of the cord, cervical spondylosis or cervical cord tumour. A neural lesion is confirmed by the presence of muscular weakness, sensory loss and depression or loss of the knee or ankle jerk. Muscle wasting usually has the same significance but may be associated with extraneural disease or disuse. Nevertheless, radicular pain of recent onset may not be accompanied by any objective neurological signs.

Lesions of the cauda equina are uncommon. Tumours, notably slowly growing neurofibromas, may cause intermittent sciatic pain for months or even years before the diagnosis is established; neurological signs may be relatively late in appearing, but lumbar puncture will usually reveal a raised cerebrospinal fluid protein level and there may be a partial or complete intrathecal block. Backward protrusion of the lower intervertebral lumbar discs or of the lumbosacral disc may compress the cauda equina with unilateral or

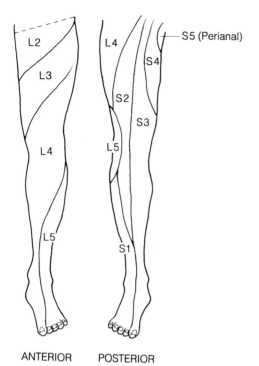

ANTERIOR   POSTERIOR

Fig. L.3. Areas of reduced sensation to pinprick in lumbosacral root lesion.

Sciatica is usually unilateral, occasionally bilateral and rarely alternating. Examination reveals a stiff lumbar spine with tenderness at the level of the lesion. The lumbar lordosis may be lost and there may be a scoliosis which becomes more marked with forward flexion. Areas of reduced sensation to pinprick, weakness and reflex change associated with individual root lesions are summarized in *Fig.* L.3 and *Table* L.1.

With an L5 root lesion weakness is most marked in extensor hallucis longus and with an S1 lesion calf wasting may be seen. After acute disc prolapse, the spinal fluid is often normal though there may be a slight rise in protein content. Radiographs of the lumbar spine may show significant narrowing of the affected disc space. Contrast myelography (*Fig.* L.4a) may outline the herniation unless the lesion involves the lateral recess when appearances may be normal. Localization of such herniation by CT or MRI scanning (*Fig.* L.4b) offers an improved and non-interventional diagnostic method.

Spondylosis commonly leads to pain in the neck and back and to root pains in the arm and leg, especially in the elderly. Symptoms may mimic those of an acute disc herniation but there is often a history of chronic or intermittent spinal pain, recurrent sciatica with evidence of osteoarthritis elsewhere in the spine. More than one root may be involved, either simultaneously or at different times, but objective neurological signs are usually less prominent than in younger individuals with acute disc prolapse. Spinal radiographs show variable disc space narrowing with osteophytic lipping and irregularity of the facet joints. It is important, however, to remember that such changes will be found in the majority of aged spines so that the appearance seen may not account for the symptoms.

Spinal abscesses due to tuberculosis, brucellosis or other pyogenic infections may mimic spondylotic symptoms with local pain, stiffness and sciatic radiation. Sudden onset, or exacerbation, of pain may accompany fracture of the affected vertebra(e). X-rays

bilateral sciatica. The spinal fluid may or may not show evidence of block and the protein level may be raised. Meningeal irritation from local meningitis, haemorrhage or intrathecal injections can give rise to severe bilateral sciatica, usually of short duration and obvious origin.

Posterolateral herniation of the nucleus pulposus of the intervertebral discs at L4/5 and L5/S1 spaces is the commonest cause of acute sciatica. There may be a history of an acute injury, which may be slight, or of preceding lumbago, but there may be no such history.

Table L.1. Signs associated with common nerve root lesions affecting the legs

Root	Paraesthesiae/numbness	Muscle weakness	Reflex change
L1	Groin	—	—
L2	Front of mid thigh	Quadriceps	—
L3	Front of lower thigh	Quadriceps	Knee ↓
L4	Front of lower thigh, knee and inner aspect of shin	Quadriceps and tibialis anterior	Knee ↓
L5	Back of thigh, lateral aspect of I dorsum of foot to big toe	Extensor hallucis longus	Ankle ↓
S1	Back of I lateral aspect of foot and sole	Calf wasting and weakness of plantar flexors	Ankle ↓

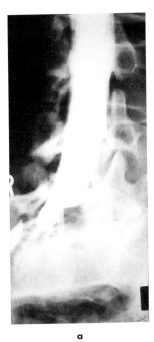

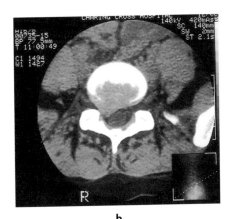

a

b

Fig. L.4. *a.* Lumbosacral disc herniation: *a.* X-ray myelogram showing disc bulge and swelling of the S1 nerve root. *b*, CT scan showing right posterolateral L5/S1 disc protrusion.

may initially be normal but a chest X-ray and a CT or MRI scan at the suspect level may be helpful in any suspicious case of sciatica.

    Osteomyelitis of the lumbar vertebrae is a rare cause of sciatica. *Fracture-dislocations* also are clinically obvious but *spondylolisthesis* (forward or backward displacement of one vertebra upon its neighbour) can only be diagnosed with certainty by radiography (*Fig.* L.5). The presence of this deformity does not prove that it is the cause of sciatic pain since it may be present without discomfort. When sciatica is caused by spondylolisthesis it is usually bilateral, severe and with marked neurological signs including motor, sensory and reflex changes. Pelvic disease rarely produces sciatica and when it does so the pelvic pathology is usually gross. However, exceptional cases will be overlooked if rectal or vaginal examination is not performed in every case of sciatica in which no cause is apparent. Acute sciatic pain occurring during parturition is usually transient and due to the pressure of the fetal head on the lumbosacral trunk as it crosses the pelvic brim. Permanent paralysis of the muscles distal to the nerve has been reported after prolonged dystocia. Persistent sciatica following parturition is usually due to herniation of a lumbar disc.

    Tumours of the sciatic nerve are exceedingly rare; the presence of other evidence of von Recklinghausen's disease — café-au-lait spots and subcutaneous

tumours — may suggest this diagnosis, symptoms being due either to increasing size of a neurofibroma or to malignant change.

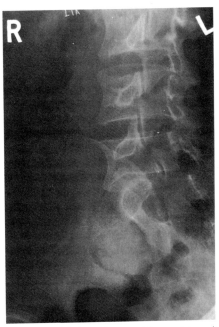

Fig. L.5. Spondylolisthesis: Fracture of the pars intermedialis shown in oblique X-ray of the lumbosacral spine.

Extraneural disease may give rise to referred sciatic pain without paraesthesiae or objective neurological signs. Sacroiliac joint disease is a major cause of such pain (*see below*). Tumours of the iliac bones and sacrum may rarely lead to sciatic pain. These can be demonstrated by X-rays, bone scintigraphy scanning, CT or MRI scanning. Benign osteoid osteomas may respond well symptomatically to aspirin.

Intermittent claudication

CAUSES

Spinal stenosis
Leriche syndrome
Iliac, femoral or popliteal stenosis or occlusion
Anaemia

The term intermittent claudication is used to describe the development of pains in the leg, usually the calf, brought on during walking, which necessitates limping or rest. It is relieved after 5–15 minutes by rest but recurs after walking a similar distance. With the passage of time the distance walked before pain becomes intolerable usually decreases, progressively restricting exercise tolerance. The condition is due to inadequate arterial blood supply to the leg muscles due to narrowing or occlusion of iliac, femoral or popliteal arteries. Atheroma with or without thrombosis is the usual culprit but embolism, Buerger's disease and, rarely, syphilitic endarteritis may also give rise to intermittent claudication. Anaemia may also lead to this symptom or may aggravate it.

Physical examination of the affected limbs is usually grossly normal although may reveal the usual physical signs of reduced blood supply to the skin of the toes and feet. However, careful examination will reveal absence of pulsation at the dorsalis pedis and posterior tibial arteries. Similarly the popliteal pulse may also be lost though femoral artery pulsation may be reduced or normal. There may however be an audible femoral bruit. After exercise the foot may appear unduly pale; with rest the returning flush of normal colour spreads gradually over its surface.

Similar symptoms, though usually bilateral, may also result from intermittent ischaemia of the cauda equina (spinal claudication). Walking produces characteristic aching in the legs sometimes with paraesthesiae in the feet. Ankle jerks may be lost during exercise. This condition is usually distinguishable from arterial disease by a history of chronic back pain usually with marked radiographic changes of spondylosis and by the presence of peripheral leg pulses with good skin perfusion. This condition is quite common, especially among the elderly. It is important since appropriate spinal surgery may provide effective cure. Myelography, CT or MRI scanning of the lumbosacral spine shows a narrow anteroposterior diameter of the spinal canal (*Fig.* L.6), usually with marked osteoarthritic changes at the intervertebral joints. Often large osteophytes at the apophyseal joints link to form bony bars compressing the cauda equina with further pressure exerted by bulging of the intervertebral disc. Symptoms arise when sufficient stenosis of the spinal canal develops to prevent dilatation of the vasa nervorum during exercise.

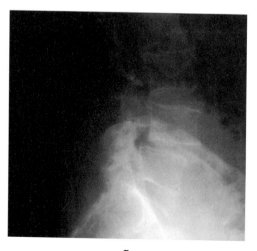
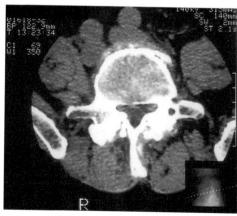

a   b

Fig. L.6. Lumbar spinal stenosis: *a*, Lateral X-ray showing spondylosis with grade 1 spondylolisthesis at L5/S1 level. *b*, CT scan showing markedly diminished anteroposterior spinal diameter and apophyseal osteophytes.

Pain in the Hip

CAUSES

Adult

Osteoarthritis
Inflammatory joint disease
Joint infection — tuberculous or pyogenic
Aseptic necrosis
Polymyalgia rheumatica
Bursitis — trochanteric
   — iliopectineal
Enthesopathy — adductor tendinitis
   — pubic tubercle

Child

Perthés' disease
Slipped femoral epiphysis
Joint infection — tuberculous or pyogenic
Juvenile chronic arthritis
Congenital hip dysplasia
Transient osteoporosis
Haemoglobinopathies — aseptic necrosis, synovitis
Familial Mediteranean fever
Henoch–Schönlein purpura
Myeloproliferative disorders

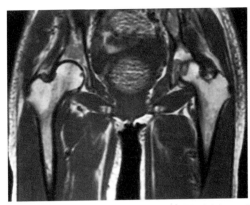

Fig. L.7. MRI showing avascular necrosis of the left femoral head.

Typically, pain from the hip joint is felt in the groin or perineum, although it may be referred to the greater trochanter. It is aggravated by weight-bearing or exercise and examination reveals restricted movements with pain, especially on rotation. In children hip disease may present with thigh or knee pain.

In children, especially, the diagnosis of hip joint disease is of great importance and requires specialist attention whenever possible. In the adult, degenerative and inflammatory arthritis, including infection, can usually be diagnosed on the basis of other clinical features and X-ray changes. A history of acute onset of unilateral hip pain may suggest aseptic necrosis, though X-rays may remain normal for up to 6 months. CT or MRI scanning may reveal a hypodense segment in the femoral head at an earlier stage (*Fig.* L.7).

Polymyalgia rheumatica may present with hip pain and, especially, inactivity stiffness. Usually there are also spinal or shoulder-girdle symptoms and the erythrocyte sedimentation rate will be raised. *Pelvic bursitis* is common and may coexist with X-ray changes of osteoarthritis of the hip. Careful clinical assessment is therefore essential. *Trochanteric bursitis* produces pain aggravated by walking and climbing stairs and there is local tenderness just behind the greater trochanter. This may produce pain when the patient lies on that side. A virtually full, painless range of hip movements is possible but pain may be aggravated by full abduction and adduction of the hip. *Iliopectineal bursitis* occasionally accompanies inflammatory hip disease, producing tenderness over the front of the hip joint, in the groin and pain on forced flexion and extension. The bursa is seen on CT examination of the hip.

Pain in the Buttock

CAUSES

Sacroiliitis — spondyloarthropathies
Infection — tuberculous or pyogenic
Primary and secondary tumours of pelvic bones
Pelvic fracture (especially due to osteoporosis in the elderly)
Osteomalacia
Paget's disease of bone
Polymyalgia rheumatica
Gluteal or trochanteric bursitis

Sacroiliac joint pain is felt in the buttock, sometimes with radiation down the back of the thigh to the knee but no further. Pain may be aggravated by standing, walking and by twisting the trunk. Inflammatory aseptic sacroiliitis may occur as part of ankylosing spondylitis, when it may be the presenting symptom, or in association with psoriasis, inflammatory bowel disease, acute anterior uveitis or Reiter's syndrome. It may occur alone especially in females. Sepsis of the sacroiliac joint may arise as a result of tuberculous or pyogenic infection. Pregnancy and trauma may lead to subluxation of one or both sacroiliac joints leading to a sensation of uncertainty in the legs or to a feeling of uselessness of the leg(s) immediately after an injury. Clinical signs of sacroiliac joint disease are notoriously unreliable. Induction of local pain by forced abduction of the flexed hips or direct pressure over the sacrum may be helpful in acute cases. Other clinical tests are of little value. X-ray changes generally appear late although in patients with sepsis other abnormalities such as pulmonary tuberculosis, a pointing cold abscess over the joint or in a gluteal fold or abscess formation elsewhere may be found. In the acute phase

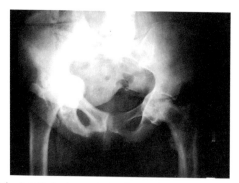

Fig. L.8. Protrusio acetabuli in Paget's disease.

the investigations of choice are radioisotope bone scanning and CT or MRI scanning.

Osteomalacia should be suspected in malnourished individuals and may give rise to a characteristic stiff gait. In the elderly, *Paget's disease of bone* may produce a local ache, although symptoms are usually due to secondary osteoarthritis and fractures through osteoporotic bone may occur with minimal trauma. Deformity at the hip secondary to softening of the bone due to Paget's disease is known as protrusio acetabuli (*Fig.* L.8). Ischial bursitis is usually associated with prolonged sitting on hard seats, producing tenderness over the ischial tuberosity.

Pain in the front of the thigh

CAUSES

Lumbar root irritation
Hip joint disease
Obturator pain
Meralgia paraesthetica
Tabes dorsalis

In most instances pain is referred from either the lumbar spine or the hip joint. Root lesions at either L2 or L3 may lead to some quadriceps wasting but without detectable sensory loss, weakness or loss of the ankle jerk. Similar features are associated with femoral nerve lesions. A root lesion at L4 produces anterior thigh pain which extends down the front of the shin and in addition the knee jerk may be reduced or lost.

Hip pain of any cause may be referred to the thigh or the knee. *Obturator pain* down the inner aspect of the thigh may arise from the hip joint, the pelvic bones or from within the pelvis. Osteoarthritis of the hip is the most common cause, though tumours of the pelvic bones or fractures in an osteoporotic

skeleton must be considered. Occasionally in females ovulation may produce brief but recurrent episodes of obturator pain; rarely obturator hernia or gross neoplastic or inflammatory disease within the pelvis gives rise to persistent pain.

Meralgia paraesthetica arises as a result of compression of the lateral cutaneous nerve of the thigh as it passes under the lateral part of the inguinal ligament. At that point it may become involved in the origin of the sartorius muscle. This compression gives rise both to numbness over the lateral aspect of the thigh and to pain. Pain develops typically on exertion and may be severe enough to produce limping (intermittent claudication) or to halt exercise. Pain is relieved by rest. Physical examination may or may not demonstrate sensory loss corresponding to the distribution of the lateral cutaneous nerve of the thigh. Symptoms may begin in middle-age especially in association with marked weight gain. Thus dieting may be sufficient to relieve symptoms though in more severe cases surgical decompression of the nerve is necessary.

The 'lightning' pains of *tabes dorsalis* most commonly affect the legs. In contrast to root pain they are usually bilateral and do not conform to any root or peripheral nerve distribution. Although the intensity may vary from trivial to excruciating the episodes are highly characteristic, being of lightning-like short duration and usually affecting an area no larger than the palm of one hand. The affected area may remain hypersensitive for hours after the paroxysm has passed. In addition to lightning pains individuals with tabes may also experience dull aching or boring pains which are persistent rather than episodic. Tabetic pains may precede all other signs and symptoms of the disease. In the presence of such symptoms special attention should be paid to the following: a history of syphilis; absent pupil reactions to light and intact convergence reactions (Argyll–Robertson pupil); loss of knee and ankle jerks; sensory impairment—loss of pain below the knees, over the trunk and inner arms and reduced postural sense peripherally; lymphocytosis in the cerebrospinal fluid; positive serological tests for syphilis in blood and CSF are usual, but not invariable.

Pain in the knee

Pain in the knee may arise because of referral from the spine or hip, ligamentous injury, internal structural derangement, inflammatory or degenerative arthritis, bursitis or underlying bone disease. The presence of soft tissue swelling or effusion indicates the presence of synovitis which may be primary or secondary to these intra-articular lesions. Bony swelling indicates

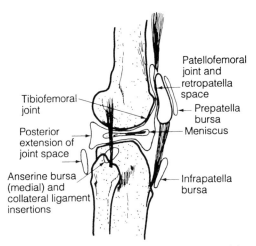

Patellofemoral
joint and
retropatella
space

Tibiofemoral
joint

Prepatella
bursa

Posterior
extension of
joint space

Meniscus

Anserine bursa
(medial) and
collateral ligament
insertions

Infrapatella
bursa

Fig. L.9. Possible sites of origin of pain in and around the knee joint. (Reproduced with permission from Dieppe, Doherty, MacFarlane and Maddison (1985) *Rheumatalogical Medicine.* Churchill Livingstone, Edinburgh, p. 387, figure 21.29.)

Inflammatory arthritis (*see* p. 203)
Trauma
Internal derangement
Infection
  —pyogenic
  —viral
Intermittent hydrarthrosis
Gout
Pyrophosphate arthropathy (pseudogout)
Synovioma
Malignant tumour of bone
  —primary
  —secondary
Scurvy
Sarcoidosis
Osteochondritis dissecans
Neuropathic (Charcot) joint
Pigmented villonodular synovitis
Synovial chondromatosis
Bursitis
Lipoma arborescens
Lipoarthritis (Hoffa's disease)
Bleeding disorders

either osteoarthritis or metabolic or malignant lesions.

In many instances isolated knee pain, in both children and adults, not associated with swelling or restriction, is transient and not explained.

Examination of the knee must establish whether symptoms arise from the tibiofemoral, patellofemoral or superior tibiofibular joint and whether or not there is synovitis or hip disease. The anatomy of the knee is illustrated in *Fig.* L.9.

Additional causes of generalized joint disease are considered elsewhere.

Causes

IN CHILDREN (UP TO 15 YEARS OF AGE)

Referred from the hip
Trauma
Chondromalacia patellae
Juvenile chronic arthritis
Infection
  —pyogenic
  —viral
Haemoglobinopathies
Osgood–Schlatter disease
Leukaemia
Rickets
Scurvy
Clutton's joints

IN ADULTS

Chondromalacia patellae
Osteoarthritis

IN CHILDHOOD

For the most part chronic arthritis in childhood is analogous to adult disease. In children under 2 years of age sepsis must be excluded with particular care. In some children mono-, pauci- (or oligo-: involvement of fewer than five joints) or polyarthritis (involvement of six or more joints) occurs, with or without systemic upset; if the condition persists for 3 months or more the term juvenile chronic arthritis (JCA) is used, arthritis being described as 'pauciarticular', 'polyarticular' or 'systemic'. A minority of children progress to develop adult seropositive rheumatoid arthritis and approximately 10 per cent of those with pauciarticular disease, mainly boys, progress to develop ankylosing spondylitis. Rheumatoid factor is almost invariably absent but antinuclear antibodies may be detected. Chronic iridocyclitis must be sought in children with JCA as this may cause painless visual loss.

Plant thorn synovitis follows the introduction of a small sharp object—often the tip of a plant thorn or a needle which penetrates the skin when the child is crawling but breaks off leaving no discernible mark. Persistent low-grade synovitis results, usually necessitating synovectomy in order to remove the foreign body. Pyarthrosis may result from penetrating injury or bacteraemia, especially in the very young child.

Clutton's joints are extremely rare today. Occurring at the age of 8–16 years, these manifestations of congenital syphilis may be misdiagnosed as cases of JCA, hydrarthrosis being present in one or both knees. Serological tests are positive. *Scurvy* is very rare but in infancy may cause intense pain on moving or touching hips or knees. Subcutaneous haemorrhages may be present elsewhere. *Leukaemia* in childhood may cause swelling of the knees and an arthropathy, usually misdiagnosed as JCA.

IN ADULT LIFE

The commonest knee disorder anywhere in the world is *osteoarthritis* which, although essentially a degenerative process, does undergo traumatic or inflammatory episodes with greater pain in the joint and sometimes effusions. Synovial fluid is clear, of high viscosity and low protein content (2 g/dl) and has a low cell count (under 2000/mm³). It may be blood-stained or contain red cells from recent injuries, detached osteophytes or from vascular synovial fringes being torn or stretched. The knees tend to be thickened in osteoarthritis. Bow-legs may predispose to degenerative changes but osteoarthritis may affect the medial compartment of the joint and cause genu varum (knock-knee). Osteoarthritis may be apparently a primary disorder or be secondary to and accompanied by other conditions, such as haemochromatosis, ochronosis, hypermobility syndromes or an inflammatory arthritis, such as rheumatoid arthritis.

Chondromalacia patellae is a premature degeneration of the patellar cartilage often occurring before the age of 30. It may be associated with a mechanical abnormality such as an unduly mobile patella. It has been considered a separate entity from osteoarthritis but tends to progress to osteoarthritis of the anterior compartment of the joint.

Rheumatoid arthritis of the knee is usually easy to diagnose as typical rheumatoid changes are present elsewhere in other joints in most cases, the changes in the hands usually being diagnostic (*see Fig. J.38*). When other joints are less obviously affected diagnosis may be more difficult. The joint or joints are painful to move, often swollen, free fluid being palpable in the joint in many cases and bursae around the knee may be affected, particularly the semimembranosus bursa (Baker's cyst) at the back of the knee, which usually communicates with the joint and acts as an over-flow tank. The joint may be tender, particularly on pressure over the medial side. In long-standing cases valgus deformity (knock-knee) is present and the muscles of calf and thigh weak and wasted. The knee may be slightly warmer than normal to the touch but not invariably (*Figs* L.10, L.11).

A similar but usually less active picture is seen in the *spondyloarthropathies*. Knees may be involved in ankylosing spondylitis, usually early in the course of the disease when spinal signs and symptoms are slight or absent, but they may also occur later when spondylitic signs are obvious, effusions sometimes becoming chronic.

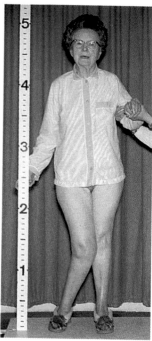

Fig. L.10. Unstable right knee from destructive rheumatoid changes.

In *Reiter's disease* knees are commonly affected early: a history of dysentery or exposure to venereal infection 7–18 days previously is common; in acute arthritis affecting the knees the possibility of psoriatic arthritis, ulcerative colitis, Crohn's disease and Reiter's disease should be kept in mind.

Trauma may be obvious from the history and from examination, but minor injuries causing damage to collateral ligaments, semilunar cartilage (usually the medial meniscus) and cruciate ligaments, usually the anterior, may cause pain, local tenderness and swelling with limitation of movements and possibly transient effusions.

A *pyarthrosis* or septic joint is usually hot and painful, the patient ill and febrile. The diagnosis may be missed if infection is superimposed on a rheumatoid joint, a not unusual occurrence. Aspiration and culture of joint fluid is obligatory. A gonococcal pyarthrosis is often accompanied by evidence of gonococcal infection elsewhere: urethra, abscesses in the skin and, in women, Bartholin's gland; endocervical and urethral swabs should be taken. Infections elsewhere in the body, usually staphylococcal, may suggest the source of the infection.

In *intermittent hydrarthrosis* effusions occur at fairly regular intervals every 1–3 weeks, lasting only a few days at a time. Effusions may be quite large, are uncomfortable but not agonizing. The fluid, if aspir-

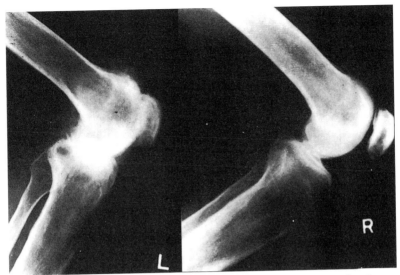

Fig. L.11. Rheumatoid arthritis. Marked active disease on the left side, right side only minimally affected.

ated, contains less than 6000 cells per mm³, mostly mononuclears. Biopsies reveal only a non-specific synovitis. Some of these cases eventually prove to be part of a polyarthritis, usually rheumatoid arthritis, but others subside spontaneously. It differs from palindromic rheumatism in being confined usually to the knees and in its fairly regular recurrence. Onset is often in adolescence.

Acute gout is uncommon in the knee but when it occurs the joint is agonizing, hot and swollen. The inflammatory fluid contains crystals of monosodium urate. The serum uric acid is almost always raised.

Acute pyrophosphate arthropathy (pseudogout) is, unlike true uratic gout, most common in the knee, crystalline deposits of calcium pyrophosphate dihydrate (CPPD) setting up intense irritation in the joint. Aspirated fluid will usually reveal the typical crystals.

A *synovioma or synovial sarcoma* is a rare but highly malignant tumour arising most commonly in the knee in the synovium or soft tissue around the joint. Pain is not always present, the condition starting as a painless, slowly growing mass which may have been present for several months before being reported. Vague mild pain in the knee may precede any obvious swelling by several months. It may become painful and tender and after a slow start increase more rapidly, and metastases are common. The prognosis is bad. Other varieties of sarcoma may occur in the knee, sarcomatous change in Paget's disease of the lower end of the femur, for instance (*Fig*. L.12), but metastatic malignant disease from elsewhere is rare in the knee.

Scurvy is rare today in adults but is seen occasionally in the elderly, alcoholics, food faddists or patients on over-restricted reduction diets. Haemorrhages, subcutaneous and gingival, suggest the diagnosis.

Sarcoidosis may present as a flitting polyarthritis affecting the knees and other joints, lasting several weeks. Joints are affected in 10–30% of patients with sarcoidosis, more often in women. Erythema nodosum and bilateral hilar lymphadenopathy suggest the diagnosis. Effusions are minimal or non-existent and no deformity is left after resolution.

Osteochondritis dissecans is due to separation of avascular fragments of bone and cartilage from the joint surface. Usually only one knee is involved, pain being slight, but aggravated by exercise. Swelling may be intermittent but the knee may become unstable. It may occur at any age but is most common in the teens. Radiographs show separation of fragments of bone from the joint surface, most commonly over the medial condyle of the femur. The condition often leads to osteoarthritis of the knee later in life.

Neuropathic (Charcot's) knee joints are today a rarity in Europe; in the past they were seen in tabes dorsalis—painless, grossly distorted unstable joints causing extraordinary types of gait. Similar neuropathic knee joints may occur in leprosy and yaws, but syringomyelia affects joints of the upper extremity and diabetes mellitus those of the feet.

Pigmented villonodular synovitis is an uncommon non-malignant condition characterized by marked synovial proliferation and the formation of grape-like masses pigmented with haemosiderin. It usually affects only one knee and though it may sometimes involve bursae, tendon sheath and less often capsule and even

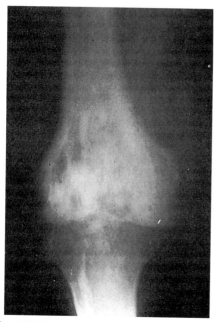

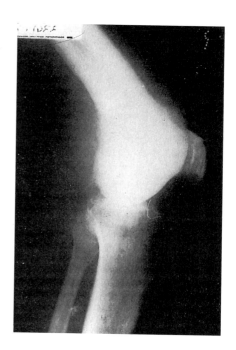

Fig. L.12. Paget sarcoma, lower end of femur.

bone it is not neoplastic but essentially a chronic synovitis, the aetiology of which is unknown. Repeated bouts of swelling without great pain with heavily blood-stained aspirate in young adults suggests the diagnosis.

Synovial chondromatosis is a benign self-limiting uncommon disorder affecting the young and middle-aged, usually males. Many nodules of metaplastic cartilage form within the synovium and are released into the joint space as loose bodies. The knee is the joint most commonly involved, usually unilaterally, the patient experiencing discomfort, stiffness, crepitus, swelling and limitation of movement associated with a grating feeling. Some of these loose bodies ossify or calcify and show up typically in radiographs.

Bursitis: There are up to seven bursae around the knee, (*see Fig.* L.9) but not all are present in every individual: (1) the prepatellar bursa; (2) the suprapatellar bursa proximal to the patella behind the quadriceps tendon in front of the distal part of the anterior surface of the femur, communicating with the joint; (3) the subcutaneous infrapatellar bursa anterior to the proximal part of the ligamentum patellae; (4) the deep infrapatellar bursa between the ligamentum patellae and anterior surface of the proximal part of the tibia; (5) the semimembranosus bursa which lies between the semimembranosus and the medial head of the gastrocnemius as they cross one another, usually communicating with (6) a bursa between the medial head of the gastrocnemius and the back of the knee joint which in turn communicates with the knee joint; and (7) the semitendinosus bursa which lies between sartorius, gracilis, semitendinosus and the tibia. Much of the swelling of a knee may be due to inflammation or injury of these bursae rather than the joint itself. In 'housemaid's knee' the prepatellar bursa is swollen and painful, in 'nun's or priest's knee' the infrapatellar bursa, and often the prepatellar also. Inflammation or injury to the semitendinosus bursa may cause pain on the medial side of the knee, not uncommon after athletic activities in persons out of training.

Lipoma arborescens is a benign lipomatous mass which occurs most often in the knee joint and is usually associated with degenerative changes; it causes pain, swelling, restriction of movement and sometimes locking, sometimes with a joint effusion. A visible swelling in the suprapatellar area may become more apparent on flexing the knee.

Hoffa's disease (lipoarthritis traumatica genu), said to be more common in acrobats and ballet dancers, often after trauma or excessive exertion, appears to arise from infrapatellar subsynovial fat becoming swollen and locked in the joint. There is tenderness below the patella but no other physical sign.

Bleeding states may cause a haemorrhagic effusion or frank haemorrhage into a joint: haemophilia, anticoagulant therapy and acute leukaemia are examples. A sudden painful effusion in an arthritic subject on anticoagulants for thromboembolic disease may be due not to the arthritis itself but to a haemarthrosis, the physician having failed to warn the patient that anti-inflammatory drugs and warfarin should not be taken together. Leukaemia itself may also cause pains in the knee from leukaemic involvement of capsule, periosteum and other joint tissues. In hypertrophic pulmonary osteoarthropathy (HPOA) periostitis, some-times with joint swelling and effusions, accompanies malignant disease or chronic infection at a distant site. Knees and ankles and other joints may become swollen and ache, and effusions may be present in the knees. New periosteal tissue is laid down on bones of forearms, legs below the knees and elsewhere and finger- and possibly toe-clubbing is present. A bronchial carcinoma is often responsible but no malignant changes are present in the joint itself. The changes usually resolve fairly rapidly after removal of the tumour.

Pain in the shin

CAUSES

Referral from the lumbar spine (sciatica)
Referral from the patellofemoral
    joint — usually osteoarthritis
Shin splints
Tabes dorsalis
Periostitis
Hypertrophic pulmonary osteoarthropathy (HPOA)

Most pain is associated with retropatellar osteoarthritis. Discomfort after activity, especially running, is characteristic of shin splints which, if chronic, may lead to radiographically detectable periosteal reaction. HPOA is discussed above.

Pain in the calf

CAUSES

Deep venous thrombosis
Ruptured Baker's cyst
Intermittent claudication
Referral from the lumbar spine (sciatica)
Muscle tension
    —psychological
    —spasticity

If swelling of the calf is also present exclusion of deep venous thrombosis by Doppler examination or venography is the first priority. Even in the presence of known synovitis at the knee demonstration of a Baker's cyst by arthrography or ultrasound does not exclude venous thrombosis.

Pain in the ankle

CAUSES

Arthritis
Ligamentous strain/trauma
Hypermobility syndrome
Achilles tendon bursitis or enthesopathy
Referral from the lumbosacral spine (sciatica)
HPOA

Pain in the foot

CAUSES

Forefoot

Gout
Hallux rigidus
Bunion/hallux valgus
Inflammatory arthritis
Bone or joint infection
Morton's metatarsalgia
Stress fracture
Ingrowing toenail
Ischaemia
Freiberg's disease

Hindfoot

Plantar fasciitis
Achilles' tendonitis/bursitis
Osteochondritis of the navicular (Kohler's disease)
Bone and joint infection

Others

Plantar warts
Stiff flat feet
Oedema
Erythromelalagia
Painful polyneuropathy

Pain in the foot usually arises locally rather than through referral from elsewhere, although root lesions may cause pain along the lateral border of the foot.

Burning pain affecting the 2nd, 3rd or 4th toes which is aggravated by exercise and relieved by rest and removing the shoe is caused by swelling and inflammation of the digital nerve ('digital neuroma'). Usually the cleft between the 3rd and 4th or 2nd and 3rd toes is affected. There may be pain on lateral compression of the metatarsals or tenderness over the adjacent metatarsophalangeal (MTP) joints but there may be no abnormal signs. Surgical excision of the neuroma is curative. Stress fracture of the 2nd, 3rd or 4th metatarsal may also produce forefoot pain which is relieved by rest.

Forefoot pain often arises through deformity (hallux valgus) at the big toe MTP joint with an overlying bunion (*see Fig.* F.46), stiffness at the same joint (hallux rigidus) with frequent strains due to walking, or inflammatory arthritis at the MTP and toe joints. Rheumatoid disease commonly affects these joints but symmetrical or asymmetrical involvement of toes and MTP joint is also characteristic of seronegative arthritis, the upper limbs being frequently spared. Lesions of the toes including hammer toes (*see Fig. F.51*) and ingrowing toenails are readily apparent. The excruciating podagra of acute gouty arthritis, with surrounding erythema and oedema, is highly characteristic. Bone and joint infections in previously normal feet are rare though opportunistic bone infections may occur in immunocompromised patients including those with human immunodeficiency virus infection.

Pain in the hindfoot is usually attributable to either plantar fasciitis, with pain and tenderness on pressure (especially standing and walking) beneath the calcaneus or Achilles' tendinitis which produces posterior heel pain. Pain at either site impairs or precludes strenuous weight-bearing exercise. Achilles' tendinitis occurs especially in athletes and plantar fasciitis is common in older, overweight, individuals. However, both lesions may occur in young adults in association with seronegative arthritis. In the case of plantar fasciitis X-rays may reveal characteristic plantar spur formation. More rarely osteochondritis of the navicular bone causes transient pain over the inner side of the foot and limb in children between 3 and 6 years. Spontaneous resolution is the rule.

Diffuse pain over the foot may be associated with stiff flat feet (all feet are flat but mobile up to the age of 3 years) and chronic oedema. Burning pain which may be continuous or intermittent may be the presenting feature of erythromelalgia. This uncommon abnormality of superficial blood vessels of the foot may occur in polycythaemia, syringomyelia or in the early stage of chronic arsenical poisoning. It may also occur in normal subjects and may affect the hands. Pain may be severe and is aggravated by heat, dependency and walking. Pain is followed by cutaneous flushing, going on to cyanosis with the pain taking on a pulsatile character. There may be extreme tenderness with oedema and hyperhidrosis. Occasionally Raynaud's phenomenon produces similar episodic pain. Painful polyneuropathy may be attributable to many causes including toxins (especially alcohol) and nutritional deficiencies (especially vitamin B) but is increasingly seen in association with HIV infection. There are usually objective neurological signs.

Andrew Keat

Leg, ulceration of

Ulceration of the leg may be classified under four headings: (1) *Non-infective ulcers*; these include those that are not due to any specific infection, but which are caused by various factors that interfere with the vitality of the part by injury, poor circulation or deficient innervation of the tissue. (2) *Infective ulcers* resulting from the direct action of a definite specific infection, e.g. tuberculosis or syphilis. (3) *Ulcerating tumours*; these are malignant tumours, which have originated in or invaded the skin. (4) Ulcers associated with leukaemic states and other blood disorders.

Non-infective ulcers

There are usually several aetiological factors at work, of which circulatory disturbance, venous, arterial or both, is the most frequent and the most important, and may alone be sufficient cause. With trauma and mild non-specific infection added, the situation is ripe for the development of an indolent ulcer. These conditions obtain in the following varieties:

1. NUTRITIONAL ULCER. Following childbirth or surgical operations, or during the course of recumbency from any disease, especially in patients over the age of 40, there is a liability to thrombosis of the deep veins of the calf. This is manifested by a slight pyrexia, a glossiness, indicative of early oedema, over one ankle joint, an area of tenderness in one calf not present on the opposite side, and pain in one calf on strongly dorsiflexing the foot with the knee straight. The condition may spread into one of the main veins of the leg, and considerable oedema of the limb follows. Such cases, if followed up for a number of years, often develop a chronic oedema, with ulceration subsequently. The ulceration is usually determined by trauma; and some slight knock causing an abrasion which would normally heal is the starting-point of a chronic ulcer.

2. An almost precisely similar condition is caused by *varicose veins* and for the same reason—namely, deficient venous return leading to oedema and circulatory insufficiency (*Fig. L.13*). Not infrequently both factors operate together, and in such cases treatment of the varicose veins is essential and may be sufficient to lead to healing of the ulcer.

These two groups of causes—deep venous thrombosis and varicose veins—account between them for the great majority of leg ulcers seen in practice.

In cases of extreme chronicity the serological tests for syphilis should be made, as this may be a factor, and a biopsy is taken from the edge of the ulcer to preclude carcinoma.

3. ULCERATION DUE TO ARTERIAL DISEASE. Arteriosclerosis and thrombo-angiitis obliterans may lead to poor circulation and so to loss of nutrition. Ulcerative conditions are common in such cases and even gangrene may result. Such ulceration can start as a

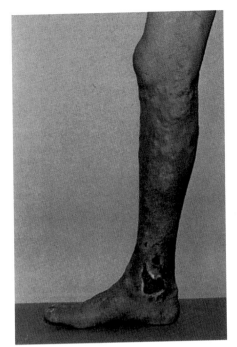

Fig. L.13. Varicose ulcer.

result of tissue infarction in large or small blood vessels (arteries or arterioles) due to many causes, thrombotic

or embolic. Ulcers over the shin are not uncommon in advanced rheumatoid arthritis, particularly in Felty's syndrome (rheumatoid arthritis with splenomegaly and neutropenia and a tendency to sepsis) (*Fig.* L.14). They also occur in polyarteritis nodosa, scleroderma, systemic lupus erythematosus and allergic vasculitis.

It is important to note, that in the elderly, arterial and venous disease may frequently co-exist. An apparent varicose ulcer that fails to respond to adequate treatment may well be associated with arterial obstruction. The digital pulses should always be examined and, if necessary, the Doppler probe used to investigate the peripheral arterial flow in the legs.

4. LYMPHATIC OBSTRUCTION also leads to loss of nutrition, and ulceration may result. The best instance is seen in elephantiasis due to *Filaria bancrofti*. In Great Britain elephantiasis is rare. Other instances that may be cited are swellings of the leg following a badly united fracture and the cicatricial contractions of extensive burns.

5. DEFICIENT INNERVATION leads to loss of nutrition. Examples are seen in infantile palsy; rubbing of the boot or pressure of an instrument is liable to be followed by an obstinate ulcer. In cases of hemiplegia, even when the patient is lying on a water-bed, ulceration in the form of bed sores will occur much more rapidly on the paralysed side than on the other. Perforating ulcer of the foot is a well-known sequel of

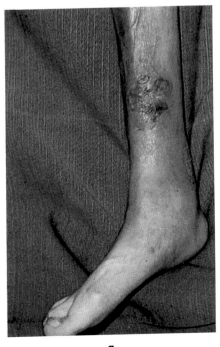

a

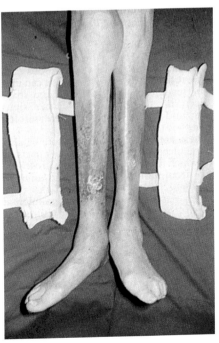

b

Fig. L.14. *a*. Typical shin ulcer in rheumatoid arthritis. This woman with Felty's syndrome has recurrent shin ulcers due to trivial injuries. She wore these shin pads (*b*) to prevent their recurrence. (*Dr F. Dudley Hart.*)

leprosy, *tabes dorsalis* and *diabetes mellitus*. It should be remembered that the comonest cause of a peripheral neuropathy in the Western World is diabetes, while in the whole of the world it is leprosy.

6. TRAUMA, unless it is continuous, is not alone sufficient to cause an ulcer in healthy people, in whom any abrasion usually heals without trouble. Old ladies, with thin atrophic skin, may lacerate the tissues over the shin, and the poor blood supply may result in necrosis and subsequent ulceration of the damaged skin. Interference with the normal contraction of scar tissue may also retard healing, as when the lesion is situated over and adherent to a bone. Self-inflicted trauma may be seen producing a leg ulcer or ulcers in hysterics and in the so-called Munchausen syndrome.

7. PHYSICAL AGENTS. Burns due to heat or to radium need no elaboration, nor do the ulcers which result from the inadvertent permeation of the subcutaneous tissues by the sclerosing fluids used for the injection of varicose veins. Cold is a factor in the production of ulcerating chilblains, but here once again deficiencies of circulation play a part. Self-inflicted trauma may be seen producing a leg ulcer or ulcers in hysterics and in the so-called Munchausen syndrome.

8. DIABETES MELLITUS needs special mention. In this disease ulceration and gangrene are prone to occur because the resistance of the sugar-laden tissues to infection is lowered, because the arterioles may be occluded by diabetic microangiopathy and because there may be anaesthesia of the foot due to diabetic neuropathy.

9. Varicose or syphilitic ulceration of the leg may be simulated by a *malingerer* who for some reason desires to make out that he is ill; nitric acid or other corrosive may have been rubbed into the leg, or a coin bandaged firmly against the skin, and the diagnosis may be obscure unless the circumstances of the case are well known. Sometimes the diagnosis is suggested by the rectangular or other definite shape of the ulcer itself.

10. BLOOD DYSCRASIAS. Ulcers of the leg may also occur in sickle-cell anaemia, thalassaemia, polycythaemia rubra vera, thrombotic thrombocytopenic purpura and hereditary spherocytosis, all of which should be considered where the aetiology is not evident. Ulceration of the leg, particularly on the lateral aspect, may occur in leukaemia.

Infective ulcers

The legs may be attacked by any form of acute infective ulcer such as *anthrax* or *glanders*, but such an event is rare. *Pyoderma gangrenosa*, frequently affecting the legs but sometimes involving skin elsewhere, may complicate ulcerative colitis or Crohn's disease (*see below*). The chief ulcers that belong to this group are chronic, and due to syphilis or tuberculosis.

SYPHILITIC ULCERS are the result of gummas which have formed in the subcutaneous tissues. These ulcerated gummas tend to occur in the upper part of the leg and, if in the lower part, on the outer aspect; they are almost always circular, and present a punched-out appearance; they are generally multiple and tend to run into each other, so that the ulcer has a serpiginous outline. They are today rarely seen. Diagnosis can in most cases be made on the distribution and shape of the ulcer; on the presence of other signs of syphilis; and by finding a positive blood serological reaction.

There are rare cases of subacute or chronic sores and ulcers of the leg, as of other parts of the body, which have been shown microscopically to arise from various skin fungi. *Blastomycosis, sporotrichosis* and *actinomycosis* of the skin are examples of this group. They are granulomatous eruptions sometimes associated with subcutaneous abscesses and multiple sinuses, sometimes simulating tertiary syphilitic lesions; their exact nature is determined by means of the microscope. Another fungus infection, one occurring in a tropical climate, is *Madura foot*, where the whole foot may become broadened, swollen and distorted by the formation of suppurating granulomatous tissue.

TUBERCULOUS ULCERS usually follow the formation and bursting of tuberculous abscesses, starting either in the subcutaneous tissue or in a bone, and the history may help materially in diagnosis. The ulcer is very chronic, and is characterized by undermining of the skin for a considerable distance from the edge. Lupus vulgaris, a form of primary tuberculosis of the skin, is not often found on the leg, though it may occur there as in any cutaneous area. A useful guiding rule is that lupus never starts later than the age of 20 and lasts for years, whereas a gumma starts at a later period and tends to heal spontaneously. In lupus the chief characteristic is the presence of minute, semi-transparent nodules at the margin of the ulcer and in the skin around, resembling apple jelly.

Leg ulcers may also be seen in amoebiasis, chancroid, diphtheria, leprosy, yaws, tularaemia, osteomyelitis, kala-azar and granuloma inguinale, all of which should be considered, particularly in recent immigrants. The so-called 'phagedenic ulcer' of feet or legs in a chronic lesion caused by mixed bacterial infection that occurs in persons suffering from neglect or starvation.

DYSPROTEINAEMIAS. Leg ulcers may be seen in association with cryoglobulinaemia and macroglobulinaemia.

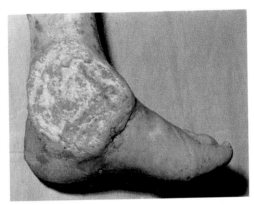

Fig. L.15. Marjolin's ulcer. (*Mr Nils Eckhoff.*)

PYODERMA GANGRENOSUM. In this condition, often associated with ulcerative colitis or Crohn's disease, the ulcers may be multiple and cover large areas of the leg. The ulcers tend to have ragged blue-red overhanging edges and necrotic bases. They often start as pustules or tender red nodules, often from minor trauma.

Ulcerating tumours

EPITHELIOMA may develop in a simple varicose ulcer that has existed for many years (Marjolin's ulcer). The

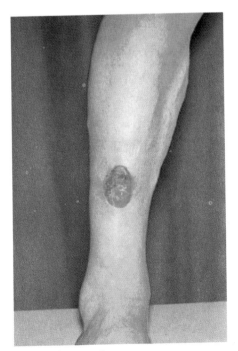

Fig. L.16. Malignant melanoma.

change may be very slow, or rapid. The ulcer spreads, the edges become heaped-up, everted and indurated (*Fig.* L.15). The groin lymph nodes become enlarged, and if the disease is allowed to progress the bone is attacked. If any doubt arises as to a change in the character of an ulcer, a piece from the edge should be removed for histological examination. The appearance of bare bone at the base of a varicose ulcer should always arouse the gravest suspicion that malignant change has taken place.

RODENT ULCER (*see also Fig.* F.21) usually attacks the face, though it may rarely be found on any part of the body.

MALIGNANT MELANOMA may ulcerate and bleed (*Fig.* L.16).

SARCOMA, starting in the deeper tissues or bone may fungate through the skin and give rise to an irregular breaking-down mass, which is obviously malignant, but may be mistaken for epithelioma unless there is previous knowledge of a malignant bony or soft tissue tumour or unless histological examination is made. Hodgkin's disease and mycosis fungoides may also be associated with ulcers of the leg.

Harold Ellis

Lips, affections of

The lips form an important mucocutaneous junction and their proper function is important for feeding and communication. They have a very rich nerve supply and hence inflammation can cause disproportionate irritation and pain. The lips are also of considerable cosmetic, psychological and emotional importance. (*See Table* L.2.)

MACULES

Macular affections around the lips include flat *moles*, *freckles* and the multiple tiny dark freckles seen in *Peutz–Jegher's syndrome*. Multiple lip telangiectases are seen in *hereditary haemorrhagic telangiectasia* and sometimes with severe liver disease.

PAPULES

The commonest papules on lips are probably plane *warts*, but *lichen planus* papules have a predilection for the lips, as well as plaques of *discoid lupus erythematosus*. *Pyogenic granuloma* can form at this site and in older patients *venous lakes* are commonly seen. The lip can be the site of a primary *syphilitic* chancre. *Actinic cheilitis* is common on the lower lip, especially in seafarers and agricultural

Table L.2. Affections of the lips

Macules
Flat mole (junctional naevus)
Freckle (ephelide)
Peutz–Jegher's syndrome
Telangiectasis
   hereditary haemorrhagic telangiectasia
   liver disease

Papules
Plane warts
Lichen planus
Discoid lupus erythematosus
Pyogenic granuloma
Venous lake
Syphilitic chancre
Actinic cheilitis
   ±solar keratosis
   ±squamous-cell carcinoma

Swollen lips
Trauma, thermal insult
Angio-oedema
Melkersson–Rosenthal syndrome
Crohn's disease
Erosions
Impetigo
Herpes simplex
Hand-foot-and-mouth disease
Secondary syphilis
Erythema multiforme
Fixed drug eruption
Zinc deficiency
Acrodermatitis enteropathica
Pemphigus

Thickening
Atopic dermatitis
Lip-rubbing

Cheilitis
Candidiasis
Contact dermatitis
Lip-licking

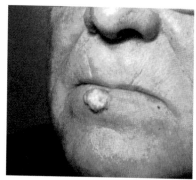

Fig. L.17. Squamous cell carcinoma. (*Dr Richard Staughton.*)

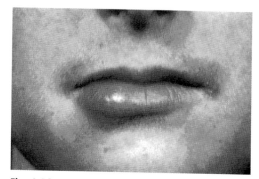

Fig. L.18. Granulomatous cheilitis. Crohn's disease. (*Dr Richard Staughton.*)

EROSIONS

Erosions on lips occur in acute infections such as *impetigo* in children, *herpes simplex*, which may be recurrent in adults, *hand-foot-and-mouth disease* and secondary *syphilis*. Erosive dermatoses which affect the lips include *erythema multiforme* (Stevens–Johnson syndrome) and *fixed drug eruption* (codeine and sulphonamides). Chronic erosions around the lips are seen in *zinc deficiency, acrodermatitis enteropathica* and *pemphigus*.

THICKENED LIPS

Thickening of the skin around the mouth is a characteristic feature of *atopic dermatitis* due to rubbing of the lips with the backs of the hands.

CHEILITIS

When inflammation is confined to the lips, search should be made for occult *candidiasis*, especially in those with dentures and iron deficiency. Chronic *contact dermatitis* can occur at this site, e.g. nickel dermatitis from sucking hairpins, lipstick dermatitis, toothpaste dermatitis and rather surprisingly nail

workers. The appearance is of atrophy with greyish plaques often surmounted by crusts in cold weather. *Solar keratoses* appear and invasive *squamous-cell carcinoma*, nearly always of the lower lips (*Fig. L.17*) must be detected early as metastases can quickly occur.

SWOLLEN LIPS

Swollen lips can follow trauma and thermal insult, or be part of an *urticaria*, as *angio-oedema*. The *Melkersson–Rosenthal syndrome* comprises permanently oedematous thickened lips (granulomatous cheilitis) with recurrent facial palsy and scrotal tongue. Granulomatous cheilitis is occasionally seen in Crohn's disease (*Fig. L.18*).

varnish dermatitis. Irritation from excessive *lip-licking* can often be observed in patients with cheilitis and may sometimes be the primary cause.

Richard Staughton

Liver, enlargement of

In adults the liver is about $\frac{1}{36}$; but at birth it is $\frac{1}{24}$ to $\frac{1}{18}$ of the whole body weight, so that in infants and young children it is relatively larger than adults. The normal liver is therefore usually palpable in children. In thin people with lax abdominal muscles the liver may be palpable about 1 cm beneath the costal margin and it descends to meet the fingers on deep inspiration. In clinical practice palpation of the liver is an unreliable indicator of actual liver size and the most accurate way of determining this is by percussion. Hepatic dullness extends from the 5th intercostal space in the right nipple line to the 7th intercostal space in the midaxillary line then downwards to the right costal margin.

In health the edge of the liver is firm and uniform and the surface feels smooth. If the liver is transposed the right lobe is small and the left large. A tongue-like projection of the right lobe may protrude from its lower right hand part. This projection, known as *Riedel's lobe* is more common in women than in men. It may cause difficulty of diagnosis, being confused with a mobile kidney, gallbladder or tumour.

Many conditions unconnected with the liver cause an apparent alteration in its size. In emphysema the liver is easily palpable but percussion will reveal that the organ is merely displaced. Deformities of the chest due to rickets or curvature of the spine may depress the liver as may a right subphrenic abscess. It is unusual for enlargement of the liver to lead to upward extension of hepatic dullness because the weight of the liver causes it to descend. Elevation of the upper limit of hepatic dullness occurs when local hepatic disease involves the diaphragm. The best example is an amoebic abscess which may elevate the diaphram. A hydatid cyst may have a similar effect. Loss of hepatic dullness occurs in emphysema, principally because of displacement of the liver. Free gas in the peritoneum or distension of the colon may also do this.

Hepatoptosis or *wandering liver* are terms applied to a liver which is found in an abnormal position. This is rare but does occur after therapeutic pneumoperitoneum at laparoscopy. It is usually an asymptomatic condition although the patient may complain of a dragging sensation and heaviness in the right upper quadrant of the abdomen. The liver which is displaced may be thought to be enlarged.

Table L.3. Causes of hepatic enlargement

Congenital
Riedel's lobe
Polycystic disease

Hepatitis
Acute
  Viruses
  Drugs
  Alcohol
Chronic
  Lupoid
  Hepatitis B and C infection

Venous congestion
Cardiac failure
Constrictive pericarditis
Budd–Chiari syndrome
Veno-occlusive disease
Haemolytic crisis

Fatty liver

Biliary disease
Extrahepatic obstruction
Sclerosing cholangitis
Primary biliary cirrhosis

Infiltration
Malignancy
Granulomatous hepatitis
Amyloidosis

Metabolic
Glycogen storage diseases
Haemochromatosis
Endrocrine diseases

Abscess
Pyogenic
Amoebic

Tropical diseases
Viral hepatitis
Protazoan infections
Helminthic infections

Cryptogenic cirrhosis

The major categories of disease associated with hepatic enlargement are shown in *Table L.3.*

CONGENITAL CAUSES

Occasionally an additional lobe of the liver, *Riedel's lobe*, projects from the lower border of the right lobe and extends as a palable mass below the right costal margin.

Polycystic disease results in gross hepatic enlargement from numerous cysts of the varying size producing a honeycomb appearance on cut section. The cysts contain clear fluid, usually without bile. Usually the whole liver is involved, but sometimes one lobe, more frequently the right, is implicated. Hepatic function is surprisingly often normal. The condition is often associated with cystic involvement of other organs, kidneys most commonly, but occasionally also pancreas, spleen, ovary and lung.

Hepatitis

Acute hepatitis is most commonly due to viral infection (hepatitis A, hepatitis B, hepatitis C, delta virus, hepatitis E, cytomegalovirus, herpes simplex, Epstein–Barr), adverse reaction to a drug, or alcohol. These are fully discussed under JAUNDICE.

Acute hepatitis is invariably associated with hepatic enlargement. The liver is moderately enlarged, usually tender but regular. There are frequently, but not invariably, signs of liver dysfunction including jaundice and in the presence of alcohol abuse there may be stigmata of chronic liver disease. The patient is usually systemically unwell, with anorexia, nausea and weight loss. There may be fever. In alcoholic hepatitis a liver bruit may be audible.

Chronic active hepatitis is also described under JAUNDICE. The usual causes are auto-immune (lupoid hepatitis), chronic hepatitis B and C virus infection and an adverse reaction to drugs. Hepatomegaly is variable in chronic hepatitis. In the early stages the liver is usually enlarged and may be tender. As the disease progresses continuing fibrosis may result in the liver decreasing in size and it becomes impalpable. Liver size can then only be ascertained by percussion. In late stages the stigmata of chronic liver disease develop and splenomegaly and ascites occur as a consequence of portal hypertension. Massive enlargement of the liver associated with hepatitis B and C-related chronic active hepatitis is usually due to a complicating primary hepatocellular carcinoma.

Venous congestion

Venous congestion of the liver results from *obstruction of flow in the hepatic vein*. This may occur at the level of the heart as a consequence either of *right ventricular failure or constrictive pericarditis*. It may occur following *thrombosis of the inferior vena cava* or of the *hepatic vein* (Budd–Chiari syndrome), or there may be an obstruction at the intrahepatic postsinusoidal level.

Venous congestion from *heart disease* causes uniform enlargement of the liver of variable degree. The liver may sometimes be massively enlarged, reaching the umbilicus. In acute heart failure stretching of the hepatic capsule leads to acute pain and tenderness in the right upper quadrant. In chronic heart failure the liver is not usually tender. The

presence of a pulsatile liver indicates *tricuspid regurgitation*, as evidenced by a pronounced v wave in the jugular neck veins, cardiac enlargement with a thrill and a pansystolic murmur at the base of the sternum are also evident. Peripheral oedema is usually severe and ascites may occur.

In *constrictive pericarditis* the liver is also considerably enlarged, ascites is often extreme particularly in relation to the degree of peripheral oedema. Jaundice may be prominent and a diagnosis of parenchymal liver disease may be made by the unwary. This should be avoided by the observation that the neck veins are engorged and that the heart is small and 'quiet'.

The *Budd–Chiari syndrome* may present acutely or chronically. Thrombosis of the hepatic vein usually occurs as a consequence of an underlying hypercoagulable state such as polycythaemia rubra vera or thrombotic thrombocytopenic purpura. In some patients the hypercoagulable state is subtle and a bone marrow examination is necessary to make the diagnosis. Anti-thrombin 3 or protein C deficiency, underlying malignancy (breast, pancreas, lung) or consumption of oestrogens in a relatively high dose are other causes. In the acute disease sudden, painful, massive hepatomegaly develops. Liver decompensation follows and is characterized by jaundice, ascites and splenomegaly due to portal hypertension and (in severe cases) coagulopathy, portasystemic encephalopathy and death. Some surviving patients progress to chronic liver disease associated with marked hepatomegaly, ascites and variceal gastrointestinal bleeding. Rarely the Budd–Chiari syndrome develops insidiously without an initial acute phase. An isotopic liver scan shows diffuse poor uptake, sparing the caudate lobe. The disease is confirmed by hepatic venography and liver biopsy.

Intrahepatic veno-occlusive disease may also occur in hypercoaguable states and presents with painful hepatomegaly. The classical cause is the ingestion of certain plant toxins especially bush tea.

The liver may enlarge suddenly and painfully as a response to venous congestion from *haemolysis*. Haemolytic crises in sickle-cell anaemia and thalassaemia are the best examples.

Fatty Liver

The liver may be enlarged because of excessive deposition of fat droplets. The commonest cause is *alcohol abuse. Protein malnutrition, diabetes mellitus, obesity* and *jejuno-ileal bypass* are others.

The liver is uniformly enlarged, firm but not tender. Signs of hepatic decompensation are absent unless there is pre-existing ethanolic damage.

In acute fatty liver of pregnancy, microvesicular deposition of fat occurs throughout the liver cells. This is a condition which develops in late pregnancy and is associated with liver failure characterized by encephalopathy, coagulopathy and renal failure. The liver is grossly enlarged and tender. The prognosis is poor but Caesarean section and removal of the baby is life-saving.

Biliary disease

Biliary obstruction (cholestasis) can be due to disease affecting the extrahepatic biliary tract, the intrahepatic bile ducts and ductules or the canaliculi.

Extrahepatic biliary obstruction is most commonly due to gallstones within the bile duct or to malignant tumours, either in the pancreas, gallbladder or secondary deposits or within the bile duct itself. Benign strictures following operative trauma or sclerosing cholangitis, chronic pancreatitis or infestation by ascaris lumbricoides are less common causes. Patients presenting with extrahepatic obstruction due to impacted gallstones present with right upper quadrant abdominal pain and fluctuating jaundice. The liver is tender and moderately enlarged. A common consequence of choledocholithiasis is infection of bile leading to pain, jaundice and fever with rigors (Charcot's triad).

Biliary infection is unusual in patients with malignant extrahepatic biliary obstruction; such patients present with progressive painful jaundice and the depth of jaundice is usually greater than that associated with gallstones. The liver is uniformly enlarged unless there is metastatic malignant disease. When the obstruction is distal to the cystic duct the gallbladder is also distended and palpable. Courvoisier's law which states that 'in a patient with obstructive jaundice a palpable gall bladder is unlikely to be due to stones', is often true. However, the distended gall bladder may not be clinically palpable. Patients with malignant extrahepatic biliary obstruction may have other evidence of neoplastic disease; weight loss is often pronounced. Back pain may occur as a consequence of vertebral or coeliac plexus erosion by tumour. Ascites with a high protein content may be present. The patient with an ampullary tumour may be anaemic because of chronic blood loss from the tumour. Extrahepatic biliary obstruction is considered more fully in under JAUNDICE.

Congenital malformations of the biliary tract are associated with hepatomegaly. In biliary atresia there is failure of development of the extrahepatic biliary tree and the infant develops progressive jaundice and liver failure associated with marked hepatomegaly. The diagnosis is made by radio-isotopic HIDA scan and hepatic transplantation or portoenterostomy (Kasai operation) are life-saving. Other congenital abnormalities of the biliary tree include choledochal cyst, congenital dilatation of the intrahepatic ducts (Caroli's disease), and congenital hepatic fibrosis. *Choledochal cyst* characteristically presents in young women with a triad of jaundice, pain and an abdominal mass. Poor drainage of the biliary apparatus results in recurrent cholangitis and the disease predisposes to the development of cholangiocarcinoma. Primary repair of the cyst is necessary. The cysts may occasionally be intrahepatic when they have to be differentiated from simple cysts or polycystic disease which may be part of a spectrum of polycystic syndromes affecting the liver, pancreas and kidneys. Such cysts do not communicate with the biliary tree. *Caroli's syndrome* is a rare condition associated with intrahepatic cystic dilatation of the bile ductules. Recurrent infection may lead to jaundice and hepatomegaly.

Biliary strictures affecting both the intra- and extrahepatic tree are characteristic of *sclerosing cholangitis (Fig.* L.19). This may occur as a consequence of recurrent biliary sepsis, usually associated with bile duct trauma. It may alternatively be a primary condition commonly associated with ulcerative colitis. In primary sclerosing cholangitis males predominate and the disease is extremely variable in its presentation. It is likely that the majority of patients are asymptomatic for many years. Others present with recurrent jaundice

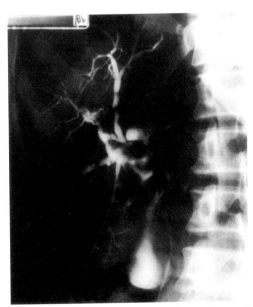

Fig. L.19. Percutaneous cholangiogram showing the typical appearances of intrahepatic primary sclerosing cholangitis in a patient with ulcerative colitis. The biliary tree is beaded with irregularly narrowed ducts.

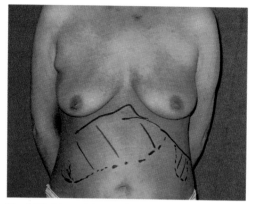

Fig. L.20. Primary biliary cirrhosis. Late disease demonstrating hepatosplenomegaly, ascites and skin pigmentation.

and cholangitis. Examination reveals firm hepatomegaly and in those patients who progress to cirrhosis this may be irregular and associated with other evidence of chronic liver disease. The treatment of sclerosing cholangitis is unsatisfactory. The condition is reviewed more fully under JAUNDICE.

Chronic intrahepatic cholestasis occurs in *primary biliary cirrhosis*. This is a condition of middle-aged women in which the bile ductules are destroyed by a cell-mediated auto-immune process. The disease is extremely variable in its presentation but it progresses slowly in the majority of patients. Many patients are asymptomatic; the characteristic symptom is that of pruritus. Others present at a late stage with hepatic decompensation or variceal haemorrhage. In the late stages the woman presents with jaundice, xanthelasmata and hepatomegaly which is often marked, irregular and firm (*Fig.* L.20). Splenomegaly and ascites are common and there may be evidence of other auto-immune disease such as thyroiditis, systemic sclerosis or Addison's disease. In common with all chronic cholestatic conditions, pigmentation due to deposition of melanin in the skin develops. Defective copper excretion may occasionally lead to Kayser-Fleischer rings (*see Fig.* J.10). The diagnosis is suggested by cholestatic liver function tests in a woman and is confirmed by the presence of circulating anti-mitochondrial antibodies and a typical liver biopsy appearance characterized by destruction and paucity of bile ductules, granulomata and evidence of fibrosis or cirrhosis.

Other cholestatic conditions are also associated with hepatomegaly, jaundice and pruritus. Rare patients present with *benign recurrent cholestasis* in which severe jaundice and pruritus relapse and remit from birth. Liver biopsy shows only evidence of

cholestasis without liver damage. Certain *drugs*, particularly chlorpromazine, tricyclic antidepressants and chloropropamide are associated with cholestasis. Cholestasis may also occur as a non-specific response to severe systemic illness, particularly following operations; the cause is unknown and resolves as the general condition of the patient improves.

Hepatic infiltration

The liver parenchyma may be infiltrated by malignant cells, granulomata or by amyloid.

The commonest of these is *secondary carcinoma*, usually arising from the gastro-intestinal tract, breast, bronchus and kidney (*Fig.* L.21). Symptoms do not develop until very late and comprise right upper quadrant abdominal pain and jaundice. Examination reveals irregular hepatomegaly. The liver is hard and sometimes extremely large, extending into the pelvis. Sudden painful enlargement may be due to bleeding into a secondary deposit. Ascites is common and is associated with a high protein content. There may be evidence of primary disease and it is important in all patients presenting with hepatomegaly to examine the breasts, thyroid and prostate as specific therapy may affect progression both of the primary and of the secondary diseases.

Secondary deposits from **malignant melanoma**, either from a cutaneous or choroid of the eye primary, may produce massive hepatomegaly ('beware of the glass eye and the elnlarged liver').

The diagnosis of secondary malignant infiltration is strongly supported by ultrasound or CT scanning of the liver but should always be confirmed by guided needle biopsy or cytology. Once a diagnosis has been achieved it is usually pointless to seek the primary tumour because cure is impossible. The only excep-

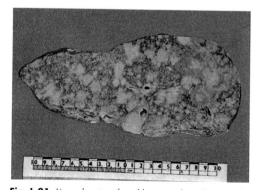

Fig. L.21. Liver almost replaced by secondary deposits. The primary site was a carcinoma of the breast.

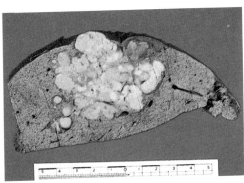

Fig. L.22. An unusual primary hepatoma arising in a previously normal liver.

tions are those of tumours which might be amenable to hormonal therapy or chemotherapy (prostate, breast, thyroid) and the occasional patient who has a solitary hepatic secondary deposit from a colonic carcinoma. In this situation it may be reasonable to embark upon a colonic resection. Rarely secondary deposits are suitable for hepatic resection.

It is important to differentiate secondary deposits in the liver from a *carcinoid tumour*. These commonly arise from the small bowel or appendix and may replace large amounts of the liver. A proportion secrete polypeptides and present with the *carcinoid syndrome* which only occurs when the tumour has spread to the liver. Such patients present with flushing and watery diarrhoea and may develop chronic pigmentation of the hands and face. The tumours are often extremely slowly growing and considerable palliation can be achieved either by the use of somatostatin and its analogues, or interferon, by embolization of the tumour via the hepatic artery, or by surgical removal.

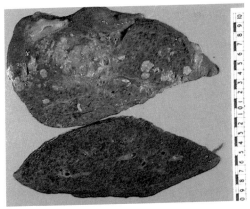

Fig. L.23. Multiple hepatomas in a cirrhotic liver.

Primary hepatocellular carcinoma is comparatively rare in Britain but is the commonest hepatic malignancy worldwide. It is associated with chronic infection with hepatitis B or C and usually develops in cirrhotic patients (*Figs* L.22, L.23). Other causes of cirrhosis, particularly long-standing alcoholic cirrhosis and, treated haemochromatosis also predispose to the tumour. Patients present with weight loss, abdominal pain and massive hepatomegaly. The liver is greatly enlarged and may or may not be tender. The tumour mass is hard, irregular and sometimes associated with a bruit. There is usually evidence of chronic liver disease. Ascites may either be due to underlying portal hypertension from cirrhosis or as a direct consequence of the primary liver cancer in which event the protein concentration is high (>30 g/l). The diagnosis is made by the finding of increased concentration of circulating alpha-fetoprotein, by liver biopsy or by angiography. The prognosis is very poor.

Haemangiomas of the liver are relatively common, probably occurring in as many as 10 per cent of livers. They are usually asymptomatic. Angiosarcomas occasionally arise from these benign tumours and they are associated with ingestion of plant toxins (aflatoxins), or chronic infestation with liver fluke. Massive enlargement of the liver occurs and health rapidly deteriorates. A liver bruit is often present. The prognosis is very poor.

Benign tumours of the liver are unusual. Adenomas occur in association with the use of oestrogens and in pregnancy. These are usually asymptomatic but may present acutely with massive intraperitoneal bleeding.

Lymphoma may cause hepatomegaly in a variety of ways. The liver may be infiltrated in Hodgkin's disease or non-Hodgkin's lymphoma. The liver is then irregularly enlarged and non-tender. There may be other evidence of lymphoma such as splenomegaly and lymphadenopathy. In other cases infiltration is diffuse and the liver is then smooth, regular, firm and only moderately enlarged. Some patients with lymphoma present as granulomatous liver disease showing little or no hepatomegaly but cholestatic liver function tests. Occasionally patients present as extrahepatic biliary obstruction from lymph node masses particularly arising in the region of the porta hepatis. Lymphoma may present as the Budd–Chiari syndrome as previously described. Occasional patients present with cholestatic jaundice without obvious extrahepatic biliary obstruction and without infiltration. The liver is then enlarged, the patient deeply jaundiced and a biopsy merely shows evidence of intrahepatic cholestasis.

Sarcomas of the liver are extremely rare and cannot be differentiated clinically from carcinoma.

The liver may also be infiltrated in *amyloidosis*. This may either occur as a primary disease or in association with myelomatosis or chronic suppurative disease. The liver is extremely large, smooth, firm and non-tender. In addition the spleen may be enlarged and there may be proteinuria because of renal involvement. The diagnosis may be made by liver biopsy although this can be dangerous because rarely the procedure may cause the rigid liver to split.

The liver may be infiltrated by *granulomata*. There are a wide variety of causes of which the most important are sarcoidosis, tuberculosis, lymphoma, and an adverse reaction to drugs.

The liver is frequently involved in *sarcoidosis* when the alkaline phosphatase concentration is often increased. Symptoms and signs of liver disease are rare and hepatomegaly occurs in only about 20 per cent of patients. Those with enlargement of the liver are often West Indian. The liver may then be considerably enlarged, irregular, and it is usually firm but non-tender. There is often splenomegaly and other features of sarcoidosis including pulmonary infiltration and hypercalcaemia may be evident.

Tuberculosis is also associated with granulomatous liver disease and the liver is commonly somewhat enlarged in this disease. It is usually firm, modestly enlarged but non-tender.

Chronic infection with *schistosomiasis* causes granulomatous infiltration of the liver. The liver is enlarged, firm and non-tender. Pre-sinusoidal portal hypertension causes splenomegaly and oesophageal varices develop. Hepatic synthetic function is maintained until a late stage and jaundice is relatively mild.

Syphilis is now an extremely rare disease in the Western hemisphere. It is associated with hepatomegaly in the secondary stage and in addition tertiary syphilis and the formation of gummas lead to the formation of an irregular rather hard liver similar in appearance and feel to that of cirrhosis.

Metabolic causes

A variety of metabolic, genetic and endocrine disorders are associated with the development of hepatomegaly.

Glycogen storage diseases cause hepatomegaly from birth. Lipid storage disorders such as *Gaucher's disease* are associated with massive hepatosplenomegaly and growth retardation while *Niemann-Pick disease* may have neurological associations including mental retardation.

Haemochromatosis and *haemosiderosis* are disorders associated with accumulation of iron within the liver. Haemosiderosis is commonly associated with multiple blood transfusions often required for haemolytic disorders such as thalassaemia. Iron accumulates within Kupffer's cells. Hepatic function is well maintained and the liver is only moderately enlarged. In contrast, haemochromatosis is a genetic syndrome inherited as an autosomal recessive gene. The condition is associated with alcohol abuse, probably because this also enhances iron absorption. The disease is rare in premenopausal women because of menstrual blood loss. Patients present with hepatomegaly due to cirrhosis. The liver is firm and considerably enlarged. There may be evidence of portal hypertension including splenomegaly, ascites and a proportion of patients present for the first time as a variceal haemorrhage. Iron is also deposited in the skin producing dusky pigmentation. Deposition also occurs in endocrine glands accounting to the common association with diabetes. Marked feminization manifest as gynaecomastia, absent body hair, testicular atrophy and decreased need for shaving are prominent features. Although relatively unusual the diagnosis of haemochromatosis is important because the prognosis is greatly improved by venesection. The diagnosis is made by demonstrating an increased serum ferritin concentration and by liver biopsy. Massive hepatomegaly associated with haemochromatosis may be due to the development of hepatocellular cancer which is a relatively common late complication.

Acromegaly is associated with hepatomegaly without evidence of liver dysfunction. The liver is modestly enlarged but soft. Thyrotoxicosis may also be associated with hepatic enlargement and deranged liver function tests.

Liver abscess

Liver abscesses are either a consequence of bacterial infection or amoebiasis. Pyogenic liver abscess follows portal pyaemia due to diverticulitis, appendicitis, subphrenic abscess, or inflammatory bowel disease. It may complicate biliary disease, usually choledocholithiasis, but sometimes an infected endoprosthesis, sclerosing cholangitis or ampullary tumour. Pyogenic abscesses are commonly multiple and rarely large. They are associated with modest painful hepatomegaly with marked constitutional disturbances including fever with rigors, and jaundice.

An amoebic abscess may be single and large. It commonly follows a history of dysentery and the majority occur in the right lobe. Men are affected more often than women. The patient presents with swinging pyrexia, associated with rigors and tachycardia, a considerably enlarged and very tender liver; there may be a sympathetic pleural effusion.

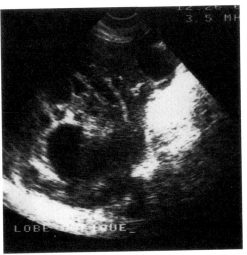

Fig. L.24. Ultrasound examination of the liver demonstrating multiple pyogenic abscesses of the right lobe of the liver.

The diagnosis of liver abscess is made by ultrasound and confirmed by guided aspiration and culture of pus (*Fig*. L.24). Small multiple abscesses may respond to systemic antibiotic therapy and relief of the underlying cause (viz. relief of biliary obstruction, irradication of the primary intra-abdominal sepsis). Larger abscesses are drained either by a percutaneous wide-bore catheter or by formal surgical drainage.

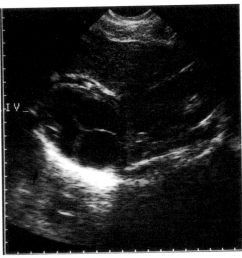

Fig. L.25. Ultrasound examination of the liver revealing classical appearances of hydatid cyst with multiple daughter cysts.

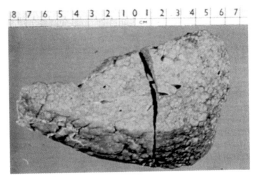

Fig. L.26. Cirrhosis of the liver.

Tropical diseases

A variety of tropical and sub-tropical diseases are associated with hepatomegaly. These include viral hepatitis, protozoan infections including malaria, schistosomiasis, Kala-azar, hydatid and infestations with liver flukes and ascaris lumbricoides.

Acute painful hepatomegaly occurs during the crises of malaria.

Large hydatid cysts can occur within the liver but these are usually asymptomatic and cause no disturbance of liver function. The cysts may achieve considerable size, they are rounded and smooth, and there may be a thrill perceived on percussion (ballottment). The diagnosis is made by plain abdominal X-ray if the cysts are calcified. Ultrasound appearances are extremely characteristic and daughter cysts are often seen (*Fig*. L.25). Needle aspiration is contraindicated because this may cause infection and spillage of cysts within the peritoneal cavity. About one quarter of the patients demonstrating eosinophilia. The Casoni complement fixation test is usually positive.

Cryptogenic cirrhosis

A proportion of individuals present with well-established cirrhosis and hepatomegaly without an obvious cause. The majority of these are women and there is no evidence of exposure to alcohol or the hepatitis B or C virus. The smooth muscle antibody and antinuclear factor are negative but there is no evidence of metabolic or congenital liver disease. The clinical findings are variable but include the stigmata of chronic liver disease, evidence of portal hypertension and portosystemic encephalopathy. The size of the liver is variable, ranging from barely palpable to moderately enlarged. The organ is firm, irregular and non-tender (*Fig*. L.26).

K. R. Palmer

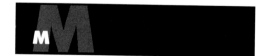

Melaena

Melaena is the term applied to the black bowel motion resulting from haemorrhage which has occurred in the gastrointestinal tract at a high enough level for chemical alteration to take place. It may also occur after swallowing blood derived from haemoptysis or epistaxis. Melaena stools are black, tarry, with a treacly or sticky consistency, rendering it difficult to flush down the toilet. It has been shown by feeding healthy volunteer medical students with increasing aliquots of their own blood, that between 50 and 80 ml are sufficient to cause a melaena stool.

Black or dark stools, simulating melaena, may occur after taking iron preparations by mouth (the iron being converted to the sulphide form), bismuth preparations, licquorice or following the ingestion of charcoal biscuits, black cherries, bilberries or red wine in large quantities, or by the excretion of large amounts of bile pigments. The characteristic thick sticky nature of melaena stools is generally easily differentiated from other causes of black stools, but the diagnosis can be confirmed by laboratory investigation of the stool for the presence of blood.

Melaena is most commonly due to bleeding from the stomach or duodenum, or more rarely from the oesophagus. In such situations it is generally associated with haematemesis (*see* p. 151) before the melaena is apparent. If melaena occurs alone from these sources, it generally indicates that the rate of bleeding is relatively slow. Melaena is as serious as haematemesis as an indication of upper gastric haemorrhage; patients with melaena should be investigated and managed as urgently as those with haematemesis. It is possible to judge the severity of a gastrointestinal bleed from the patient's description of the stools.

A detailed account of symptoms such as faintness, sweating and collapse, together with the general assessment of the patient's haemodynamic state allows the clinician to assess the severity of the gastro-intestinal bleed leading to the development of mel-aena. Upper gastrointestinal endoscopy may be required and blood transfusion may be necessary.

The great majority of patients with melaena will have bled from lesions situated in, or proximal to, the duodenum. The commonest cause (perhaps more than 85% of patients) is from duodenal or gastric ulceration, acute gastric erosions and peptic oesophagitis. Bleed-ing from haemorrhagic erosions associated with the use of non-steroidal anti-inflammatory drugs (NSAIDs) is an increasingly common cause of melaena, especially in elderly patients.

Lesions distal to the duodenum generally give rise to dark or bright red blood in the stools rather than melaena. However, melaena may occur in the relatively uncommon group of causes of the small intestinal bleeding, which include mesenteric thrombosis or embolism, leiomyoma, leiomyosarcoma, or haeman-gioma of the upper small intestine, the Ehlers–Danlos syndrome, peptic ulcer in a Meckel's diverticulum, Crohn's disease of the small intestine, haemorrhage in typhoid fever from an ulcerated Peyer's patch in the ileum, angiodysplasia of the small intestine, blood dyscrasias resulting in oozing from the intestinal mucosa, or the use of anticoagulant therapy.

Rarely melaena may be associated with small intestinal ulceration in coeliac disease or secondary to drug-induced damage to the small intestine, a rare but increasing occurrence.

R. I. Russell

Menorrhagia

Menorrhagia signifies excessive menstrual flow, or undue prolongation of the time during which it takes place. The patient is free from bleeding during the intermenstrual periods, the term Metrorrhagia or Irregular Uterine Bleeding (q.v.) being reserved for bleeding which occurs between the periods. Careful distinction between these symptoms often serves to distinguish very important conditions, and they should not be confounded with one another. Pure menor-rhagia is an important symptom of many well-defined conditions which do not, as a rule, give rise to irregular bleeding. Both these terms must be limited carefully to patients who menstruate, and must not be used for bleeding after the menopause.

The diagnosis of menorrhagia may be difficult because of the absence of anaemia or other signs of severe menstrual blood loss. The diagnosis has to be accepted when the patient complains of having to use more than a dozen and a half pads per menstrual period or when she loses clots or has flooding. Experiments using radioactive chromium to label red cells show that some women may suffer excessive menstrual loss without becoming anaemic, while others who do not bleed so heavily may show all the signs of a severe iron-deficiency anaemia due to chronic blood loss.

Excess of menstrual loss in women without abnormal physical signs is believed to be endocrine in origin and is called *dysfunctional menorrhagia*. Acute endometritis of gonococcal or pyogenic origin tends to cure itself owing to the shedding of the endometrium during menstruation. *Tuberculous endometritis* a rare

Table M.1. Causes of menorrhagia

1. Dysfunctional menorrhagia	2. In the generative system	3. Circulatory and other systems	4. In the nervous system
At puberty	Fibromyomas	Uncompensated valvular disease of the heart	Excessive coitus
At maturity without obvious lesions	Salpingo-oophoritis (chronic)	Cirrhosis of the liver	Prevention of conception
In relation to the menopause, and in the years preceding	Endometriosis	Emphysema of the lungs	A single excessive period
Hypothyroidism	Adenomyoma	Chronic alcoholism	Fright
	Tuberculous endometritis		Violent emotion
	Intrauterine contraceptive device	The blood itself	Sudden changes of temperature
		Deficient coagulability	Cold bath
	Acute infectious diseases	Scurvy	Dancing
	Influenza	Purpura	Hunting
	Typhoid	Leukaemia	Gymnastics
	Cholera		Bicycling, etc.
	Scarlatina	High blood pressure	
	Variola	Arteriosclerosis	
	Malaria		
	Diphtheria		
	Measles		

cause of infertility in the UK. It is due to spread from the Fallopian tubes and is therefore associated with menorrhagia due to the tuberculous salpingo-oophoritis. If a tuberculous infection is suspected the uterine curettings should be examined for the typical tubercles and the organism isolated by culture. Causes of menorrhagia are given in *Table* M.1.

1. Dysfunctional menorrhagia

Menorrhagia of puberty is mainly due to hypofunction of the anterior pituitary body, with consequent failure of ovulation and therefore no corpus luteum. The ovaries contain unruptured Graafian follicles, there is increased oestrogen production, and a lack of the luteal hormone progesterone. These cases often right themselves in time as the pituitary gradually assumes its normal cyclic activities.

Menorrhagia of mature women without obvious lesions of the generative or other systems is thought to be due to an imbalance between the secretion by the ovary of oestrogen and progesterone, with an increase in oestrogen and a complete lack of or a deficiency of progesterone. When there is a complete absence of progesterone in the second half of the menstrual cycle the cycle is referred to as *anovular*, drawing attention to failure of ovulation and formation of a corpus luteum. The condition may be diagnosed by a study of basal temperature charts, there being no postovulatory rise in basal temperature, or by examination of endometrial curettings, which show evidence only of oestrogenic hypertrophy. Sometimes the ovaries become cystic and the endometrium undergoes polypoidal thickening with a characteristic microscopic appearance known as 'Swiss cheese' endometrium or 'cystic glandular hyperplasia'. This condition is known as *metropathia haemorrhagica* (Schröder's disease). Bouts of amenorrhoea of some weeks are followed by prolonged irregular bleeding, a symptom-complex which does not properly come under the heading 'menorrhagia'.

Menorrhagia in relation to the menopause and in the years preceding is the result of increasing failure of the ovarian functions and consequent upset in balance between the secretion of oestrogen and progesterone.

Polymenorrhoea is the name given to a form of irregular and excessive menstruation in which the cycle is shortened from the usual 28 days to 21 days or even less; this is due to disturbed balance of internal secretions, causing ovulation to occur too early in the cycle; in some cases two corpora lutea have been found at the same stage of development; in many cases fibroids are present.

The function of the thyroid gland can influence the menstrual loss. Menstruation is less or non-existent in cases of hyperthyroidism but menorrhagia occurs as the result of hypothyroidism.

2. Generative system

In considering this, some diseases will be easy to discover, others will require some special method of examination. For instance, of all the causes of pure menorrhagia, *fibromyoma* (fibroids) of the uterus stands out as the only important growth associated with this symptom, and a simple bimanual examination, as a rule, suffices to show that such a tumour exists. The chief characteristics of a fibromyoma of the uterus are these: the uterus itself is enlarged and in almost every instance the enlargement is asymmetrical, the typical shape of the organ being altered according to the number and size of the fibroids it contains; as there may be more than one tumour in the uterus, its shape may be exceedingly irregular; the consistence of the tumour is hard and unyielding as a rule, but pathological changes in these tumours are common, some of them leading to softening, others to cystic changes. The tumour and cervix always move together if the organ can be moved at all. The only difficulty in diagnosis, as a rule, lies in distinguishing a fibromyoma of the uterus from an ovarian cyst, and sometimes this is difficult, for it is not always possible to say that a given tumour is actually the enlarged uterus. It must be remembered, however, that the symptom under discussion is menorrhagia, and ovarian tumours almost never give rise to it. Ultrasound scanning is helpful in the diagnosis of fibroids because it is possible by the method to determine if a pelvic swelling is both uterine and solid. If, however, it appears that a swelling is extra-uterine and cystic a diagnosis of ovarian cyst will be made, but it still may be a fibroid which has undergone cystic degeneration and is attached to the uterus by a pedicle (subperitoneal fibroid). If doubt still exists a uterine sound passed into the uterus can be used to determine if the cavity is longer than the normal of 6 cm. Pregnancy must be excluded, of course, before a sound is passed into the uterus. Fibroids that are submucous or intramural enlarge the uterine cavity; ovarian cysts and subperitoneal fibroids do not. Adenomyoma of the uterus produces enlargement as a rule, but cannot be distinguished from fibromyoma until after removal.

Chronic salpingo-oophoritis (in the form of a pyosalpinx, a hydrosalpinx, a tubo-ovarian abscess or chronic interstitial salpingitis) and *ovarian endometriosis* both give rise to menorrhagia due to pelvic congestion, but dysmenorrhoea, pelvic pain, dyspareunia and backache are usually more prominent symptoms. In either case a firm tender swelling in the pouch of Douglas is felt on bimanual palpation. It is often not possible to differentiate between these two conditions until the pelvis is inspected at laparoscopy or even until a laparotomy is performed. Examination of the uterine curettings will reveal a tuberculous origin of the pelvic inflammation.

Retroversion and retroflexion of the uterus may be associated with menorrhagia but, in the absence of other causes, an endocrine imbalance is the reason for the excess menstrual loss, the abnormal position of the uterus merely being coincidental.

Intrauterine contraceptive device. There is almost always some increase of the menstrual blood loss with the use of these devices, and in some cases the loss amounts to menorrhagia.

Exanthemas. The various exanthems are likely to cause menorrhagia but the symptom only occurs during the acute phase of the disease, the periods becoming normal again with improvement in the general condition.

3. Circulatory and other systems

Any lesion of the heart, liver or lungs which leads to back pressure in the venous system may in theory cause hyperaemia of the pelvic organs and consequent excessive menstrual losses. However, it happens very occasionally that menorrhagia is caused by uncompensated valvular lesions of the heart, cirrhosis of the liver or emphysema of the lungs.

Anaemia. The quality of the blood itself may be a cause of menorrhagia if it is deficient in calcium salts or other factors, leading to retardation of the coagulation-time. Modern methods of estimating coagulation-time enable us to distinguish these cases with some certainty, and thus point out a line of treatment. Often, however, there is an underlying cause, such as an endocrine imbalance, which is responsible for both the menorrhagia and the anaemia. Removal of the cause then cures the anaemia.

Thrombocytopenia. Severe menorrhagia may complicate this condition. As soon as it is cured the period loss becomes normal.

4. The nervous system

The nervous system alone is never a cause of menorrhagia. Emotional upsets such as are liable to occur at the time of the menopause may be connected with an endocrine cause of menorrhagia but usually are coincidental.

N. Patel

Metrorrhagia (irregular uterine bleeding)

Metrorrhagia means loss of blood from the uterus between the menstrual periods, and the term should be applied strictly only to irregular haemorrhages during menstrual life. It may be used for losses of actual blood or for blood-stained discharges in which mucus is mixed with blood. There has been a tendency of late to refer only to MENORRHAGIA (q.v.) and to *metrorrhagia*, including all types of irregular vaginal bleeding, whether they occur during menstrual life, before puberty, after the menopause, or during pregnancy. For the purposes of discussion irregular vaginal

Table M.2. Causes of irregular bleeding during menstrual life

1. Generative system	2. Endocrine

Malignant growths:
  Carcinoma of cervix
  Carcinoma of body of uterus
  Sarcoma
  Chorionic carcinoma
  Carcinoma of Fallopian tube
  Carcinoma of the ovary
	Dysfunctional uterine bleeding
	Metropathia haemorrhagica
	Irregular shedding of the endometrium
	Oestrogen withdrawal bleeding
	Break-through bleeding from contraceptive pill
	Granulosa-cell tumour

Benign growths:
  Submucous fibroid
  Fibroid polyp
  Mucous polyp
  Endometrial polyp	

Inflammatory lesions:
  Erosion of cervix
  Endometriosis
  Tuberculosis of uterus	

bleeding will be considered here under three headings: (*A*) Irregular bleeding during menstrual life; (*B*) Irregular bleeding before puberty and after the menopause; (*C*) Irregular bleeding during pregnancy.

A. Irregular bleeding during menstrual life

Causes of irregular bleeding are given in *Table* M.2.

1. Lesions of the uterus and cervix

Those lesions that give rise to metrorrhagia are well defined as a rule, as in the case of carcinoma of the cervix uteri, when the cervix is replaced by a mass of friable growth which bleeds readily on being probed or touched with the finger. A growth of the body of the uterus is more difficult to diagnose and in all instances microscopical examination of material removed by curettage is required; in fact, with the exception of obvious mucous polyps, fibroid polyps and advanced growths of the cervix, all the growths of the uterus require a preliminary histological examination for their exact diagnosis.

The curetted material must be obtained after cervical dilatation, with a sharp curette, and the larger the fragments removed the more easy will be the histologist's work. Anaesthesia is frequently given, except in the case of cervical growths. A Danish suction machine (the Vabra) or similar device can be used safely on patients in the outpatient department for diagnostic purposes. The curettings obtained are quite satisfactory for histology. In doubtful cervical growths following colposcopic examination, a rectangular shaped biopsy should be cut out, including some normal tissue if possible. If malignant cells have been seen in a vaginal or cervical smear and the cervix looks grossly normal, intraepithelial diseases of the cervix will be suspected. Several small biopsies of the cervix may be taken from areas which appear abnormal under the colposcope.

Carcinoma of the body of the uterus, carcinoma of the cervical canal, early carcinoma of the cervix, sarcoma of the uterus, chorionic carcinoma, some sloughing fibroids and tuberculous endometritis can be distinguished from one another only by investigations carried out on these lines. The fact that all these lesions produce metrorrhagia and may give rise to haemorrhage on coitus, walking, straining at stool, or bimanual manipulation of the uterus, makes it imperative that there should be histological confirmation of the nature of the lesion before making an exact diagnosis.

Fibromyoma usually causes menorrhagia. Fibroids only produce irregular bleeding when they are submucous and in process of extrusion, when they are infected and sloughing, or when they are actually polypoid. The reason for this is that in these conditions the tumours are always partly strangulated by uterine contractions, and therefore in a state of gross venous congestion; hence they bleed more or less constantly, without provocation. The occurrence of irregular bleeding in a person who is known to have fibroids almost always means one of these conditions, and, commonly, extrusion of the tumour from the uterus. On the other hand, it must not be overlooked that carcinoma may develop in the endometrium with a fibroid also present, or that a fibroid may become sarcomatous, or that a sarcoma may arise *de novo* in the uterus and invade a pre-existing fibroid. Rapid enlargement of a uterus, with irregular haemorrhage, is also very suspicious of a sarcoma, but as it is not uncommon for several fibroids to be present in the same uterus, it is also common for rapid enlargement to occur as a result of cystic changes in one of them, whilst haemorrhage may take place due to extrusion of another.

A *carcinoma of the body of the uterus* rarely produces much enlargement of the organ, and any increase in size is not very rapid. Normally the postmenopausal uterus shrinks considerably in size; thus a uterus of a size which would be regarded as normal in a younger woman indicates abnormal enlargement in a women past the menopause.

Chorionic carcinoma, fortunately a very rare condition, follows hydatidiform mole in about 5 per cent of the recorded cases, and it always follows pregnancy, never having been seen in the uterus where pregnancy could be excluded, although the pregnancy may have occurred some years before. It is associated with profuse bleeding and the rapid development of a foetid discharge due to decomposition of blood and necrosing tissues *in utero*. Carcinoma of the body of the uterus rarely produces foul discharges until the condition is advanced. Secondary deposits of chorionic carcinoma appear as small plum-coloured ulcerating nodules in the vagina and secondaries in the lungs cause haemoptysis. The patient rapidly becomes ill with pyrexia and profound anaemia. A raised level of chorionic gonadotrophin is found in the urine. The diagnosis depends upon the finding of masses of trophoblastic cells in uterine curettings without any evidence of villous formation.

Clear-celled adenocarcinoma of the vagina occurs in teenage girls following high doses of stilboestrol taken by their mothers during pregnancy. The practice, though rare in Great Britain, was common in Boston, USA, some years ago, and the vaginal growths are appearing there now. They tend to occur in areas of vaginal adenosis.

The differential diagnosis of bleeding due to *carcinoma*, erosion and *tuberculosis of the cervix* is often difficult in the early stages. Erosions of the cervix do not as a rule cause bleeding; if there has been irregular bleeding or the cervix bleeds during examination malignancy should be suspected. In advanced cancer the friable hardness of the growth distinguishes it at once from the tough leathery hardness present in erosions. In the former, the growth can be broken down with the finger; in the latter, the soft velvety erosion can be scraped off the tough leathery and fibrous cervix beneath. Whenever there is doubt, colposcopy should be carried out. Tuberculosis of the cervix is usually mistaken for carcinoma, but the difference is clear enough in microscope sections. On occasions sectional biopsy of the cervix reveals a 'carcinoma in situ' or pre-invasive carcinoma. In this condition the epithelial cells throughout the whole depth of the cervical mucosa have the typical appearance of cancer cells but no invasion of the deeper tissues of the cervix has taken place. This condition has been known to become a true cancer, although many years may elapse before this takes place. Only a small proportion of the cases of carcinoma in situ of the cervix becomes invasive cancer even if left untreated. The small possibility of true cancer supervening, however, makes treatment desirable in most cases. They are usually found in the first place by routine cervical smears (*Fig.* M.1).

Mucous polyps and *fibroid polyps* are common causes of intermenstrual bleeding, and are usually quite definitive growths. The mucous polyp is soft, strawberry-red in colour, pedunculated, and contains cystic spaces filled with glairy mucus. It rarely gives rise to a malignant growth. The fibroid polyp is hard, and shows the glistening whorled appearance so well known in fibromyomas on section. These growths are liable to infection and sloughing, and are then apt to be mistaken for carcinoma or sarcoma. The microscope alone will enable the difference to be made out.

2. DYSFUNCTIONAL UTERINE BLEEDING

Although modern techniques of ovarian steroid estimation in serum allow serial measurements to be made of hormone levels throughout the menstrual cycle, no clear pattern has emerged to explain the mechanism underlying dysfunctional uterine bleeding, except, perhaps, in the case of metropathia haemorrhagica (*see below*).

Dysfunctional bleeding may occur at any age between puberty and the menopause, but 50 per cent occur between the ages of 40 and 50, about 10 per cent at puberty, and the remainder between these ages. Then bleeding is more commonly menorrhagia, although the interval between the bleedings may be shortened. Particularly is this the case in this type of bleeding occurring at the time of puberty and the menopause. The bleeding may be profuse or only slightly in excess of normal. In other cases intermenstrual bleeding occurs, continuing for days or weeks. It is usually preceded by amenorrhoea for some weeks. In a large proportion of these cases ovulation fails to occur. Schröder was able to demonstrate the absence of corpora lutea and the persistence of unruptured follicles in the ovary. This state of excess oestrogen secretion affecting the endometrium leads to marked endometrial hyperplasia (Schröder's disease or metropathia haemorrhagica (*see* p. 259). In other

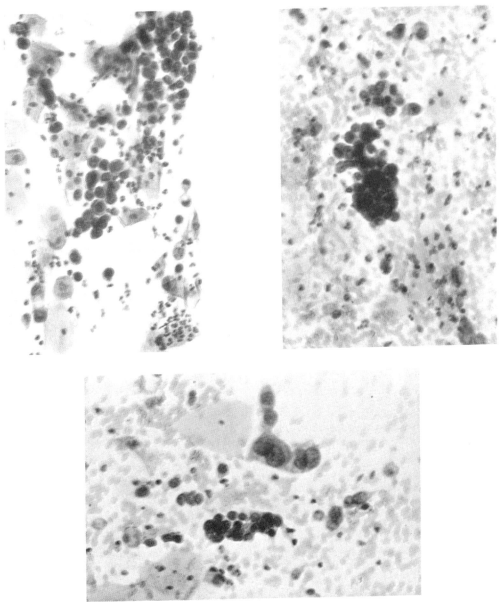

Fig. M.1. Abnormal cervical smear from carcinoma in situ. (Dr J. Vale.)

cases, however, there is no endometrial hyperplasia present; indeed, the endometrium may be atrophic; again in others the endometrium may be in the secretory phase so that we know ovulation has taken place. In such cases a quantitative imbalance of the sex hormones is assumed, although the cause may lie in the uterine musculature or its autonomic nerve supply. It may be that the close relationship between the pituitary and ovarian functions is disturbed, leading to a temporarily excessive drop in the oestrogen level in the blood because of the inhibition of excessive action of the pituitary gonadotrophins. In other cases it is thought that the endometrium is unable to respond to the stimulation of the ovarian or pituitary hormone in a normal manner (those cases with atrophic endometrium). In other cases irregular shedding of the endometrium takes place leading to prolongation of the desquamative phase of the menstrual cycle. In these cases menstruation is very prolonged, and a late curetting in the bleeding phase reveals islands of secretory endometrium, when normal regenerated endometrium should be found.

There are no gross abnormal physical signs to be found on pelvic examination in cases of dysfunctional bleeding. The diagnosis largely depends on the history and when in doubt curettage. Amenorrhoea followed by prolonged irregular bleeding may be caused by pregnancy and abortion (threatened or incomplete), or by the menopause followed by carcinoma of the body of the uterus. When pregnancy is unlikely, curettage may be indicated to make the diagnosis.

Oestrogen withdrawal bleeding. Women commonly take oestrogen preparations to control menopausal symptoms or to prevent conception. Irregular uterine bleeding may occur while the drugs are being taken or following their withdrawal. In cases where there is doubt curettage should be carried out.

Bleeding associated with ovulation. It is not uncommon for women to bleed very slightly about midway between the periods at the time of ovulation. When this is accompanied by lower abdominal pain (*Mittelschmerz*) the diagnosis is easy.

Bleeding due to granulosa-cell tumour of the ovary. When irregular bleeding occurs in the presence of an ovarian swelling the possibility of a granulosa-cell tumour arises. Removal of the tumour and histology reveal its nature. The presence of an intrauterine lesion and a non-secreting ovarian tumour must not be overlooked.

B. Irregular bleeding before puberty and after the menopause

The causes of irregular bleeding before puberty and after the menopause are given in *Table M.3*. The bleeding which occurs from the vagina occasionally in newborn infants is usually due to a high concentration of oestrogen in the fetal circulation. It is usually trivial, but a fatal case has been reported. Bleeding later in childhood may be due to sexual precocity when secondary sexual characteristics will be in evidence; or

due to a new growth such as an embryonal rhabdomyosarcoma (sarcoma botryoides). Vaginoscopy under anaesthesia (and biopsy if a lesion is found) is essential.

After the menopause the differentiation of *malignant growths*, *polyps* and *senile endometritis* can only be established by uterine curettage. Carcinoma of the body of the uterus (endometrial adenocarcinoma) is the commonest malignant growth after the menopause. In any doubtful case routine dilatation and curettage of the uterus must never be omitted. Senile (atrophic) vaginitis must not be overlooked as a possible cause; the vaginal walls at the fornices become inflamed and form granulation tissue which may bleed if the surfaces rub together; the surfaces may be partly adherent, and the separation brought about by the examining finger may cause bleeding. Pyometra, or distension of the uterus with pus, may cause haemorrhage, with a foul discharge; although it is almost always due to malignant growth, it may be only the result of infection. The only growth of the ovary which produces uterine haemorrhage is the granulosa-cell tumour. This may occur at almost any age. (*See* Pelvis, Swelling in.)

C. Irregular bleeding during pregnancy

In relation to a recent pregnancy, haemorrhage may result from simple subinvolution, from retained products of conception, or from chorionic carcinoma. The differentiation of these conditions can be established only by exploration of the uterine cavity, with, if necessary, the assistance of the microscope. Such conditions may be termed 'secondary postpartum haemorrhage' in cases occurring within a few days of delivery.

Haemorrhage from the pregnant uterus almost always means separation of the placenta or of the embryo from its attachments, but malignant growth of

Table M.3. Causes of irregular bleeding

Before puberty and after menopause	During pregnancy
Uterine bleeding in the newborn	Threatened, inevitable or incomplete abortion
Malignant growth of the uterus	Carneous mole
Polyps	Hydatidiform mole
Senile endometritis	Antepartum haemorrhage
Senile atrophic vaginitis	Secondary postpartum haemorrhage
Pyometra	Subinvolution
Granulosa-cell tumour of ovary	Chorionic carcinoma
Oestrogen withdrawal bleeding	Extrauterine gestation
	Malignant growth of cervix or vagina
	Erosion
	Polyps

the cervix, erosions and polyps may have to be considered. Haemorrhage from a pregnant uterus is never due to malignant growth of the body of the organ, because pregnancy is impossible with this lesion. There are, however, two great difficulties in connection with pregnancy haemorrhages; these are to differentiate: (1) the uterine haemorrhage which occurs along with *extrauterine gestation* from that due to *threatened abortion*; and (2) the bleeding of *placenta praevia* from that due to the *separation of a normally situated placenta*.

In the first case, arising very early in pregnancy, generally when only one menstrual period has been missed, or is overdue, the external haemorrhage occurs when the extra-uterine gestation is separated from its tubal or other attachments and is converted into a tubal mole, when it becomes extruded from the fimbriated extremity of the tube, or when the tube ruptures, events which cause acute pain in the lower part of the abdomen, faintness, and possibly collapse from internal haemorrhage. Along with these the uterus will be found not obviously enlarged, whilst there is some sort of swelling in one or the other posterior quarter of the pelvis. Even if no actual swelling can be defined, bimanual palpation will elicit very marked tenderness, which may be excruciating, due to the presence of blood clot in the peritoneal cavity. In the case of ectopic gestation the abdominal pain is severe. It is often referred to the shoulder. It is much more severe than that experienced in an intrauterine abortion and it almost always precedes the onset of vaginal bleeding; on the other hand the vaginal blood loss in an inevitable abortion is much more than that in ectopic gestation, which is usually scanty. Haemorrhage due to threatened abortion cannot be diagnosed unless the presence of an intra-uterine pregnancy can be established; therefore we must look for the definite signs of a normal pregnancy, which in the early months will be: amenorrhoea, morning sickness, breast swelling, darkening of the nipple, dark secondary areola around the nipple, enlargement of the uterus, Hegar's sign, and blue discoloration of the cervix and vaginal walls. Hegar's sign consists in extreme softening of the upper part of the cervix and lower part of the uterine body associated with the as yet unsoftened vaginal portion and globular tense fundus; it is found from the 6th to the 8th week. Ultrasound scanning is very useful because the pregnancy sac can be visualized in the uterus and the size of the embryo measured to make sure of the duration of the pregnancy. The presence of a live fetus can be demonstrated by the beating of the heart with the aid of real-time ultrasound and means that the outlook for continuation of the pregnancy is good. Absence of a pregnancy sac in the uterus with a

mass outside of the uterus (sometimes seen to contain a pregnancy sac) make the diagnosis of ectopic pregnancy a certainty. In the case of a positive pregnancy test using methods employing detection of low level of BHCG and a negative ultrasound scan for intrauterine pregnancy, laparoscopy would be advisable to exclude the diagnosis. The diagnosis of inevitable abortion depends upon finding some part of the uterine contents presenting through the dilating cervix. Incomplete abortion is diagnosed by the continuation of bleeding or seeing that not all the products of conception have been passed. Retained products are then confirmed on ultrasound scanning.

If repeated small haemorrhages occur into the chorio-decidual space in early pregnancy a carneous mole results. Unless it is removed by suction or by curettage it may be retained in the uterus for weeks or even months before it is expelled spontaneously (missed abortion). While it remains in the uterus there is a brown or blood-stained vaginal discharge with bleeding intermittently and the uterus ceases to enlarge. On examination the uterus is found to be smaller than it should be for the estimated duration of pregnancy. A pregnancy test may be negative but it is not always so.

A hydatidiform mole should be suspected when rapid increase in size of the uterus occurs during the early months of pregnancy, associated with uterine bleeding. Most cases have a uterus which is larger than would be expected for the dates, but in one-third it is smaller. Sometimes vesicles are passed and the diagnosis is clear. If not, the finding of a high level of chorionic gonadotrophin in the blood or urine and the characteristic 'snow-storm' appearance on ultrasound scanning makes the diagnosis certain. In a normal pregnancy up to 100 000 IU of chorionic gonadotrophin (HCG) are passed in the urine daily. Five times this amount is passed in the presence of a hydatidiform mole. If bleeding continues after evacuation of a hydatidiform mole chorionic carcinoma should be suspected. Chorionic gonadotrophin continues to be produced by the remaining chorionic tissue and high titres are found in blood and urine. Uterine curettage may reveal the malignant tissue unless it is buried deep in the myometrium, in the pelvis or at a remote site such as the lungs. In fact all patients who have a hydatidiform mole removed should be followed up for 2 years with regular urine tests for the beta subunit of HCG, in case of post-molar trophoblastic disease (chorionic carcinoma) develops.

Bleeding due to *placenta praevia* generally does not occur until 30 weeks of pregnancy. Antepartum haemorrhage is likely to be due to placenta praevia if the fetal presenting part is high above the pelvic brim or there is a malpresentation such as a breech or a transverse lie. If the fetal head is engaged in the pelvis antepartum haemorrhage cannot be due to placenta praevia and must therefore be due to accidental haemorrhage, provided that incidental causes such as carcinoma or polyp on the cervix can be excluded. The diagnosis of antepartum haemorrhage has been made much easier with the aid of ultrasound scanning because the placental echo can be seen clearly and the relation of the edge of the placenta to the internal os can be accurately determined. It is not uncommon for a low-lying placenta found in the mid-trimester to be seen on serial scanning to move wholly into the upper uterine segment as term approaches.

N. Patel

Micturition, frequency of

Many urological diseases may present as frequency of micturition. The symptom does not necessarily imply an organic abnormality, but how frequent is 'frequent'? If the normal bladder contains some 300–500 ml, and the amount of urine produced during the day is of the order of 1500 ml, the 'normal' person should pass urine between three and five times daily. As the patient will pass urine less frequently if fluid intake is reduced and insensible loss increased, so will the patient pass urine more frequently if the fluid intake is increased and insensible loss reduced. Frequency is a symptom which we have all experienced during periods of stress, classically before examinations or interviews, but this reflex nervous polyuria may be exaggerated in hysterics. Frequency is also modified by the rate at which the bladder fills, which relates not only to the quantity of fluid drunk but its quality; while water itself is diuretic, the addition of caffeine or theophylline in tea or coffee, or alcohol, will stimulate the urine output. The consequent rapid filling of the bladder will provoke the stretch reflex to a degree that is far less easily controllable than during slow filling and stretching.

Increased frequency may also relate to general medical conditions, in particular diabetes mellitus, diabetes insipidus and chronic nephritis.

Assuming that there is no systemic disorder, continuing frequency relates to: (1) a small bladder capacity; (2) inflammation of the bladder; (3) reduced bladder emptying.

Reduced bladder capacity

Bladder capacity can be reduced by a large intraluminal object such as a large stone or large tumour. These conditions lead simply to a small amount of available effective capacity, the same mechanism that exists in outflow tract obstruction when bladder emptying is incomplete. True reduction in bladder capacity occurs when there is fibrosis of the bladder wall, which may be secondary to the chronic sepsis associated with long-term catheter drainage, tuberculous cystitis or infiltration of the bladder wall with an advanced tumour.

Small bladders may be acquired by habit, where 'habit frequency' is more common in women, especially the older age group, who make use of every opportunity to empty their bladders lest they should run into difficulty with incontinence. After some years of practising this habit the bladder is no longer capable of distention and frequency becomes the rule by day and night.

Bladder contraction also occurs after radiotherapy and as this treatment modality has become more effective in achieving cure in many conditions, such as testicular tumours, some ovarian carcinomas and localized prostatic carcinoma, postradiation fibrosis in the increasing number of survivors becomes a reality, although perhaps a small price to pay for cure of the primary condition.

Inflammation of the bladder

Primary inflammatory conditions of the bladder will give rise to frequency by day and night as will inflammatory processes involving the bladder secondarily, as in pelvic inflammatory disease. Acute appendicitis may also influence bladder behaviour in the short term while carcinoma in adjacent structures, such as the uterus, rectum and colon, may occasionally present as frequency. Diverticulitis of the sigmoid colon can of course increase frequency from the secondary inflammatory changes but it is surprising how infrequently this symptom arises, considering how frequently colovesical fistulae develop in apparently unheralded fashion.

Reduced bladder emptying

Outflow tract obstruction in males and females also gives rise to increased frequency by day and night. Nocturia may be the presenting feature of outflow tract obstruction in the male related to prostatic hypertrophy, bladder neck stenosis and detrusor sphincter dyssenergia. It should be borne in mind that this symptom is least affected and corrected by surgical removal of the obstruction.

The presence of a stone in the lower third of the ureter may precipitate reflex frequency of micturition while impaction of the calculus at the uretero-vesical junction may precipitate the most intense frequency, associated with pain in the glans penis or labia and the passage of but a few drops of urine at a time. When a stone is lodged within the bladder, frequency may be a feature by day as the patient moves around and the stone irritates the trigone. This symptom is often relieved at night as the stone rolls back into the bladder proper, an area far less sensitive to stimulation from the sharp points of the calculus.

Lynn Edwards

Micturition, hesitancy

The classical presenting features of outflow tract obstruction are frequency, nocturia, reduction in the flow rate and hesitancy. In hesitancy, the patient feels the desire to pass urine, presents himself in an appropriate place and yet finds that seconds, or even minutes, elapse before the flow starts. Sometimes it is necessary for the male patient to sit down before the stream is initiated.

A distinction must be made between hesitancy and difficulty of micturition. Hesitancy implies a definite time lag between the intended start of micturition and the appearance of the urine at the urethral meatus. In difficulty, the flow is reduced and can often be augmented by abdominal straining. Abdominal straining during the waiting period of hesitancy can often prolong the waiting time.

Difficulty of micturition is caused by: (1) poor bladder contractility and (2) obstruction to outflow.

Poor bladder contractility

Reduced contractility is relatively common in diseases of the nervous system, particularly spinal cord lesions producing a lower motor neurone lesion, such as transverse myelitis, tabes, multiple sclerosis, tumour of the spinal meninges or cord, syringomyelia and secondary deposits in the vertebrae. The level of the lesion is critical and it must involve the cord at the level of the sacral reflex arc. If the lesion is higher than this, the characteristics are of an upper motor neurone lesion, which are frequency, urgency and incontinence secondary to reflex micturition.

Systemic disturbances are also responsible for difficult emptying, for example when there is a peripheral autonomic neuropathy as in diabetes mellitus. Such a neuropathy can often exist in the absence of physical signs of a peripheral diabetic neuropathy. Small vessel disease within the pelvis may reduce the vascular supply to the sacral reflex arc. A lower motor neurone type of lesion is found following prolonged periods of chronic retention when proper detrusor tone is never regained following the surgical relief of the outflow obstruction. A prolonged period of cath-

eter drainage under these circumstances can sometimes cause sufficient restoration of muscle tone to allow normal emptying to occur.

Difficulty of micturition is often seen in herpes zoster lesions affecting the sacral reflex. The same applies to herpes genitalis, a condition which is transmitted by intercourse and which is becoming relatively common in younger women.

Outflow obstruction

Hesitancy and difficulty in women may be secondary to pelvic tumours which push the bladder out of the pelvis and therefore stretch the urethra. It occurs with uterine fibroids or with a retroverted pregnancy. Direct involvement of the urethra by vaginal carcinoma or by a primary urethral carcinoma is rare. Stricture of the urethra in women is far more common than might be suspected and is dealt with fully under (URINE, RETENTION OF). Urethral strictures rarely give rise to true hesitancy in that urine can be felt entering the posterior urethra early enough but the urine then trickles though the stricture zone. A feeling of presence in the urethra proximal to the stricture is often felt. The same symptom is experienced when a stone is impacted along the urethra, or when a well organized blood clot has entered the urethra from a bladder lesion. When there is a urethral obstruction, straining often increases the strength of the stream.

Prostatic enlargement secondary to inflammatory changes can also give rise to hesitancy but pain will also be a feature in these conditions.

Hesitancy and difficulty are rarely observed in children as primary complaints but both may be observed when there is a meatal stenosis or a tight phimosis. In the latter ballooning of the foreskin occurs during micturition.

Lynn Edwards

Mouth, pigmentation of

The oral mucous membrane contains melanocytes in the basal layer, as a result of neuroectodermal migration in the fetus, which are similar to those present in the skin. Therefore, any condition which causes abnormal pigmentation in the skin can produce similar changes in the oral cavity, although the effects are usually not as marked. The following are important causes of oral pigmentation.

Melanotic naevae

These occur less often than in the skin, with the hard palate and the buccal mucosa being the most commonly involved site. As in the skin, they represent a collection of the normal melanocytes but instead of being evenly distributed in the basal layer, the cells are aggregated together. Depending on their position in relation to the basement membrane, they give rise to junctional naevae, compound naevae, intramucosal naevae and blue naevae. The lesions are generally small, well circumscribed, macular or slightly raised. The majority are pigmented with varying shades of brown, blue or black. The lesions are twice as common in females as in males and tend to occur in middle age.

Malignant melanoma

This is a rare tumour of the oral mucous membrane with a slight male predominance, again occurring in middle age (*Fig.* M.2). They are mostly found in the upper jaw, especially the palate, followed by the gingival mucosa. It is more common in the Japanese, Indian and African races and one-third are preceded by a history of oral pigmentation. As in the skin, any oral pigmented lesion which increases in size or changes its surface characteristics or colour and starts to bleed, should be suspected as being a malignant melanoma. Growth of the lesion is followed by destruction of the underlying bone and loosening of the teeth, with rapid spread to the regional lymph nodes. If malignant change is suspected then a wide excision of the lesion should be carried out. Rarely the mouth may be involved with secondary deposits from a cutaneous melanoma.

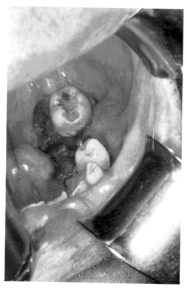

Fig. M.2. Malignant melanoma of the floor of the mouth.

Melanotic neuroectodermal tumour of infancy

This pigmented lesion is invariably noted within the first 6 months of life, the majority of which occur in the anterior maxilla. The tumour grows rapidly in size with underlying bone destruction, and displacement of the developing teeth. The correct diagnosis is essential as the tumour is benign and responds well to simple enucleation.

Peutz–Jegher's syndrome

This inherited condition is characterized by intestinal polyposis involving the small bowel and melanotic spots of the face and mouth, with occasionally the hands and feet also being affected. Although it is an inherited condition, a family history will not always be found. There are multiple freckles on the face, especially around the mouth (circum-oral pigmentation) (*Fig.* M.3), the eyes and the nose. The polyps in the intestine rarely become malignant as they are hamartomas in origin. Not infrequently a polp acts as the head of an intussusception, so that the patient presents with acute intestinal obstruction.

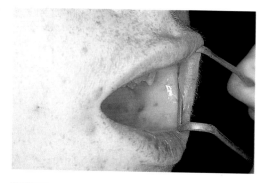

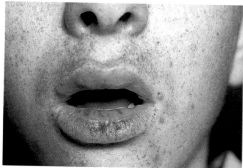

Fig. M.3. Pigmentation of the mouth.

Addison's disease

This condition is caused by bilateral destruction of the suprarenal glands, the most common cause previously being infection with tuberculosis. Today it is usually caused by auto-immune destruction or an opportunist infection in immuno-deficient patients and more recently, this has been demonstrated in patients suffering from AIDS. The skin becomes pigmented early on in the disease, especially the exposed areas, while the oral cavity shows patchy melanotic pigmentation, which varies in colour from light brown to black. If this disease is suspected then the diagnosis will be verified by measuring the blood pressure which is low, blood urea which is raised and serum sorium which is lowered, and performing the Synacthen test (measurement of plasma cortisol in response to injection of synthetic ACTH).

Racial

This is the most common cause of oral pigmentation which is most prevalent in the black and Indian races (*Fig.* M.4). However, 5% of Caucasian people also show pigmentation of the oral mucosa. The pigment is evenly distributed in the palate, buccal and gingival mucosa. The colour of the pigment is not necessarily related to the colour of the skin.

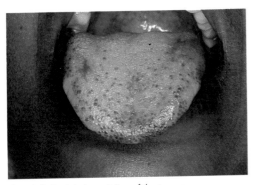

Fig. M.4. Racial pigmentation of the tongue.

Amalgam tattoo

This is a common cause of oral pigmentation and arises by small amounts of amalgam filling material gaining access to the mucosa via a small abrasion during restorative dental procedures or tooth extraction. This produces small regular or irregular areas of pigmentation in the mucosa which rarely require treatment.

Lichen planus

The inflammatory process in this condition may cause some degeneration of the basal layer of the mucous membrane and the pigment released is ingested by macrophages, causing diffuse pigmentation.

Chemicals/Drugs

The metals lead, bismuth and mercury following industrial exposure or their previous use as therapeutic agents can cause blue, brown or black lines characteristically adjacent to the gingival margin. It is felt that these metals formed sulphides following reactions with the dental plaque and were deposited in the gingival mucosa. The drugs in current use which have been reported as causing oral pigmentation are the phenothiazines, antimalarials and the oral contraceptive.

Black hairy tongue

This curious phenomena of unknown origin is characterized by overgrowth of the filiform papillae of the tongue which become stained due to proliferation of chromogenic microorganisms. Heavy smoking and the persistent use of antiseptic mouthwashes have been implicated, but in the majority of cases the cause is unknown (*Fig.* M.5).

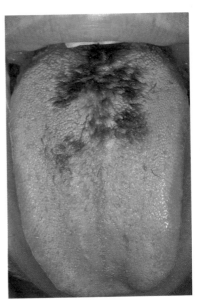

Fig. M.5. Black hairy tongue.

Oral pigmentation has also been found in thyrotoxicosis, malabsorbtion, cachectic states, disorders of iron metabolism and neurofibromatosis.

P.T. Blenkinsopp

Mouth, ulcers in

Mouth ulcers may be classified as follows:

1 TRAUMATIC
2 APHTHOUS

3   ULCERATION ASSOCIATED WITH OTHER MUCOUS MEMBRANES
  (Behçet's syndrome, Reiter's disease)
4   ULCERATION ASSOCIATED WITH SKIN DISEASE
  Lichen planus
  Mucous membrane pemphygoid
  Pemphigus
  Bullous erythema multiforme
5   BLOOD DYSCRASIAS
  Agranulocytosis
  Leukaemia
6   ULCERATION ASSOCIATED WITH GASTROINTESTINAL DISEASES
  Coeliac disease
  Ulcerative colitis
  Crohn's disease
7   ULCERATION ASSOCIATED WITH CONNECTIVE TISSUE DISORDERS
  Lupus erythematosis
8   INFECTION
  a. (Bacterial)
  Acute ulcerative gingivitis
  Syphilis
  Tuberculosis
  b. (Fungal)
  Candida
  c. (Viral)
  Herpes simplex
  Herpes zoster
  Epstein–Barr herpes (infectious mononucleosis)
  Coxsackie (herpangia, hand, foot and mouth disease)
9   TUMOURS
  Squamous-cell carcinoma
  Malignant melanoma

1. Traumatic

The diagnosis is usually easy to make because there is a definite history of trauma associated with mastication, ill-fitting dentures or other minor injury to the oral cavity. The ulcers are usually shallow and painful and heal quickly once the noxious stimulant is removed. (*Fig.* M.6). Secondary bacterial infection can occasionally occur, causing an abscess or cellulitis.

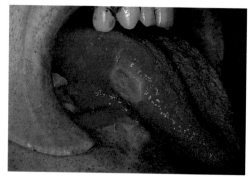

Fig. M.6. Traumatic ulcer of the tongue caused by irritation from a carious tooth.

2. Aphthous ulceration

This is the commonest form of oral ulceration and three types are recognized, depending on the size

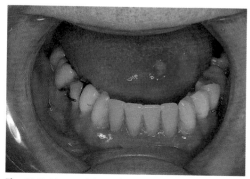

Fig. M.7. Minor aphthous ulcer of the tongue.

and number of ulcers. The term **minor aphthous ulcer** is given to ulcers less than 5 mm in diameter which occur intermittently as single ulcers or in crops (*Fig.* M.7). The ulcers take from 1 week to 10 days to heal, and in some patients new ulcers may develop before the original ones have healed so that they are never without ulceration. This type of ulceration tends to commence in childhood and early life and the attacks diminish as the patient becomes older. They are characteristically found on the buccal mucosa, in the sulcus between the jaws and the cheeks, the ventral aspect of the tongue and the floor of the mouth. This condition is often described as recurrent aphthous stomatitis (RAS). The ulcers are round and have an erythematous periphery with a pale central crater.

Major aphthous ulcers are larger and more persistent and, in addition to the previous sites, may affect the tongue and the palate. They may be up to a centimetre in size and, because of their duration, give concern that the ulcer could be neoplastic.

Herpetiform ulcers are the third variant and here the patient suffers from crops of very numerous small ulcers, which are painful and tend to coalesce into one large irregular area on an erythematous background. Anything from 10 to 100 ulcers may be present at one time.

The cause of aphthous ulceration is unknown, although an auto-immune theory has been advanced. Ten per cent of patients will have an underlying haematological deficiency, especially of vitamin B_{12}, folate or iron; 3 per cent will be suffering from coeliac disease and a few may have Crohn's disease. In some female patients the ulcers are related to the menstrual cycle and will respond to hormone therapy. There is also an association with stress and the cessation of smoking. Aphthous ulceration is thought to be a feature of AIDS, but in the majority cases the cause remains unknown.

3. Ulceration associated with other mucous membranes

BEHÇET'S SYNDROME

This syndrome consists of recurrent aphthous ulceration with also genital and ocular involvement in the form of anterior uveitis. The latter may subsequently cause impairment of vision. The disease characteristically affects young men and there may be associated disease of the skin, joints and nervous system. The cause is unknown, but viral or auto-immune theories have been put forward.

REITER'S SYNDROME

The oral manifestations of this complaint are white circinate lines on an area of erythematous mucosa. These lesions are accompanied by urethritis, arthritis and conjunctivitis. The aetiology is again unknown, but may follow infection with mycoplasma or Shigella.

4. Mouth ulceration associated with skin disease

LICHEN PLANUS

Lichen planus is a common condition affecting both the skin and the mouth, although it can affect either in isolation. There are several types of oral lichen planus, with the erosive type being characterized by large, irregular areas of mucosal ulceration; the base of the ulcer is often slightly raised with a covering of white to yellow slough (*Fig.* M.8).

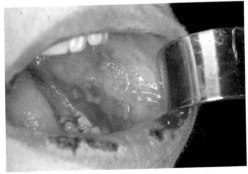

Fig. M.8. Erosive lichen planus affecting the cheek.

Examination of the mouth elsewhere often demonstrates white lacey striations or a desquamative gingivitis. The aetiology of lichen planus is obscure, but it may be mediated by an immunological process, liver disease, drugs (e.g. methyldopa) or in the graft-versus-host reaction (marrow transplantation).

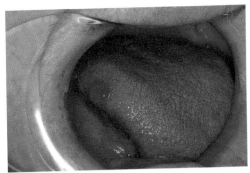

Fig. M.9. Bulla formation on the tongue in a patient with mucous membrane pemphigoid.

PEMPHIGUS AND PEMPHIGOID

Pemphigus and pemphigoid both may produce oral lesions which commence as bullae when the epithelium separates from the basal layer in pemphigus, and when the epithelium and basal layers separate from the underlying mesoderm in pemphigoid. As a result, the bullae in pemphigus are far more fragile and rupture quickly whereas the bullae in pemphigoid are more resiliant (*Fig.* M.9).

In pemphigus there are circulating auto-antibodies against the intercellular attachments of the squamous epithelium but in pemphigoid circulating auto-antibodies are not detectable. They can, however, be found in the basement membrane zone using immunofluorescent techniques.

Pemphigus is a serious mucocutaneous condition, mostly affecting woman in the 40- to 50-year age group, which unless treated may be fatal. The mouth may often be affected first with small bullae or widespread ulceration and loss of the oral epithelium. The diagnosis is made by biopsy of an intact bulla and treatment is by the use of systemic steroids with replacement of fluid and protein in the acute phase.

Benign mucous membrane pemphigoid is a disease of the elderly, which affects the oral mucous membrane and the conjunctiva of the eyes. Anogenital lesions may also occur and minor involvement of the skin may be noted. Because the bullae are more rigid, they tend not to enlarge and rupture late. Once ruptured they leave areas of irregular ulceration, which is accompanied by considerable scarring. The oesophagus and nasopharynx may also be involved, but the most significant aspect of the disease is conjunctival fibrosis leading to visual disturbance.

Examination of the mouth will demonstrate several intact or ruptured bullae during the active phase of the disease and the gingivae may be severely affected with a desquamative gingivitis. Treatment is with topical steroids, although occasionally systematic steroids may be necessary.

BULLOUS ERYTHEMA MULTIFORME

Bullous erythema multiforme or Stevens–Johnson syndrome is the more severe form of erythema multiforme, invariably involving the oral cavity and can be the predominant feature of the attack. The appearance is dramatic because of the severe oral ulceration and the blood-stained and crusted lips. It tends to affect children and young adults and is probably immunologically mediated, via exposure to micoorganisms, e.g. herpes simplex and mycoplasma, or from drugs, typically the sulphonamides, non-steroidal anti-inflammatory agents, phenytoin and penicillin.

Examination of the skin will demonstrate either extensive erythema, or a macular rash with target lesions exhibiting central bullae formation or ulceration. There is a conjunctivitis, leading to corneal ulceration. In the mouth diffuse inflammation leads to vesicle formation followed by widespread erosions and haemorrhage. Epistaxis commonly occurs. Treatment of the minor case is with topical steroids, but the more severe attack may require systemic therapy. Tetracycline antibiotics should be given if infection with mycoplasma is suspected.

5. Blood dyscrasias

Blood dyscrasias have been discussed under Gums, Bleeding, but ulceration of the gingivae is also common, caused by acute local bacterial infection secondary to the abnormal white cell function.

However, it should be remembered that the ulceration may be due to acute ulcerative gingivitis or acute herpetic gingivostomatitis which has arisen *because* of a blood dyscrasia.

6. Ulceration associated with gastrointestinal diseases

Whilst coeliac disease, ulcerative colitis and Crohn's disease can be associated with recurrent aphthous

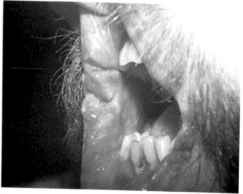

Fig. M.10. Oral mucous membrane showing typical 'cobblestone' appearance in a patient with Crohn's disease.

ulceration, these conditions may also show distinctive oral signs. Crohn's disease characteristically produces a 'cobble stone' thickening of the buccal mucosa with hyperplastic folds and fissuring (*Fig.* M.10). Painful ulcers, which are slow to heal, may also be present. Inflammatory bowel disease may also produce the condition of pyostomatitis vegetans, which is characterized by soft hyperplastic mucosal folds between which fissures and ulcers may form.

7. Ulceration associated with connective tissue disorders

Approximately 20 per cent of patients with discoid and systemic lupus erythematosis will show oral ulceration. There may be areas of erythema with erosions and, in some areas, these may resemble lichen planus due to minor striae formation. Frank ulceration may also be present.

The differential diagnosis may be difficult to make but here the lesions often occur on the hard palate, which is rare in lichen planus. The diagnosis is made by biopsy and immunofluorescent studies. Antinuclear antibodies should be looked for in the serum and a history of arthritis and skin rashes should be elicited, particularly an erythematous rash of the face in the butterfly distribution.

8. Infection

BACTERIAL

Acute ulcerative gingivitis
Bacterial infection of the oral mucous membrane is rare in normal circumstances, the most important example being acute ulcerative gingivitis, which is associated with large numbers of Vincent's organisms (*Treponema vincentii* and *Fusiformis fusiformis*).

There is haemorrhage, inflammation and the formation of painful, shallow ulcers at the crest of the gingival margin. This eventually leads to destruction and flattening of the interdental papillae. Infection is associated with pre-existing periodontal disease and also any condition reducing host immunity. Patients with leukaemia, AIDS, or those receiving chemotherapy are, therefore, all susceptible and infection may follow an episode of acute herpetic stomatitis.

Acute ulcerative gingivitis in the severely debilitated patient may progress to the destructive condition of *cancrum oris*. This is rare in the developed world, apart from those patients who are immunosuppressed but, still occurs in the Third World as a result of malnutrition and severe viral infections, e.g. herpes and measles. Small areas of gangrene appear in the lips, cheeks or other oral structures, which rapidly progress to larger areas of slough and extensive loss of facial tissue (*Fig.* M.11).

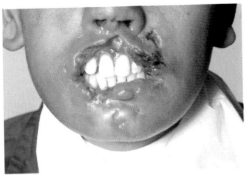

Fig. M.11. Cancrum oris in a patient with acute leukaemia.

Syphilis

The oral cavity may be involved rarely, during the primary stage, to produce a chancre on the lips or the tip of the tongue. Secondary lesions known as the mucous patch are now seldom seen, because of modern effective treatment. Here there is an erosion in the mucous membrane of a few centimetres with a yellowish slough surrounded by erythema. When these areas coalesce they give an irregular shaped ulcer known as the 'snail track' ulcer.

The tertiary stage of syphilis, now rarely seen, produces the gumma, which is a deeply punched-out ulcer caused by central necrosis. These may typically affect the tongue or the palate and in the latter, perforation will produce a central oronasal fistula.

Tuberculosis

With the successful treatment of tuberculosis, oral lesions are rare but, when they do occur, are usually found in the tongue and lips. The ulcer typically shows undermined edges and a granulating floor. The mode of infection is thought to be expectoration of tubercle bacilli from a primary focus in the lungs, which then become implanted in the oral cavity.

B. FUNGAL

Candida (Thrush)

This infection is caused by the yeast-like fungus, *candida albicans*, which invades the epithelium, causing erythema of the epithelium and a yellow soft plaque, that can be easily removed. This leaves an area of haemorrhagic mucosa or ulceration.

C. VIRAL

The majority of acute infections of the oral mucosa are viral in origin. They tend to effect the younger age groups and are normally associated with constitutional symptoms of fever, malaise and enlarged and tender cervical lymph nodes.

Herpes simplex

The primary infection invariably involves the mouth with many small vesicles, approximately 2 mm in diameter, which are regular in shape and size. The mouth is generally inflamed and in areas the ulcers coalesce to produce irregular raw erosions and a yellow slough (*Fig.* M.12).

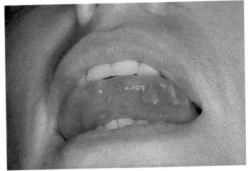

Fig. M.12. Primary herpes infection of the oral cavity.

The gingival mucosa is red and swollen and may bleed even in the absence of ulceration. Herpetic stomatitis may be an opportunist infection and can be severe in immunocompromised patients and patients with AIDS. The lesion of reactivation is known as secondary herpes. The virus which has been quiescent in the trigeminal ganglion becomes active once more, to produce a cold sore or herpes labialis in the distribution of the infected nerve.

Herpes zoster

Herpes zoster causes chicken pox in the patient who has not been exposed to the virus and mouth ulcers are common in this condition. The virus again remains quiescent in the trigeminal ganglion and on reactivation causes painful ulceration within the exact anatomical distribution of the nerve (*Fig.* M.13).

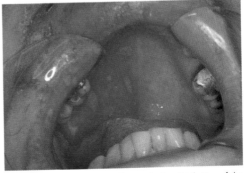

Fig. M.13. Herpes zoster infection in the distribution of the maxillary branch of the trigeminal nerve.

This condition is known as herpes zoster or shingles and on occasions can be an indication of a more serious underlying disease. Again the picture is of erythema, small regular ulcers and pain within the distribution of the nerve affected. If the ophthalmic branch is involved then care needs to be given to the cornea. The infection may be complicated by post-herpetic neuralgia.

Epstein–Barr virus

Infectious mononucleosis (glandular fever) is caused by the Epstein–Barr virus. There may be characteristic petechiae of the soft palate and pharynx, which are often considered diagnostic.

The patient has a sore throat, the lymph nodes are enlarged and occasionally there is extensive ulceration of the faucies. Ampicillin should not be given for the sore throat as this exacerbates the condition.

Coxsackie

Mouth ulcers arise from infection with the coxsackie virus which causes a febrile illness, lymphadenopathy and ulcers in the region of the soft palate. The ECHO virus causes hand, foot and mouth disease which is a highly infectious condition characterized by small vesicles, leading to ulcers on the hands, the feet and in the mouth. Both these latter infections are trivial conditions and are self-limiting.

9. Tumours

Squamous-cell carcinoma is the most common malignant tumour of the oral cavity and is associated with excessive smoking and alcohol consumption. It is a common tumour in the Indian sub-continent, where it occurs in betel nut chewers and smokers of bidis (native cigarettes).

The clinical picture of oral carcinoma is very varied but in the advanced case is obvious. There is a friable mass arising in the mucous membrane with a rough, irregular surface, which bleeds easily. There is usually deep, irregular central ulceration with an infected slough at its base (*Fig. M.14*). Radiographs may show associated bone erosion.

The early lesion may be more difficult to diagnose, showing only an area of erythema or hyperkeratosis, slight roughening of the mucosa and shallow ulceration.

Unfortunately many oral carcinomas are still diagnosed late and therefore, any ulcer which does not heal within 3 weeks, or does not obviously fall into one of the other categories should be submitted to a biopsy.

Other tumours of the oral cavity, both benign and malignant, including malignant melanoma (*see Fig. M.2*), can undergo ulceration due to trauma or

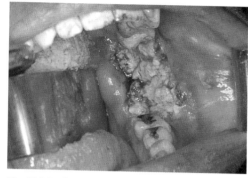

Fig. M.14. Ulcer in the left retro-molar region arising in an extensive squamous-cell carcinoma.

ischaemic necrosis; these are described under Jaw, Swelling of.

P. T. Blenkinsopp

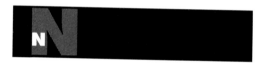

Nasal deformity

Nasal deformity can be congenital, acquired or developmental. The skeleton of the nose consists of bone in the upper third and cartilage in the lower two thirds. The septal cartilage should articulate with the columellar cartilages which form the division between the nostrils.

Congenital abnormalities of the nose are rare. Arhinia (absence of the nose) is almost unknown and a bifid nose is rarely seen (*Fig. N.1*). The more usual type of congenital nasal abnormality is the bony cartilaginous hump. Many regard this as a sign of distinction but others dislike it and want it corrected by cosmetic

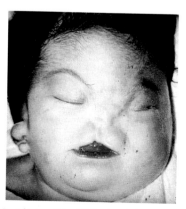

Fig. N.1. Arhinia—This child had multiple craniofacial and other abnormalities and has since died.

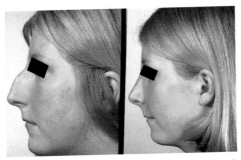

Fig. N.2. Bony cartilaginous hump. Congenital bony cartilaginous hump (a). Corrected by rhinoplasty (b).

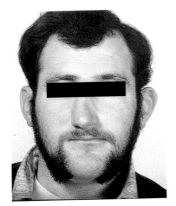

Fig. N.3. Fractured nasal bones.

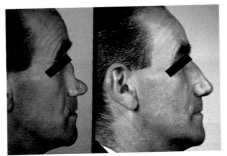

Fig. N.4. Saddle nose—The cause of this was a submucous resection operation for a septal haematoma (a). Corrected by the insertion of a bone graft (b).

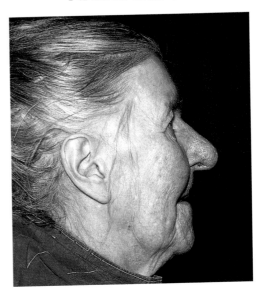

Fig. N.5. Rhinophyma.

by a severe blow, a commoner clinical situation is for a green-stick fracture to occur in childhood. During growth spurts, the nose then apparently grows squint. The patient may either present with a squint nose or nasal obstruction due to internal derangement of the septal cartilage.

Severe trauma to the nose, or a septal excision operation carried out with excessive zeal, can cause a saddle nose (*Fig.* N.4). This does not usually cause nasal obstruction and is corrected by inserting a bone graft into the nasal dorsum. A saddle nose can also be caused by congenital syphilis, but this is almost unknown now. The most usual cause of a saddle nose in conjunction with a systemic illness is polychrondritis or a nasal granuloma such as Wegener's granulomatosis.

The skin of the nasal tip is normally thicker than the skin of the nasal dorsum due to an increased volume of sebaceous tissue. A relatively common development abnormality of this part of the nose is for the sebaceous tissue to hypertrophy with age, producing an ugly deformity of the tip of the nose known as rhinophyma (*Fig.* N.5).

A. G. D. Maran

Nasal discharge

The causes of nasal discharge are listed in *Table* N.1.

CONGENITAL

Choanal atresia by blocking the posterior choana prevents the normal nasal mucus stream from reaching the pharynx, so that anterior nasal discharge is the

rhinoplasty (*Fig.* N.2). The commonest acquired nasal deformity is the fractured nose. Severe trauma fractures the nasal bones and this presents as an obvious deformity, accompanied by epistaxis and bruising of the eyes (*Fig.* N.3). It is easily seen on X-ray, although X-rays are unreliable in the primary diagnosis of a fractured nasal bone because of the multiple vascular markings in normal nasal bones.

The nose is the most prominent part of the face in the Caucasian and is frequently struck during falls in childhood. While the septal cartilage can be fractured

Table N.1. Conditions causing nasal discharge

Congenital
Choanal atresia

Infective
Acute rhinitis
Sinusitis
Enlarged adenoids (pharyngeal tonsil)
Caseous rhinitis
Atrophic rhinitis
Fungus infections
Chronic infective granulomas
  Syphilis
  Tuberculosis
  Leprosy
Rhinoscleroma

Trauma
Foreign body
Rhinolith
Inhaled irritant gases or vapours
Fractured anterior fossa
Excessive cold

Hypersensitivity
Vasomotor rhinitis
Perennial nasal allergy
Seasonal nasal allergy (pollinosis)
Nasal polyps

Neoplastic
Carcinoma
  Nasal fossa
  Nasopharynx
  Sinus
Malignant granuloma
Wegener's granuloma

Old age
Senile rhinorrhoea

result. Infections ensure that the discharge is muco-purulent at times.

INFECTIVE.

The common cold and the prodromal stages of the infectious fevers give rise to clear mucoid discharge. When and if secondary bacterial infection follows the discharge becomes increasingly purulent. Purulent discharge, either unilateral or bilateral, occurs in sinusitis, the origin of the discharge indicating the sinus or sinuses involved. The maxillary sinuses open into the middle meatus, so pus is seen there and on the floor of the nose. Pus from the anterior ethmoids is also found in the middle meatus but that from the posterior ethmoids or sphenoid comes down the postnasal space. If the pus is especially foul smelling it has probably arisen in the maxillary antrum as a result of dental infection. Caseous sinusitis or rhinitis follows inspissation of pus and possibly fungus infection. The material is whitish, cheesy and foul smelling. Even more foul smelling are the crusts and dry discharge of atrophic rhinitis. In these patients the nasal fossae are unduly wide and the mucosa thin and devoid of mucus cells. The especially disgusting odour is called 'ozaena'.

Pathogenic fungi and yeasts cause nasal infection and discharge, mainly in tropical countries but, of course, nowadays occasionally in this country in immigrants and returning travellers.

To summarize the nasal symptoms of the main fungal diseases: *Rhinosporidiosis* predominantly affects the nasal mucosa where the characteristic lesion is a bleeding polyp containing the sporangium from which spores spread via the lymphatics. It chiefly affects the peoples of Sri Lanka or India. *Phycomycoses* cause serious disease often starting with granuloma-tous lesions in the nose and considerable mucoid discharge. This fungus occurs in tropical areas.

Aspergillus infection, sometimes contracted from captive birds, is characterized by a watery mouldy smelling discharge and a greyish membrane on the mucosa.

Actinomycosis, showing the typical 'sulphur gran-ules', rarely but sometimes affects the sinuses and nose. There is a woody mass and multiple sinuses from which the pus exudes.

Candida albicans occurs commonly in the mouth and occasionally in the nose in the young and those in a poor state of general health. The white patches can be removed without bleeding.

The pathology of fungus diseases is complex. Many start with nasal discharge and bleeding. Diagnosis is by identifying the fungus in scrapings or by biopsy.

Secondary syphilis affects the nose, causing a simple catarrhal rhinitis; the diagnosis is usually suggested by other lesions. *Tertiary syphilitic gum-mas* affect the nose very commonly with destruction of bone and cartilage; secondary infection causes offensive discharge and there is bleeding and often the later development of atrophic rhinitis.

Lupus vulgaris is probably the commonest tuber-culous infection of the nose. There is nasal discharge and the typical lesion, a reddish firm nodule, is found at the anterior end of the nasal septum which may later perforate.

Leprosy occurs in the nose as almost the earliest sign of the disease. Nodular thickening of the mucosa with inflammation and obstruction are associated with discharge. Later perforation of the septum and destruc-tion of tissue allows for secondary infection and very offensive discharge.

Rhinoscleroma is a progressive granuloma begin-ning in the nose in an atrophic form with ozaena. Nodules later form and there is considerable scarring. Diagnosis is by biopsy and by the identification of the Frisch bacillus and Russell bodies.

AIDS is associated with a watery nasal discharge which is frequently found concomitantly in the disease.

TRAUMA

A unilateral nasal discharge in an infant or child is pathognomonic of a foreign body, often a piece of foam rubber or paper inserted into the nasal fossa. Small hard objects may remain in the nose for some time before symptoms occur. A rhinolith may develop in these circumstances if calcium salts are deposited around the foreign body.

A clear watery discharge following a head injury must lead to thoughts of a fracture of the anterior fossa or cribriform plate with cerebrospinal fluid rhinorrhoea. Such a discharge will increase on leaning the head forward or on compression of the jugular veins. The presence of sugar in this fluid confirms that it is cerebrospinal fluid. This can be confirmed by isotope tests.

HYPERSENSITIVITY

Copious clear mucoid nasal discharge almost as freely flowing as water is present in nasal allergy and may be associated with violent attacks of sneezing, lacrimation and conjunctival injection. The diagnosis is confirmed by the history and by RAST and PRIST tests. Nasal allergy is liable to be confused with less non-specific vasomotor rhinitis, which is also very common. Numerous factors are present in the aetiology of this troublesome condition and these include changes of environmental temperature and humidity, mechanical irritation from dusts and vapours, psychological factors, pregnancy and drug reactions. The patient with vasomotor instability not infrequently carries a box of paper tissues. The diagnosis is made after excluding nasal allergy.

NEOPLASTIC

Malignant nasal disease may cause nasal discharge, sometimes relatively clear to start with but later almost always offensive and thick. The presence of blood must always raise the question of malignancy. The growth may be in the nasal fossa, sinus or in the nasopharynx. Nasal discharge stained with blood occurs and when one of the sinus ostia becomes blocked infection follows. If an undue amount of blood is found in a sinus undergoing lavage when there has been no undue trauma the sinus must be carefully investigated for a growth. Diagnosis is by a CT scan and biopsy.

Malignant or non-healing granuloma, sometimes called 'midline granuloma', is a slowly progressing ulceration of the face starting in the region of the nose. The chronic inflammatory reaction naturally produces discharge. They may represent a special form of malignant lymphoma and must be differentiated from Wegener's granuloma by their clinical and histological characteristics.

Wegener's granuloma affects kidneys, lungs and respiratory tract including the nose. The lesions are giant-celled granulomas and there is never the gross destruction seen in malignant granuloma.

OLD AGE

Senile rhinorrhoea, due probably to the failure of the vasomotor control of the mucosa, is common and sometimes distressing in the elderly. There are no physical signs apart from the nasal drip.

Although nasal discharge may be of various different characters, the cause can usually be arrived at by the history and simple clinical examination. Three clinical situations, however, require special management.

A unilateral, blood-stained discharge might be the prodromal bleed of an epistaxis but the possibility of a tumour or granuloma of the nose or sinuses must be ruled out by nasal endoscopy and flexible endoscopy of the nasopharynx.

A clear nasal discharge after trauma is cerebrospinal fluid rhinorrhoea until proved otherwise. Although assessment of sugar content of the discharge with a clinistix is a useful indicator, a definitive diagnosis cannot be made without assessment by CT scan and injection of fluorescein or radioactive albumin to the CSF with subsequent measurement in the nose.

A. G. D. Maran

Nasal obstruction

All the conditions mentioned in the section on nasal discharge are likely to cause nasal obstruction owing to the associated inflammation and oedema of the mucous membrane. There are, however, some disorders which simply cause a blockage of one or both nasal passages and are less commonly associated with discharge.

These can be listed (*see below*) and should be read in conjunction with the list of the causes of nasal discharge.

CONGENITAL
Choanal atresia
  Bilateral
  Unilateral
Deviated nasal septum
INFLAMMATORY
Adenoids (pharyngeal tonsils)
Trauma
Haematoma of septum
Deviated nasal septum

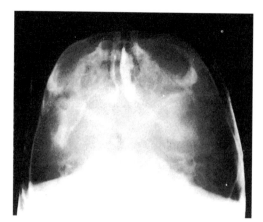

Fig. N.6. Bilateral choanal atresia. Radiograph of infant's skull with radio-opaque fluid outlining the nasal fossae. The fluid is held up by the membranous obstruction to the posterior choanae.

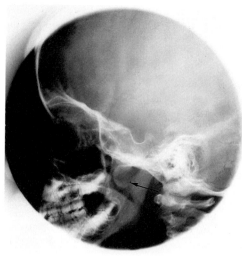

Fig. N.7. Enlarged adenoids in a child, indicated by the arrow (*Mr Roger Parker.*)

HYPERSENSITIVITY
Vasomotor rhinitis
Atopic rhinitis
Rhinitis medicamentosa
NEOPLASTIC
Benign tumours
   Papilloma
   Fibroma
   Osteoma
   Fibroangioma of puberty
   Teratoma
   Nasal polyps
Malignant tumours
   Nasopharyngeal carcinoma
   Squamous carcinoma of the nose and sinuses
   Adenocarcinoma of the nose and sinuses
   Malignant melanoma of the nose and sinuses
   Transitional cell carcinoma of the nose and sinuses

Choanal atresia (*Fig.* N.6), when bilateral, causes complete nasal obstruction at birth and must be relieved at once if the infant is to live. Unilateral choanal atresia is sometimes not discovered until later. Soft rubber or plastic catheters are often employed to assess the patency of the nasal fossae. Malleable silver probes bent into a smooth curve with a radius of about 5 cm are preferable and can be passed painlessly along the floor of the nose. They do not kink and curl up like the thin soft catheters and by palpation it is possible to say if the blockage is fibrous or bony in nature.

Many deviated nasal septa originate at the time of birth when the infant's skull is compressed as it passes through the birth canal. The components of the bony septum are forced out of alignment and, during the development of the nose and upper jaw until about 18 years of age, the septum gradually deviates. The angles of maximum deviation are along the cartilage/vomer and ethmoid/vomer junctions and at the lower border of the vomer where it meets the maxillary and palatine crests.

This deviation can be seen with a nasal endoscope. It will often be found that the inferior turbinate in the concavity of the deviation will have hypertrophied, thus increasing the obstruction. It is important to remember that the spur of the deflected septum may obscure other pathology behind.

Adenoid enlargement is probably the commonest cause of nasal obstruction in childhood. These lymphoid masses, (the pharyngeal tonsils), usually regress at about 8–10 years of age but may cause nearly complete obstruction in the young. It is sometimes possible to see them with a postnasal mirror in co-operative children. If there is doubt as to the size of adenoids a soft-tissue lateral radiograph is helpful (*Fig.* N.7).

Trauma frequently causes nasal obstruction without discharge. Immediate mucosal swelling and depressed nasal bones after a blow may cause very considerable blockage. A haematoma of the septum is characteristic as there is a swelling, soft to gentle palpation, on each side. This may resolve spontaneously but the pressure may cause cartilage necrosis and later a collapsed septum or infection may supervene with a septal abscess and an increased likelihood of cartilage necrosis. Though not dissimilar in appearance the abscess is more tense and the nose is very tender. Both must be evacuated. The deviated nasal septum following trauma is more likely to show a corrugated appearance as the component parts of the septal skeleton may overlap and the fibrosis after fracture may lead to considerable anatomical abnormality and difficulty in corrective surgery.

Vasomotor rhinitis has been mentioned in the section dealing with nasal discharge, but it commonly occurs without discharge, causing nasal obstruction. Not infrequently patients notice that at one time one nasal passage is more obstructed and within hours the problem is worse on the other side. This alternating obstruction is merely an exaggeration of the normal nasal cycle which passes unnoticed in those with clear noses but becomes obvious in the partially obstructed. On examination, the inferior turbinates may be enormous and in chronic cases show a 'mulberry' appearance.

Rhinitis medicamentosa may be the cause of very acute nasal obstruction. The nasal mucosa is very red, swollen and the turbinates rather firm to palpation. The condition is caused by rebound vasodilatation following the too-frequent use of constrictor drops which have to be used more and more often to obtain relief. There is often some psychological instability in these patients.

Atopic rhinitis is seasonal if associated with a grass allergy (hay fever) or episodic if associated with other contact allergens (cats, dogs, etc.). The release of histamine and other related substances from the degranulated mast cells cause mucosal oedema, vasodilatation and hypersecretion. The patient will always be aware of the cause and conversely, if he is not, the diagnosis is probably not atopic rhinitis; it is more likely to be vasomotor rhinitis.

Benign nasal tumours are not common but cause nasal obstruction and can nearly always be seen on nasal examination in the outpatients. Papillomas may arise on Little's area at the anterior end of the nasal septum. They are typically wart-like in appearance and bleed easily. Fibromas and osteomas are rare. The bleeding nasal fibroma, almost confined to adolescent boys, is a fibroangioma and usually arises from the roof of the nasopharynx. Torrential haemorrhage may occur if the surface is breached. Benign teratomas of the nasopharynx occur. The simplest is the 'hairy nasal polyp' which is usually a pedunculated dermoid. It can be seen hanging below the level of the soft palate or in the postnasal space. Other dermoids and teratomas are more complex and usually associated with extensive deformities of the head.

Nasal polyps are very common and are of unknown aetiology. They are not due to atopy as was formerly thought. They are known to be associated with aspirin sensitivity and over 50 per cent of patients have associated asthma. They are probably the result of an abnormality of arachidonic acid metabolism with either an excess of leukotrienes or a deficiency of prostaglandins. They must be removed surgically and their recurrence rate is significantly lowered by the continual use of steroid nose drops.

Malignant tumours of the nose, as opposed to the sinuses, are rare. Tumours nearly always begin in the ethmoid or maxillary sinuses and it is only when the tumour exists from the sinus 'box' that the patient gets symptoms which may be related to the eye, the cheek, the palate and alveoli or the nasal cavity, depending on where the tumour comes out of the box.

A. G. D. Maran

Nasal regurgitation

Regurgitation of food through the nose may be only a temporary accident, the result of an unsuccessful attempt to stave off a sneeze, a cough or a burst of laughter when the mouth is full of food or fluid; or it may result from an explosive return of gas from the stomach or oesophagus, particularly after drinking gassy fluids. Pathological regurgitation of food through the nose results from three main groups of causes:

PERFORATIONS OF THE PALATE

Congenital
  Cleft palate
  Congenital short soft palate
Trauma
  Oro-antral fistula after dental extraction
  Palatal fenestration following surgery for malignancy of maxillary antrum
  Gunshot wounds
Inflammatory
  Destruction or perforation of palate due to syphilis, tuberculosis or leprosy
Malignant disease

FIXATION OF THE PALATE

Post-infection scarring
Post-traumatic scarring

PARALYSIS OF THE PALATE

Post-diphtheritic paralysis
Damage to the nucleus of the 10th nerve
  Postero-inferior cerebellar artery thrombosis
  Tumours of the medulla
  Bulbar palsy
  Poliomyelitis
  Landry's ascending paralysis
Posterior fossa lesions
  Tumours
  Syphilitic meningitis
  Glomus jugulare tumour
  Hydrocephalus
Extracranial lesions
  Malignant disease
  Post-tonsillectomy weakness

Examination of the roof of the mouth and the soft palate should be sufficient to determine the causes of regurgitation in the first group. Congenital short soft palate may be suspected but is less easy to assess without cine-radiography to demonstrate palatal competence. An oral-antral fistula (usually postsurgical) is revealed by direct inspection. In these cases usually only a small amount of food or, more usually, liquid comes through the nose.

Fixation of the palate may occur from the scarring of syphilis, lupus or leprosy (now all uncommon in the Western world), scarring after extensive palate surgery in severe cleft-palate cases and, rarely, palatal scarring after badly performed tonsillectomy. These fix the palate so that it cannot be drawn up to close the nasopharynx.

In the majority of the third group, where palatal paralysis is present due to vagal innervation involvement, other symptoms and signs will be present with 10th nerve paralyses of the larynx and paralysis of the 5th nerve and other nerves depending on the extent of the lesion. Diphtheritic paralysis may involve the soft palate alone and usually recovers in time.

Malignant disease of the nasopharynx is characteristically silent and insidious — palatal palsy (sometimes part of 'Trotter's triad' of deafness, trigeminal pain and palatal palsy) may be an early sign and is due to local infiltration rather than to involvement of the nerve-trunks.

Paralysis of the palate, when bilateral, may be difficult to notice at rest but it remains immobile on phonation and is even more obvious if the patient is made to gag. In addition the patient is unable to blow up a balloon. When the paralysis is unilateral the normal side is drawn up like a curtain and the uvula is displaced to the normal side.

Harold Ellis

Nausea

Nausea is the unpleasant sensation experienced by patients who are usually about to vomit. The causes of nausea are therefore very similar to that of vomiting and are listed on p. 412. Nausea is characterized by an unpleasant, 'sick' feeling with a revulsion for food and abdominal fullness. The patient feels that he is about to vomit but does not actually do so. Other sensations or phenomena which accompany nausea are a desire to swallow, a certain amount of sweating, hypersalivation and lightheadedness.

When the patient is nauseated there is an associated decrease in gastric tone and an inhibition of gastric peristalsis with increased duodenal tone. Nausea may result from unpleasant or frightening emotional experiences, from a variety of psychological causes, from stimuli arising from intra-abdominal viscera or a variety of visual, oral, olfactory or tactile sensations which are unpleasant, and from stimulation of the labyrinths.

Although nausea is intimately bound with the act of vomiting, there are certain circumstances when nausea is more prominent than the vomiting. This occurs, for example, with certain *drugs* such as salicylates, digoxin, non-steroidal anti-inflammatory agents, opiates, oral contraceptive pill, some antibiotics and many of the cancer chemotherapeutic agents. Nausea may be a prominent feature of *motion sickness*. Early morning nausea is a feature of *pregnancy, anxiety states* and *alcoholism*. Nausea may have *psychogenic* origins and this is seen, for example, in people who are averse to certain foods and feel nauseated on sitting at table, the nausea which occurs in certain stressful situations many of them of a domestic or social reason. Patients with *migraine* may suffer intense nausea and not necessarily vomit. Intense nausea is one of the earliest features of *viral hepatitis* and precedes other features of the disease such as abdominal pain and the development of icterus. Patients in severe *right-sided heart failure* with hepatic congestion will also complain of nausea.

Ian A. D. Bouchier

Neck, stiff

The important causes of stiff neck may be classified as follows:

Congenital

Congenital torticollis or wryneck
Congenital deformities, e.g. Klippel–Feil

Acquired

ACUTE

Exposure to cold
Positional
Intracerebral and subarachnoid haemorrhage
Cerebral tumour

Infective

Reflex spasm due to adenitis from otitis media, tonsillitis, etc.
Abscess in the neck

Traumatic

Fractures of cervical spine
Dislocations of cervical spine

Subluxations of cervical spine
Strains of cervical spine
Injuries to muscles and soft tissues

Degenerative

Acute painful episode in cervical spondylosis

Malignant

Multiple myeloma
Primary or metastatic neoplasm

Acute systemic infections

Meningitis
Typhus
Brain abscess
Poliomyelitis
Psittacosis
Arbovirus infections (e.g. sandfly fever)
Leptospirosis
Tetanus, etc.

Hysteria

CHRONIC

degenerative

Cervical spondylosis

Arthritic

Chronic juvenile arthritis (Still's disease)
Rheumatoid arthritis
Ankylosing spondylitis
Other spondylarthropathies

Infective

Tuberculous disease of the spine

Post-traumatic

Untreated acute traumatic lesions
Contractures following burns, nerve injuries, etc.

Congenital

With the exception of congenital lesions, contractures and possibly some late cases of untreated injury and a few cases of arthritis, all these conditions are usually painful at some stage.

Congenital torticollis or wry neck is due to a contraction of the sternocleidomastoid muscle on one side, generally considered to be the result of an injury during labour, possibly ischaemic in nature. The muscle stands out as a tight band in the neck, and its contraction leads to a characteristic deformity. The head is pulled down towards the affected side, and the face and chin are tilted towards the opposite shoulder. (*see Fig.* S.39). The movements of the head are necessarily restricted owing to the shortening of the

muscle, and in long-standing cases this leads to a marked asymmetry of the face. The consequences are not limited to the head and neck, for the spine shares in the general obliquity, and shows marked lateral curvature in old cases.

In the Klippel–Feil syndrome there is a congenital fusion of one or more cervical vertebrae resulting in a short, thick stiff neck, the head set low on the shoulders. Other coexisting abnormalities are common: undescended scapulae (Sprengel's deformity), platybasia, etc.

Acquired

Exposure to cold or sleeping in a cramped position may give rise to a transient stiff neck associated with no other symptoms. There is generally a distinct history of the patient waking up in the morning with a stiff neck, and the diagnosis is made by exclusion.

A cold draught on the neck when driving in a car or from air-conditioning may result in an acutely painful stiff neck for a short time.

Cerebral or subarachnoid haemorrhage. Conscious patients who have had intracranial bleeding usually complain of headache and stiffness of the neck, and after subarachnoid haemorrhage the main physical sign is marked neck rigidity and pain on trying to move the head. A brain tumour may cause a stiff neck by causing meningeal irritation from bleeding into the subarachnoid space, by direct meningeal involvement or by causing cerebellar herniation through the foramen magnum.

Inflammation of the lymph nodes. Infection of the cervical nodes and the cellular tissues of the neck may cause local stiffness, whether the infecting focus be a boil or carbuncle, or a carious tooth, an inflamed tonsil, pediculosis capitis, or other similar cause. In a mild case the neck can be moved, but movement is painful and therefore it is held stiffly. With a more severe reaction reflex muscle spasm is present.

Injuries to the neck. These vary from soft-tissue injuries and strains to fractures and dislocations. Although some are rapidly fatal, subluxation may occur without cord involvement, the only symptoms being stiffness and pain. Readily missed cases and permanent disability may result if the condition is not diagnosed and treated. The deformity is rendered more obvious when the spine is X-rayed in the flexed position, and may be missed in extension.

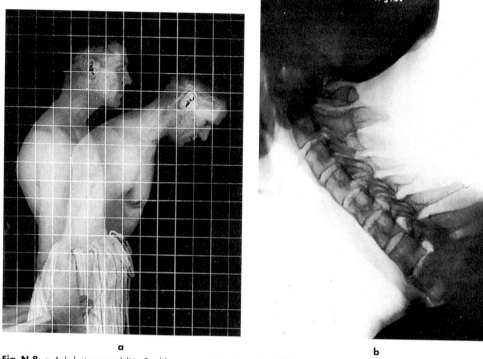

Fig. N.8. *a.* Ankylosing spondylitis. Double-exposure showing neck in full flexion and extension. *b.* Radiograph of same patient showing typical anterior ligamentous calcification.

New growth. A secondary deposit in one of the cervical vertebrae may cause progressive stiff neck, and generally much local pain on movement; the diagnosis may suggest itself when the patient is known to have had a primary neoplasm elsewhere, especially a carcinoma of the breast, lung, prostate, kidney or the thyroid gland; cases of primary new growth of the vertebrae (apart from multiple myeloma deposits), are fortunately rare.

Acute systemic infections. Many acute infections are accompanied by a stiff neck (meningism), particularly in children; pneumonia, once a common cause in childhood, is now much less so. Fever is almost always present. Meningitis from any cause, bacterial or viral, almost always causes some neck rigidity. Neck stiffness may be an early prodromal sign in paralytic or non-paralytic poliomyelitis and changes in the cerebrospinal fluid are found. Phlebotomus (sandfly) fever, an arbovirus infection, presents as fever, malaise, myalgia and sometimes headache, in some cases with findings of an aseptic meningitis. Stiffness of the neck may be an early sign of tetanus, but other signs, such as trismus (inability to open the mouth due to tonic contraction of the jaw muscles) rapidly appear.

In hysteria. A theatrical and over-dramatic symptom of neck stiffness is accompanied by other features of hysteria but not by any objective physical signs of organic disease.

Chronic

Degenerative. The commonest cause of stiffness of the neck is degenerative disease of bone, joint and cartilage, i.e. cervical spondylosis. This is a common disorder of the group of patients over 60 years of age. Pains are commonly referred from the painful stiff neck into the occiput and out towards the shoulders.

As few radiographs of the neck are normal in this age-group care should be taken in relating radiological findings to symptoms.

Arthritis. Stiffness of the neck is less common in rheumatoid arthritis of adult life than in chronic juvenile arthritis (Still's disease). It is more common, however, in cases of ankylosing spondylitis, where the neck and head may be held in a completely fixed position (*Figs* N.8, N.9). A similar picture may more rarely be seen in the spondylarthritic varieties of psoriatic arthropathy, Reiter's disease and the arthrop-

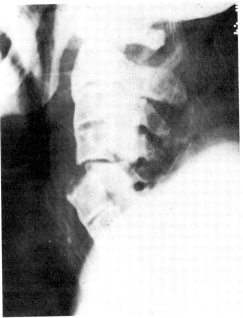

Fig. N.9. A broken neck in ankylosing spondylitis. Such rigid necks are more prone to such traumatic lesions than are normal supple ones. (*Courtesy of the Gordon Photographic Museum, Guy's Hospital.*)

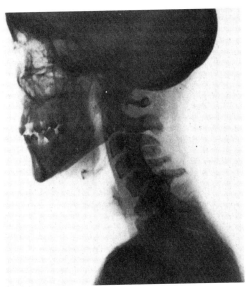

Fig. N.11. Cervical tuberculosis showing collapse of bodies of 6th and 7th cervical vertebrae. (*Dr T. H. Hills.*)

athy associated with ulcerative colitis and Crohn's disease.

Atlanto-axial subluxation in rheumatoid arthritis is not uncommon in advanced cases and leads to stiffness of the neck and a characteristic posture (*Fig. N.10*). Such subluxation occurs, but less often, in ankylosing spondylitis.

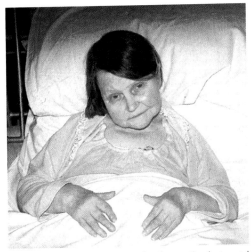

Fig. N.10. Advanced rheumatoid arthritis with atlanto-axial subluxation.

Cervical caries (*Fig.* N.11). The greatest care must be taken not to overlook tuberculous disease of the cervical vertebrae as a cause of reflex muscular rigidity of the neck. Pain and rigidity are among the earliest signs; the pain is increased by the least movement, and the child—for it is generally a child that is affected—takes the greatest precaution to avoid any movement, even holding the head between the two hands. The position of the head varies; it is most often held very stiff and straight, the natural backward curve of the neck being lost. In the late stages there may be an angular or lateral curve.

Post-traumatic. A neck may remain stiff from previous injuries. The diagnosis will be given by the history, but nervous overtones may cause persistence of symptoms, particularly in medico-legal cases where compensation is involved.

Harold Ellis

Neck, swelling of

See also THYROID ENLARGEMENT

Anatomy

The neck on either side is divided into anterior and posterior triangles by the sternocleidomastoid muscle arising from the sternum, sternoclavicular junction and medial third of the clavicle below and being inserted into the mastoid process of the temporal bone above.

At the upper end of the anterior triangle the digastric muscle defines the lower borders of a subsidiary space known as the 'digastric triangle', and at the lower end of the posterior triangle the posterior belly of the omohyoid muscle defines the upper border of a subsidiary space known as the 'supraclavicular fossa'.

The sternocleidomastoid muscles are enclosed within the deep cervical fascia which splits to embrace them. If even a part of a mass in the neck overlaps either border of the sternocleidomastoid muscle then, by putting one or other of these muscles into contraction, the relation of the mass to the sternoclei-domastoid muscle and so to the deep fascia can readily be determined. This method is applicable to practically all masses in the neck except the majority of those situated in the midline. The right sternocleidomastoid muscle is put into contraction by rotating the head to the left while resistance is applied to the chin and vice versa; both sternocleidomastoids are made to contract when the forehead is pressed forwards against resistance.

Lumps in the neck arising from structures super-ficial to the deep cervical fascia are not specific to the neck. Thus, sebaceous cysts, lipomas, carbuncles and so on are common, particularly in or deep to the skin at the back of the neck. It is the masses deep to the deep cervical fascia which have particular relevance in

regard to the neck and it is the differential diagnosis of these that must be considered.

It is conventional to divide swellings in the neck into midline swellings and lateral swellings, but this is a little misleading as nearly all so-called 'midline swellings' deviate slightly to one side or the other. They can, however, be divided appropriately into masses arising from unpaired midline structures and masses arising from paired lateral structures.

1. Masses arising from unpaired midline structures

A.   THYROGLOSSAL CYST

The thyroid gland is developed from an epithelial-lined duct which grows downwards from the region of the foramen caecum of the tongue, passing close in front of and then behind the hyoid bone, and so towards the site of the adult isthmus from which the lateral lobes expand. A cyst may form in any part of this track by failure of obliteration of the duct, but the most common site is at the lower border of the hyoid bone, anterior to the thyrohyoid membrane. These cysts usually appear at about puberty and enlarge to a variable size slightly to one or other side of the midline. They are fluctuant, globular masses which, if super-

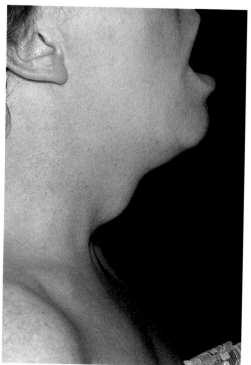
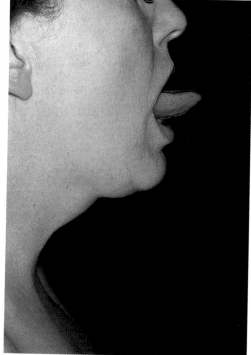

Fig. N.12. Thyroglossal cyst showing elevation on protruding the tongue.

ficial, may transilluminate. If the jaw is held open and the tongue steadily protruded, the swelling will rise in the neck, demonstrating its attachment to the hyoid bone (*Fig*. N.12). These cysts occasionally become infected and may rupture, leading to a fistula.

B.   SWELLINGS ARISING FROM THE ISTHMUS OF THE THYROID GLAND

All those pathological conditions described on page 373 and giving rise to swellings of the thyroid gland can arise in the isthmus. It should be repeated once more that practically all thyroid swellings move up and down on deglutition owing to their intimate relation to the larynx and upper part of the trachea, the movements of which they following during this act.

C.   PHARYNGEAL POUCH (*Fig*. N.13)

At the back of the inferior constrictor muscle of the pharynx there is a triangular area (Killian's dehiscence), between the upper border of the transversely running fibres of the cricopharyngeus below and the lower border of the obliquely running fibres of the thyropharyngeus above, where the wall is deficient in muscle. Through this defect, a pouch of mucosa, covered only by the fascia propria of the pharynx, may protrude. This pouch gradually enlarges, usually towards the left side of the neck, and tends to fill up when food or fluid is swallowed. At first this is just a nuisance and gives rise to an uncomfortable feeling on swallowing together with a rapidly developing swelling which may be emptied by pressing on the mass. Later, the mass becomes sufficiently large to press upon the oesophagus, against which it lies, to produce severe dysphagia with inanition.

Diagnosis is confirmed by a barium swallow which outlines the pouch and and which also demonstrates any constriction or deviation of the adjacent oesophagus (*Fig*. N.13).

Food is apt to stagnate within the pouch and this leads to diverticulitis which may spread giving rise to pharyngitis or oesophagitis, and so adding to the burden of dysphagia. This condition may appear at any age, but usually arises during the 3rd and 4th decades. Treatment, after attention to the nutritional needs of the patient, is by surgical excision.

D.   RARE CASES OF SWELLING ARISING IN MIDLINE STRUCTURES

i. Subhyoid bursa, a cystic swelling arising behind the hyoid bone and indistinguishable clinically from a thyroglossal cyst.

ii. Perichondritis of the thyroid cartilage.

iii. A carcinoma of the larynx, trachea or oesophagus penetrating the walls of these viscera and protruding to one or other side.

iv. The so-called 'Delphic lymph node', which lies in the midline on the thyrohyoid membrane, may enlarge in carcinoma of the thyroid gland and may be the first evidence of this disease.

v. Laryngocele (*Fig*. N.14).

2.   Masses arising from paired lateral structures

A.   LYMPH NODES

The commonest swellings in the neck are undoubtedly due to pathological processes arising in the cervical lymph nodes, usually secondary to some inflammatory or neoplastic process in one of the organs which they drain, but sometimes, as in the lymphomas, appearing to arise primarily within these nodes.

The distribution of the lymph nodes in the neck is variable, but the general disposition is as follows. In

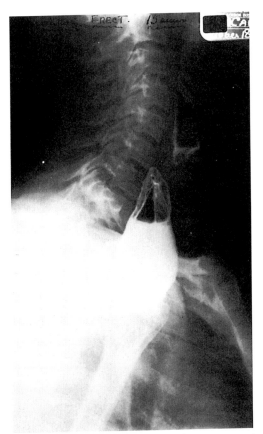

Fig. N.13. Pharyngeal pouch filled with barium. Lateral view.

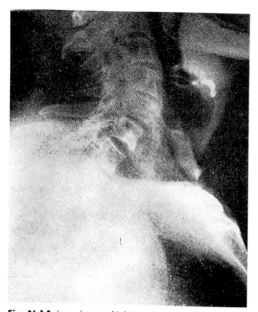

Fig. N.14. Lateral view of left-sided laryngocele.

the upper part of the neck there is a horizontally disposed system consisting of the submental, supra-hyoid, submandibular and upper deep cervical groups. The names of these groups indicate suffi-ciently their situation except for the upper deep cervical group which is situated in relation to the internal jugular vein where it is crossed by the posterior belly of the digastric muscle. One important node of this group — the jugulo-digastric node — is particularly significant in relation to pathological conditions of the tongue and tonsil. These nodes all drain from before backwards.

In addition to the horizontal system, there is a vertical system ranged along the internal jugular vein. At the upper end there is the upper deep cervical group, common to both systems, and at the lower end the lower deep cervical group with subsidiary groups in between. The lower deep cervical group of lymph nodes is in relation to the internal jugular vein where it is crossed by the posterior belly of the omohyoid, and one large node of this group — the jugulo-omohyoid node — is again of significance in relation to patho-logical processes in the tongue, receiving lymphatics from this organ without the interposition of any intervening lymphatic nodes; so that, for instance, a carcinoma of the side of the tongue can give rise to secondary deposits in the supraclavicular fossa, where this node is situated, without the enlargement of any of the systems in the upper part of the neck. It remains to mention the Delphic node on the thyrohyoid mem-brane already referred to.

B.   THYROID SWELLINGS

These, which are the second commonest cause of swellings situated laterally in the neck, are fully described on page 373. Nearly all these swellings move up and down with deglutition, by which property they may be recognized. There are, however, some exceptions to this rule. If the mass is very large and fills one or both anterior triangles and perhaps the midline as well, there may not be room for the thyroid to move on deglutition. Again, in certain types of carcinoma with infiltration of the pretracheal muscles the growth may not move on deglutition. This is because the larynx, which causes the thyroid to move, cannot itself do so as there is no elasticity left in the infiltrated pretracheal muscles. Indeed it is this tether-ing of the larynx by infiltration of the surrounding structures which leads to dysphagia in carcinoma of the thyroid, as can readily be appreciated by anyone who attempts to swallow while holding down his thyroid cartilage by placing a finger on its upper border. Sometimes in a nodular goitre the excursion of the mass on swallowing or on coughing may be so considerable that it rises up from 'plunging down' into the superior mediastinum or retroclavicular spaces during these movement. This so-called 'plunging goi-tre' is only a type of retrosternal or retroclavicular goitre with an abnormally free range of movement. Its very mobility argues that it will probably be a simple matter to deal with surgically.

C.   MORE RARE CASES OF SWELLING LATERALLY PLACED IN THE NECK

i. *Branchial cyst.* This is a congenital condition believed to arise in the remains of the second branchial cleft and giving rise to a cystic swelling in the lateral part of the neck. Another theory is that it represents cystic degeneration within a lymph node. The condi-tion may arise at any age, but usually occurs in young people and is rare after the age of 40 (*Fig.* N.15). The swelling, which varies in size, usually protrudes into the anterior triangle from the deep surface of the upper part of the sternocleidomastoid muscle. It is usually rather soft and fluctuates readily, but it is generally too deeply situated to demonstrate trans-lucency. Occasionally these cysts become infected, when the differential diagnosis from breaking-down tuberculous nodes may be difficult.

Ordinarily the sternocleidomastoid muscle tends to spread over and be attached to a mass of breaking-down tuberculous nodes, whereas it is inclined to go into spasm and retreat from an inflamed branchial cyst. However, the diagnosis can usually be determined by aspiration, which will yield either tuberculous pus or,

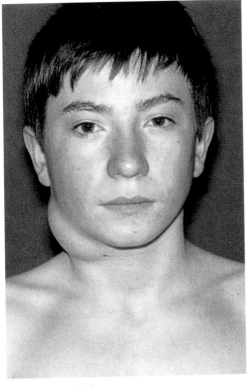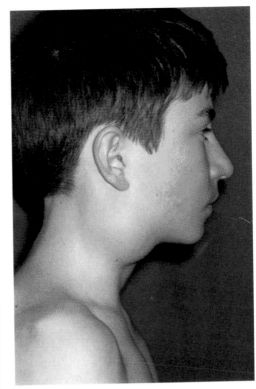

Fig. N.15. Branchial cyst.

on the other hand, purulent fluid containing numerous cholesterol crystals, which is typical of an inflamed branchial cyst.

Although not strictly a swelling in the neck, it should be mentioned here that the unobliterated second branchial cleft, instead of forming a cyst, may communicate with the exterior, usually just medial to the sternal head of the sternomastoid muscle below and into the pharynx in the supratonsillar fossa above, forming a *branchial fistula*.

ii. *'Sternocleidomastoid tumour.'* As a result of birth or intra-uterine injury, some fibres of the sterno-mastoid muscle may be torn and a haematoma appears in this muscle. This gives rise to a lump which may persist and prevent the proper development of the muscle, leading to torticollis (wryneck).

iii. *Cervical rib.* Another congenital abnormality which may give rise to a swelling in the supraclavicular fossa is cervical rib. The swelling may be due to the rib itself or there may be a pulsatile swelling due to a 'post-stenotic' dilatation of the subclavian artery.

iv. A rare congenital abnormality is *cystic hygroma*, a lymphangiomatous condition arising usually in the supraclavicular fossa of infants. It forms a soft, fluctuating, translucent and painless swelling

which may grow rapidly. These masses are liable to attacks of infection.

v. *Aneurysm and arteriovenous fistula*. The large vessels of the neck are liable to the same pathological changes as vessels elsewhere. Aneurysms may occur in the cervical part of the subclavian artery, or the carotid arteries. A penetrating injury of the neck, as by a metallic fragment, may damage both the carotid artery and the internal jugular vein, leading to an arteriovenous fistula.

vi. *Carotid body tumour.* This is a rare lesion arising in the chromaffin tissue situated at the bifurcation of the common carotid artery. It appears at any time after infancy as a very firm 'potato-like' tumour in close association with the carotid sheath so that pulsation is usually, but not invariably, transmitted to it (*Fig.* N.16). Its steady growth over a period of years serves to distinguish it from tuberculous cervical adenitis with which it may readily be confused. Carotid angiography demonstrates the diagnostic splaying apart of the internal and external carotid arteries at their origins by the tumour mass at the bifurcation.

vii. *Swellings of the submandibular salivary gland* arise in the digastric triangle and are described

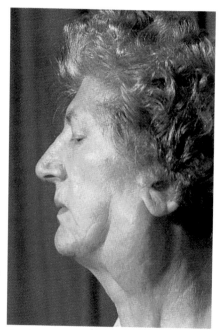

Fig. N.16. Carotid body tumour. (*Professor G. Westbury.*)

on page 340. Ludwig's angina is an acute inflammatory process of the cellular tissue around the submandibular gland, usually arising from the floor of the mouth or the teeth. The physical signs extend into the floor of the mouth and give rise to considerable oedema which, without treatment, may spread to the glottis and demand tracheotomy.

viii. *Actinomycosis* is a chronic inflammatory swelling of the cellular tissue about the angle of the mandible. The diffuse induration with the eventual development of multiple sinuses and the accompanying trismus should make the diagnosis obvious.

Late in the disease, 'sulphur granules' containing the streptothrix may be discharged, but the diagnosis should not await bacteriological confirmation which may be equivocal in the early stages.

ix. *Spinal abscess*. In certain cases of tuberculosis of the cervical spine, the abscess may track from the retropharyngeal region laterally, and present as a fluctuant mass in the upper part of the posterior triangle and deep to the insertion of the sternocleidomastoid muscle. The accompanying stiffness of the neck, together with the general evidence of a chronic infection, should alert the examiner to this possibility. Xrays of the cervical spine will confirm the bony lesion. If untreated, the abscess breaks down, discharges and forms multiple sinuses in the apex of the posterior triangle.

Harold Ellis

Nipple, abnormalities of

Deformities of the nipple may be classified as follows:

Congenital

Congenital absence
Supernumery
Congenital inversion
Bifid nipple

Acquired

Acquired inversion
Plasma cell mastitis
Mammillary duct fistula
Duct ectasia
Tumour
    Retro-areolar carcinoma
    Paget's disease

Congenital abnormalities

Rarely there can be complete absence of the development of the breast and the nipple. This may be associated with failure of development of the pectoral muscles when the condition is known as Holland's syndrome. Supernumery nipple areolar complexes are quite common, running down the milk line from the subclavicular area across the lateral part of the abdomen, ending in the region of the anterior superior iliac spine (*Fig.* N.17). Congenital inversions of the nipples are common and must be distinguished from the acquired inversion of the nipple associated with either carcinoma of the breast or duct ectasia. A bifid nipple is a rare but well-recognized entity.

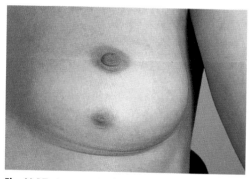

Fig. N.17. Accessory nipple.

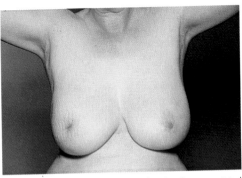

Fig. N.18. Nipple inversion and skin dimpling associated with a carcinoma of the right breast.

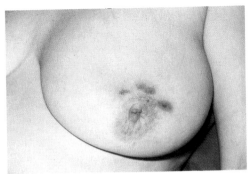

Fig. N.21. Multiple mammillary fistulae.

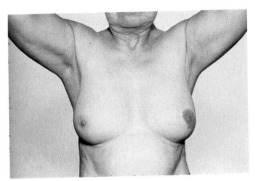

Fig. N.19. Paget's disease of the left nipple.

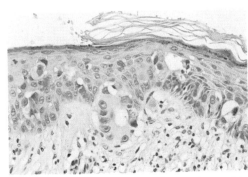

Fig. N.20. Histological appearance of Paget's disease of the nipple.

Acquired abnormalities

Acquired inversion of the nipple may be a consequence of duct ectasia/plasma cell mastitis syndrome (*see section on* BREAST LUMP). In this condition the inversion of the nipple is usually bilateral, central and slit-like. Apart from this, acquired inversion of the nipple is usually of sinister significance and may represent a retro-areolar carcinoma, or even the first sign of a cancer in one of the outer quadrants of the breast (*Fig.* N.18).

Paget's disease of the nipple (*Fig.* N.19) is a relatively rare presenting sign of carcinoma of the breast and may be an eczematous condition affecting the nipple and areola. This is usually associated with an intraduct element of carcinoma invading along the terminal portions of the lactiferous ducts to infiltrate the dermis of the nipple and areola. If this eczematous condition is unilateral and not associated with patches of eczema elsewhere on the body, then it should be treated seriously by an immediate biopsy. The histological appearance is characteristic, with foamy cells with large atypical nuclei seen scattered throughout the dermis and subdermal layers (*Fig.* N.20).

Mammillary duct fistula is a sequel of periductal mastitis and presents as a discharging sinus at the areolar margin (*Fig.* N.21). This complex of diseases is described under BREAST LUMPS.

Michael Baum

Nipple, discharge from

Discharge from the nipple may be divided into three classes:

1. Normal discharges

A discharge of milk from the breast during pregnancy is not uncommon, especially in multiparae; both then and during lactation it is usually of small amount except when the child is put to the breast, but occasionally the flow at other times may be sufficient to be distressing.

2. Normal discharges at abnormal times

A secretion similar to colostrum sometimes occurs from the breasts of both sexes in the newly born and again at puberty; it is due to endocrine stimulation but it may predispose to a true infective mastitis, when the breast, already tender and swollen, becomes hot and red, and the discharge may change from being clear to purulent.

Occasionally the normal secretion of milk during lactation is prolonged for many months or years after the stimulus of suckling has been removed. This is probably due to some endocrine abnormality and, apart from being a serious nuisance and sometimes a source of anxiety to the patient, has no sinister significance. It usually resolves spontaneously and unpredictably after a varying period with or without the aid of endocrine therapy. Women with prolactin-secreting tumours of the anterior pituitary may present with galactorrhoea and amenorrhoea.

3. Abnormal discharges

A.   SEROUS FLUID

A discharge of serous fluid from the nipple is a common accompaniment of duct ectasia or epithelial hyperplasia.

B.   PIGMENTED FLUIDS

i. *Green fluid.* When the colour is due to melanin or pigments other than derivatives of haemoglobin, its admixture with yellow serum gives to the resultant discharges a green colour of varying shades. If the discharge is very dark, dilution with water will disclose the green colour. In cases of real difficulty the discharge may be submitted to spectroscopic or chemical assay for haemoglobin. Such discharges have precisely the same significance as the non-pigmented serous discharges discussed above.

ii. *Haemorrhagic.* Blood-stained discharges can usually be recognized on sight; the colour is red to black, and again if there is real doubt the final arbiters are the microscope and the chemical test. Blood-stained discharges are indicative of duct papilloma, epithelial proliferation, and intraduct carcinoma, in that order of frequency.

The nipple should be examined through a magnifying glass and a bead of blood or a speck of clot may reveal from which of the twenty or so ducts the bleeding is arising. Such evidence is important in determining from which section of the breast the bleeding is originating. Having examined the nipple thus, it should be wiped clean and (with the breast rendered moderately tense by an assistant if available) the tip of the finger is pressed on to the breast at successive sites, working spirally from the nipple, and paying particular attention to the subareolar region, where the source of the bleeding lies in the majority of cases. By this means it will be found possible to cause blood to issue from the nipple on pressure over quite a restricted area, whereas pressure elsewhere has no effect. If the affected duct has been previously identified the significant area will be found to lie in the segment of the breast drained by that duct, and the pathological region is confirmed. The segment of the breast affected should be removed by local operation, and the pathological condition causing the bleeding determined by naked-eye inspection and histological study. Further treatment depends upon the nature of the lesion so determined. Solitary papillomas adjacent to the nipple are the commonest cause of this symptom, and if removed in this way bleeding seldom recurs.

Should it be impossible to localize the origin of the bleeding, and with care and practice this is most unusual, the diagnosis depends on an assessment of probabilities. The younger the patient the more likely is the cause to be benign; the older the patient the more likely is to be malignant. Mammography is valuable in demonstrating or excluding an occult neoplasm as the source of the haemorrhage. Where the discharge of pigmented fluids from multiple ducts associated with duct ectasia is profuse and embarrassing, total excision of the subareolar duct system (Hadfield's operation) will affect a cure.

4.   Grumous material

The discharge of 'cheese-like' material or material having the consistency of toothpaste or putty, grey or green in colour, indicates the condition known as 'comedo mastitis'. This is another variant of the duct ectasia/periductal mastitis complex (see p. 58).

5.   Pus

Pus, or pus mixed with milk, generally indicates acute suppurative mastitis; the other signs of inflammation or abscess are well marked as a rule, so that there is no difficulty in arriving at a diagnosis. A *tuberculous lesion* also causes a discharge of pus, and it may simulate carcinoma; the discharge may contain demonstrable tubercle bacilli, but specific bacteriological culture, together with a radiograph of the chest, will very likely be required before a positive answer on the nature of the infection can be given.

Michael Baum

Oedema, generalized

Generalized oedema is due to an increase in the volume of extracellular fluid. This is brought about by excessive renal tubular reabsorption of sodium and water; the mechanism of this reabsorption is complex and the renin–angiotensin–aldosterone system is only one of the factors involved. The accumulation of fluid in the extravascular space which causes oedema is determined by the relationship between the hydrostatic and oncotic pressures in the capillaries and the interstitial tissue. Thus, a rise in capillary hydrostatic pressure due, for example, to venous obstruction and a fall in capillary oncotic pressure, as a result of hypoalbuminaemia, increases the net movement of fluid from the capillaries to the tissues. When sufficient fluid has been transferred in this way — at least 5 litres in adults — clinically detectable oedema results. Another factor concerned in the transfer of fluid across capillary walls is their permeability; in practice, an increase in this is more important in the production of localized rather than generalized oedema. Impairment of the lymphatic drainage of tissues is also a cause of localized oedema (see ARM; LEG, OEDEMA OF). In any patient with generalized oedema, fluid may also accumulate in serous cavities in the form of ascites and pleural or pericardial effusion.

Gravity determines the fact that, in any situation in which sodium and water retention occurs, the oedema fluid tends to accumulate in the dependent parts of the body. This tendency is so marked that, even in normal subjects, a little ankle oedema is common following prolonged periods of immobility in the seated position. It is particularly common during long journeys by air and, sometimes, by train or coach; it is probable that this is mainly due to a reduction in lymphatic drainage which is critically dependent on muscular activity. Also, in about 90 per cent of pregnant women, slight oedema is present at term and is, in fact, associated with a more favourable outcome to the pregnancy than when no oedema is present. The pathological situations in which generalized oedema most commonly occurs are heart failure and renal, hepatic and, less often, gastrointestinal disease. These, and other less common causes of oedema, are discussed below.

Heart failure

The oedema of *heart failure* is typically dependent, affecting particularly the ankles and, in recumbent patients, the sacral region. Despite this clear evidence of a hydrostatic component in determining the site of the oedema, the rise in central venous pressure in heart failure is a minor factor in the production of the oedema, compared with the reduction in renal blood flow and glomerular filtration rate and the increase in tubular reabsorption of sodium and water. These mechanisms operate whatever the cause of the heart failure but, in cor pulmonale, an additional factor may be a movement of fluid from the cells to the interstitial tissue; this is believed to occur in order to provide more buffers for the associated respiratory acidosis. The oedema is usually symmetrical but, sometimes, it is more marked in the left leg than the right; this is thought to be due to pressure on the left common iliac vein by the right common iliac artery as it crosses it. It is heart failure which is the mechanism of the oedema of so-called 'wet' beri-beri, due to a dietary deficiency of thiamine, and also of the oedema seen commonly in severe anaemia from any cause.

Renal disease

Slight transient generalized oedema is a characteristic feature of *acute poststreptococcal glomerulonephritis* but this is not due to the proteinuria, which is of no more than moderate severity. It is in the *nephrotic syndrome* that hypoalbuminaemia, due to heavy proteinuria, is severe enough to lower the intracapillary oncotic pressure to a level at which oedema occurs. In this condition the urinary protein loss is usually more than 3 g per 24 hours and the serum albumin below 30 g per litre. It is probable that the hypovolaemia resulting from massive loss of fluid from the capillaries stimulates the renin–angiotensin–aldosterone system and this leads to renal retention of sodium and water. The oedema is usually dependent but, in children, it may be as prominent in the trunk and face as in the legs (*Fig. O.1*); the external genitalia are commonly very swollen. Spontaneous disappearance of the oedema is not necessarily a good sign as, with advancing renal failure, the fall in glomerular filtration rate may markedly reduce the amount of protein lost.

There are numerous conditions which can cause the nephrotic syndrome. In children, by far the commonest cause is *minimal change nephropathy*, in which, as the name implies, the glomeruli are nearly normal on light microscopy but show characteristic changes on electron microscopy; clinically the most typical feature is the complete remission produced by steroid therapy. In adults, *membranous* and *proliferative nephropathy* are at least as common as the minimal change lesion and these three conditions together represent about three-quarters of all cases of the nephrotic syndrome. Less common causes include *focal glomerulosclerosis*, a condition of unknown

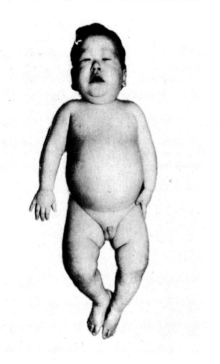

Fig. O.1. Massive oedema and ascites in the nephrotic syndrome. (*Dr. P.R. Evans.*)

aetiology with patchy glomerular scarring without previous inflammatory changes, *systemic lupus erythematosus, amyloidosis* and *diabetic nephropathy*; oedema is quite common in diabetics even in the absence of heavy proteinuria, perhaps due to microvascular disease. There is also a recognized association of the nephrotic syndrome with *malaria* due to *Plasmodium malariae* and with *malignant disease*, especially adenocarcinoma and lymphoma. The high venous pressure of *constrictive pericarditis* is also known occasionally to cause the nephrotic syndrome which has also been seen in *cyanotic congenital heart disease*. Renal vein thrombosis *per se*, however, is no longer thought to be a cause but rather a complication of the nephrotic syndrome. A number of *drugs and other substances* are known to cause a membranous glomerular lesion and proteinuria heavy enough to cause oedema; these include mercurials, gold, penicillamine and captopril. A specific allergy is probably responsible for the nephrotic syndrome associated with certain foods, pollens, penicillin, bee stings and poison ivy.

Liver disease

Fluid retention is common in hepatic failure in which it is due to impaired protein synthesis and consequent hypoalbuminaemia. The changes in renal function are similar to those in the nephrotic syndrome. Both oedema and ascites can occur, often together, but one can be present without the other. Any form of cirrhosis may be the underlying disorder but *cryptogenic* and *alcoholic cirrhosis* and *chronic active hepatitis* are those most likely to be associated with oedema.

Protein-losing enteropathy

Protein may be lost from the body not only in the urine but also via the gastrointestinal tract. Marked hypoalbuminaemia can develop, causing oedema and, sometimes, ascites and pleural effusion. This situation arises particularly with *intestinal lymphoma* and *giant hypertrophic gastritis (Menetrier's disease)* but has been seen in many other disorders such as *coeliac disease, ulcerative colitis, Crohn's disease, tumours of the stomach and colon* and *intestinal allergies*.

Other causes of oedema

Oedema, more or less generalized, is a recognized feature of a number of other conditions, all rather rare in Britain. *Malnutrition*, of course, is far from rare in developing countries where it is an all too common cause of oedema. It is usually due to dietary deficiency of protein, causing hypoalbuminaemia, and is a constant feature of kwashiorkor. A condition affecting emotionally labile women of reproductive age is known, non-committally, as *idiopathic oedema*. The distribution of the oedema is curious, affecting particularly the face, hands, breasts, thighs, buttocks and abdominal wall and, hardly ever, the ankles. The aetiology is unknown but in some cases it may follow the use of diuretics in an attempt to lose weight; in that case it would be described as 'rebound' oedema. Oedema of the face, hands and ankles sometimes occurs at *high altitudes*. It may or may not be accompanied by the more severe manifestations of acute mountain sickness, such as pulmonary oedema, and is relieved by a spontaneous diuresis on return to a lower altitude. Very rarely oedema may occur in diabetics on first being given *insulin*; this resolves completely in a week or so.

Peter R. Fleming

Oliguria

The volume of urine which constitutes clinically significant oliguria varies with the pre-existing state of the kidneys. With a urine volume of less than 400 ml per 24 hours even a normal kidney is unable to concentrate the glomerular filtrate sufficiently to

Table O.1. Causes of oliguria

Renal circulatory insufficiency

Primary renal disease
Acute tubular necrosis
Acute cortical necrosis
Drugs and poisons
Acute interstitial nephritis
Acute glomerulonephritis
Vascular lesions, e.g. accelerated hypertension
Other causes, e.g. hepatorenal syndrome, mismatched
  blood transfusion

Obstructive
Calculi
Pelvic tumours
Retroperitoneal fibrosis

oliguria. Other mechanisms operate in so-called 'cardiogenic' shock following myocardial infarction, acute pancreatitis and septicaemia, often due to Gram-negative organisms. All these conditions can also cause acute tubular necrosis, a poorly defined pathological entity but a diagnosis which is made when renal function does not improve rapidly following restoration of normal renal perfusion. It is clearly important not to delay the recognition that this change for the worse has taken place and a useful indication may be provided by estimation of the urinary sodium concentration. With oliguria due to renal circulatory insufficiency this is typically low, around 20 mmol per litre, whereas in acute tubular necrosis with oliguria it will be about three times that level.

prevent a rise in plasma urea and creatinine. Much larger volumes may be needed to maintain homeostasis if renal function has been impaired for any reason. Oliguria is present in most, but by no means all, cases of acute renal failure of which the causes, summarized in *Table* O.1, are conventionally classified as prerenal, renal and postrenal. Although these categories are not entirely mutually exclusive, it is important to identify, in any individual patient, the dominant factor causing renal failure because the management is very different for these three groups. It is also important to decide whether the condition from which the patient is suffering is acute renal failure with previously normal kidneys or an acute exacerbation of chronic renal disease. The latter is more likely if the patient is very anaemic, shows evidence of long-standing hypertension, has biochemical or radiographic evidence of osteodystrophy or, most significantly, the kidneys can be shown to be shrunken by plain X-rays of the abdomen or ultrasound scanning.

Renal circulatory insufficiency (prerenal uraemia)

This situation arises whenever the renal blood flow falls steeply. It is most commonly due to a fall in cardiac output secondary to a reduction in circulating blood volume. The implication of a diagnosis of prerenal uraemia is that normal renal function will be restored as soon as the circulatory abnormality has been corrected. The cause of the circulatory failure is usually obvious. External loss of fluid is a common cause; severe diarrhoea and vomiting, haemorrhage, burns and previous polyuria in diabetes mellitus or Addison's disease are all well-known causes of, usually transient,

Renal causes of oliguria

ACUTE TUBULAR NECROSIS

As has been said, this is an imprecise term and will be used here to designate only those cases of acute, usually oliguric, renal failure due to those circulatory disorders described above under prerenal uraemia. Other specific disorders causing a similar clinical syndrome will be discussed separately. In practice the diagnosis will usually be made in patients under observation and treatment for the causative condition. The symptoms are those of uraemia, i.e. anorexia, nausea and vomiting, perhaps muscle cramps and a 'flapping' tremor. Bleeding into the skin and gastrointestinal tract and fits can occur. Hypertension is unusual and suggests a different cause for the renal failure. The plasma creatinine will rise progressively unless effective treatment is started and dangerous hyperkalaemia, especially when there has been much tissue destruction, is common. Improvement can usually be expected in 6 weeks or less and, if this does not occur, renal biopsy may reveal that the damage is severe, perhaps in the form of acute cortical necrosis. In such a case recovery is very slow and may be incomplete.

ACUTE CORTICAL NECROSIS

This condition may follow insults similar to those which cause acute tubular necrosis. It is a recognized feature of severe obstetric emergencies such as antepartum haemorrhage, eclampsia and septic abortion. Irreversible renal damage occurs but the changes may be patchy and, therefore, compatible with some recovery. Radiography may show shrunken kidneys with cortical calcification as early as 2 months after the onset.

ACUTE RENAL FAILURE DUE TO DRUGS AND POISONS

Many drugs are known to damage the kidneys and cause acute renal failure. Some do so by causing acute interstitial nephritis (*see below*). Others, such as the aminoglycoside antibiotics, amphotericin, colistin, polymyxin B and radiographic contrast media, do so by other mechanisms. Heavy metals, organic solvents, particularly carbon tetrachloride, paraquat, snake bite and mushroom poisoning can also cause acute renal failure.

ACUTE INTERSTITIAL NEPHRITIS

This is a common cause of acute oliguric renal failure and is most often due to drugs. Those most commonly implicated include the non-steroidal anti-inflammatory drugs, the penicillin and cephalosporin groups of antibiotics and diuretics but many other drugs are known to cause this syndrome occasionally. The same type of renal damage is occasionally caused by bacterial and viral infections.

ACUTE GLOMERULONEPHRITIS

Some reduction in urine volume is common in most cases of acute nephritis and severe oliguric renal failure is a common feature, particularly in adults, of the more rapidly progressive forms of glomerulonephritis which are discussed under HAEMATURIA on p. 155.

VASCULAR LESIONS

Renal infarction, if extensive, may cause acute renal failure; *renal vein thrombosis* is much less likely to do so except in infants. The fibrinous necrosis of *accelerated (malignant) hypertension* as well as the similar vascular damage seen occasionally in *systemic sclerosis* together with intravascular coagulation occurring in the *haemolytic-uraemic syndrome* of children, *thrombotic thrombocytopenic purpura* and the rare *idiopathic post-partum renal failure* are all rare causes of oliguria and renal failure.

OTHER CAUSES OF ACUTE OLIGURIC RENAL FAILURE

Renal failure may complicate hepatic failure from any cause; the term *hepatorenal syndrome* is applied, particularly, to the acute renal failure which may follow surgery in patients with obstructive jaundice. Muscle damage is an important contributory cause of renal failure following trauma and *rhabdomyolysis* in the absence of trauma can also cause renal damage. This can be due to acute myositis, either idiopathic or in association with viral infections, prolonged convulsions or marathon running, malignant hyperpyrexia following general anaesthesia, carbon-monoxide poisoning and a number of other conditions. It is probably the myoglobinuria which is responsible for the renal damage but the mechanism by which this occurs is unclear. Similar damage can occur, as a result of intravascular haemolysis as in *malignant malaria* or following a *mismatched blood transfusion*. In *myelomatosis* acute renal failure may occur, probably due to hypercalcaemia as well as the specific renal lesion of that condition. Finally, obstruction of the renal tubules by crystals of *urate*, during treatment of leukaemia and similar conditions or following starvation, is a rare but important and preventible cause of acute oliguric renal failure

Postrenal (obstructive) causes of oliguria

Unlike primary renal disease, obstructive lesions below the renal papillae more commonly cause total anuria than oliguria and this is sometimes a helpful differential diagnostic feature. Also the rate of deterioration, clinical and biochemical, is slower with obstructive than with renal lesions. Conventionally the term 'anuria' is applied to obstruction in the ureters or above; obstruction to outflow from the bladder is termed urinary retention (*see* URINE, RETENTION OF). It goes without saying, therefore, that obstructive anuria can occur only if the outflow from both kidneys or from the only functioning kidney is obstructed. In a patient with acute renal failure and anuria, or severe oliguria, it is clearly important to distinguish between an obstructive cause which can usually be quickly dealt with surgically and a primary renal cause in which other treatment is required. The situation is not always clear-cut. For example, chronic calculous disease may cause severe renal damage and chronic renal failure without much in the way of symptoms as well as acute anuria from obstruction; or chronic ureteric obstruction by spread from a uterine carcinoma might be complicated by pyonephrosis and Gram-negative septicaemia causing acute tubular necrosis.

Calculous disease is the commonest cause of obstructive anuria. It is rare for this to occur as a result of simultaneous obstruction of both ureters by calculi; it is more common to find that one kidney has been severely damaged by chronic disease and that there is a calculus in the other ureter. Exceptionally the blockage of one ureter may cause reflex anuria in the other kidney. The patient will usually complain of pain in the acutely obstructed kidney with renal colic and may feel a constant desire to micturate despite the empty bladder. If the patient has total anuria, it is necessary to confirm the diagnosis and localize the obstruction. Radiographic examination of the kidneys and ureters is essential, perhaps tomography to demonstrate a small or poorly radio-opaque calculus. At cystoscopy the ureteric orifice on the affected side may be congested and show ecchymoses; ureteric catheterization may localize the calculus precisely (*Fig. O.2*).

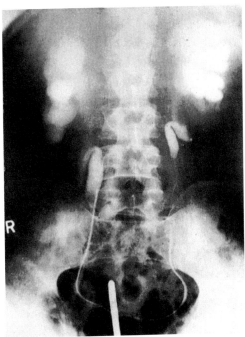

Fig. O.3. Bilateral hydronephrosis due to retroperitoneal fibrosis involving the ureters.

Sulphonamide crystalluria with blockage of both ureters is now very rare although the need for a high fluid intake in patients on these drugs remains.

Peter R. Fleming

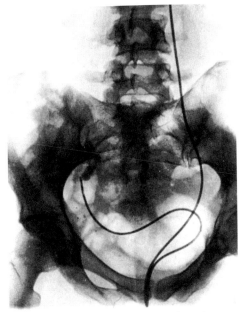

Fig. O.2. A radiograph showing the tip of a radio-opaque catheter obstructed by a calculus in the right ureter.

Other causes of anuria from ureteric obstruction include *vesical carcinoma*; in such cases it is likely that the diagnosis will already have been made and chronic partial bilateral ureteric obstruction will have caused hydroureter and hydronephrosis with severe renal damage. A similar situation can arise in *carcinoma of the uterine cervix* but occasionally anuria may be the presenting feature. Other *pelvic or abdominal tumours* can also cause bilateral ureteric obstruction and *ligation of both ureters* is an occasional complication of extensive pelvic surgery for malignant disease. *Retroperitoneal fibrosis* is a rare cause of bilateral ureteric obstruction; in most cases no cause can be found but there is a recognized association with retroperitoneal lymphoma, abdominal aortic aneurysm and exposure to methysergide, used in the prophylaxis of migraine; the ureters are seen to be displaced medially on urography (*Fig. O.3*).

Otorrhoea

Otorrhoea (aural discharge) may arise from the external meatus or the middle ear itself. In rare cases discharge of fluid may originate in nearby structures. It is important to note the duration of the discharge, whether it is continuous or intermittent, its character, colour, amount and whether it is inoffensive or offensive.

Careful aural toilet with a sucker and examination with a good light are necessary for a diagnosis.

The various causes of discharge may be listed (*Table O.2*).

External meatus

Wax (cerumen) is so variable in colour and consistency that it may be mistaken for other substances. It may be present in small flakes only which, by epithelial movement, are carried out of the meatus. It may collect in hard masses or may be semi-liquid and yellow

Table O.2. The causes of otorrhoea

External meatus
Wax
Localized boils or furuncles
Otitis externa
  Reactive—eczematous or atopic
  Infective
    Bacterial
    Fungal
    Viral
  Malignant
Trauma—blood
Salivary fistula (rare)
Branchial fistula (very rare)

Middle ear
Acute otitis media
Chronic otitis media
  Tubotympanic otitis media
  Attic disease
Mastoiditis
Mastoid cavity infection
Tuberculosis
Malignant disease
Eosinophilic granuloma
Wegener's granuloma (very rare)
Fracture of temporal bone
  Cerebrospinal fluid
  Blood
Radionecrosis

in colour when it can truly be called a discharge. In children, perhaps as a result of fungal infection, the wax may form as a yellowish-grey material with the consistency of toothpaste, completely blocking the meatus and causing deafness. Keratosis obturans is a condition where wax and desquamated squamous epithelium forms an adherent mass in the bony meatus, sometimes even causing bony erosion. This condition may be associated with bronchiectasis and sinusitis. In most cases, however, wax causes no symptoms at all until water from swimming or bathing makes it swell to occlude the meatus and cause sudden deafness.

Otitis externa is a common disease and is sometimes a straightforward allergic reaction. The sorts of things that incite an allergic eczematous reaction are hairsprays, perfumes and ear drops, especially those containing neomycin. Some wax solvents can also cause enough irritation to create an eczema.

The most common cause of otitis externa, however, is a breakdown in the migratory mechanism of the skin of the deep meatus. Elsewhere in the body where skin epithelium divides, movement, clothes, friction and washing get rid of the dead skin. The external meatus is one-and-a-half inches long, therefore is not exposed to any of these factors and so a different

mechanism must exist to get rid of the dead epithelium. The epithelium in the area has the property of migrating dead skin from the deep meatus to the wax glands in the outer half-inch of the ear canal. If, for any reason, this migratory process breaks down, then dead epithelium collects in the deep meatus. This acts as an excellent culture medium for bacteria if it is moistened with water from bathing or from a swimming pool. Secondary bacterial infection occurs and creates the symptoms of pain and discharge. Treatment consists of removing the dead epithelium and keeping the ear in a sterile condition until the migratory process recovers in a number of months.

The overuse of ear drops can lead to the fungal otitis externa. This usually presents as moist, whitish debris like damp blotting paper. *Aspergillus niger* infection will show black spots; the other common fungus is *Candida albicans*.

Two types of viral infections can cause an otitis externa. The commonest is a herpetic infection which causes severe pain and may sometimes be accompanied by facial paralysis (Ramsay–Hunt syndrome). The other type is myringitis bullosa haemorrhagica, which is often seen in conjunction with the flu virus. Blood blisters form on the drum and lead to a serosanguinous discharge and bouts of severe pain.

In many cases it is not possible, because of the oedema, to see the tympanic membrane. It is most important, however, to differentiate between otitis externa and otitis media as soon as possible and it must be remembered that as the discharge of the latter may set up a secondary otitis externa both conditions may coexist. The pain of external otitis is chiefly felt on moving the pinna, while in otitis media it is pressure above and behind the ear that is painful. If in addition to the characteristic pain the patient has good hearing and a positive Rinné test, even though the meatus may be almost completely occluded, the condition is not otitis media. If the meatus is completely blocked efforts must be made to clear a very small air passage to the drum, so that this most important differentiation can be made.

Malignant otitis externa is caused by *Ps. pyocyaneus* and is a very severe, sometimes fatal infection which occurs in elderly, immunocompromised and nearly always diabetic patients. Green purulent discharge and much oedema precede osteomyelitis of the temporal bone and base of skull.

Salivary fistula leading into the cartilaginous meatus may follow injury that involves the ear, the temporo-mandibular joint and the parotid gland. Discharge may be caused by a first branchial arch sinus, which classically communicates with the bony cartilaginous junction and may travel into the parotid and underneath the facial nerve.

Middle ear

Acute otitis media rarely gives rise to discharge until the tympanic membrane ruptures with sudden relief from pain. There may be a little blood followed by mucopurulent discharge which may be profuse and may continue for some days before (in most cases), stopping spontaneously. If the meatus is carefully cleaned the discharge will be seen to be pulsating as it comes out of the perforation. The pus is usually inoffensive and mucopurulent and the organism is a streptococcus, pneumococcus or haemophilus.

In chronic suppurative otitis media (CSOM) it is of great importance to differentiate between the safe tubotympanic otitis media and the potentially serious attic disease. Tubotympanic otitis media is often accompanied by an anterior or a central perforation of the pars tensa of the drum. There is a constant moist discharge, usually related to a blocked Eustachian tube. There is a mucositis of the mucosa of the middle ear and often an accompanying otitis externa. It is a very difficult condition to eradicate and should be kept under control with ear drops and occasional antibiotic therapy. If the perforation in the drum can be closed the ear dries up.

Attic disease is due to cholesteatoma. The origin of cholesteatoma is not known but it may be related to childhood serous otitis media that remains untreated. It is also a disease related to poor socioeconomic circumstances. It is a collection of keratin which has enzymes in its matrix that can dissolve bone. The cholesteatoma, therefore, destroys the attic region of the middle ear and can extend into the mastoid, may paralyse the facial nerve and make form a fistula into the lateral semicircular canal. It can also erode the floor of the middle fossa, causing an extradural abscess or even a brain abscess and meningitis. It is essential to make the diagnosis of cholesteatoma and have it eradicated by mastoid surgery.

Aural polyps develop from granulation tissue which, in turn, signifies an underlying osteitis of the tympanomastoid bone. Polyps may bleed easily to the touch and must be distinguished from glomus tumours. Glomus tumours usually present, however, with no previous history of chronic otitis media where its polyps are nearly always associated with long-standing ear problems. The presence of a polyp usually indicates that the patient will have to undergo some form of mastoid surgery at some time.

Acute mastoiditis may complicate a case of acute otitis media. The mastoid air cells are filled with pus as well as the middle ear, so that if after cleaning the meatus it immediately refills with pus. Mastoid infection is now much rarer than previously because of better social environments and more aggressive treatment of ear disease in children.

Malignant disease presents with granulations in the middle ear and deep meatus and a blood-stained mucopurulent discharge. Diagnosis is by biopsy as in the case with Wegener's granuloma. Eosinophilic granuloma (or histiocytosis X) affecting the ear presents with granulomatous polyps and discharge. Osteolytic skeletal lesions in skull and elsewhere give an indication of the diagnosis but biopsy is also required.

Osteoradionecrosis occurring months or years after radiotherapy in the area of the ear may present with suppuration following sequestration of dead bone. There is also atrophy of the organ of Corti and deafness.

Blood and cerebrospinal fluid, both originating from outside the middle ear but presenting as a middle-ear discharge, may result from trauma. Simple trauma to the meatus or a ruptured drum usually bleeds slightly. The drum may be damaged by direct trauma from a penetrating injury. Otitic barotrauma, air pressure changes in diving, aircraft or bomb blast injuries, may rupture the membrane, the tear being usually in the posterior half of the drum. It may also be ruptured by syringing. More serious trauma with fractures of the temporal bone, often so fine that they do not show on X-ray, lead to bleeding and, if the meninges are torn, a cerebrospinal fluid leak.

A. G. D. Maran

Pelvis, pain in

In practice, pelvic pain can usually be classified under six headings, namely:

(1) *Deep-seated pain*
(2) *Referred pain*
(3) *Spasmodic pain*
(4) *Backache or sacralgia*
(5) *Mid-cycle ovulation pain (Mittelschmerz)*
(6) *Pain related to varicosity*

All women at some time experience pelvic pain associated with events such as menstruation, ovulation or sexual intercourse. Although only a few women seek medical advice for such pain, it is the commonest reason for laparoscopy examination in the UK. In many of these cases a cause is not found. It is recognized that the incidence of anxiety and depression is high in women with unexplained pelvic and abdominal pain but it is necessary to carry out a detailed examination to exclude the other causes of pain.

1. DEEP-SEATED PAIN is aching in character, continuous, and may be acute in onset or chronic in duration. It is the result of congested blood vessels and oedema of the pelvic organs, most commonly the result of inflammation. In acute inflammation the pain is severe, elicited by lower abdominal pressure and thereby made worse. Infection of the pelvic organs gives rise to *local peritonitis*, and hence the severe pain. Chronic dull aching pain is caused by chronic salpingo-oophoritis (pyosalpinx, hydrosalpinx, ovarian abscess or chronic interstitial salpingitis), whether gonococcal, tuberculous or pyogenic in origin or following labour or abortion, by endometriosis of the ovaries and by chronic pelvic appendicitis or sigmoid colon diverticulitis. It may also occur as the result of infection of the pelvic cellular tissue, parametritis, following labour or abortion. More severe pain may be due to a twisted or infected or ruptured ovarian cyst or to a ruptured ectopic pregnancy.

Sometimes there is no evidence of infection or other disease to account for chronic pelvic pain. Although congestion due to unrelieved sexual stimulation is suggested as the reason there are not always good grounds for saying this. It is unlikely that retroversion or retroflexion of the uterus causes pelvic pain; they may occasionally give rise to backache. Culdocentesis (puncture and aspiration of the pouch of Douglas), ultrasound scanning and laparoscopy are used to diagnose pelvic lesions, but generally a careful history and examination make such procedures unnecessary. When no lesion is found but the patient still complains these procedures may be used to exclude pathology.

2. REFERRED PAIN may appear to arise in the pelvis when the true cause lies elsewhere, pain being referred through spinal segments T10–L3, as, for instance, from a spinal tumour, or in tabes dorsalis.

3. SPASMODIC PAIN in the pelvis is nearly always due to painful uterine contractions when it is of genital origin. The exception to this is the spasmodic pain which occurs in connection with *tubal gestation*, as a rule in the few days which precede tubal abortion or rupture of the tube. The only way to diagnose between this tubal pain and that due to uterine contractions is by a careful consideration of the history of the case, and the finding of a definite tubal swelling by bimanual palpation. Even then the diagnosis may be difficult. Laparoscopy is indicated when doubt persists. Spasmodic pain due to *uterine contractions* is caused by: the onset of abortion or labour; spasmodic dysmenorrhoea (p. 83); attempted expulsion from the uterus of a growth such as a fibromyoma; 'after-pains' following

labour; the presence of a contraceptive device in the uterus.

The differential diagnosis of these conditions is easy, but it may be difficult to be sure that the pelvic pain has a uterine origin, for sometimes spasmodic pain may be referred to the pelvis from such relatively distant causes as appendicitis, intestinal, renal or bilary colic, leaking gastric ulcer, ruptured tubal gestation, twisted ovarian pedicle, haemorrhage into a Graafian follicle, leakage or rupture of an ovarian cyst or pyosalpinx, dyspepsia or flatulent distension of the bowels.

4. BACKACHE or SACRALGIA (*see also* BACK, PAIN IN) is a common complaint in many cases of pelvic disease, but as a sole symptom is most unlikely to be due to a pelvic lesion. It is true that in such cases the pain may be worse at the time of menstruation but the same applies to those cases which have an orthopaedic origin. Before the pelvic contents can be suspected there should be present other symptoms of pelvic disease, and it will be found, almost invariably, that the backache is only a secondary or minor complaint. The presence of such conditions as (1) a heavy congested retroverted uterus with prolapse; (2) large, or impacted ovarian or fibroid tumours; (3) a retroverted gravid uterus impacted in the pelvis; (4) a pelvic haematocele; (5) pelvic endometriosis or chronic salpingo-oophoritis make the association more likely, particularly if the backache is low down. Most backaches in women are at a high level in the small of the back or lumbar region and are of orthopaedic origin; pain arising in the pelvic organs is at a lower level in the back, over the sacrum. Sometimes a large cervical erosion with surrounding parametritis is the only finding, and in many of these cases adequate treatment of the erosion cures the backache. Pelvic congestion, the result of coitus interruptus or other unsatisfactory sexual relationship, particularly if a retroversion is present, may be responsible. A backwardly displaced uterus, however, without some other complicating factor is hardly ever the cause of backache. In some cases where slight prolapse is present in addition, if the uterus is replaced and a ring inserted, the backache will be cured. Dyspareunia is often present in such cases owing to the prolapse of one or both ovaries. The back should be examined and any abnormal posture, limitation of movement, tenseness of the back muscles or tender areas should be noted. In such cases an orthopaedic cause is more likely, although a pelvic cause may be responsible for the assumption of abnormal postures to secure comfort. In cases of impacted tumours the pain may be due to actual pressure on the sacral nerves at their exits, in which case pain will be felt down the inner sides of the thighs and back of the legs. In advanced cases of

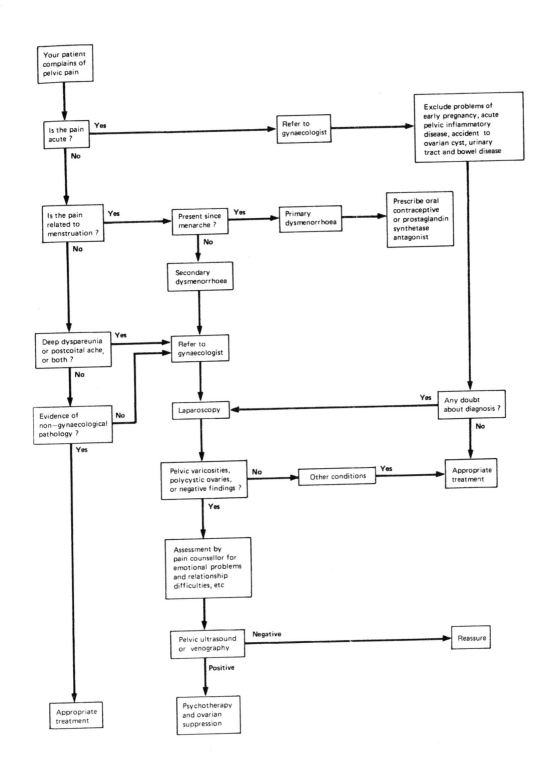

Fig. P.1. Algorithm for diagnosis of pelvic pain. (Reproduced with permission from Beard R. W. et al. (1986) Pelvic pain in women. British Medical Journal **293**, 1161.)

carcinoma of the cervix, backache is a complaint, but it is always associated with pain in the buttock, due to involvement of the sacral plexus, and the pain radiates down the legs. Secondary deposits in the lumbar spine may be the cause.

Probably not more than a very small minority of backaches are of genital origin. It may result from some urinary irritation due to oxalates or coli bacilluria; it may accompany a calculus in the ureter or some lesion of the renal pelvis, though as a rule, in renal cases, the pain is situated rather higher up. Caries of the spine low down, growth in the spine or in the spinal cord membranes, might also cause it, or it may result from inflammation or strain of the sacro-iliac joint, displaced disc, rectal growth, haemorrhoids, proctitis or scybala. Injuries to the lumbar spine, including strain and subluxation as well as damage of a minor character to the erector spinae and other muscles causing muscle fatigue, have to be remembered in this connection. A correct diagnosis cannot be made without a complete examination of all adjacent structures, combined with careful urinary analysis.

5. MID-CYCLE OVULATION PAIN (MITTELSCHMERZ). Some women habitually experience some dull pain in the midline or in one or other iliac fossa at about the time of ovulation about 14 days before the next period. In others the pain may be experienced for a few cycles only. Occasionally slight vaginal bleeding accompanies the pain. The timing of the pain and the absence of any abnormal pelvic findings usually make the diagnosis clear.

6. PAIN RELATED TO VARICOSITY. Recent work suggests that in some women with pelvic pain it is possible to demonstrate congestion of the pelvic veins using examinations such as pelvic venography. These women tend to be in their early thirties and the pain is often described as dull and aching with sharp exacerbation. The diagnosis is made based on history, and on clinical examination, tenderness could be elicited at a point located two-thirds from the junction of anterior-superior spine to the umbilicus. Initial results suggest that progesterone therapy in this group of patients helps to alleviate the problem (*Fig. P.1*) indicates the algorithm for diagnosis of pelvic pain.

N. Patel

Penile sores

Sores on the penis may be present on the thin mucous covering of the glans or prepuce, or on the cutaneous surface of the body of the penis; they are more common in the former situation.

Ulceration in the neighbourhood of the glans penis may be due to:

Balanitis
Herpes genitalis
Soft sore
Granuloma venereum (inguinale)
Lymphogranuloma inguinale (venereum)
Chancre
Epithelioma
Papilloma
Gummatous ulceration
Tuberculous ulceration
Injury, for example from a bite

Balanitis

If inflammatory processes have been allowed to continue beneath the prepuce, ulceration and excoriation of the mucous membrane covering the glans penis or lining the prepuce will occur, accompanied by a stinking, purulent discharge. Multiple shallow ulcers are formed, rapidly coalescing and causing considerable discomfort. The prepuce often becomes swollen and oedematous, preventing retraction, so that a condition of phimosis occurs, or, if retraction has taken place, the analogous state of paraphimosis, almost strangulating the end of the penis and even causing it to become gangrenous. Care must be exercised in diagnosing a simple balanitis from one accompanying acute gonorrhoeal urethritis or an underlying syphilitic or soft chancre. The so-called balanitis circinata is part of Reiter's syndrome, occurring in association with urethritis, arthritis, conjunctivitis (often slight and transient) and buccal ulceration. In Behçet's syndrome also ulcerative penile and scrotal lesions may occur in association with buccal ulcers. With an acute urethritis there will be a history of infection and pain along the course of the urethra during micturition; the intracellular gonococcus may be identified in a Gram-stained smear of the discharge.

If a chancre exists under the swollen phimosed prepuce there is often a tender spot about the corona or at the fraenum. With a soft sore consecutive sores may appear about the orifice of the prepuce, while the inguinal nodes are much more likely to be inflamed or to suppurate than with simple balanitis. A syphilitic chancre obscured by a phimosis can usually be felt distinctly under the skin, and causes a comparatively small amount of discharge, while the inguinal nodes become enlarged but do not suppurate. The interval of about 4 weeks from the time of the possible source of infection until the appearance of the sore will suggest, and the finding of spirochaetes (*Treponema pallidum*) in the fluid expressed from the ulcer will prove, the diagnosis. In later cases, enlargement of the inguinal nodes, secondary cutaneous rash, sore throat and positive serological reactions will be present.

A form of balanitis which is frequently very obstinate to treatment may occur in patients with diabetes mellitus. The main causative organism is *Candida albicans*. Phimosis appearing in an adult male is often due to unsuspected diabetes; the urine should always be tested for sugar.

Herpes genitalis

Herpes may attack the genital organs as part of a herpes zoster which is unilateral. This is a rarity compared with herpes simplex, which is now regarded as an important sexually transmitted disease. Recent work has implicated *Herpes simplex virus* Type 2 in the aetiology of uterine cervical cancer. The disease begins as a patch of erythema on the inner surface of the prepuce or on the glans penis, followed by vesicles and pustules; the latter become rubbed by the clothes, and form small ulcers. Herpes of the genital organs tends to recur, so that a previous history of a similar attack is often forthcoming. If seen during the vesicular stage no difficulty will be met with in the diagnosis; but if suppuration has followed, it must be diagnosed from a venereal sore. Soft chancres are usually deeper, with marked edges; their bases are sloughing, and they are usually accompanied by a bubo, which is exceptional with herpes. A syphilitic chancre is usually single, indurated and raised, and is accompanied by the typical multiple, discrete nodes in the inguinal region. It should be remembered that syphilis may become inoculated upon a herpetic patch or that herpes may appear in an area already infected with syphilis.

Soft sores or chancroids

Soft sores or chancroids of the penis occur almost invariably from infection during sexual connection. The incubation period is short, a vesicle occurs in 2 days, and this breaks down rapidly to form a rounded or oval ulcer with undermined edges and a yellowish sloughing base. The ulcers appear usually on the mucous surface of the glans, fraenum or corona, and are multiple, direct inoculation occurring from each ulcer to the contiguous part. They may cause rapid destruction of tissue, perforating the fraenum or spreading over the surface of the glans. The soft sore must be differentiated from others occurring on the glans, and above all from a syphilitic chancre, and serum from the edge of the lesion should be examined for *Haemophilus ducreyi* (Ducrey's bacillus) as well as by dark-ground illumination for *Treponema pallidum*. At the same time it must be remembered that besides the infection with chancroid, a simultaneous infection with syphilis may have taken place, so that a soft sore

may ultimately become indurated and assume the character of a primary syphilitic lesion. The chancroids are multiple, are accompanied by a good deal of thin, purulent discharge, and by a painful swelling of the inguinal nodes, usually of one side, which have a marked tendency to suppurate. On the other hand, a syphilitic chancre is single, is raised and indurated, has little discharge, and is accompanied by enlarged but firm and indolent nodes in both inguinal regions; the incubation period of a syphilitic chancre is from 21 to 28 days. The multiple ulcerations caused by herpes are more superficial, and rarely cause a bubo.

Granuloma inguinale

Granuloma inguinale (granuloma venereum) is a chronic granulomatous ulceration which may affect the perineum and the inguinal regions as well as the penis. It occurs in tropical countries and is mildly contagious. The lesion on the penis starts as a papule which appears after a few days' or weeks' incubation period and breaks down to form a superficial ulcer. Examination of the discharge shows intracellular capsulated bacteria known as Donovan bodies (*Donvania granulomatis*). Lymph nodes are not involved.

Lymphogranuloma venereum

Lymphogranuloma venereum (lymphogranuloma inguinale) is also commoner in the tropics, and is a chronic condition characterized by a small initial lesion on the penis with marked glandular enlargement in the groins and severe constitutional disturbances. The nodes tend to break down and form sinuses. The lesion on the penis appears, after an incubation period of about a week, as a vesicle, papule or ulcer, and it tends to disappear by the time the lymphatic nodes are enlarged. It is due to a filter-passing organism which is a member of the *Chlamydia* group and can be diagnosed by complement fixation reactions, demonstration of specific skin reactivity (Frei's test), and a biopsy of the primary lesion or lymph node. It must be distinguished from chancroid and from granuloma venereum. Rectal stricture and effusions into joints are other lesions caused by this disease.

Chancre

Chancre—the initial lesion of syphilis—generally appears on the penis, and is most common in the neighbourhood of the fraenum or coronary sulcus. A chancre appears about 25 days after infection as a reddened patch, which becomes raised above the surface of the mucous membrane, with distinctly indurated margins. The central part breaks down into

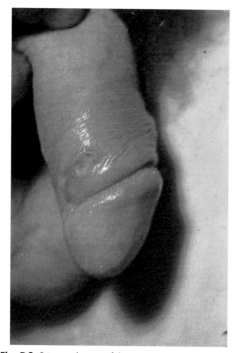

Fig. P.2. Primary chancre of the penis.

an ulcer (*Fig.* P.2), discharging a thin, purulent fluid, and at the same time the inguinal nodes of both sides become palpable, slightly enlarged, but discrete, and with no tendency to suppurate. The chancre increases but slowly in size, or may occasionally become smaller without any treatment, and after a further lapse of from 4 to 6 weeks the typical secondary symptoms make their appearance: namely, a roseolar rash on the chest, abdomen, face and thighs, general adenitis, and mucous patches about the faucial pillars and tonsils, accompanied by low pyrexia. The diagnosis of the primary lesion of syphilis frequently presents no difficulties, the indurated character of the sore, the date of its appearance after infection, and the presence of firm, indurated nodes in the inguinal region being distinctive. If the character of the sore is not distinctive it is necessary to differentiate it from other lesions of the penis. Careful search must be made by dark-ground illumination for the *Treponema pallidum* in the serum expressed from the sore; negative serological reactions in the early stage of the disease are not reliable. If the sore is syphilitic, the secondary manifestations of the disease will follow, provided that the doubtful ulcer is not treated as a chancre.

A chancre may be simulated by an inflamed soft sore; soft sores are, however, frequently multiple, appear within a few days of infection, and are accompanied by painful enlargement of the inguinal lymphatic nodes, which are particularly prone to suppurate. It must not be forgotten that a double infection may have occurred, so that a soft sore may show little inclination to heal or, becoming indurated, may present the features of a chancre after about 3 weeks, followed later by the symptoms of constitutional syphilis.

Epithelioma of the penis in the early stage may be confused with syphilitic chancre. In epithelioma there is no history of infection; it occurs usually in elderly uncircumcised patients, and there is frequently a greater destruction of tissue than in syphilis. The inguinal nodes are not enlarged until the sore has been present for some weeks, and there are no secondary lesions such as the faucial ulceration and cutaneous rash. Diagnosis is confirmed by histological examination of a biopsy specimen.

Perhaps the greatest difficulty in the diagnosis of a chancre is experienced when it is hidden beneath an inflamed and phimosed prepuce. There is a purulent and foul discharge from beneath the oedematous and swollen prepuce; the inguinal nodes are enlarged from the associated sepsis. If a chancre is present it can frequently be felt as an indurated area under the prepuce, while if it has been present for some time the secondary lesions of syphilis may be present. If any doubt exists as to whether an indurated subpreputial area is an early epithelioma or a syphilitic sore, the prepuce should be split up along the dorsal aspect under anaesthesia, the ulceration inspected, a small piece submitted to microscopical examination if necessary or some serum expressed from the ulcer examined on a dark stage for *Treponema pallidum*.

Epithelioma

Epithelioma (squamous-celled carcinoma) is the commonest form of malignant growth of the penis (*Fig.* P.3). It arises most frequently from the inner aspect of the prepuce, or from the mucous membrane of the glans, as a small, raised ulcer with friable, irregular edges. It is rarely present before the age of 40, and frequently occurs on the site of previous ulceration or long-standing irritation; it is unknown where circumcision has been performed in infancy, although later circumcision does not confer this near-total immunity. An *epitheliomatous ulcer* increases in size gradually in spite of various forms of treatment, and with it is frequently associated enlargement of the inguinal lymph nodes. At first the nodes may be enlarged from septic infection, but later from malignant infiltration. An epitheliomatous ulcer may in some cases be confused with a chancre; but the friable, irregular edges of the former, the liability to bleed, and the

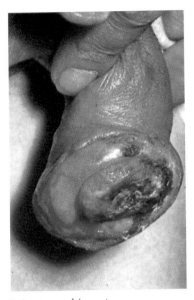

Fig. P.3. Carcinoma of the penis.

gradual progressive increase in size in spite of treatment, in an elderly patient, together with the extensive induration of the base, should give rise to grave suspicion of malignant disease. Microscopical examination of a small biopsy removed from the edge of the ulcer will give direct evidence of epithelioma.

Carcinoma of the penis may also occur in a *papillary form* which grows to produce a large cauliflower excrescence. In this type any enlargement of the inguinal nodes is more likely to be due to infection than to metastasis.

Papillomas

Papillomas (venereal warts or condylomata acuminata) occur on the glans and contiguous surface of the prepuce and are most frequently found on the corona. They are simple papillomas, usually multiple, and are distinguished from epithelioma by the absence of jyin-duration in the base.

Gummatous ulceration

Gummatous ulceration of the penis occurs today with great rarity, resulting from the disintegration of a small gumma of the glans or prepuce, frequently in the position of an old scar. A gumma begins as a small, elevated nodule, which, if left untreated, softens and discharges its contents, leaving an ulcer bounded by thin edges and with a yellowish, sloughy base.

Tuberculous ulceration

Tuberculous ulceration of the penis is rare, and is generally associated with advanced tuberculous infiltration elsewhere. Tuberculous ulcers are usually shallow, with thin overhanging edges, painful and multiple. The diagnosis is clinched by discovering tubercle bacilli in films made from the discharge.

Injury

Injury is an uncommon cause of a penile sore.

Harold Ellis

Penis, pain in

Pain in the penis is a symptom which occurs not only in association with lesions of the penis or urethra, but also as a referred pain from disease of the prostate, bladder or kidney. Penile pain may be present either during or immediately after micturition, or may be entirely independent of the act. If pain is felt only during micturition there is probably some inflammatory lesion of the urethra or prostate; if it occurs immediately after the flow of the urine it suggests some lesion in the urinary bladder; pain present quite apart from micturition may be due to various diseases of the penis, bladder, ureter or kidney.

The term 'pain', too, is a relative quantity, varying with the nervous susceptibility of the patient, for what is pain in one may be merely discomfort in another, so that the patient's description may have to be discounted to a certain extent by the clinician.

A. Causes of pain in the penis experienced during micturition

1. DISEASES OF THE URETHRA

acute inflammation, gonorrhoeal or other
the passage or impaction of a calculus
stricture of the urethra
injury of the urethra
foreign body in the urethra

2. DISEASES OF THE PROSTATE

acute prostatitis
prostatic carcinoma
prostatic abscess

3. DISEASES OF THE BLADDER

acute cystitis
vesical calculus
papilloma
pedunculated carcinoma

1. diseases of the urethra

The commonest cause of pain in the penis *during* micturition is acute inflammation of the urethra, usually gonorrhoeal, but may result from other organisms, and this is particularly common following catheterization (*see* URETHRAL DISCHARGE). In the earliest stages of an acute urethritis, before any marked urethral discharge is apparent, there is usually a sense of smarting or tingling in the terminal urethra, more marked as the discharge increases, when it is of a burning or scalding character. The pain during micturition within a few days of sexual connection is frequently the earliest symptom of urethral infection; a purulent discharge from the urethra is usually present when the patient comes under observation.

The *passage of a calculus* through the urethra cases a sharp, cutting pain along the urethra, the cause of which is apparent when the calculus is voided. Occasionally it may happen that micturition occurs in these cases in the dark, or that urine is not passed into a vessel, so that the calculus is not actually seen by the patient; but if there is a history of previous renal descent of a stone or symptoms pointing to vesical calculus, the sharp urethral pain during micturition occurring upon one single occasion is significant of the passage of a calculus. A stone may, however, pass into the urethra during micturition and become *arrested* at some narrowed portion of the canal, usually at the membranous portion or at the distal end, when a sudden, sharp pain is felt in the urethra, and at the same time the flow of urine is partially or completely stopped before the bladder has been emptied, further efforts to expel urine resulting only in a forceless stream; the whole length of the urethra should be examined by passing the finger along its course, when a stone may be actually felt; or the calculus may be seen through an endoscope or identified on a plain radiograph.

Occasionally a calculus may remain in the urethra, becoming gradually enlarged in size and causing pain on micturition. These calculi usually lie in the dilated posterior urethra behind a stricture in the bulb.

Urethral stricture occasionally causes pain in the urethra during micturition, especially if the calibre is small, and if there is septic infection or ulceration of the urethral mucosa behind the stricture, but as a rule stricture causes but little pain; gradually increasing difficulty in micturition, feeble stream and dribbling of urine from the meatus after the stream has terminated are common symptoms; the diagnosis will be confirmed by the obstruction offered to the passage of a full-sized bougie or, better, by direct observation of the urethra through a urethroscope under water distension.

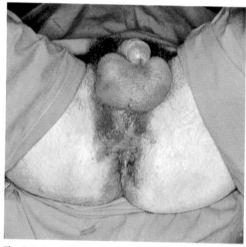

Fig. P.4. Traumatic rupture of the urethra showing blood from meatus and perineal haematoma limited posteriorly by the attachment of Colles' fascia.

Injury of the urethra may cause pain during micturition. The urethra may be injured by a fall on the perineum, by a kick or blow, or by the faulty or careless passage of instruments; it may also be injured or lacerated in association with a fracture of the pelvis. The urethra may be merely bruised, lacerated on one aspect or completely ruptured. If it is lacerated by direct injury blood usually appears at the external urinary meatus, together with a contusion in the perineum or along the course of the urethra; any attempt at micturition causes pain in the penis, while urine may or may not be expelled from the meatus, depending upon the extent of the injury, or may be extravasated into the perineal or scrotal tissues (*Fig. P.4*). As a rule there will be no difficulty in the diagnosis, but in any suspected case the greatest care should be exercised in passing an instrument into the urethra.

A *foreign body* in the urethra may cause considerable pain. In some cases the history will be clear; for instance the end of a catheter or bougie may have broken off within the urethra; but in others, especially in weak-minded individuals, no history of the insertion of a foreign body in the urethra will be forthcoming. Urethroscopy will show the foreign body; various articles have been found in the urethra, such as a wax taper, a seed of barley with its barb, a hairpin, a small shell, a nail and a glass tube used to contain hypodermic tablets.

2. Diseases of the prostate

Acute prostatitis and *prostatic abscess* both give rise to pain during micturition in addition to increased frequency and difficulty during the act. Both are usually sequelae of an acute urethritis, and whereas an acute prostatitis is accompanied by a temperature raised to 100–101°F (38°C), a prostatic abscess causes the usual rise and fall common to septic processes. The diagnosis of the two conditions is made by careful rectal examination, the acutely inflamed gland presenting a much enlarged, smooth-surfaced prominence in the rectum, while if an abscess is present a softer acutely tender area in the inflamed gland can usually be detected. An acute prostatitis may accompany a haematogenous bacterial urinary infection as distinct from a venereal urethritis.

Adenomatous enlargement of the prostate gives rise to no penile pain during micturition; but pain in the penis is present during micturition occasionally in cases of *prostatic carcinoma*, owing to the direct infiltration of the urethral mucous membrane. Prostatic carcinoma is by no means uncommon (indeed, it is the sixth commonest cause of death from cancer in the United Kingdom), and while in its general symptoms it resembles those of prostatic adenoma, there is a marked difference found on digital examination of the gland per rectum. The carcinomatous gland presents rounded areas of densely infiltrated tissue, in contradistinction to the elastic, uniform feel of the adenomatous variety; the whole gland becomes fixed and immovable, and in advanced stages distinct infiltration of the lateral pelvic lymphatics and soft tissues may be felt extending laterally from the affected organ. It is often tender on palpitation.

Care must be taken not to mistake the hard nodules felt in a prostate containing *calculi* for carcinoma; with calculous disease the gland is not fixed and is only slightly enlarged. During the passage of a catheter through the prostatic urethra distinct grating may be felt if any calculus has ulcerated the urethral wall. Radiography will distinguish the two conditions (*see Fig.* K. 15) but they may coexist.

3. Diseases of the bladder

Diseases of the bladder may cause penile pain during micturition under certain circumstances, although it is much more common to find that pain in vesical disease follows the completion of micturition. In *acute cystitis*, penile pain is present throughout micturition, due to the intense congestion of the vesical mucous membrane of the trigone and around the internal urethral orifice. The other symptoms of acute cystitis, namely suprapubic pain, pyrexia, increased frequency of micturition and the presence of pus and blood in the urine, suggest the diagnosis.

Pain during micturition in other vesical lesions is caused whenever there is sudden obstruction to the normal flow or urine by the impaction of something against the internal urethral orifice. This may occur with a small *calculus* or with a *pedunculated tumour*, whether simple or malignant, when during micturition the flow is arrested suddenly, accompanied by a shooting pain in the urethra, while after an interval of a few seconds the stream may be established. With vesical calculus the urine may be normal or may contain pus and blood if the bladder has become infected; there is penile pain after micturition, and the stone will be seen both on plain X-ray of the pelvis and with a cystoscope. With a simple villous papilloma there is no pain unless part of the fimbriated portion of the tumour engages in the urethral orifice during micturition, but there are usually recurrent attacks of profuse haematuria, while with a carcinoma there is increased frequency of micturition, with pain following the act and more frequent haematuria. Upon rectal examination the base of the bladder may be felt to be infiltrated, but by far the most valuable means of diagnosis between the three conditions is by cystoscopy, when a calculus or villous tumour is seen readily, whilst a pedunculated carcinoma appears as a dark red tumour covered with stunted processes.

B. Penile pain following micturition

This symptom is common to many lesions of the urinary bladder, more especially those in which there is ulceration or infiltration of the basal areas. The particular pain felt by the patient is described as a sharp pricking or tingling at the terminal part of the penis on the cessation of micturition, lasting some minutes and causing a desire to squeeze the glans. It was thought to be diagnostic of vesical calculus, but this is far from being the case, for it may be due to almost any affection of the trigone.

The common causes of pain in the penis following upon micturition are:

1.   VESICAL

Calculus
Tuberculosis
Tumour (carcinoma, papilloma)
Acute cystitis
Bilharzia

2.   URETERIC

Calculus in lower end
Tuberculous ureteritis

3.   PROSTATIC

Acute inflammation
Abscess

Calculus
Carcinoma

4. VESICULAR

Acute seminal vesiculitis

5. RECTAL

Carcinoma

6. ANAL

Fissure or ulcer
Inflamed haemorrhoids

1. Diseases of the bladder

A *calculus* in the bladder, unless it is trapped in the pouch behind an enlarged prostate or in a diverticulum, causes pain referred to the glans penis after micturition. It may exist without causing cystitis, although commonly there is some degree of pyuria when the case is first seen. There is increased frequency of micturition during active exercise or during the jolting of travelling, but not during complete rest unless cystitis is marked. The terminal drops of urine during micturition are often tinged with blood, and on some occasions there may have been a sudden stoppage of the stream during micturition. In some cases there is a history of acutely painful colic due to the descent of a stone from the kidney without the subsequent passage of a calculus in the urine. Patients subjected to vesical stone have usually reached the later part of life in this country, although bladder stones in children are still common in tropical parts, and although the symptoms are as a rule sufficiently marked to render the diagnosis easy, sometimes they may be so few that vesical calculus is unexpected, or the symptoms are so like those caused by other lesions of the bladder that error is easy. The great majority of vesical calculi are radio-opaque and can be seen on a plain X-ray of the pelvis. In such a case it is advisable to examine the interior of the bladder with a cystoscope, by which means stones can be seen, their approximate size determined, and any other conditions of the bladder accompanying or simulating calculus may be diagnosed with certainty.

Vesical tuberculosis is usually secondary to tuberculous disease in some other part of the genito-urinary tract, particularly the kidney. It causes marked penile pain after micturition, together with pyuria and a tinge of blood in the terminal drops of urine; the frequency of micturition is increased during both day and night, and is uninfluenced by rest, thus differing from the increased frequency of calculous disease. Vesical tuber-

culosis occurs in young adults and is usually associated with renal tuberculosis in which symptoms referable to the bladder are commonly present before the bladder is attacked by disease. In a young patient in whom increased frequency of micturition, pyuria and penile pain are present, a search should be made for any tuberculous focus, especially in the kidneys by excretion urography, and in the epididymes, prostate or seminal vesicles, or for marked thickening of the terminal ureter as felt per rectum, and a careful search should be made for acid-fast tubercle bacilli in the urine. The deposit from three early morning specimens should be examined, and if this is negative, search should be continued by culture. A cystoscopic examination may be necessary to determine the extent of the disease.

Vesical tumours. Carcinoma of the bladder occurs in a papillary or a solid form. Papillary carcinoma is at first non-infiltrating, while the solid nodular and ulcerative types and adenocarcinoma are infiltrating. They begin most commonly in the base of the bladder, except the urachal adenocarcinoma, which arises in the dome; the submucous coat and the muscular wall become infiltrated by malignant cells so that contraction of the bladder during micturition causes pain referred to the terminal portion of the urethra. All forms occur in elderly patients, mostly men, and give rise to increased frequency of micturition during both day and night, and to haematuria. They also often give rise to renal pain when the infiltration has extended to the ureteric orifice in bladder.

The incidental cystogram of intravenous urography (*Figs* P.5, P.6) may sometimes afford visual proof of the deformity the new growth is producing or of a filling defect in the otherwise regular contour of the bladder.

Under anaesthesia the base of the bladder may be felt per rectum to be thickened, or lymphatic infiltration may be felt in the lateral pelvic space, and a cystoscopic examination, together with biopsy, will usually clear up the diagnosis.

Whereas solid infiltrating growths of the bladder give rise to penile pain after micturition from the direct infiltration of the vesical walls, the pedunculated papillary carcinoma and the simple villous papilloma may occasionally give rise to sharp penile pain during micturition from blocking of the internal urethral orifice by a process of growth. The occurrence of this, together with attacks of profuse haematuria, is suggestive of a pedunculated growth. On cystoscopic examination the carcinomatous pedunculated tumour is seen to be covered by blunt, stunted processes, whereas the innocent villous papilloma presents much more delicate fimbriae.

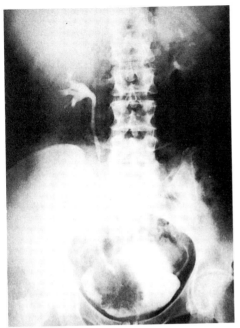

Fig. P.5. An intravenous pyelogram and cystogram taken 20 minutes after injection. There is a filling defect on the right sides of the bladder due to a large benign papilliferous tumour. Both kidneys are normal.

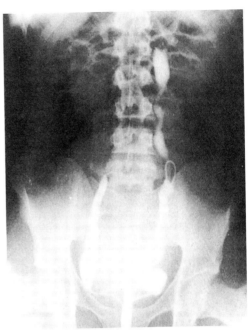

Fig. P.7. Dilatation of ureters following stricture of their lower ends in a case of vesical schistosomiasis. From a man of 20 who lived in East Africa. Demonstrated by retrograde pyelography.

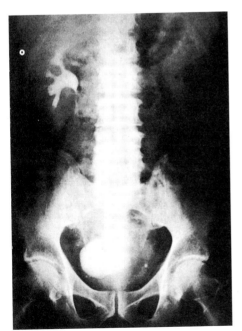

Fig. P.6. An intravenous pyelogram and cystogram taken 20 minutes after injection. There is a solid defect in the left side of the bladder caused by an infiltrating carcinoma. The left ureter is obstructed and there is no function in the obstructed left kidney.

Acute cystitis causes tingling pain in the penis after micturition from the inflammatory infiltration of the trigonal area. The mode of onset, the character of the pain and other symptoms of cystitis will point to the cause of the pain.

Bilharzia haematobia gives rise to clinical symptoms very similar to those of vesical tuberculosis. The history of residence in an infected district (e.g. Egypt or East Africa), microscopical examination of the urine for ova, and the typical cystoscopic appearance of the bladder establish the diagnosis.

Radiographs may show calcification of the bladder or ureters and pyelography often demonstrates stricture formation and gross dilatation of the ureters (*Fig.* P.7).

2. Ureteric lesions

Ureteric lesions not infrequently produce pain in the glans penis after micturition, and may cause considerable difficulty in the diagnosis from vesical disease.

When a *calculus* becomes impacted in the narrowed terminal or intramural portion of the ureter, symptoms are produced almost exactly similar to those of vesical calculus or tuberculosis, namely increased frequency of micturition, pain in the glans penis after

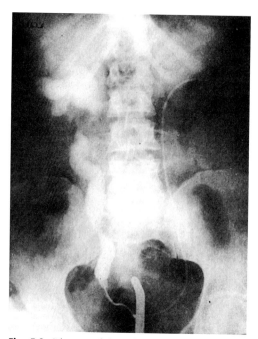

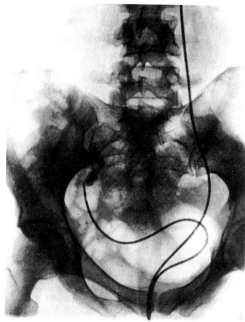

Fig. P.8. Dilatation of the right ureter due to a calculus impacted at its lower end (retrograde pyelogram).

Fig. P.9. A radiograph showing the tip of a radio-opaque catheter obstructed by a calculus in the right ureter.

micturition, and a small amount of pus and blood in the urine. Intimate knowledge of the history of the illness will often be of value in these cases; the first attack of pain is usually described as being sudden, and felt in the renal angle posteriorly, passing forwards above the iliac crest and spine and finally becoming localized at the situation of the external abdominal ring. The calculus may become impacted in the terminal inch of the ureter, when, in addition to this pain, there will be increased frequency of micturition and penile pain, and possibly haematuria. With ureteric calculus there is usually aching pain in the kidney of the affected side from the dilatation of its pelvis. The diagnosis of these cases is not difficult if a careful inquiry is made into the history and symptoms, and so long as it is remembered that increased frequency of micturition and penile pain may be caused by ureteric impaction of a calculus; a good radiographic examination of the pelvic areas may show the shadow of a stone. Indeed, some 90 per cent of these calculi are radio-opaque but, when small, may mimic phleboliths or be obscured by gas shadows or underlying bony structures (*Fig.* P.8). The stone itself may be felt occasionally as a small, painful nodule on pelvic examination, especially in women. A cystoscopic examination also affords valuable information, not only in excluding vesical lesions, but by giving a distinct indication of ureteric calculus by the marked congestion and dilatation of the blood vessels in the immedi-

ate vicinity of the ureteric orifice. An intravenous pyelogram may demonstrate obstruction of the ureter and confirm that the calculus lies in its lumen. A small bougie passed into the ureter may meet with obstruction in its passage; a stereoscopic radiograph of the pelvis with an opaque bougie passed into the ureter will show the shadow to be in the immediate line of the ureter (*Fig.* P.9).

Ureteritis descending from infection of the renal pelvis may give rise to slight penile pain and to increased frequency of micturition, and thus simulate vesical disease before the bladder is actually infected. This is seen most commonly in the *tuberculous* form, but is present in a less marked degree with infection by other organisms, of which the most common are *Escherichia coli communis* and *Streptococcus faecalis*. In the non-tuberculous form the ureter may be felt per rectum to be slightly thickened, but the cystoscopic appearance of the inflamed ureteric orifice is distinctive. In *descending tuberculosis* from the kidney, the ureter may be felt as a firm, infiltrated cord on the bladder base, the penile pain and increased frequency of micturition are more marked, the kidney may be felt enlarged and tender, and tubercle bacilli will be found in the urine. Apart from this, typical changes in the ureteric orifice are seen on cystoscopic examination, the orifice being pulled up or retracted or horseshoe-shaped, and usually occupying a position slightly above and outside the situation of the normal orifice, due to the actual shortening of the ureter by infiltration of the submucous coats. The rigid 'golf-hole' ureteric orifice is a late manifestation caused by contraction of scar tissue around it and in the ureter above it.

3. Diseases of the prostate

These often cause pain in the penis immediately following micturition. This is seen most commonly with acute inflammation or abscess in the gland as a sequela of acute gonorrhoea or septic urethritis. In either case there is penile pain, sometimes associated with erection, but little difficulty will be experienced in the diagnosis on due consideration of the symptoms and upon rectal examination.

Prostatic calculi are not uncommon there may be a single calculus or a nest of them in the prostate. They may ulcerate into the urethra so that small calculi may be passed in the urinary stream, or some may pass back along the dilated prostatic urethra into the bladder. If a calculus projects from the prostate into the urethra it causes pain in the penis after micturition. A diagnosis of prostatic calculus is often made by the grating sensation imparted to a catheter in traversing the prostatic urethra, whilst on rectal examination the calculus may be felt as an isolated hard nodule in the gland (where it may mimic prostatic carcinoma), or, if more than one is present, by the crepitation of one upon another on digital pressure in the rectum. A radiograph of the pelvis will show the shadows of prostatic calculi at the level of the upper part of the pubic symphysis (*see Fig.* K.14).

4. Diseases of the seminal vesicles

These are seldom present without accompanying disease of the prostate of bladder. Acute vesiculitis may follow urethritis and give rise to pain after micturition, but in most cases it will be associated with prostatitis. Similarly, tuberculous nodules in the vesicle will be associated with foci in the epididymis, prostate or bladder.

5, 6. Diseases of the rectum and anus

These may occasionally give rise to penile pain following micturition, apart from any infection of the bladder or prostate. Thus an infiltrating carcinoma in the anal canal, an anal fissure or an inflamed haemorrhoid may occasionally cause pain in the penis, but in each the local symptoms of the trouble will be the more marked, and little difficulty will be found in the diagnosis if a local examination is made with care.

C. Pain in the penis apart from micturition

Under the above divisions the symptom of penile pain has been considered in relation to the act of micturition, and it remains to consider some conditions giving rise to pain in the penis *apart from urination*. These include certain local lesions of the penis and urethra, and also the pains referred from disease elsewhere. Although a local lesion may cause little more than discomfort in many patients, in some it is described as pain, the degree of which depends upon the nervous susceptibility of the individual. Thus penile pain may be present with *acute urethritis*, with *balanitis* in association with *phimosis*, with *paraphimosis*, or with the *lymphangitis* of the organ due to a septic sore or abrasion of the skin or mucous membrane. In some instances *herpes* of the prepuce or penile skin causes distinct pain. Any infiltration of the cavernous tissue of the penis causes pain during erection of the organ; thus during an attack of acute urethritis the symptom known as *chordee* arises from this cause. It may occur in a chronic form in Peyronie's disease (chronic indurative cavernositis), a condition of unknown aetiology but similar to, and sometimes associated with, Dupuytren's contracture and retroperitoneal fibrosis. In this condition erection is not only painful but may be accompanied by lateral deviation of the organ. Another condition causing the same trouble arises from the organization of a haematoma in the cavernous tissues of the penis following upon a local injury, due either to external violence or arising during forcible attempts at coitus. A similar condition may arise spontaneously in blood diseases, especially *lymphatic* or *myelocytic leukaemia*.

Epithelioma of the penis on rare occasions and in advanced disease gives rise to pain in the organ.

Pain may be felt in the penis in some cases of *renal colic*, in which case it is classed as a referred pain. Thus in the acute colic accompanying the passage of a calculus, blood clot or debris of caseous material, aching pain may be felt in the penis quite apart from the increased desire to pass urine. Penile pain is, however, only a minor detail in the presence of the severe pain in the loin, and along the course of the ureter, and is often only lightly alluded to or revealed on direct questioning of the patient.

Finally, pain in the penis may be based on an anxiety state or some other mental cause rather than organic disease.

Harold Ellis

Perineal pain

Pain in the perineum is a symptom often mentioned by patients in giving their history of some affection of the genito-urinary apparatus or of other organs, but usually only as a dull aching, of which little notice is taken, as it is generally of minor degree in comparison with other more striking symptoms. The complaint of perineal pain *per se* does not convey much information to the clinician, and it is practically never present as the only symptom in a case. It may be a manifestation of an anxiety state.

Aching in the perineum is frequently present in diseases of the following organs:

PROSTATE

Acute or subacute inflammation
Abscess
Chronic prostatitis
Tuberculosis
Calculus
Adenomatous enlargement
Carcinoma

SEMINAL VESICLES

Acute inflammation
Tuberculosis

TESTICLE

Congenital misplacement in perineum

URINARY BLADDER

Cystitis
Tuberculosis
Calculus
Carcinoma

URETHRA

Gonorrhoea
Injury and rupture
Stricture with extravasation or urethral abscess
Fistula
Calculus impacted in bulbo-prostatic portion

ANAL AREA

Haemorrhoids
Fissure
Follicular abscess
Carbuncle
Ulcer
Carcinoma

VAGINA

Acute inflammation
Inflammation or abscess of Bartholin's glands
Cystocele
Epithelioma

CUTANEOUS DISEASES

Intertrigo
Diabetic inflammation
Condylomas

From the foregoing list it will be seen that aching in the perineum occurs with numerous different lesions, but other symptoms discussed elsewhere are in almost every case more marked. In prostatic disease it is an indication of inflammation rather than of enlargement. In clinical practice it is most commonly found to be due to chronic inflammation of the prostate gland. Examination of the secretion expressed after prostatic massage will show the presence of many pus cells.

Harold Ellis

Perineal sores

Ulceration may be present in the perineum as the result of:

1 Cutaneous inflammation or injury
2 Urethral suppurations or fistulas
3 Prostatic suppuration
4 Anal fistula
5 Syphilis
6 Granuloma venereum (inguinale)
7 Lymphogranuloma inguinale (venereum)
8 Epithelioma and other cutaneous cancers
9 Carcinoma of the urethra

1. Cutaneous inflammation or injury

An ulcer in the perineum may result from *direct injury* to the area, or from inflammatory *infection of the sebaceous* or *hair follicles*. An ulcer from these causes may be placed at the centre or to one side of the perineum, is movable on the deeper parts, and shows no track into which a probe can be passed. In women, ulceration of the perineal area may be associated with *gonorrhoeal* or *septic vaginal discharge*. It may also arise from severe scratching caused by the irritation of such skin infections as *tinea cruris* or *pruritus ani*.

2. Urethral suppurations or fistulas

During the progress of an acute urethritis a glandular follicle may become infected. The suppurative process leading from this in the bulbous urethra may extend towards the perineum and open externally, leaving a small fistula which may or may not discharge urine during the act of micturition. In a similar manner urinary fistulas may result from inflammatory processes behind a urethral stricture, and in an old-standing case it is not uncommon to find a urinary calculus in the dilated portion of the urethra behind the stricture. When the urethral suppuration is acute and an abscess bursts in the perineum, the diagnosis will be obvious, and the ordinary treatment for an abscess, in addition to that of the acute urethritis, will usually suffice to cure the condition. If the perineal wound discharges urine this occurs as a rule only during the act of micturition, as there is no interference with the vesical sphincter; a stricture of the urethra, not necessarily of sufficient degree to cause severe interference with micturition, will generally be seen on endoscopic examination, the sloughy granulations behind it denoting the position of the urethral opening of the fistula.

3. Diseases of the prostate

An abscess or tuberculous focus in the prostate may occasionally discharge in the perineum, and remain as a sinus. An abscess in the prostate arises practically always from some infection in the posterior urethra, from venereal causes, or after septic instrumentation. It is accompanied by urethral discharge, or there is a history of a recent infection, whilst per rectum the prostate may be felt to be inflamed, or scarred from the shrinkage of the abscess cavity.

When a tuberculous cavity in the prostate opens in the perineum there is advanced tuberculous disease, so that little difficulty will be found in arriving at a diagnosis. A tuberculous prostate is very rarely a primary condition, but in most cases is secondary to disease in the kidney, epididymis or bladder, so that examination of these organs will in nearly all cases give evidence of tuberculous disease and indicate the nature of the perineal fistula. Palpation of the prostate per rectum may reveal the rounded nodular deposits of tubercle in the gland.

4. Anal fistula

An ulcer on the perineum may be present as the result of an anal fistula — commonly from perianal suppuration and occasionally as a tuberculous infection. The history of pain on defecation followed by the rupture of a suppurating focus and the history of passage of flatus or faecal matter from the fistula are usually present, or a probe may be passed into the fistula and felt by a finger passed into the rectum.

Perianal and perirectal abscesses, fissures and fistulas may occur in Crohn's disease, especially when the colon is involved, and less commonly in ulcerative colitis.

5. Syphilis

Syphilis may cause ulceration on the perineum either as a chancre or as mucous tubercles. A *chancre* at this site is rare. It forms a small ulcer with slightly indurated borders, indolent in character, and accompanied by slight enlargement of the inguinal lymph nodes. A chancre of the skin may not possess the usual features of a genital chancre, and is not usually diagnosed with certainty until the secondary lesions of syphilis become apparent; but an ulcer with raised, infiltrated edges, which shows no tendency to heal under aseptic precautions, should always give rise to a suspicion of syphilis. The *Treponema pallidum* should be looked for, under darkground illumination, and serological tests for syphilis performed.

Condylomas may be present about the perineum in association with active syphilis. They may extend from the anal or vulval orifice, and form oval or rounded, flat-topped, sessile masses, covered by macerated greyish epithelium, or they may be ulcerated on the surface. The accompanying signs of syphilis will indicate the diagnosis.

Soft sores may occur in the perineum as well as on the scrotum or the vulva; they are generally venereal, but are not in themselves syphilitic; they are generally multiple, are apt to be foul, and cultures from them yield Ducrey's bacillus (*Haemophilus ducreyi*).

6, 7. Ulceration of granuloma inguinale

Ulceration of granuloma inguinale sometimes attacks the perineum, and fistulas there can be caused by lymphogranuloma venereum (*see* PENILE SORES).

8, 9. Epitheliomatous ulceration

Epitheliomatous ulceration of the perineum is seen as a direct spread of a growth of the anus or vulval area, when the diagnosis presents no difficulty. An epithelioma may develop in the scar of some former cutaneous affection, particularly in long-standing fistula in ano, in which case an ulceration may exist showing the usual characteristics of a cutaneous epithelioma. The inguinal nodes may be enlarged early from the inflammatory absorption, or later by invasion with malignant disease. Other cutaneous cancers, malignant melanoma and basal-cell carcinoma, may also occur in this situation. In case of doubt a fragment may be removed for microscopical examination. In late cases of carcinoma of the urethra following urethral stricture malignant ulceration spreads to the perineum by direct extension.

Harold Ellis

Peristalsis, visible

(*See also* BORBORYGMI)

Usually visible peristalsis is pathological. However, in a number of conditions the normal movements of the bowel may be visible; these circumstances are divarication of the abdominal recti muscles, an incisional or massive umbilical hernia containing bowel, and extreme thinness of the abdominal parietes—the result of emaciation or, rarely, congenital absence of the recti. It is not uncommon to see visible peristalsis within the sac of a very large ventral or inguinoscrotal hernia (*Fig.* P.10). In all these circumstances the diagnosis can be made at inspection and the patient is otherwise symptomless. In all other situations, visible peristalsis is pathological and may be of two types, gastric and intestinal.

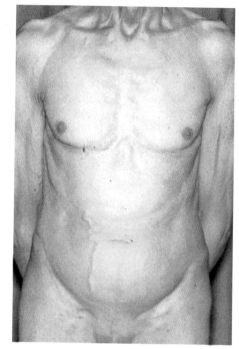

Fig. P.11. Gross gastric dilatation due to a stenosing duodenal ulcer. The stomach was visible, gave a loud splash, and showed typical gastric peristalsis.

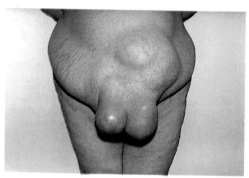

Fig. P.10. Visible peristalsis was obvious in this large thin-walled umbilical hernia.

Gastric peristalsis

Gastric peristalsis takes the form of a comparatively large swelling in the upper abdomen showing slow waves of peristalsis which progress from under the region of the left ribs, slowly downwards and to the right. This swelling indicates obstruction to the gastric outlet. There may be other signs of gastric dilatation and distension, particularly a loud succussion splash (*Fig.* P.11). Typically there is a history of the vomiting of large amounts of liquid in a projectile manner which may contain fragments of food ingested 24 hours or more previously. The diagnosis can be confirmed by the passage of a nasogastric tube, which will yield a pint or more of fluid several hours after the last food or drink has been taken; the aspirate has a typical stale, unpleasant smell and may contain recognizable particles of food eaten even several days before. A barium X-ray examination will clinch the diagnosis by demonstrating the gastric retention and dilatation. An X-ray

taken 6 or 8 hours after the ingestion of the barium is particularly valuable since this will confirm the extent of gastric holdup (*Fig.* P.12). In doubtful cases of visible gastric peristalsis, the sign may be accentuated by asking the patient to swallow several glasses of soda-water. In the normal subject no peristalsis is seen, but in cases of pyloric obstruction, previously invisible peristalsis may now become obvious.

In congenital hypertrophic pyloric stenosis of infancy not only can gastric peristalsis be seen after a drink from a bottle but the hypertrophied pylorus can often be felt. This interesting and eminently treatable condition becomes apparent not immediately, but some 4 weeks after birth.

Visible intestinal peristalsis

Visible intestinal peristalsis is a feature of advanced intestinal obstruction with the limitations discussed above. As a pathological entity it will not occur alone but is accompanied by colicky abdominal pain, abdominal distension, vomiting and absolute constipation. The discussion of the differential diagnosis of the different causes of the symptoms will be found elsewhere. If the small intestine alone is involved, the

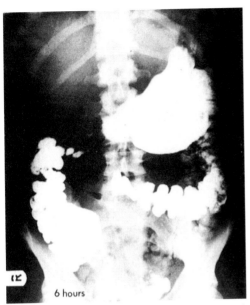

Fig. P.12. Six hours after ingesting barium this patient, with gross pyloric stenosis due to duodenal ulceration and with obvious visible gastric peristalsis, still has considerable residue in the stomach. Note that the barium which has escaped through the stenosis has already reached the splenic flexure.

waves are multiple and run more or less transversely across the abdomen—the ladder pattern; when the colon is obstructed, peristalsis takes the form of vertical waves, especially in one or both flanks, but this is much more rarely seen. Plain radiographs of the abdomen taken in the erect and supine positions are invaluable; the first demonstrate multiple fluid levels, the second the distribution of gas shadows within the dilated loops of bowel which will often enable the clinician to determine whether small or large bowel is obstructed. (*See also* p. 63 and *Figs* C.1, C.2.)

Harold Ellis

Pilimiction

Pilimiction, that is the passage of hairs in the urine, a rare condition which almost invariably signifies that the patient has a pelvic dermoid cyst that has become inflamed, thereafter opening into the bladder and discharging its contents via the urinary passages, has been observed in men, but it is less uncommon in women. Subacute or acute cystitis accompanies the event with vesical pain, frequency of micturition and pyuria. The obvious fallacy in diagnosis arises from the possibility of contamination in the urine of hairs which were not, as supposed, passed per urethram.

Harold Ellis

Pneumaturia

The passage of gas per urethram, either with or independently of urine, is a rare but striking peculiarity, particularly when it occurs in males. It may be due to one or other of two distinct groups of causes, namely:

1 Communications between the rectum, sigmoid colon, caecum, vermiform appendix or other part of the alimentary canal and the bladder, ureter or renal pelvis, either directly or via an intermediate gas-containing abscess cavity.
2 Infection of the bladder or other part of the urinary tract by gas-producing microorganisms.

When the cause lies in the first group, the patient is apt to pass faecal material as well as gas. It should be added, however, that the passage of gas without faeces per urethram by no means excludes a fistulous communication between some part of the alimentary canal and the urinary tract: the fistula may be of such a character that while gas can traverse it faeces cannot. It may also happen that a lesion such as appendicitis or, most commonly, acute sigmoid diverticulitis has led to the formation of a local abscess which, owing to infection by the *Escherichia coli*, contains gas; this abscess may open into the bladder and cause the discharge of pus and gas, but no faeces, per urethram. The same applies to similar abscesses which though not arising primarily in connection with the bowel nevertheless contain gas from infection by the *E. coli*—for instance, a suppurating hydatid or ovarian dermoid cyst, or a pyosalpinx. Rectal, vaginal, abdominal, barium-enema X-ray, intravenous pyelographic and cystoscopic examinations may yield the diagnosis, but on occasion doubt will persist as to whether the gas is finding its way into the urinary passages from some external source, or whether it is being produced in situ, for certain organisms, notably *E. coli* and *Aspergillus aerogenes*, produce gas when they grow in urine, as may various *yeasts* in patients with glycosuria.

If no sign of a fistulous communication between any part of the bowel or a gas-containing abscess cavity with the urinary tract can be distinguished on cystoscopic examination, it may be with confidence presumed that the pneumaturia is due to infection. Such patients are usually elderly female diabetics with considerable glycosuria. The infecting organisms are usually *E. coli.*, *A. aerogenes*, *yeasts* or combinations of these.

The urine in such a case contains pus, sugar, and albumin. It may be acid, and not foul-smelling or ammoniacal; on the other hand, it may sometimes be so foul and faeculent as to arouse unwarranted suspicion of a communication between the colon and the bladder. A cystoscopic examination will serve to exclude a fistulous opening into the bladder, but it may be much more difficult to exclude a similar communication with the higher parts of the urinary tract, especially the renal pelvis. Such a condition is very rare, so that urinary infection is the more probable unless there is a known or recognizable cause for communication between the bowel and the renal pelvis, such as a carcinoma.

Harold Ellis

Popliteal swelling

Popliteal swellings may be divided into:

1. FLUID SWELLINGS

Bursa
Morrant Baker's cyst
Varicose veins
Abscess
Aneurysm

2. SOLID SWELLINGS NOT CONNECTED WITH BONE

Enlarged lymph nodes
Malignant tumours
Innocent tumours

3. SOLID SWELLINGS CONNECTED WITH BONE

Exostosis
Sarcoma
Periostitis
Separation of the epiphysis

1. fluid swellings

BURSAE

There are four primary bursae associated with muscles and tendons around the posterior aspect of the knee. Communications between two bursae and between a bursa and the knee joint are common.

The semimembranosus bursa on the posterior aspect of the knee is often enlarged. When the leg is extended it stands out as a tense fluctuating swelling on the inner side of the popliteal space: on flexion it disappears completely. It may be found enlarged in young athletes and cause no symptoms whatever. On account of its fairly frequent communication with the knee joint it may be distended when that joint is the seat of an effusion, acting, as it were, as an overflow tank. Where the joint condition is an acute one the bursa may be very tender. In rheumatoid arthritis it is

common for fluid to pass from joint into bursa but not in the reverse direction, a ball-valve mechanism apparently operating.

The bursae under either of the two heads of the gastrocnemius muscle or those connected with the insertion of the semitendinosus may be enlarged similarly, but these are rare.

MORRANT BAKER'S CYST

This is a herniation of the synovial membrane and only occurs in connection with chronic inflammatory changes in the joint, most commonly in rheumatoid arthritis, but the semimembranosus bursa is usually also affected and is also distended. The extension from the joint tends to spread along fascial planes and may point at varying distances from its origin. The 'cysts' may be multiple. Such extensions of the knee joint may sometimes rupture and cause an inflammatory reaction in the calf muscles which may be mistaken for a deep venous thrombosis. Arthrography may be of help in diagnosis.

VARICOSE VEINS

Varicose veins, varices of the small saphenous vein, are often present in the popliteal space; the diagnosis presents no difficulties, as the veins in the lower part of the leg will also be varicose. They become much more obvious when the patient stands.

These are the most common causes, the conditions which follow being much more rarely encountered.

ACUTE ABSCESS

This is recognized by the signs of acute inflammation; the skin is red and oedematous, the pulse and temperature are raised, and the swelling is very painful. The knee is kept flexed in order to minimize the tension of the part. The abscess may be caused by suppurating lymphatic nodes or by suppurative periostitis or necrosis of the lower end of the femur. In the former case the abscess will be superficial, and in the latter deep to the popliteal vessels.

ANEURYSM OF THE POPLITEAL ARTERY

This gives rise to an expansile pulsating tumour, the pulsation being synchronous with the heart's beat. Pressure on the femoral artery above will cause a diminution in size of the swelling and cessation of pulsation. The pulse at the ankle on the affected side may be smaller than that on the opposite, and delayed.

If a stethoscope be placed over the swelling a distinct bruit can be heard.

The complaint of the patient will probably be of pain, which may be referred down the leg if either the tibial or the common peroneal nerve is pressed on, or in the site of the swelling if the bone is eroded. Varicose veins are almost always present on account of pressure on the popliteal vein. Owing to its pulsatile character an aneurysm is not often mistaken for anything else, but every swelling that pulsates is not an aneurysm. A soft vascular sarcoma growing from the end of the femur may be pulsatile, and over it a bruit may be heard, but the tumour is not as compressible as an aneurysm is and the effects on the distal pulse are not so marked. A radiograph will usually settle the question at once. Distinction must also be drawn between a tumour that pulsates and a tumour to which pulsation is communication. For instance, an abscess or a solid swelling lying over the popliteal artery may appear to pulsate, but the movement is heaving in character and not expansile. In the rare event of an aneurysm having become filled with clot it might be taken for a solid tumour growing either from the soft parts or from the bone. Finally the aneurysm may present on the medial side of the lower end of the thigh, anterior to the tendon of the sartorius. The diagnosis and exact configuration of the aneurysm can be confirmed by arteriography or the non-interventional Doppler duplex ultrasound scan.

2. Solid swellings not connected with bone

ENLARGED NODES

It is not common to find the popliteal nodes enlarged from any cause. It is possible that they may become infected with pyogenic organisms from a sore on the back of the leg.

TUMOURS

Tumours are rare. They may be innocent, e.g. *lipoma* and *neurofibroma*; or *sarcomatous*, starting in the connective tissue of the popliteal space, or attached to one of the muscles. The innocent tumours are of long history and well defined; the malignant, rapidly growing and infiltrating.

A lipomatous mass, either in the popliteal fossa or on the medial aspect of the knee, is not infrequently present in osteoarthritis of this joint, and is part of the general fatty infiltration which gives rise inside the joint to the *lipoma arborescens* of the synovial membrane. Exact delineation of these tumours can be

made by MRI scanning and pathological diagnosis established by biopsy.

3. Solid swellings connected with bone

In all cases of bony tumour a radiograph should always be obtained.

INNOCENT TUMOURS

Cancellous exostoses may be found, generally in children and young adults, growing from the region of the epiphysial cartilage of the femur. There may be others in other parts of the skeleton, and sometimes several members of the family are similarly affected. The swelling is of slow growth, well defined and rarely gives any trouble. It is most often found at the inner side of the popliteal space. There is one thing that may be confounded with it, namely, *ossification of the insertion of a tendon* or muscle. The adductor longus muscle is the one most commonly affected (rider's bone).

Osteoclastoma is prone to occur in the bones around the knee joint and may cause an asymmetrical expansion of the cortex presenting in the popliteal fossa. Usually expansion of the bone can be detected on other aspects and the shell may be so thin in some places if the condition is advanced that 'eggshell crackling' can be elicited. The radiographic appearances are typical—the expansion and thinning of the cortex, the absence of new bone formation and the trabeculation. The epiphysis is involved in the process but the articular cartilage is seldom perforated (*see Fig.* B.26).

MALIGNANT TUMOURS

These include osteosarcoma, fibrosarcoma arising from the fibrous periosteum and metastases from neoplasm elsewhere. Here, as in giant-cell tumour, enlargement of the bone is not usually confined to the popliteal space. The diagnosis from inflammatory lesions can be very difficult even with a radiograph, and is often impossible without. The type of osteosarcoma which shows a palisade of bony spicules perpendicular to the line of the cortex is easily diagnosed by radiography, but it must be remembered that a sarcoma may present itself with an obvious clinical swelling and yet with little or no radiographic changes. This usually but not always denotes a *fibrosarcoma of the periosteum*, particularly if a thin line of periosteal new bone is laid down. Occasionally a small central area of erosion with a clinical swelling may indicate the presence of a bone sarcoma of the osteolytic type. Although there may be marked swelling, there is usually less effusion into the joint than is the case if the lesion is inflammatory. Computerized tomography is useful in providing accurate anatomical delineation of the tumour mass. Serological tests and a biopsy of the diseased part should be done in all doubtful bone lesions. A *gumma* is indicated by dense sclerosis around the lesion, clear-cut central softening without erosion, and regular bone formation. For further details and illustrations *see* the article on BONE, SWELLING OF.

PERIOSTITIS

Popliteal necrosis with abscess formation may give rise to a large swelling. The signs of inflammation will usually be well marked and accompanied by constitutional symptoms and leucocytosis. Chronic periostitis, or chronic abscess of the bone, or central necrosis, may be extremely difficult to distinguish from a malignant growth. A radiograph should be taken, and if necessary an incision made down to the tumour for a piece to be removed for histological examination.

SEPARATION OF THE EPIPHYSIS

In the somewhat rare accident of separation of the lower epiphysis of the femur the lower fragment becomes displaced backwards, forms a prominence in the popliteal space, and presses on the vessels sometimes to a dangerous extent. It is unlikely that such a condition would present itself as a doubtful popliteal swelling for diagnosis.

Harold Ellis

Priapism

'Priapism' (*see also* PENILE PAIN) signifies erection of the penis, persistent, of troublesome degree and not necessarily accompanied by sexual desire. Though generally spoken of in connection with the male sex, a precisely similar affection may occur in the female clitoris. The symptom is not often by itself of diagnostic importance. Though it may be due to a considerable number of different conditions, the ultimate cause is usually thrombosis in the vascular spaces in the cavernous tissue which are found to contain thick black grumous blood.

The important causes are:

1 After injury to the upper dorsal region of the spinal cord. The damage may have produced fracture-dislocation of the spine with paraplegia, in which case the diagnosis will be obvious; short of this, however, a minor degree of injury, with contusion and small haemorrhages into the substance of the cord, may be followed by painful priapism, persisting sometimes for weeks before recov-

ery occurs. Cerebrospinal syphilis or tumour may also rarely be responsible.

2 In leukaemia; apart from obvious change in the penis—cavernous haemorrhage or the like—priapism has been noted in both myelocytic and lymphatic leukaemia even before the other symptoms and signs have led to a haematological diagnosis. The cause of the priapism in leukaemia is obscure, but the diagnosis is suggested by the concomitant splenomegaly and/or lymphadenopathy and is confirmed by the haematological findings.

3 Sickle-cell anaemia.

4 New growths of the urethra, either primary or secondary to carcinoma of the bladder or testis.

5 Trauma with haematoma formation.

Chronic intermittent priapism is the term used to describe frequently repeated erections which are of long duration but lack the persistence of true priapism. The attacks occur in the night and may or may not be associated with sexual desire. They are due to nerve irritation arising from lesions of the central nervous system or from local lesions in the posterior urethra, prostate or seminal vesicles. In elderly men they are frequently associated with enlargement of the prostate.

Seldom will priapism be the only symptom in the case; the diagnosis will be made from the history and from the other symptoms.

Harold Ellis

Pruritus ani

Pruritus ani, the sensation of itching around the anal verge, is a common symptom. In more than half the patients, no obvious cause can be found (idiopathic pruritis) but in every case the following checklist should be considered:

1 The pruritus may be the result of a general disease associated with itching. Examples are lymphoma, advanced renal failure, severe jaundice and diabetes mellitus. The latter is often associated with *Candida albicans* infection (thrush) and this may occur, of course, in the nondiabetic patient. Moreover, *Candida* is often a secondary invader on any moist and excoriated skin and so may well not be the primary cause of the condition.

2 The localized itching may be due to a skin disease which happens particularly to affect the perianal region. Examples are scabies, where characteristic lesions may be seen elsewhere in the body, notably between the fingers and on the anterior aspects of the wrists, pediculosis pubis, where the parasites may be noted in the anal region, as well as in their usual site in the pubic hairs, and fungal infection. The latter is particularly to be thought of where the skin lesion has a well-defined border at its lateral extent. Other lesions may be found between the toes and in the groin and proof may be obtained by examination of scrapings from the affected skin.

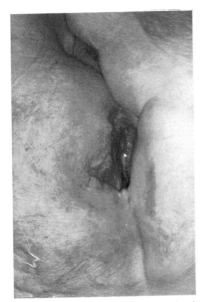

Fig. P.13. Severe pruritus ani extending forward to the vulva in a young girl with extensive Crohn's disease of the distal colon and rectum.

3   Any cause within the anus or rectum which produces moisture and sogginess of the anal skin is liable to cause pruritus ani. These lesions include prolapsing piles, prolapse of the rectum, anal fissure, anal fistula, anal papillomata or condylomata, carcinoma or benign tumours of the rectum, colitis or colonic Crohn's disease (*Fig.* P.13). Anal incontinence due to sphincteric injury may result in constant soiling of the perianal skin. Careful inspection of the anal verge, digital examination of the anal canal, proctoscopy and sigmoidoscopy, where necessary, will rapidly expose the underlying cause of this condition.

Excessive sweating, especially in hot weather and in hairy men, may be associated with pruritus ani, especially in subjects who wear thick and rough undergarments.

Pruritus ani is unusual in children and, when it occurs, a well-recognized cause is infestation with threadworms (*Enterobius vermicularis* or *Oxyuris vermicularis*). Characteristically the worms migrate to the anal verge especially at night and scratching results in auto-infection. The parasite is white and about 6 mm long with the thickness of cotton thread. The parasites may be noted at the anal verge or seen at proctoscopy. If the diagnosis is suspected but no parasites immediately seen, a wash-out of the rectum with normal saline should be inspected against a black background when the white parasites can be detected. It should be noted that threadworm infection may also occur in adults.

Idiopathic pruritus is diagnosed when no obvious cause can be found. A number of theories have been suggested, which include allergy, that the original cause has now disappeared but the pruritus has persisted because of continued scratching of the anal region by the patient, irritation of the perianal skin by faecal contamination even when no gross soiling is evident, or some psychogenic cause.

Harold Ellis

Ptosis

Ptosis is the term applied to drooping of the upper eyelid with inability to elevate it to the full extent (*Fig.* P.14). The commonest form is a congenital defect and if the pupil is in consequence covered urgent surgical correction is indicated to prevent amblyopia. The acquired kind is usually caused by *paralysis of the III nerve*, when it may also be associated with paralysis of other ocular muscles, either external or internal.

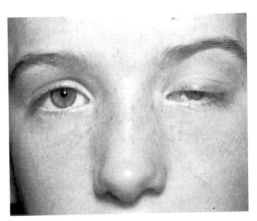

Fig. P.14. Ptosis.

In *paralysis of the cervical sympathetic*, slight ptosis may be associated with diminution in the size of the pupil on the affected side, retraction of the eyeball or 'enophthalmos' and absence of facial sweating—Horner's syndrome (*Fig.* P.15). Ptosis occurs in *myasthenia gravis* and is diagnosed using the Tensilon test.

Ptosis, associated with oedema and infiltration of the lids, is also found in *inflammatory disorders* of the

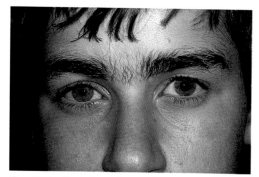

Fig. P.15. Horner's syndrome affecting the right side, showing ptosis and small pupil. This followed an upper thoracic sympathectomy by the cervical route.

conjunctiva and upper lids. Gross oedema may occur in angioneurotic oedema. It also follows direct injury of the elevating muscle or its nerve supply following lid laceration or blunt trauma.

Congenital ptosis is often bilateral, and associated with smoothness of the upper lids and absence of all the usual cutaneous folds. The levator palpebrae may be absent or ill-developed, and efforts to open the eye are made by the occipito-frontalis muscle.

In the condition called 'jaw winking', movements of the jaw, especially lateral movements, cause the lid to rise.

S. T. D. Roxburgh

Ptyalism

Ptyalism means excessive secretion of saliva. It is not always easy to determine if there really is excess, or if the patient is merely allowing the normal volume of saliva to dribble from the mouth. Thus the difficulty may be solely that of swallowing the normal secretion, as in bulbar paralysis. There may be both excess of secretion and difficulty in swallowing, as in mercurial stomatitis. In other instances there is too much secretion but no difficulty in swallowing, as in functional or hysterical ptyalorrhoea. The first step towards ascertaining the cause is to inquire as to any *medicine* or *drug* the patient may be taking orally or applying externally.

Mercury was the most important of these when the drug was used in the treatment of syphilis; its effects were worst when the mouth was not kept clean. Iodides, bromide and arsenic were in the past often responsible.

If the salivation is not attributable to any drug it may be the result of one of the many forms of *general stomatitis*.

The nature of a severe stomatitis will be ascertained by local examination; by bacteriological examination of swabbings from the mouth; by serological tests for syphilis; or by microscopical examination of a fragment of the affected tissues. Tuberculous stomatitis is one of the rarer but severe forms; it may be primary but is more often associated with pulmonary tuberculosis.

If drugs and general stomatitis can be excluded, local examination may still serve to detect a cause acting by reflex irritation of the 5th nerve, especially:

A jagged carious tooth
A stump left beneath a dental plate
A broken or ill-fitting dental plate
A foreign body impacted in the gum
An ulcerating tumour of the oral cavity

If appropriate examination serves to exclude these, the salivation, apparently rather than actually increased, may be found to result from *mechanical difficulties in swallowing* (*see* DYSPHAGIA). The excessive salivation seen in many cases of advanced carcinoma of the oesophagus results from the oesophago-salivary reflex; a constant excess flow of saliva is secreted in an attempt to 'swallow' the obstructing bolus of tumour in the gullet.

In the absence of an obvious local structural lesion, apparent salivation may be due to inability to swallow, as in cases of:

Parkinsonism
Bulbar paralysis
Pseudo-bulbar paralysis
Bilateral facial paralysis
Myasthenia gravis
Hypoglossal nerve paralysis

It is only in bulbar and pseudo-bulbar paralysis that the dribbling of much saliva is a prominent symptom. Pseudo-bulbar paralysis, being of cortical and not of medullary nuclear origin, does not exhibit wasting of the tongue.

Slovenliness and lack of cerebral control are responsible for the slobbering and salivation of some elderly or mentally handicapped patients.

Harold Ellis

Pupils, abnormalities of

Abnormalities of the pupil may be classified as irregularities in shape or irregularities in size and movement.

1. Irregularities in shape

The normal pupil is circular or slightly oval with its longer axis horizontal. Its outline may become irregular due to an adhesion between the iris and the lens, most commonly the result of previous iritis. Such adhesions are most evident when the pupil is dilated. A similar irregularity sometimes occurs in association with the persistence of a pupillary membrane, a congenital defect in which the adhesions are distinguished from inflammatory adhesions by the fact that they arise from the anterior surface of the iris at a slight distance from the pupil and not from the posterior surface or the extreme edge.

Irregularities in the shape of the pupil may result from injury, such as rupture of the sphincter and tearing of the root of the iris from its ciliary attachment, referred to as iridodialysis, dislocation of the lens, or partial adherence to an old perforated corneal ulcer. A concussion injury may cause a dilatation of the pupil, regular or irregular, and with or without associated loss of reflex movement. Rarely a traumatic meiosis may be seen. Irregularity of shape after injury may give an important clue as to whether perforation of the globe has occurred, since incarceration of the iris in a corneal wound will necessarily cause distortion of the pupil.

The circular shape of the pupil is lost in coloboma or as a result of surgery in the form of iridectomy.

2. Irregularities in size and movement

Pupillary size and equality are dependent on a balance between the action of parasympathetic nerve fibres which innervate the constrictor of the pupil (carried by the third cranial nerve) and of the sympathetic fibres responsible for pupillary dilatation (the cranial sympathetic supply). Slight inequality in the size of the pupils (anisocoria) is observed frequently and may be of no pathological significance. Pronounced difference in the size of the pupils is likely to be symptomatic of an organic lesion. In cases where the abnormal pupil is the smaller, the condition is usually due to hyperaemia of the iris resulting from iritis, paralysis of the cervical sympathetic or the use of a miotic drug such as pilocarpine. In cases where the abnormal pupil is the larger, the dilatation is usually due to stimulation of the sympathetic (the so-called 'reverse Horner syndrome'), the use of a mydriatic such as atropine, paralysis of the fibres of the third cranial nerve, or increased ocular tension, as in glaucoma.

The pupil varies in size depending on age. In infancy it is small and it becomes larger during young adult and middle life. It becomes small again in old age. As a general rule the pupil is smaller in hypermetropic and larger in myopic eyes. In pontine haemorrhage there is bilateral pupillary constriction.

Variations in pupillary movement may occur spontaneously as in hippus, when the pupils are seen to constrict and dilate together without any obvious stimulus being applied. This is simply an exaggeration of physiological movements of the pupil. Otherwise movements of the pupil occur as a result of one of the pupillary reflexes of which there are four:

i   The light reflex.
ii   The near reflex (accommodation).
iii   The reflex to sensory stimulation.
iv   Psychic reflexes.

The reflex to light and the near, or accommodation, reflex both cause pupillary constriction on each side; the sensory and psychic reflexes cause pupillary dilatation. The former reflexes are mediated by the

Table P.1. Pupillary disorders

Unilateral	Light reaction	Associated signs
IIIrd nerve palsy	Negative	Ptosis (may be complete) External ophthalmoplegia
Horner's syndrome	Poor dilatation to shade	Ptosis (always partial) Anhidrosis Enophthalmos
Holmes–Adie syndrome	Slow reaction	Constriction to methacholine
Bilateral Argyll Robertson	Negative	Depigmented iris
Metabolic coma	Positive	Coma
Midbrain compression	Negative	Coma plus or minus lateralizing signs
Pontine stroke	Negative	Coma Hyperventilation Hyperpyrexia

third cranial nerves and the latter two by the sympathetic supply to the iris. Some abnormalities of the pupil and their reflexes are illustrated in *Table* P.1.

A third nerve palsy results in dilatation of the pupil with absence of response to both direct and consensual light stimuli and to accommodation. Damage to the sympathetic supply to the head results in a Horner's syndrome with a small pupil in association with ptosis. The pupillary light reflex and the accommodation reflex are preserved. However, the pupil will have some impairment of dilatation in response to shading the eye. The Adie pupil seen as part of the Holmes–Adie syndrome is characterized by a large pupil which reacts slowly on accommodation and shows incomplete response to a bright light. The pupil will usually constrict to dilute (2.5 per cent) methacholine indicating supersensitivity. The Adie pupil is thought to result from degeneration of postganglionic neurones in the ciliary ganglion. It is most commonly seen in young women in the second and third decades of life and is usually asymptomatic though occasionally photophobia may be a symptom. The pupil gradually becomes smaller with the passage of time. Argyll–Robertson pupils are typically small and irregular and may be bilateral or unilateral. There is loss of the pupillary light reflex but often preservation of the accommodation reflex. They occur most often in neurosyphilis but sometimes also in diabetes. Damage to the afferent limb of the pupillary light reflex, as in an optic nerve lesion, results in an afferent pupillary defect. Complete transection of the optic nerve results in ipsilateral loss of the direct light reflex, with loss of the consensual light reflex in the opposite eye. In these circumstances the pupils are often equal. Less severe damage to the optic nerve may result in minor impairment of the pupillary light reflex which may be detected only by the so-called 'swinging flashlight' test. A bright light is shone into the affected eye and maintained until the pupillary constriction is static, then into the unaffected eye with a similar reaction. But, when the light is once more shone into the affected eye, the pupil may initially dilate before constricting. This lag in response is diagnostic of a partial optic nerve lesion.

N. E. F. Cartlidge

Pyuria

Pyuria means no more than the presence of pus in the urine. It will be present when there are infective processes affecting the urinary tract, in some chronic non-infective conditions such as bladder carcinoma in situ and interstitial cystitis, and occasionally following the rupture of an abscess outside the urinary tract into the system. The quantity of pus may vary; when present in large quantities it forms a thick, grey or yellow sediment. The sediment of urate crystals is usually pink or red in colour and clears when the sample is warmed to body temperature; the sediment of phosphate is cleared by the addition of acetic acid: pus in the urine will be unchanged by both these tests.

When the urine is alkaline, pus cells tend to aggregate either into a dense viscid deposit or into large clumps, the deposit or clumps separating to leave a slightly turbid supernatant. On microscopy, pus cells are seen as rounded multi-nucleated bodies about twice the size of a red cell. As pus cells are, in fact, protein, dip-stick testing is almost invariably positive for this substance; this test will also be positive if there are abnormally large numbers of epithelial cells in the sample so that microscopy of a urine sample is the only reliable simple test for the presence of pus.

The site of the pus-producing lesion cannot be determined simply by examination of the urine. The general and specific history of the individual case are essential although, in general, vesical lesions are often consequent upon renal lesions, particularly when these are infective. For example, when a pyelitis arises as a result of haematogenous spread, the initial symptom may be frequently due to cystitis. In time, the hyperpyrexia, rigors and sweating attacks of pyelitis become manifest, together with severe loin pain on the affected side. A pyonephrosis need not necessarily present with pyuria if outflow from the kidney is blocked for one reason or another, such as a stone.

Special Investigations

Imaging

If the patient is investigated during an acute illness associated with pyuria, imaging investigations of the urinary tract may give specific answers with regard to the site of the pus. The kidney which is the seat of acute pyelitis will appear larger on *ultrasound examination* and the fluid in the collecting system will appear less transonic than normal urine, implying turbidity.

Urography during an acute episode of pyelitis may show spasm of the collecting systems on the affected side, or dilatation if there is sufficient oedema of the pelvi-ureteric junction to obstruct the outflow of urine; complete cessation of renal function is occasionally observed in acute interstitial bacterial nephritis.

Cystoscopy

Instrumentation of the lower urinary tract has little to commend it during an acute illness as the risk of septicaemia is considerable. However, following appropriate antibiotic therapy and resolution of gross infection, cystoscopy under further intravenous antibiotic cover may give useful information.

It is most likely that the bladder will be the source of pyuria but if the viscus is normal on cystoscopy, inspection of the two ureteric orifices may yield valuable information.

A **ureterocele** is seen as a bulge above and lateral to the ureteric orifice, disappearing as the pressure inside the bladder increases with filling.

A **refluxing ureter** is wider than it should be and often placed far lateral. The ureteric efflux may be thick and turbid, and exuding like toothpaste from the orifice if the urine production from that side is diminished.

The ureteric orifice may be oedematous if pyelitis has extended along the whole length of the ureter as secondary ureteritis.

The ureteric orifice in **chronic tuberculosis** is characteristically 'golf-ball' in appearance.

Tiny nodules resembling sand granules are seen around the orifice in **schistosomiasis**.

The areas above and lateral to the orifices are those characteristically affected by early **carcinoma** in situ, looking very much like inflammatory patches.

Interstitial cystitis (Hunner's ulcer), presents as a red vertical line on the posterior wall of the bladder; this line extends into a split as the bladder is distended and rivulets of blood are seen on the back wall of the bladder, falling down as a curtain into the area behind the trigone.

The following is a classified list of the causes of pyuria:

A   FROM DISEASES OF THE URINARY ORGANS
1   RENAL
Pyelitis
Pyelonephritis
Renal abscess
Renal papillary necrosis
Pyonephrosis
Tuberculosis
Calculus
Medullary sponge kidney

2   URETERIC
Calculus
Megaureter
Ureteric foreign body
Vesico-ureteric reflux

3   VESICAL
Cystitis
Tuberculosis
Calculus or foreign body
Ulcer—simple or epitheliomatous
Tumour—sloughing papillary or solid carcinoma
Diverticula
Bilharzia haematobia

Trichomoniasis
Carcinoma in situ
Interstitial cystitis

4   URETHRAL
Urethritis
   specific
     gonococcal
     chlamydial
     trichomonal
     monilial
     non-specific
Stricture
Calculus or foreign body

5   PROSTATIC
Prostatis, acute or chronic
Prostatic abscess
Calculus
Prostatic epithelial tumour

6   VESICULAR
Seminal vesiculitis, acute or chronic vesicular abscess

B   FROM DISEASES OUTSIDE THE URINARY ORGANS
Leucorrhoea
Balanitis with phimosis
From the extension of inflammatory processes to the bladder, or the rupture into the bladder or urethra of an abscess such as:
   Prostatic abscess
   Appendicular abscess
   Iliac or pelvic abscess
   Abscess due to colonic diverticulitis
   Psoas abscess
   Pyosalpinx
   Carcinoma of the uterus, rectum, caecum, sigmoid or pelvic colon
   Ulceration of the small intestine, tuberculous or dysenteric

A. URINARY TRACT PYURIA

The kidneys

Recurrent attacks of **pyelitis** are commonest in childhood, during pregnancy and after childbirth. In childhood, pyelitis secondary to reflux often remains undetected and therefore untreated; **chronic pyelonephritis** in later life is a serious complication.

The kidneys may be infected: (1) *through the blood stream*—It is surprising that they are not infected more frequently, remembering the enormous renal blood flow and the oft-repeated transient bacteraemia associated with normal eating; (2) *by direct spread from the bladder* which can occur if there is vesico-ureteric reflux; (3) *by infections ascending through peri-ureteric lymphatics* from an infected bladder or from a para-vesical structure; or (4) *by direct spread* from the bladder along submucosal planes.

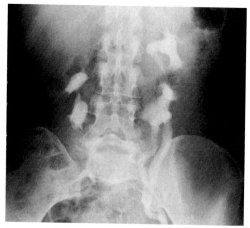

Fig. P.16. Horseshoe kidney. The classical malrotation is shown on this intravenous pyelogram. The picture is complicated by a duplex left kidney with distal obstruction of both ureters.

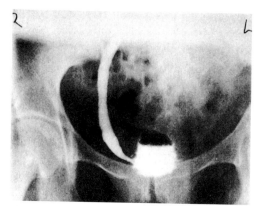

Fig. P.17. Vesico-ureteric reflux shown during a voiding cystogram.

Outflow tract obstruction will predispose to ascending infection, particularly if the bladder has to contract violently in order to expel urine. This explains the occasional association of pyelitis with **prostatic hypertrophy** and almost certainly accounts for the increase of incidence of **pyelitis in pregnancy**. It is unusual for both kidneys to be affected simultaneously but it is certainly true to say that once a kidney is damaged it is more likely to be a seat of infection on subsequent occasions.

Congenital abnormalities in themselves will not predispose towards sepsis, but if there is interference with free drainage in a **horseshoe kidney** (*Fig.* P.16), an **ectopic kidney** or a kidney with a degree of **pelvi-ureteric junction obstruction**, it may be the seat of infection more frequently than a normal system. A **duplex kidney** may become infected in one or other of its moieties.

Vesico-ureteric reflux arises because the intramural course of the ureter is short and the normally acute 'ureterovesical angle' is lost. The normal 'hydraulic valve' which prevents reflux is not therefore present and there is no obstruction to the retrograde passage of urine. At the same time, acute cystitis may in itself alter the efficiency of this ureterovesical angle so that reflux can occur secondary to the primary cystitis.

Cystoscopy of a patient with reflux often shows a small saccule or shallow diverticulum above and lateral to the ureteric orifice. It seems more likely that this is part of the original maldevelopment than a traction diverticulum.

Megaureter in children is a condition in which the whole of the ureter may be dilated, although the condition more commonly affects the distal ureter

only. A megaureter may be obstructed or non-obstructed, and may reflux or may not; paradoxically, an obstructed megaureter may also reflux, with relative obstruction to the passage of urine from upper tract to bladder but a facilitated passage from lower tract to upper.

Megaureter is physiological during pregnancy, either as a result of direct obstruction from the gravid uterus or secondary to the progestogen effect of a maintained pregnancy. Whatever the aetiology of megaureter the resulting stasis predisposes to sepsis, stone formation, squamous metaplasia, and so on.

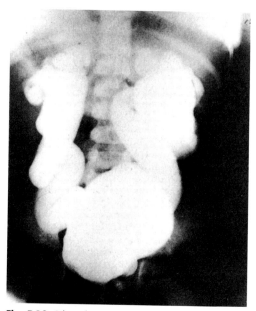

Fig. P.18. Bilateral vesico-ureteric reflux with gross hydroureter due to congenital valve of the posterior urethra in a boy of 5 years.

as is the increasingly common multiple-resistant *Staphylococcus aureus* (**pyogenes**).

The symptoms of **acute pyelitis** are severe. There is loin pain, symptoms of an associated acute cystitis, hyperpyrexia, tachycardia, rigors and sweating. The urine is turbid, opalescent, may be bright red from haematuria, positive for protein and microscopy reveals large numbers of free bacteria with pus cells and red cells. The patient may be oliguric because of fluid loss.

While examination reveals a high white cell count and ESR, urography may show reduced function on the affected side; calculi will almost always show up as radiopaque bodies overlying the urinary tract.

Chronic pyelitis is dangerous because there may be few symptoms early in the course of the disease. Slight stinging during micturition and vague pain in the renal areas may be ignored and general malaise, lassitude secondary to anaemia, a low-grade persisting pyrexia and hypertension are often presenting features. The urine classically has a specific gravity of 1010, the blood urea and plasma creatinine are raised and creatinine clearance significantly diminished. Excretion urography may be impractical because of poor renal function but delayed films will show irregularity and blunting of the calyces, cortical atrophy and a reduction in renal size. The physical signs of hypertension may be manifest.

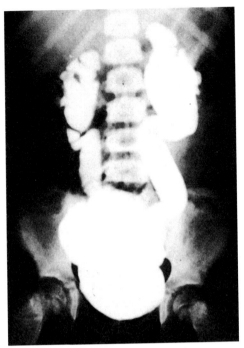

Fig. P.19. Bilateral vesico-ureteric reflux in the megaureter megacystis syndrome.

Reflux may occur in severe cases of outflow tract obstruction where the intravesical pressure rises to a level that overcomes the resistance of the most normal ureteric orifice.

Reflux is demonstrated by a micturating cystogram (*Fig.* P.17), by radioisotope investigation during micturition and also by ultrasound assessment. Reflux is sometimes severe enough to cause gross distention of the upper urinary tract especially when there is congenital outflow obstruction as in urethral valves (*Fig.* P.18).

The congenital megaureter megacystis syndrome arises because of improper development of the urinary tract and the ureteric orifices are widely patent (*Fig.* P.19), a similar picture may be seen in severe chronic retention when dilatation of the bladder and ureters has occurred beyond the point of recovery when the obstruction is relieved.

PYELITIS

Haematogenous pyelitis arising as an entity separate from other urinary tract pathology is not unusual following acute febrile illness or secondary to suppuration elsewhere in the body. The organisms responsible are usually *Escherichia coli*, *Proteus* and *Klebsiella*; *Pseudomonas* is common as a hospital-based infection

RENAL ABSCESS

Renal abscesses follow acute haematogenous infections and are initially situated in the peripheral area of the cortex. There are general symptoms and signs of a systemic abscess, with acute tenderness in the loin, developing into a mass with an overlying hyperaemic skin. It is rare for renal abscesses to discharge spontaneously through the skin as they are usually seen and treated well before this happens. Occasionally they may discharge into nearby viscera, the ascending or descending colon and the second and third parts of the duodenum, depending on the side affected. It is uncommon for a left-sided abscess to involve the tail of the pancreas. An abscess may occasionally follow a renal infarct.

RENAL PAPILLARY NECROSIS

Renal papillary necrosis is common in **diabetics**. It is now rarely seen following **phenacetin abuse** as the substance was withdrawn following the discovery of the association between its abuse and renal failure. The renal papillae undergo avascular necrosis and separate from the kidney. They may be passed as sloughs, in which case the patient may present with ureteric colic, or retained within the pelvicalyceal system, where they calcify. An acute bacterial infection often supervenes and presentation with an acute pyelitis or cystitis is not unusual.

Urography shows several changes depending on the severity of the process; in the early stage, a line of contrast can be seen crossing the base of each papilla; as the papilla sloughs it may be seen as a filling defect within a dilated calyx; later still a triangular zone of calcification lying within the pelvicalyceal system is readily apparent. Bilateral renal papillary necrosis can lead to progressive renal failure and death from uraemia.

PYONEPHROSIS

In pyonephrosis, the urine within an obstructed pelvicalyceal system becomes infected, usually secondary to congenital pelvi-ureteric junction or impaction of a stone at the junction. Obstruction of a ureteric orifice by stone or tumour, or ureteric involvement from a primary bladder or primary uterine carcinoma, are less common causes of pyonephrosis. The symptoms are not as severe as those of an acute pyelitis and more gradual in their onset. Examination almost invariably shows tenderness in the affected loin, together with a palpable renal mass.

Radiological examination often reveals the presence of a stone while renal function is rarely preserved. The quickest way of proving the diagnosis is by establishing a nephrostomy under local anaesthesia and ultrasound control; this will not only allow aspiration of pus for diagnostic and therapeutic purposes but will also provide drainage of the system. Nephrectomy is usually required together with appropriate management of the precipitating cause.

RENAL TUBERCULOSIS

This disease, once commonplace, is now relatively rare and there must always be the danger that the diagnosis will be missed unless it is remembered that all cases of persistent sterile and acid pyuria must be considered as tuberculosis until disproved by the examination of no fewer than three early morning urine samples. Even this number may be insufficient to exclude the diagnosis with certainty and as many as 12 could be reasonably cultured for tubercle bacilli if the clinical suspicion of the disease is relatively high.

The miliary form of tuberculosis, once seen in childhood, is now extremely rare; it is not associated with urinary symptoms. Renal tuberculosis, however, is still very much a reality, the kidney at first being attacked by a tuberculous infection on a microscopic basis, the resulting small tuberculous nodules even-

tually coalescing to form an area of caseation, which then bursts into the renal pelvis by direct ulceration into a calyx. The transitional cell lining of the pelvis and ureter are subsequently infected with tubercle bacilli, becoming thickened by submucosal infiltration and by oedema.

The symptoms prior to discharge into the urinary tract may be very slight; aching in the loin may be the only symptom and albuminurea the only finding once the septic focus has discharged. The symptoms mimic a low-grade pyelitis and cystitis; aching in the renal area increases, while frequency of micturition, discomfort while passing urine and polyuria occur.

The urine is pale, acid, of low specific gravity and turbid; tubercle bacilli may sometimes be found after appropriate acid-fast staining of a centrifuged sample.

Cystoscopy may show areas of oedema within the bladder and sometimes small tubercles are visible, while the ureteric orifice is usually oedematous and pouting into the bladder. The 'golf-ball' change is seen in long-standing disease when fibrosis has caused contraction of the orifice. Digital examination per rectum or per vaginam may reveal thickening of the bladder wall and pencil-like thickened ureters are occasionally felt as they hook their way into the bladder base.

Urography may show reduced renal function on one side, together with cavities, ureteric dilatation, and a thick-walled bladder. The caseating areas occasionally undergo calcification, these areas being poorly defined, contrasted with the clear-cut margins or a renal calculus. Calcific caseous debris is sometimes seen passing along the ureter, with a dilated column of contrast proximal. Renal tuberculosis should be considered strictly in relation to the rest of the genito-urinary system, the male frequently having lesions in the bladder, epididymis, prostate and vesicles while the female may have tuberculosis secondarily in the Fallopian tubes. Evidence of former disease in the spine, joints, chest or mesenteric lymph nodes may also be noted.

RENAL CALCULUS

The symptoms of stones will depend on their site, size and pathological effects (*Fig. P.20*). Renal stones may be asymptomatic. A stone floating free within the renal pelvis may cause intermittent obstruction and loin pain; a stone in the ureter presents as acute ureteric colic. Macroscopic haematuria is rare but microscopic bleeding is almost invariable. Secondary infection is most likely to occur if calculi impact at a narrow area — a calycine neck, the pelvi-ureteric junction, the ureter as it crosses the iliac vessels or at the uretero-vesical junction. Ninety per cent of renal calculi are

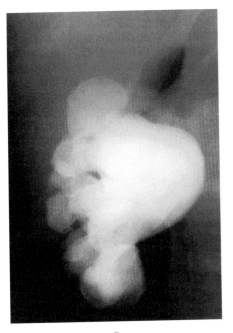
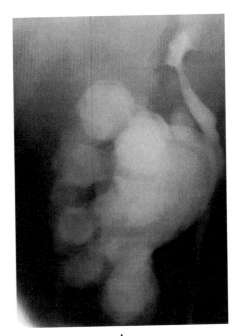

a

b

Fig. P.20. Staghorn calculus. *a*, plain X-ray. *b*, after contrast—the calculus fills the whole of the lower moiety of a duplex kidney. The small upper moiety is remarkably normal.

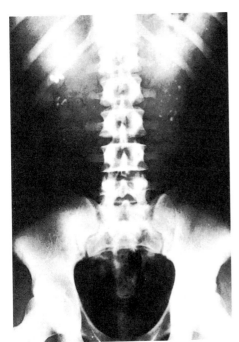
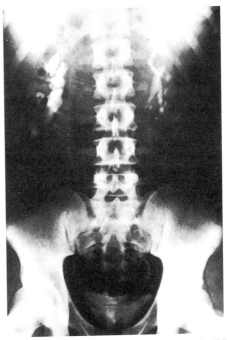

Fig. P.21. Multiple small bilateral renal calculi in a case of medullary sponge kidney shown on the preliminary plain X-ray.

Fig. P.22. Excretion pyelogram in the same case as *Fig.* P.21, showing caliceal saccules which contain the stones. From a boy of 16.

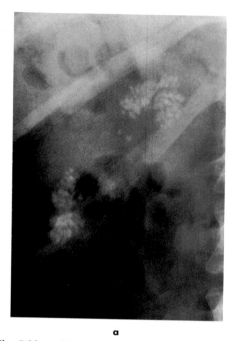
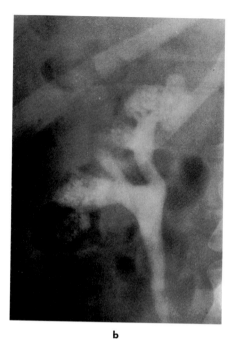

a **b**

Fig. P.23. Medullary sponge kidney. *a*, Plain X-ray showing nephorocalcinosis. *b*, after contrast—'bouquet of flowers' appearances of upper and lower groups of calices.

radio-opaque; all stones are shown on ultrasound of the kidneys or on CT scanning.

MEDULLARY SPONGE KIDNEY

This is a congenital abnormality which probably represents a minor form of polycystic kidneys. The condition is not always bilateral and is often associated with the unusual physical sign of body hemihypertrophy. Unless the family history is known, the condition usually presents as renal angle pain, pyuria, supervening upper tract sepsis and ureteric colic. The stones may erode into the pelvicalycine system and from there make their way along the ureter. The radiological changes are pathognomonic of the condition, showing the typical 'bouquet of flowers' sign (*Figs* P.21–P.23).

Ureteric disease

URETERIC CALCULUS

Most ureteric calculi will pass of their own accord once they have passed the pelvi-ureteric junction. This is the rule in 95 per cent of cases if the stone is less than 1 cm in diameter. It is probable that acute ureteric colic is the most severe pain known to man (or woman), the severe pain starting on the affected side radiating upwards to the renal area and downwards towards the bladder and into the testicles or labia. It is

surprising how many ureteric stones are, in fact, asymptomatic and present as an incidental finding. Complete blockage of a ureter by a calculus is unusual but, if it happens, it can result in a nonfunctioning and atrophic kidney. The lower down the ureter the stone impacts, the more lower urinary tract symptoms will be manifest; a stone impacting very near to the bladder can exactly mimic an acute cystitis, with supervening pyelitis, except that there is no pyrexia unless the obstructed and retained urine becomes infected.

Calculi are well demonstrated by urinary tract ultrasound; most stones show on plain X-rays; ultrasound will also give an accurate picture of the degree of upper tract dilatation.

URETERIC FOREIGN BODIES

It might seem inappropriate to discuss foreign bodies within the ureter but with the increasing frequency of endoscopic stone surgery, iatrogenic foreign bodies are now introduced with increasing regularity. One of the disadvantages of overvigorous ultrasound stone destruction is fragmentation of the metal probe-tip; these metal fragments may embed in the mucosa of the ureter and predispose to pyuria.

It should be noted that non-absorbable suture materials should never be used to close surgical incisions in the ureter; they form an excellent nidus for calculus formation.

Vesical diseases

Pyuria will be present in any lesion of the bladder which is associated with inflammation. This applies to acute and chronic bacterial infections, parasitic infections, the presence of stone, primary and secondary malignant disease, squamous metaplasia, leucoplakia and interstitial cystitis.

CYSTITIS

Cystitis may be acute or chronic and, while both forms are usually associated with infection by a micro-organism, a true infective cause is not essential as any process which produces congestion of the bladder will give rise to cystitis.

In **acute cystitis** the mucosa of the bladder is oedematous and congested, leading to epithelial desquamation, pyuria, haemorrhage, the development of small abscesses within the mucosa and occasionally to areas of ulceration. The changes are sometimes sufficiently severe to cause sloughing of the whole of the mucosa of the bladder, with profuse haemorrhage.

The symptoms of acute cystitis are well known: there is frequency, urgency, dysuria, perineal pain and pain in the suprapubic area, haematuria and pyuria. The diagnosis of an acute bacterial cystitis depends on the positive culture of an infective organism.

While the precipitating cause may be evident in some cases, such as lower tract instrumentation, over-vigorous intercourse, or acquired urethritis, many cases cannot be attributed to a specific event. An attack of **acute abacterial cystitis** may exactly mimic a true cystitis; the inflammatory agent in these cases must be a chemical irritant which is irrigated into the bladder by the turbulent urine flow associated with distal urethral stenosis in women. A causative organism can never be found, but red cells and pus cells are frequently present on urine testing. The condition is most frequently seen in young women after they become sexually active, but is also common in perimenopausal women. The name 'honeymoon cystitis' is often given to the condition but it seems rather inappropriate nowadays. Because of the common incidence of the condition at the extremes of reproductive life it seems reasonable to postulate distal urethral stenosis as a very real aetiological factor, the stenosis arising because of the hormone imbalances which occur at these two stages of a woman's development.

Chronic cystitis may follow an improperly or inadequately treated acute episode. While the symptoms are less severe, increased frequency or micturition, pyuria, and a persisting alkaline urine are noted. It is often seen with some form of urinary obstruction or retention and is sometimes found in cases of urinary incontinence, of whatever cause. The main differential diagnosis is from pyelitis, which can also cause increased frequency of micturition with pyuria, but the urine is usually acid, pale, generally turbid and has little inclination to form a deposit; an important second diagnosis is tuberculous cystitis.

The differential quantities of pus and protein present in the urine can act as a useful diagnostic test—in upper tract infections there is more albumin than the pus will account for, and on microscopy casts of varying kinds of forms are found in addition to pus cells; in cystitis, the amount of albumin is far less and the cellular elements do not form casts in themselves. At cystoscopy, the bladder wall is red, smooth and oedematous; in pyelitis, the cystoscopic appearance of the bladder is normal apart from possible modifications in the appearances of the ureteric orifices, the efflux of which is often cloudy as it contains more particulate matter.

TUBERCULOSIS

This is part of a tuberculous infective process affecting the whole of the urinary system, together with the reproductive system of both sexes. Frequency is the predominant presenting symptom, by day and by night, associated with a minor discomfort usually felt at the end of the urethra. A few drops of terminal haematuria are often observed. Pyuria is constant. **Vesical calculus** and **vesical carcinoma**, particularly carcinoma in situ present in a similar fashion. **Bladder calculi** are usually found in older patients with symptoms of outflow tract obstruction or a history of previous lower urinary tract instrumentation and catheterization. Calculi in the bladder often give pain only on movement; haematuria in calculous disease is observed throughout the stream and is often a more regular occurrence than with carcinoma.

The symptoms of bacterial cystitis may supervene in both calculus and carcinoma, accompanied by frequency, urgency and painful micturition by day and night. Vesical carcinoma may be felt per rectum, especially when the patient is thin and the tumour is extensive. The early stages of tuberculous cystitis are characterized cystoscopically by the appearance of greyish tubercles in the submucosal coat of the bladder, particularly around the ureteric orifice; at this stage frequency of micturition may be the only symptom but as the disease progresses, the tubercles enlarge, coalesce and eventually ulcerate, by which time pus and blood will both be present in the urine; tubercle bacilli should show up on special staining. The bladder becomes extremely small, with micturition occurring every 15 minutes or so throughout the 24 hours.

As a general diagnostic rule, any patient with increased frequency of micturition and a 'sterile' acid urine (sterile that is, on routine culture), should be considered as suffering from tuberculosis until disproved; as noted previously, as many as 12 negative early morning sample cultures may be required before the clinical suspicion of tuberculosis can be dismissed. Tuberculosis within the bladder is often associated with tuberculosis in the Fallopian tubes, vas, epididymis, prostate and seminal vesicles.

Tuberculosis in the bladder usually arises secondarily from an infection in the upper tract. A caseous lesion, however small, in the kidney ruptures and discharges its contents into the renal pelvis so that the urothelium of the pelvis, the ureter and the bladder become affected in turn. The primary site may similarly be within the epididymis, infection ascending through the vas deferens to affect the bladder, seminal vesicles and prostate. Prostatic tuberculosis is rare but may involve the bladder by direct ulceration. As with simple infective pyelitis, renal tuberculosis may present with lower urinary tract symptoms; the amount of blood present in the urine is usually less than if the bladder is chiefly involved and blood will, of course, be noted and found throughout the urinary stream. In renal tuberculosis there may be tenderness in the loin, while the kidney may be more readily palpable than usual and the distal end of the lower ureter can sometimes be felt on rectal or vaginal examination.

It is not, however, critical to establish whether the kidneys or the bladder are the primary sites of the disease and in many cases it is impossible to do this. Intravenous urography or ascending ureterography may give useful information with regard to the state of the upper tract; cystoscopy in renal tuberculosis may show pathological changes surrounding one ureter but not the other. The affected ureter is primarily oedematous, the wall is thickened and patulous; later on, the orifice becomes rigid and patent, representing the 'golf-hole', and drawn up towards the affected kidney by fibrotic shortening of the ureter. The final stage of vesical tuberculosis is a small thick-walled bladder (the 'golf ball').

VESICAL CALCULUS

Calculus in the bladder often presents as simple bacterial cystitis and under these circumstances there is little that will distinguish cystitis from many other form except, perhaps, the urine may be loaded with crystals. An increase in the amount of blood after exercise is noted frequently, while pyuria is usually constant. Haematuria may occur after exercise, as it does in joggers.

The constant symptoms of vesical calculus are frequency and discomfort during the daytime, especially when erect and moving, penile pain after micturition and haematuria. Except for those patients who have had indwelling catheters or complex lower urinary tract surgery, vesical calculus is almost always secondary to sepsis and stasis from outflow obstruction. Management must not only aim to remove the calculus but also to eliminate the source of obstruction. A suspected calculus will almost always show on plain pelvic X-ray or ultrasound. It may not always be possible to determine whether a stone lies within a diverticulum except by cystoscopy.

Stones which form in the upper tract and pass into the bladder without producing the symptoms of ureteric colic are almost always small enough to pass per urethram, unless the bladder outlet is obstructed. Radiolucent stones within the bladder, such as uric acid stones, are unusual as they accumulate calcium once within the viscus and take on a laminated appearance; if a pure uric acid stone is present within the bladder, it will not show on plain X-ray but will probably be detected as a filling defect at urography.

ULCERATION OF THE BLADDER

This occurs secondary to chronic cystitis, following traumatic cystoscopy, secondary to a long-standing stone and as a consequence of radiotherapy for pelvic malignancy. **Hunner's ulcer (interstitial cystis)** is a disease peculiar to women, causing severe frequency, pain on micturition, urgency with incontinence, and occasional haematuria. The diagnosis is established cystoscopically when a vertical ulcer is usually observed on the posterior bladder wall; the ulcer splits as the bladder is distended, resulting in a curtain of blood rivulets falling down the posterior wall. Biopsy of the area, usually taken to exclude malignancy, shows chronic inflammatory changes with a heavy mast-cell infiltrate. Calcium encrustation occurs, so that pyuria and calcific debris are often seen. The bladder capacity in this condition is relatively small and therapy often consists of forcible distention.

Tuberculous ulceration, **malignant** ulceration and ulceration secondary to **radiotherapy**, have similar presenting symptoms of frequency, haematuria, urgency and additional pain at the termination of micturition. The cystoscopic appearances of these different ulcers are not always easy to distinguish and multiple biopsies are often necessary in order to establish the diagnosis with certainty.

MALIGNANT ULCERATION OF THE BLADDER

Malignant ulceration of the bladder and papillary transitional cell carcinoma of the bladder are common conditions, giving rise to irregular haemorrhage, which is often profuse and almost always painless. Well-differentiated tumours tend to protrude into the bladder lumen, supported by a pedicle of rather narrow size, which accounts for the fact that the surface is often necrotic and ulcerated, giving rise to pyuria in conjunction with haematuria. The pathognomonic symptom is painless haematuria but increased frequency can occur if the tumour, or tumours, are sufficiently large to disturb bladder capacity. Pain is unusual unless infection is secondary. Tumours are often multiple because of the 'field change' that occurs within the whole of the transitional cell lining of the urinary tract—the urothelium.

When tumours are less well-differentiated and situated near the ureteric orifices, there may be ureteric obstruction and loin pain secondary to distention of the affected upper tract. Diagnosis can almost always be established preoperatively by a combination of urography and ultrasound examination of the urinary tract.

Endoscopic examination of the bladder with biopsy is conclusive, and with the advent of continuous-irrigation instruments the presence of a bleeding lesion offers no handicap to the endoscopist.

When the tumours are large, clumps of the frond-like tumours may separate and be present in the urine; cytological examination of voided samples is relatively unsatisfactory if the tumour is well-differentiated as the cells are barely different from normal bladder epithelial cells. As soon as relative de-differentiation occurs, cytological examination of the urine is a useful diagnostic and monitoring tool.

It is probably true to say that the more poorly differentiated a transitional cell carcinoma, the more solid-looking it becomes. The solid carcinomas are nodular, sessile, often solitary and involve the trigone rather than affecting the lateral walls. Ureteric obstruction is a frequent complication and early invasion of the muscle wall occurs. The presence of a mass on bimanual palpation reveals that the tumour is probably beyond the scope of endoscopic resection, while fixity to the pelvis implies inoperability.

DIVERTICULUM OF THE BLADDER

A bladder diverticulum may give rise to intermittent or persistent and excessive pyuria together with increased frequency, pain and difficulty with micturition. The last symptom relates to the outflow tract obstruction. A common symptom is that bladder emptying is often followed quickly by the need to empty the bladder again; as the bladder 'empties' it expels as much urine into the diverticulum as it does through the urethra, so that when the sphincter apparatus has closed, urine flows back into the bladder cavity from the distended diverticulum.

The diagnosis is established by urography or ultrasound, but the size of the orifice into the bladder is rarely established without endoscopic examination. A cystogram gives a reasonable idea of the size of the diverticulum but an exaggerated impression may be obtained because of the magnification seen on this kind of X-ray, and the relatively forceful distention which occurs during the examination.

SCHISTOSOMIASIS

This causes pus in the urine when the small submucosal nodules, the 'sandy' patches, ulcerate into the bladder. Ova are often observed in the urine, together with pus and blood, but microscopic examination of a 'squashed rectal-snip' is pathognomonic. Complement fixation testing is specific. In advanced cases, calcification, appearing as a ring in the bladder wall, may show on plain X-ray while urography shows upper tract dilatation, due to the presence of uretero-vesical stricture. Complication of the disease process by carcinoma is all too common and is to some extent related to the duration of the disease; the consequent bladder carcinoma frequently affects young people.

TRICHOMONIASIS

This condition is relatively rare in males but may be acquired from an infected partner. The pyuria is relatively symptom free but trichomonads are found on staining the urine, or motile organisms are seen in centrifuged urine deposits. They can also be found in urethral discharge, semen, or fluid massaged from the prostrate.

Urethral causes

Urethral pyuria will be caused by any condition which causes a purulent urethritis. A profuse discharge, together with a history of recent unprotected sexual contact, are enough to provide the diagnosis but urethritis may be secondary to cystitis as well as the converse. The symptoms of urethritis are discharge, urethral pain and occasional initial haematuria; if there is also increased frequency, suprapubic pain and bleeding throughout the stream, cystitis is probably present as well. The pyuria of urethritis is usually confined to the initial sample of urine; in cystitis, the mid-stream sample will be contaminated as well. Urethral calculi, foreign bodies, and self-inflicted urethral trauma will also cause purulent urethritis.

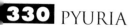

Prostatic causes

Acute prostatitis presents with increased frequency, perineal and suprapubic pain, discomfort on micturition, pyuria and even acute retention. Prostatitis may arise by haematogenous spread or may complicate cystitis or urethritis. Rectal examination reveals a large prostate which is exquisitely tender, to the degree that touching the oedematous gland causes acute reflex contraction of the external sphincter and straightening of the hips.

Prostatic abscess usually follows an acute urethritis which has affected the posterior urethra and caused an acute prostatitis. It may be secondary to a sexually transmitted infection, such as gonorrhoea or chlamydia, and may also follow instrumentation of the urethra. The prostate is intrinsically infected subclinically and endoscopy can trigger this infection, however carefully performed. Acute prostatitis may result in the formation of an abscess, almost always unilateral, which may discharge spontaneously into the urethra, bladder or rectum unless de-roofed by transurethal resection. Acute prostatitis presents with increased frequency of micturition, perineal and hypogastric pain, fever, rigors and difficulty with micturition. The abscess can be felt as a soft area within the tender and oedematous prostate.

Prostatic calculi are frequent but prostatic abscesses complicating calculi are relatively unusual, as are abscesses related to genito-urinary tuberculosis. Involvement of the prostate is a very late manifestation of this disease, presenting as increased frequency, perineal pain, difficulty with micturition and a sudden episode of initial haematuria.

Pyuria is invariable following prostatic surgery whether covered by prophylactic antibiotics or not; the healing cavity of a prostatectomy, carried out transurethrally or retropubically, can take as long as 8 weeks to epithelialize and pyuria during the whole of this period is common.

Vesicular causes

Seminal vesiculitis often accompanies acute prostatitis and often causes persistent symptoms following gonococcal or non-specific urethritis. It is a very rare complication of prostatectomy but an abscess may develop if the openings of the vesicles are involved in the cicatrization process postoperatively. Tuberculous vesiculitis also occurs.

The symptoms of vesiculitis are pain in the bladder area, in the perineum, and in the low back. Pyuria may be scant but if the channels between the vesicle and urethra are free it may be profuse; haematospermia is not infrequent while ascending inflammation of the vas and acute epididymitis are often associated. The inflamed vesicle can be felt above the prostate on rectal examination. While massage can produce a bead of pus at the urethral meatus, it is difficult to distinguish this sign from the similar phenomenon encountered in acute prostatitis.

B. PYURIA CAUSED BY DISEASES OUTSIDE THE URINARY SYSTEM

The commonest cause of pyuria is the improper collection of a sample, in that the urinary meatus, in the male or female, is improperly cleaned prior to collection. If the sample has been connected appropriately, pyuria can occur by secondary inflammatory changes within the bladder, prostate or urethra, from septic foci or malignant processes outside. In the male, retained secretions behind a phimosis can result in pyuria; and an excess of physiological discharge in the female may do the same. If there is persistent doubt with regard to the presence of pyuria in a woman, suprapubic fine-needle aspiration of a bladder, well distended with urine, is a relatively safe method of establishing the diagnosis with certainty.

The presence and spread of inflammatory processes outside the urinary tract into the urinary passages will cause pyuria, as will the **rupture of an extra-vesical abscess**. When the symptoms suggest urinary trouble, such as increased frequency, urgency, pain on micturition and haematuria, and are followed by the sudden appearance of a quantity of pus in the urine, there is a strong possibility of the rupture of an extra-urinary abscess into the bladder or urethra or very rarely into the ureter, provided that the sudden emptying of a renal abscess or pyonephrosis can be eliminated. This spontaneous discharge is often associated with a relief of the primary symptom. The history will often give some indication of the primary diagnosis, of which the most frequent are prostatic abscess, appendix abscess, pyosalpinx, psoas, iliac and pelvic abscess and an abscess around a carcinoma or diverticulitis of the colon, the last of these being the commonest of all.

Pyuria in acute appendicitis. If the appendix is in its usual position the bladder is rarely affected, but if the appendix passes downwards across the pelvic brim it is not unusual to find that the patient complains of frequency and pain on micturition when appendicitis occurs. If the appendix is severely inflamed it may adhere to the bladder and both pus and blood may be present in the urine; if cytoscopy is carried out, a localized area of congestion will be seen on the right lateral wall. Very occasionally, a small abscess may develop in the adhesions between the appendix and the bladder, and if this abscess discharges into the bladder pyuria results and an entero-vesical fistula is established. Diagnosis in the case of a dependent appendix is difficult; the pain is much lower in the pelvis than is usual with appendicitis while the lower urinary tract symptoms point to a bladder disorder; the onset of the condition is, however, gradual and there is an elevation of temperature and pulse rate with right-sided abdominal rigidity; none of these is present in acute cystitis and the possibility of an alternative acute intra-abdominal lesion has to be considered. A right-sided pelvic abscess arising from a burst appendix may rupture into the bladder. The usual history of acute appendicitis is accompanied by the presence of a mass in the right iliac fossa or the pelvic space, bimanually palpable if in the later. Pyrexia continues and is associated with rigors. If the abscess discharges into the bladder, the fever resolves and a large quantity of pus appears in the urine. Rectal examination reveals not only the tenderness of acute appendicitis but considerable thickening relating to the thick wall of the abscess cavity.

Pyosalpinx may cause cystitis by direct spread of the inflammatory process to the bladder and may eventually rupture. There has usually been a history of profuse vaginal discharge associated with constant aching in the pelvic region and in the lower back; there are often frequent attacks of severe pain and malaise at variable intervals, together with an intermittent pyrexia. Periods may be profuse, frequent, and more painful than usual, while vaginal examination reveals fullness or a mass in one or both vaginal fornices.

Psoas and iliac abscesses may rupture into the bladder, and the former has been known to discharge into a ureter. There is a swelling in the iliac fossa and sometimes in the inguinal region, and clinical and radiological evidence of spinal osteomyelitis, together with lateral displacement of the psoas shadow.

Diverticulitis of the pelvic colon often becomes adherent to the bladder and if peridiverticular abscesses form these may rupture into the bladder, causing pyuria and formation of an entero-vesical fistula. Pneumaturia, the passage of flatus per urethram, is pathognomonic but it is surprising how rarely it occurs; the appearance of solid faecal particles in the urine is more common; when air is passed in the urine the stream hisses or whistles. The main differential diagnosis of pneumaturia is an acute cystitis with a gas-forming organism, particularly in diabetic patients. A colo-vesical fistula occurs far more frequently following rupture of a peridiverticular abscess than by direct extension of a colonic carcinoma.

Carcinoma of the pelvic structures often involves the bladder by direct extension. This is particularly true of carcinoma of the cervix and of the rectum but may also happen from carcinoma of the sigmoid colon or caecum. Spread of disease to the bladder occurs relatively late and the symptoms of the primary condition have usually given a clear indication of the diagnosis before pyuria results. Involvement of the bladder is first shown by frequency, dysuria, and urgency, while the presence of blood and pus in the urine are late features, representing ulceration through the whole thickness of the bladder wall. Utero-vesical and vesico-vaginal fistulae may result from extension of primary tumours from either of these two structures into the bladder; the pathognomonic symptom is continuous incontinence by day and night. It is hardly likely that this incontinence will need to be distinguished from that secondary to an ectopic ureter as this will be evident from birth. Penetration of the bladder by a carcinoma of the rectum or colon will give rise to pneumaturia and the passage of pus, blood and faecal debris in the urinary stream. Occasionally the urine flow passes in the other direction and the urine output falls while the passage of watery stools, alternating with reasonably well-formed motions may occur.

Tuberculosis, or **dysenteric ulcers** of the intestines and **caecal actinomycosis** are rare causes of pyuria. In the last of these, the fungus, instead of infiltrating the skin and pointing in the groin externally as it usually does, extends downwards into the pelvis and opens into the bladder or rectum; the diagnosis depends on the discovery of ray fungi in the urine and it is unlikely that they would be found unless specifically sought. Actinomycosis of the kidney is usually mistaken for tuberculosis until the fungi are discovered by microscopy.

The commonest causes of the intermittent appearance of large amounts of pus in the urine are pyonephrosis, diverticulum of the bladder and vesico-colic fistula. The presence of a persistent low-grade pyuria which cannot be explained otherwise may indicate carcinoma *in situ* of the bladder or urinary tract tuberculosis.

Lynn Edwards

Rectal bleeding

Bleeding from the rectum is one of the commonest symptoms and also the most commonly mismanaged. The majority of patients with rectal bleeding are found to have haemorrhoids as the underlying cause. Haemorrhoids are cushions of erectile tissue containing extensive arteriovenous anastomoses and when traumatized arterial bleeding results. Usually the bleeding is of a minor nature; there is light staining of the lavatory paper following defaecation. Rarely profuse bleeding leading to hypovolaemic shock can occur. The possibility of a neoplasm must always be a consideration irrespective of the age of the patient. Although the incidence of rectal carcinoma is highest in the sixth and seventh decades it is not uncommon in younger age groups. The presence of malignancy must be considered particularly when there are constitutional symptoms or there is a history of recent irregularity of bowel function. Profuse mucous discharge in association with bleeding is consistent with a villous adenoma or carcinoma and a history of bloody diarrhoea is most consistent with a diagnosis of inflammatory bowel disease.

Approximately 80 per cent of rectal neoplasms are within range of digital examination and a per rectal examination should be conducted in all patients with rectal bleeding. If a lesion is palpated an assessment should be made of its mobility and fixity to surrounding tissues. A highly mobile lesion is indicative of a benign adenoma whereas any degree of fixity is strongly suggestive of invasion and hence of malignancy. Haemorrhoids, in contrast, are not usually palpable and not tender on palpation in the absence of strangulation. Undue local tenderness suggests the presence of underlying fissure, infection (intersphincteric abscess) or haematoma.

Sigmoidoscopy is an essential step in the exclusion of (a) carcinoma and (b) inflammatory bowel disease and where there is dispute over the macroscopic appearances biopsy is mandatory. The presence of oedema, erythema or a shallow discrete ulcer, usually confined to the anterior rectal wall, are features which may be indicative of the solitary rectal ulcer syndrome. This is a benign condition associated with excessive defaecation straining and can readily be confused with carcinoma on its sigmoidoscopic appearances.

The diagnosis of haemorrhoids largely rests on the appearances at proctoscopy. Most commonly the right anterior haemorrhoid is noted to be enlarged and congested and is the putative cause of bleeding since it is rare to see the active bleeding source at the time of the examination.

Patients with a history of blood mixed in with the stool or where there is a major loss of altered or of venous blood may require more detailed investigation which will include barium enema and colonoscopy. If angiodysplasia is to be excluded arteriography may be necessary.

As with bleeding from any source, there is always the possibility that the patient has a bleeding diathesis. These days, the commonest cause of this is anticoagulant drugs.

Finally rectal bleeding may be readily confused with bleeding from the upper gastrointestinal tract and small intestine; this is dealt with under MELAENA.

Classification of major causes of rectal bleeding

ANAL CAUSES

Haemorrhoids
Anal fissure
Anal fistula
Perianal haematoma
Condylomata
Trauma
Malignancy
  Squamous carcinoma
  Adenocarcinoma
  Paget's disease
  Malignant melanoma
  Bowen's disease
  Basal cell carcinoma

RECTAL CAUSES

Angiodysplasmia
Ischaemia
Infective (e.g. tuberculosis)
Inflammatory (e.g. ulcerative colitis)
Solitary rectal ulcer syndrome
Trauma
Neoplasia
  Adenoma
  Carcinoma
  Malignant melanoma

COLONIC CAUSES

Diverticular disease
Infective (e.g. dysentery)
Inflammatory
Angiodysplasia
Intussusception
Ischaemia
Neoplasia
  Adenoma
  Carcinoma

GENERAL CAUSES

Clotting deficiencies
Anticoagulants
Uraemia

(See under MELAENA for other causes particularly related to disorders in the upper gastrointestinal tract and small intestine.)

M. M. Henry

Rectal discharge

Secretion from sweat glands in the perianal area and from the anal glands is a common and normal phenomenon which rarely gives rise to significant problems. Profuse mucous secretion, however, often causes considerable discomfort and pruritis ani as a consequence of inflammation of the perianal skin. Such secretion is commonly observed with *haemorrhoids* particularly where there is a combination of *prolapse* with a weak internal anal sphincter. More serious *pelvic floor disorders* (e.g. complete prolapse, solitary rectal ulcer syndrome) may be responsible for profuse and sometimes blood-stained mucous secretion which can be incapacitating. *Inflammation* of the rectal mucosa from ulcerative colitis or Crohn's disease of the rectum may similarly produce a mucous discharge which is usually blood-stained and accompanied by diarrhoea. The existence of *neoplasia* should always be suspected since copious secretion is a particular feature of villous adenomas of the rectum in which the potassium loss may be sufficient to induce hypokalaemia. Carcinoma may also be a cause of mucous secretion although bleeding is usually a more prominent feature and there may be constitutional symptoms.

A purulent discharge is usually caused by *anal* and *perianal sepsis*. On inspection of the perineum, a small opening discharging pus to the side of the anus is highly suggestive of fistula. The diagnosis can be confirmed by palpation and observation at proctoscopy of the internal opening. Ulcerating and purulent perianal lesions should raise the possibility of Crohn's disease, anal tuberculosis or of sexually transmitted disease (e.g. AIDS, syphilis, gonorrhoea). Where there is doubt, bacteriological examination of the pus and histological examination of the biopsy from the perianal skin should be performed. Anal neoplasms and condylomata can be responsible for an offensive purulent discharge; the diagnosis is apparent on inspection but biopsy is always mandatory even if simple condyloma is diagnosed since malignant development can occur with this lesion.

Classification of major causes of rectal discharge

DISCHARGE OF MUCUS

Haemorrhoids
Rectal prolapse
Solitary rectal ulcer syndrome
Villous adenoma
Carcinoma rectum
Proctitis

DISCHARGE OF PUS

Anal fistula
Perianal Crohn's
Anal tuberculosis
Anal neoplasms
Anal fissure
Syphilis
Gonorrhoea
Condyloma accuminata
AIDS

M. M. Henry

Rectal mass

Every medical practitioner should be aware of the importance of conducting a digital examination of the anal canal and rectum in all patients with anorectal symptoms since the majority of rectal neoplasms are well within reach of the examining finger. The relevance of performing a rectal examination as part of a general examination in a patient without rectal symptoms is less clear. Since rectal cancer is a common malignancy in patients aged over 60 years, a strong argument can be made that all patients in this age group should undergo rectal examination as part of any general physical examination. Clearly, if there are urinary symptoms, a digital assessment of the prostate is highly relevant and similarly digital examination of the rectum (and, where relevant, vaginal examination) may be valuable in patients with pelvic or perineal symptoms.

Digital examination of the rectum should be conducted, where possible, with the patient lying in the left lateral position and should not be attempted until a full inspection of the perineum has been conducted to exclude fissure or other pathology which might give rise to severe pain on palpation. Initially, a digital assessment is made of anal sphincter tone which may be increased in the presence of fissure and decreased in functional disorders such as anorectal incontinence. Each quadrant of the anus and rectum should be examined sequentially. Within the anus, lesions may extend caudally from the rectum and vice versa. In the normal state, haemorrhoids are not palpable and no specific structure is palpated until the examining finger reaches the rectum. In women, the cervix frequently projects into the anterior rectal wall and is readily palpable; this is frequently mistaken by some clinicians for a rectal neoplasm; a vaginal pessary or tampon may also confuse the unwary. In men, the prostate is easily palpable anteriorly. Laterally, the ischial spines may be palpated and this may be of value in the location of the pudendal nerves (to provide a pudendal nerve blockade). Posteriorly, the 'shelf' created by the levator ani, and in thin subjects, the bony coccyx may be palpable.

Intrinsic lesions

If a mass is perceived on digital examination, it is not always possible to decide on palpation alone if the lesion is intrinsic or extrinsic. The differentiation may only be possible after sigmoidoscopy and histological examination of biopsy material. The consistency and mobility may closely relate to the diagnosis. Hence, a *benign villous adenoma* will feel soft, fleshy and highly mobile. In contrast, a *carcinoma* may feel hard with obvious fixation of the mucosal lesion to the underlying muscle or perirectal fat. Sometimes nearby *extrarectal lymph nodes* containing secondary tumour deposits may be palpable.

A circumferential stenosis of the rectum may be seen following *trauma* (e.g. previous surgery) or be a complication of: (*a*) *infection* (e.g. lymphogranuloma); (*b*) *inflammation* (e.g. ulcerative colitis) or (*c*) *ischaemia*. Digital examination under these circumstances is usually accompanied by marked tenderness and pain. *Anal neoplasms* may extend into the lumen of the anus and upwards into the rectum, in which case there may be a marked stenosis and the examination will cause pain.

Extrinsic lesions

Rectal examination is a simple clinical means of diagnosing the presence of *pelvic pus* or *pelvic tumour*. A tender mass in the presence of oedematous rectal mucosa suggests a collection of pus whereas a hard, fixed extrinsic mass in which there is no mobility of the rectal wall or uterus would be strong evidence in favour of pelvic malignancy. Infection may arise secondary to gynaecological or intestinal sepsis, most commonly sigmoid colon diverticulitis, but may be secondary to an anal fistula where pus has tracked superiorly to create a collection above the levator musculature. Such fistulas are important to recognize since their treatment is complex. *Benign enlargement of the prostate* may give rise to symmetrical hypertrophy of the gland in which the midline sulcus is preserved. *Malignant enlargement* gives rise to a mass which is denser, asymmetrical and the midline sulcus is invaded.

A mass which is clearly situated posterior to the rectum arises in the potential space ventral to the sacrum and coccyx bounded distally by the levator ani and proximally by the pelvic peritoneal reflection. The important primary distinction is whether the lesion is solid or cystic; this may require ultrasound examination for confirmation. The majority of solid lesions are *chordomas* and a cystic lesion is usually one of the following: (*a*) *epidermoid cyst*; (*b*) *mucus secreting cyst*; (*c*) *teratoma*; (*d*) *teratocarcinoma* or (*e*) *meningocele*. Neurogenic and osseous tumours are rare in this region. Clinically, presacral masses usually present with a history of low back pain radiating to the rectum and buttocks. Pressure on the bladder may lead to urinary retention and constipation is a frequent symptom. On sacral radiographs, presacral lesions may show up as an area of calcification with rarefaction of the sacrum; if there is bony destruction malignancy should always be suspected. A barium enema should always be performed to exclude colonic communication with the mass and similarly, communication with the subarachnoid space should be excluded by CT, MRI or lumbar myelography.

Classification of major causes of rectal masses

INTRINSIC CAUSES

Rectal neoplasia
  Benign
    Polyps
    Leiomyoma
  Malignant
    Carcinoma
    Carcinoid
    Leiomyosarcoma
    Lymphoma
    Melanoma
Anal neoplasia
  Benign
    Condylomata
    Polyps
  Malignant
    Adenocarcinoma
    Squamous carcinoma
    Melanoma
    Bowen's disease
    Paget's disease
    Basal cell carcinoma
  Infection
    Lymphogranuloma
    Tuberculosis

EXTRINSIC CAUSES

Infection
  Pelvic abscess
  Anal fistula with supralevator extension
Tumour
  Secondary spread to pelvis/pouch of Douglas
  Carcinoma prostate
Gynaecological causes
  Carcinoma body uterus
  Carcinoma cervix
  Carcinoma ovary
  Fibroid uterus
  Ovarian cyst
  Pyosalpinx
  Ectopic gestation
  Endometriosis
  Presence of vaginal pessary or tampon
Presacral lesions

PRESACRAL (RETRORECTAL) CAUSES

Congenital
  Epidermoid cyst
  Teratoma/carcinoma
  Meningocoele
  Chordoma
Causes arising from bone/cartilage
  Osteogenic sarcoma
  Ewing's sarcoma
  Osteochondroma
  Myeloma
  Giant cell tumour
Neurological causes
  Neurofibroma/sarcoma
  Neurilemmoma
  Ependymoma
  Neuroblastoma
Miscellaneous
  Lymphoma
  Lipoma
  Fibroma/sarcoma
  Haemangioma

M. M. Henry

Rectal tenesmus

Rectal tenesmus is a non-specific term employed to describe a state in which there is either difficulty with, or repeated, painful and sometimes *futile* defaecation. A similar condition has been described affecting micturition and is referred to as urinary tenesmus (or strangury). The repeated defaecation is often accompanied by the passage of mucus and/or blood and this collection of symptoms should be distinguished from the symptom of diarrhoea. In the latter, there is either a complaint of stool of loose consistency or there is increase in frequency, but, in contrast to patients with tenesmus, defaecation is usually productive of stool.

As with all rectal symptoms, there may be a sinister underlying cause and a full clinical assessment, which includes digital examination of the anus/rectum and sigmoidoscopy, is essential.

Inflammatory and infective causes (proctitis)

Proctitis (*see* RECTAL ULCERATION) may be inflammatory (e.g. ulcerative colitis, Crohn's disease) or infective in origin. The tenesmus may be associated with constitutional symptoms (e.g. malaise, weight loss, anorexia) and with severe diarrhoea. In patients with ulcerative colitis, the bleeding may be substantial, so leading to severe anaemia. The diagnosis is readily made by sigmoidoscopy, biopsy and, where relevant, by stool culture. Less commonly perianal sepsis (e.g. fistula) can cause tenesmus. The diagnosis is suggested either by the presence of extreme tenderness on digital examination of the anus or by the presence of a sinus/fistula opening in the perianal region.

Neoplastic causes

Benign (e.g. villous adenoma) or malignant lesions of the rectum or anus frequently cause tenesmus. An extensive villous adenoma of the rectum is notorious as a cause of excessive secretion of rectal mucus, which is sufficiently rich in potassium to lead to hypokalaemia. Adenocarcinoma of the rectum may similarly be responsible for the secretion of mucus but to a lesser degree. Rectal bleeding is a more pronounced feature in the history; the bleeding may be bright or dark red, may be mixed in with the stool, and accompanies defaecation. In the case of advanced malignancy the rectal symptoms may be accompanied by constitutional symptoms, such as weight loss. Squamous carcinoma of the anal margin should be recognizable on simple inspection of the anal verge and examination of the inguinal region may reveal lymphadenopathy in the presence of metastatic spread to the regional nodes.

Mechanical causes

Tenesmus occasionally results from a poorly understood condition in which the pelvic floor and external anal sphincter musculature fail to relax or may actively contract during attempted defaecation. Under normal circumstances these muscles relax reflexly to enable easy passage of the faecal bolus through the anal canal. This condition is usually diagnosable only either by conventional electromyography or by defaecography and may be associated with a solitary rectal ulcer as seen on sigmoidoscopy (*see* RECTAL ULCERATION). The cause is usually not known, but occasionally pelvic floor 'spasticity' is identified in patients with multiple sclerosis and the symptom of tenesmus may be the first symptom noted by patients with demyelinating diseases.

Minor anorectal disorders, particularly in an acute presentation (e.g. perianal thrombosis), may cause tenesmus since the lesion within the anus may cause stimulation of anal sensory receptors at and below the dentate line which gives rise to a false impression that there is faecal matter present within the anus and lower rectum.

M. M. Henry

Rectal ulceration

Normally a diagnosis of rectal ulceration will be made from the macroscopic appearances of the rectum at either sigmoidoscopy or radiologically at barium enema. Only under certain circumstances (*see below*) will an ulcer be palpable.

The clinical distinction between inflammatory bowel disease and infection can rarely be made on macroscopic appearances alone. Hence ulcerative colitis or shigella infection may both give rise to: (*a*) shallow ulceration; (*b*) granular appearances; (*c*) haemorrhagic friable mucosa and (*d*) oedematous mucosa in the rectum. The presence of pseudopolyps is more closely allied to ulcerative colitis but these rarely occur in the rectum and are more a feature of colonic disease. Bacterial infections tend to be of more sudden onset and are often associated with severe abdominal pain. Patients with ulcerative colitis develop symptoms usually over a prolonged period and rarely complain of significant abdominal pain. The presence of multiple yellowish-white plaques varying in size from a few millimetres to 15–20 mm in diameter may be suggestive of pseudomembranous or antibiotic-associated colitis. The latter condition is now recognized to be a toxin-mediated disease induced by *C. difficile* following exposure to antibiotics. The organism is a component of the normal flora of approximately 30 per cent of healthy adults but exogenous infection can probably occur as well.

Where ulceration is observed sigmoidoscopically, a portion of mucosa should be biopsied in most instances. Unfortunately, the discrimination between infection and inflammation is not always possible on the microscopic appearances alone; particularly in the early stage of inflammatory disease. The diagnosis in these patients will depend on bacteriology of the stool. If the stool culture is negative, the microscopic appearances will be important in the distinction between Crohn's proctitis and ulcerative colitis. The presence of granulomas, fissures, transmural inflammation and an anal lesion would provide strong evidence in favour of Crohn's disease. A non-specific microscopic inflammation may also be a feature of post-irradiation proctitis (following, for example, the treatment of cervical or prostatic cancer by radiotherapy), and can often only be distinguished by the history alone. The list of infective agents which can give rise to a proctitis is legion; only the more important are listed below. If rare organisms are cultured such as the protozoan cryptosporidia or viruses (e.g. cytomegalovirus, herpes simplex), the possibility of immune deficiency (e.g. AIDS, leukaemia) should always be considered.

Ischaemia rarely affects the rectum but when present is usually prevalent in older age groups, is of sudden onset and is associated with profuse bleeding and abdominal pain. The diagnosis is confirmed by barium enema in which the characteristic appearances of 'thumb-printing' are observed principally in the descending and sigmoid colon.

The ulcer of the solitary rectal ulcer syndrome and the ulcerating lesion associated with some rectal carcinomas are often both readily palpable on rectal examination. Both may feel indurated with fixity to extrarectal tissues and the sigmoidoscopic appearances can be identical. Adequate biopsy is essential to enable the diagnosis to be made since the presence of carcinoma will require radical surgical measures. Ulceration may rarely be traumatic in origin either as a result of self-mutilation or because digitally assisted evacuation is the only means by which the voiding of rectal contents can be achieved.

Classification of major causes of rectal ulceration

Inflammatory
  Ulcerative colitis
  Crohn's disease
  Radiation
Infective
  Shigella
  Salmonella
  Campylobacter
  Tuberculosis
  Gonococcal
  Amoebiasis
  Pseudomembranous colitis (*Cl. difficile*)
  Lymphogranuloma
  Schistosoma
  Syphilis
  Herpes simplex
  Enterovirus
  Cytomegalovirus
Solitary rectal ulcer syndrome
Trauma
Malignant ulcer
  Carcinoma
  Leukaemia
Ischaemia

M. M. Henry

Regurgitation

In regurgitation the patient is aware of food that is passed from the oesophagus into the mouth. There is therefore relaxation of the upper oesophageal sphincter to allow the contents of the oesophagus to enter the mouth. It is important to distinguish between regurgitation, reflux and vomiting. In vomiting the food passes through open lower and upper oesophageal sphincters and is the consequence of forceful contractions of the abdominal wall and the stomach muscles. Reflux is the passage of food from either the duodenum or the stomach into the oesophagus. If the food fails to pass the upper oesophageal sphincter, then the patient is said to be suffering from gastro-oesophageal reflux. If, however, the food passes into the mouth then the term regurgitation can be used. Thus reflux and regurgitation are often used synonomously. While regurgitation can be regarded as a classical symptom of oesphageal disorder, it is not necessarily so and this is seen to best effect in infants where regurgitation can be a common and normal phenomenon and is related to the passage of gastric contents into the child's mouth.

Patients who complain of regurgitation will often indicate that there is a postural element with the symptom being most marked by change of position, particularly when bending forward and often on physical exercise. The symptom occurs classically in *achalasia* (or achalasia of the cardia, or cardiospasm). In this motor disorder of the oesophagus there is a reduction in the number of ganglion cells which innervate oesophageal musculature. This is particularly so in the region of the lower oesophageal sphincter. The patient is usually between 20 and 40 years of age and classically describes dysphagia, painful swallowing and regurgitation. The regurgitation of food into the mouth at night time can be associated with inhalation pneumonia and bronchopneumonia. Halitosis may be a symptom. The diagnosis is made manometrically when reduced contractions in the body of the oesophagus will be noted. The resting pressure in the lower oesophageal sphincter is usually elevated and fails to fall, as is normal with swallowing. A poorly contracting, dilated oesophagus will be seen on barium swallow with the non-relaxing lower oesophageal sphincter giving the appearance of a 'beak' on the X-ray. Oesophagoscopy is usually unnecessary but is useful to exclude the association of a squamous carcinoma of the oesophagus which is a recognized complication of achalasia.

Gastro-oesophageal reflux is often known as reflux oesophagitis. The two terms are not necessarily synonymous because reflux into the oesophagus from the stomach is not necessarily associated with inflammation. By definition in reflux oesophagitis there is the regurgitation of fluid from the stomach into the oesophagus. The cause for the reflux is not always clear.

Reflux is associated with a reduced tone in the lower oesophageal sphincter which has inappropriate relaxation. In addition to this it has been claimed that the secondary peristaltic clearing mechanisms in the oesophagus are inadequate. In other words instead of

refluxed material being promptly cleared back into the stomach it remains for a longer period than normal in the oesophagus thereby causing symptoms and possibly inflammation. It is controversial whether in patients with severe reflux there is an element of ineffective clearing of the oesophagus. Reduced lower oesophageal sphincter pressure has been seen following ingestion of fat and alcohol. Smoking also tends to cause relaxation of the oesophageal sphincter as do drugs such as morphine, pethidine and diazepam. Carminatives such as coffee will cause a temporary relaxation of the sphincter.

Whether or not a *sliding hiatus hernia* is associated with regurgitation is a much more controversial issue. It is true that regurgitation, gastro-oesophageal reflux and a hiatus hernia may coexist, but the two conditions can exist independently and many authorities believe that the position of the lower oesophageal sphincter in relation to the diaphragm is irrelevant in the genesis of the symptoms from hiatus hernia. Patients with a sliding hiatus hernia in which the gastro-oesophageal junction lies in the thorax above the diaphragm complain of heartburn, dysphagia and reflux. A small percentage of the patients may actually have a haematemesis. The hiatus hernia may be diagnosed on endoscopy or on a barium swallow and meal. Evidence of reflux may be obtained by various tests in which the oesophageal pH is measured. There are tests available to measure oesophageal pressures, sphincter function, and the ability of the oesophagus to clear material in its lumen. It must be emphasized, however, that the demonstration of a hiatus hernia is no guarantee that it is the cause of oesophageal reflux or of the symptoms.

A picture very similar to achalasia is produced by *Chagas' disease* due to *Trypanosoma cruzi* which is encountered in South and Central America. The disease is characterized by a megaoesophagus, megacolon and severe cardiac dilatation and dysfunction. It is the cardiac complications of the disease which usually brings the patient to medical attention but occasionally the oesophageal symptoms may be dominant and they are then identical to that of classic achalasia.

Other motor disorders which may occasionally cause dysphagia include the *collagen vascular disorders* such as *scleroderma*, *diabetes mellitus*, and *alcoholic neuropathy*. In these conditions reflux or regurgitation is not a prominent feature, dysphagia or heartburn being more frequently the predominant symptoms.

It is well worth stressing that in many patients who have a complaint of reflux as manifested by heartburn or occasionally regurgitation of food into the mouth, no clear aetiological factor can be determined. Tests of oesophageal motor function and 24-hour monitoring of oesophageal pH will very often not demonstrate any evidence of abnormality despite the patient complaining of quite severe symptoms. These are important considerations in deciding whether or not a patient with the symptoms of regurgitation and who has a hiatus hernia demonstrated should be subjected to surgery.

Ian A. D. Bouchier

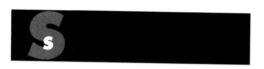

Salivary glands, pain in

Pain in one or other of the major salivary glands is associated with enlargement of the affected organ itself (*see* SALIVARY GLANDS, SWELLING OF). For practical purposes, this symptom is confined to the parotid and submandibular salivary glands. Painful enlargement of the sublingual gland is rare; it is occasionally seen as a manifestation of mumps, together with painful enlargement of the other glands, and in the unusual condition of an advanced carcinoma of the gland itself or invasion from adjacent structures. This gland will not be considered further.

The painful salivary swellings may be classified thus:

PAROTID GLAND

Mumps (epidemic parotitis)
Acute bacterial suppurative parotitis—postoperative, dehydration, following radiotherapy
Parotitis association with duct obstruction (calculus, trauma)
Carcinoma (primary or spread from another focus)

SUBMANDIBULAR GLAND

Mumps (rare)
Inflammation Associated with duct obstruction
Carcinoma

MUMPS

Mumps (epidemic parotitis) is a viral disease which is transmitted by droplet infection. It is the commonest cause of a painful parotid swelling.

Children are most often affected. There is usually prodromal fever with malaise. Only one gland may be involved, or both may be affected simultaneously, or one gland may become enlarged after the other. The swelling progresses for several days with marked tenderness of the gland and thickening of the overlying skin. There is characteristic uplifting of the lobe of the ear and stiffness of the jaw. Rarely, the submandibular

glands may also become swollen and this may also unusually implicate the sublingual glands.

After 7–10 days, the swelling gradually subsides. There may be an associated acute orchitis, which may be bilateral, and which may proceed to testicular atrophy. A rare complication is pancreatitis.

ACUTE SUPPURATIVE PAROTITIS

Acute parotitis as a complication of major surgery is now quite unusual (*Fig.* S.1): This is because it results from postoperative dehydration in a patient with poor oral hygiene and septic dental stumps. Nowadays this condition is usually obviated by adequate fluid replacement and by both pre- and postoperative oral care. Acute parotitis is also occasionally seen as a complication of the severe dehydration in conditions such as typhoid fever and cholera. Radiotherapy to the parotid region may result in damage to the gland, reduction in its secretion and a propensity, therefore, for ascending infection to occur.

On examination the whole of the gland is enlarged with a tender red swelling of the side of the face. This may progress to overlying cellulitis. Pus can be expressed from the parotid duct on the affected side. Because of the dense overlying fascia, which confines the enlarged gland, pain may be intense. There are the associated features of severe infection with pyrexia and toxaemia.

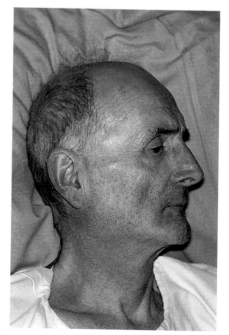

Fig. S.1. Acute postoperative right-sided parotitis following gastrectomy for gastric carcinoma.

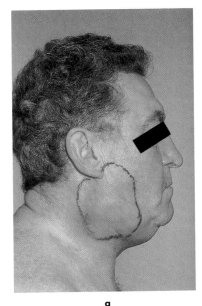

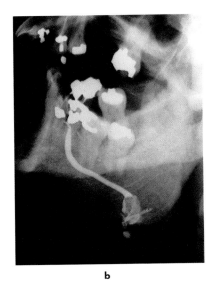

Fig. S.2. *a*, Parotitis secondary to calculus obstruction. The outline of the gland has been marked with a skin pen. Note that the whole gland is diffusely enlarged. This is in contrast to a tumour of the gland, which produces a localized swelling. The overlying skin is reddened. *b*, Sialogram of the submandibular salivary duct. This demonstrates a large filling defect produced by an impacted calculus. (*Westminster Hospital.*)

PAROTITIS ASSOCIATED WITH DUCT OBSTRUCTION

Obstruction of a salivary duct, from any cause, results in a typical syndrome in which the gland becomes painful and swollen at meal times, due to the increased secretion of saliva being unable to discharge through the duct. Between meals, as the saliva gradually escapes, the swelling and pain subside. Frequently, inflammation of the obstructed gland occurs as a result of ascending infection from mouth organisms. Under these circumstances, there may be the associated features of infection (*Fig. S.2a*) and there may be a discharge of pus from the mouth of the duct.

Although less common than in the submandibular duct, calculi in the parotid duct are not rare. They tend to be smaller and less radiopaque than in the submandibular duct or gland so that only larger ones are seen on a plain X-ray of the region. A sialogram may be necessary to identify the stone, which will then be seen as a filling defect.

Other causes of parotid duct stenosis are trauma from the irritation of an adjacent tooth stump or, occasionally, from traumatic division of the duct, for example following a knife laceration of the cheek.

SUBMANDIBULAR CALCULUS

Calculi are the commonest cause of a painful swelling of the submandibular gland and account for some 95 per cent of all salivary stones. There are several reasons for the comparative frequency of stones in the submandibular gland and its duct. Its secretion contains more mucus than the parotid duct so that it is more viscid. Its duct is longer and slopes upwards from the gland so that there is more tendency for a small concretion to remain within the duct. Furthermore, its orifice, being on the floor of the mouth, is more exposed to trauma than that of the parotid duct. The aetiology of these stones remains subject of debate. Their size varies from minute to the size and shape of a date stone. Numbers vary; there may be a single stone in the duct or the gland itself may contain numerous stones throughout a dilated duct system (sialectasia).

The classical story of swelling and pain associated with food is elicited in the history. The gland itself can be felt as a tender enlargement on bimanual palpation with one finger below the angle of the jaw and the other in the sulcus between the tongue and the mandible. Occasionally a calculus can be seen to extrude through the duct orifice at the side of the base of the fraenulum linguae. At other times it may be

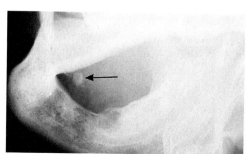

a

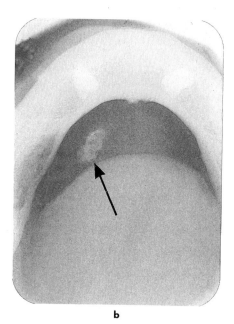

b

Fig. S.3. Radio-opaque submandibular salivary calculus demonstrated on an oblique lateral view of the mandible (*a*), and, in another case (*b*), on a floor of mouth view. In both cases, the stone has been arrowed. (*Addenbrooke's Hospital.*)

palpated along the course of the duct in the floor of the mouth or stones may be felt in the gland itself. Pus may be expressed from the duct orifice by pressure on the gland.

Submandibular calculi are nearly all radiopaque and can be visualized on a plain X-ray of the floor of the mouth (*Fig.* S.3). Occasionally a sialogram may be needed to confirm the presence of a calculus in the gland itself (*Fig.* S.2b).

CARCINOMA OF THE SALIVARY GLANDS

In its late stages, a carcinoma of the salivary gland (commonest in the parotid, less often seen in the submandibular gland and rare in the sublingual gland)

will invade adjacent tissues and produce severe pain. Invasion of a salivary gland from an adjacent tumour, for example a carcinoma of the floor of the mouth, a squamous carcinoma of the overlying skin or a malignant melanoma, will be associated with intense pain.

Harold Ellis

Salivary glands, swelling of

The salivary glands are subject to swelling due to inflammation and new growth in the same way as any other organ. In common with other externally secreting glands they are also subject to swelling resulting from retention of secretion. This most commonly occurs as a result of blockage of a duct by a stone. Parotid swelling with fever, often with lacrimal adenitis and uveitis (Mikulicz's syndrome) may occur in leukaemia, Hodgkin's disease, tuberculosis, systemic lupus erythematosus and sarcoidosis. Confusion in diagnosis may result from the close proximity of the lymphatic nodes; in the case of the submandibular gland, the lymphatic nodes may be right in the centre of the salivary tissue. The different salivary glands do not exhibit the same liability to each lesion, the submandibular for instance being the most liable to calculus formation, while inflammatory lesions are only common in the parotid. Mumps is the commonest cause of all parotid swellings; it may occasionally involve other glands than the parotid, but this is a rare exception and usually occurs only after the parotid is first attacked. Here, as in all diagnosis, it is important to decide the exact anatomical site of the lesion before considering its pathology. For example, swelling of the loose tissues over the jaw from alveolar inflammation may mimic parotitis. A useful point in this connection is that a generalized parotid swelling tends to lift the auricle away from the head and inspection of the orifice of Stensen's duct within the mouth will usually reveal some abnormality (*see Fig.* S.1). If lymphatic nodes are suspect as a site of swellings, the presence of other enlarged nodes or of a primary lesion should be sought.

Sialography may prove helpful. Radiopaque contrast is injected into the appropriate orifice (Wharton's or Stensen's, the lingual ducts are not suitable for injection). The branching system of ducts is well visualized in the radiograph. Blockage by a stone or by growth, sialectasia (dilatation and beading of the duct system, especially in the parotid gland), or the presence of a fistula is the lesion most likely to be demonstrated in this way (*see Fig.* S.2b).

The lesions of the salivary glands are summarized in *Table* S.1.

Table S.1. Lesions of the salivary glands

Salivary gland	Acute unilateral enlargement	Acute bilateral enlargement	Chronic unilateral enlargement	Chronic bilateral enlargement
Parotid	Non-specific infective parotitis (rarely bilateral)	Mumps. (One side usually appears first, second commonly appears 24–36 hours later, but occasionally up to 4–5 days later)	(1) Progressive—growth or inflammation. May involve part of gland only; differentiate from preauricular adenitis by searching area drained, etc. (*see below*)	Sarcoidosis
		Both of these show signs of inflammation with much pain. In both, orifice of Stensen's duct is red and pouting	(2) Intermittent—sialectasia (calculus uncommon)	
Submandibular	As for parotid, but both very rare. *N.B.* Inflammation of submandibular lymphatic nodes common		(1) Progressive—growth (rare) (2) Intermittent—stone. Swelling occurs at meal-times when the flow of saliva is stimulated, but the gland is permanently swollen when condition is of long standing. Stone may be palpable in duct and will show on X-ray. Orifice of duct inflamed	
Sublingual	Uncommon. Ranula was originally thought to be due to retention of secretion in this gland, but retention in adjacent simple mucous glands is the more probable explanation			
All glands	Mikulicz's syndrome—characterized by chronic painless swelling of all the salivary glands and the lacrimals. This occurs in Hodgkin's disease, tuberculosis, leukaemia, sarcoidosis and systemic lupus erythematosus			

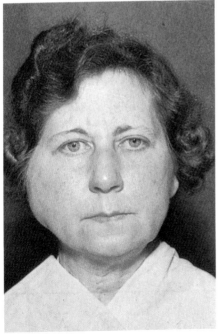
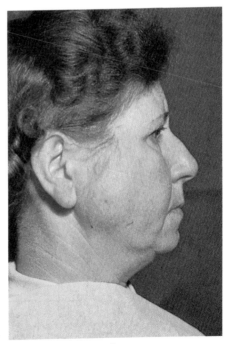

a   b

Fig. S.4. Mixed parotid tumour (pleomorphic adenoma). (*Courtesy of the Gordon Museum, Guy's Hospital.*)

Parotid tumours

The histology of salivary tumours is complicated and will not be discussed. It is sufficient to mention the so-called 'mixed tumour', which is better termed a 'pleomorphic adenoma' (*Fig.* S.4), which is benign as a rule although locally recurrent owing to inadequate removal. Characteristically the tumour arises as a lobulated mass, noticed first when about the size of a cherry, and of variable consistency. If there is much myxomatous degeneration, the lump will appear to be fluctuant; if chiefly composed of fibrous tissue it will be hard yet elastic. The lump is painless and is typically situated between the ascending ramus of the mandible and the mastoid process, although no part of the parotid is exempt from this change and these tumours may be found as low as an inch below the angle of the mandible. Women between the ages of 30 and 50 and men between 45 and 60 are the usual sufferers and a frequent history is that the lump, over a period of years, shows a progressive slow increase in size. Involvement of the facial nerve or fixity to the skin and involvement of the cervical lymph nodes indicates that the growth is a carcinoma.

The submandibular salivary gland (but very rarely the sublingual gland), may also be the site of both the pleomorphic adenoma and carcinoma, but much less commonly than the parotid (*Fig.* S.5).

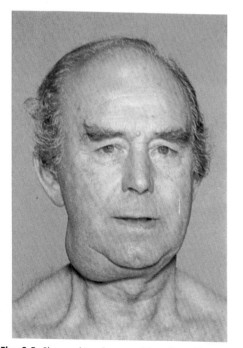

Fig. S.5. Pleomorphic adenoma of the submandibular salivary gland.

Sarcoidosis

In sarcoidosis asymptomatic enlargement of the parotid, sublingual and submaxillary glands occurs in about 6 per cent of cases. Spontaneous resolution often occurs. The glands are not tender. Facial palsy may occur with parotid enlargement. The syndrome of fever, uveitis and lacrimal and salivary gland enlargement is known as 'uveoparotid' fever or Heerfordt's syndrome.

Harold Ellis

Scrotum, ulceration of

Ulceration of the scrotum occurs in association with:

1 New growth:
   Carcinoma
   Papilloma
2 Fistula
3 Syphilis
4 Testicular disease:
   Inflammatory
   Tuberculous
   Syphilitic
   Malignant growths
5 Suppurating cysts
6 Infected haematocele
7 Irritants and corrosives, such as mustard gas
8 Behçet's syndrome, herpes simplex, candidiasis.

1. New growth

Carcinoma of the scrotum, formerly known as 'chimney-sweep's cancer', or 'tar-worker's cancer', is by no means limited to these occupations, but is certainly more common in men engaged in work in which they are exposed to much irritation from solid particles or from noxious fumes. Hence the disease is, or was, most commonly seen amongst chimney-sweeps, employees in gas works, paraffin, tar and chemical works, and coal mines and in mule-spinners in the cotton trade. It often begins as a small subcutaneous nodule, over which the skin is thinned and adherent; the nodule enlarges slowly, and the thinned covering gives way to form an ulcer with thickened irregular edges and a tendency to bleed on slight injury. The ulcerated area extends both radially and into the tissues of the scrotum, later involving the testes. The inguinal nodes become enlarged soon after active ulceration begins, at first from inflammatory causes, later from malignant infiltration and, untreated, themselves ulcerate; this indeed is the common mode of death in this condition, from repeated haemorrhages. In other cases a scrotal epithelioma begins in a *wart* or *papilloma*, which may have been present for years with only slight increase in growth (*Fig.* S.6). These soft papillomas

3. Syphilis of the scrotum

This may be present either as a primary chancre or as a mucous tubercle. A *primary chancre* in this situation is by no means easy to recognize unless other signs of syphilis are present; but the presence of a cutaneous sore which does not show much inclination to heal under antiseptic dressings should always give a suspicion of syphilis. There is often only slight induration of the ulcer compared with that of a penile chancre, but the edge is raised and of a rolled appearance. Careful search must be made under dark ground microscopic examination for the *Treponema pallidum* in the serum expressed from the ulcer. Negative serological reactions in the early state of the disease are not reliable. The inguinal lymph nodes are enlarged and discrete, and some 5 to 6 weeks after the commencement of the ulcer the usual secondary symptoms of syphilis become manifest.

Mucous tubercles may be present on the scrotum, usually on the femoral aspect. They may extend directly from the anal area. No difficulty will be met with in the diagnosis, as other signs of syphilis are obvious.

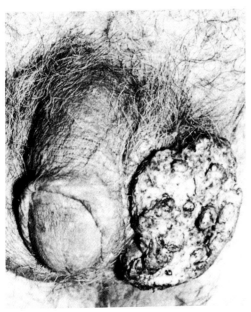

Fig S.6. Epithelioma of scrotum.

are not unusually the starting-point of malignant change, when they become more vascular, while the surface epithelium becomes thinned and easily excoriated. A small amount of foul discharge is present, often encrusted into a scab, which on removal leaves an ulcer with indurated, everted edges, with the gradual progress of a cutaneous epithelioma. Any ulcer on the scrotum, especially if indurated or readily caused to bleed, must be looked upon with extreme suspicion and immediately subjected to biopsy for microscopic examination. It is not unusual, however, for a large mass of nodes to be found in the groin when the primary lesion is very small and almost imperceptible. The scrotum must be examined very carefully in such cases lest the primary lesion be missed.

2. Fistula

Fistulas may occur in the scrotum and cause ulceration. Sinuses occur in association with tuberculosis or syphilitic disease of the testes, but fistulas may follow urine extravasation, or burrowing from rectal suppuration. An abscess may form and open through the scrotal skin from a peri-urethral abscess accompanying an acute urethritis or formed by septic infection behind a urethral stricture. In either case a small amount of urine may leak through the opening during micturition while the history of urethral discharge, or of difficulty in micturition and other symptoms of stricture, will point to the diagnosis.

4. Testicular disease

In some cases extension of disease in the testicle may involve the coverings of the scrotum, and may even perforate them to form a scrotal sore. This sequence occasionally occurs with: (1) A testicular abscess; (2) Tuberculosis of the epididymis; (3) Gumma of the testis; (4) Malignant disease of the testis.

A *testicular abscess* is somewhat uncommon, but may arise from direct extension from the urethra via the vesiculae seminales and vasa deferentia or by a haematogenous infection during the course of a specific fever, such as scarlet fever, mumps or typhoid fever. With urethral disease, the primary trouble may be due to gonorrhoea, or more frequently to a septic urethritis from the introduction of infected instruments. In cases in which the infective process extends from the urethra the epididymis is affected first, while in the metastatic cases the body of the testis usually shows the first sign of enlargement. If the vas has been divided as part of the operation of prostatectomy, or sometimes following vasectomy for sterilization, the swelling and possible abscess will occur in the upper part of the scrotum at the site of the division. These acute inflammations of the testis occasionally suppurate, when the scrotal tunics become inflamed and adherent, whilst softening occurs later, and unless surgically relieved the abscess opens through the skin, leaving an ulcer, and a sinus discharging pus. An unusual form of abscess of the testicle is caused by a *suppurating dermoid cyst* of the testicle, and may discharge through the scrotal coverings to form an ulcer.

Tuberculosis of the testicle rarely occurs as a primary disease but more often as a secondary deposit in association with tuberculosis elsewhere in the genito-urinary tract. Testicular tubercle almost always begins as a nodule in the epididymis, but in the later progress of the disease may extend into the testis proper. If the tuberculous nodule progresses rather than undergoes cure, the scrotal skin becomes adherent, thinned, and finally perforated, leaving a shallow ulcer with thin, undermined edges and discharging thin pus. The ulcer in this case is most likely to be on the posterior aspect of the scrotum. Occasionally the necrotic epididymis fungates through the opening in the scrotum, appearing as a greyish, sloughy projection from the cutaneous opening—the so-called 'hernia testis'.

A *gumma of the testis* (once common, now very rare), causes a swelling in the body of the testis rather than in the epididymis. A gumma which remains unrecognized or untreated may soften and ulcerate through the scrotal skin in a manner similar to tuberculous disease, leaving a clearly defined ulcerated area with sharply cut margins and a wash-leather-like sloughy base. Such ulcers are usually placed on the front of the scrotum. The gummatous granulation tissue may fungate through the scrotal aperture, forming a yellowish necrotic mass.

The diagnosis of these three conditions may produce some difficulty in the earlier stages (*see* TESTICULAR SWELLING), but in the advanced stage now under consideration, when an open scrotal sore is present, the diagnosis is easier.

The *opening of a testicular abscess* on the scrotum leaves a small sinus discharging pus and accompanied by a general enlargement of the organ. Preceding the rupture of the abscess there is acute pain in the testicle, with rise of temperature, rigors and general signs of suppuration, which are much diminished as soon as the abscess bursts or is incised. There is often a urethral discharge, which, however, is frequently much lessened with the onset of the acute epididymitis, with distinct thickening of the cord and aching pain in the neighbourhood of the external abdominal ring. In metastatic cases the abscess occurs during the progress of an acute fever. The general history is one of acute pain beginning in the testicle, with rapid and extremely tender swelling of the organ, followed by abscess formation.

In *tuberculosis of the testis* the progress is much more gradual. A nodule may have been present in the epididymis for some time, gradually enlarging, but causing very little pain; in some cases a nodule may have been present for months without any apparent change, and then it may enlarge rapidly, involve the scrotal tunics, and discharge its contents. By the time the disease has reached this stage it is probable that evidence of tuberculosis will be found in other organs, particularly the other testis, prostate, seminal vesicles or bladder. The affected testicle usually presents several nodules in the epididymis, tender on pressure, whilst small nodules may also be felt in the vas deferens.

The opening remaining from the discharge of a *gummatous orchitis* is usually a rounded ulcer with sharply cut edges and yellowish base. The whole testis is enlarged and practically painless. The cord is not thickened, and there is no evidence of disease in the other testicle, prostate or seminal vesicles. There is probably a history of syphilis, and other tertiary syphilitic lesions may be present elsewhere, such as gummatous periostitis.

A *hernial protrusion of necrotic testicular tissue* may be present either with tuberculous disease or from a gumma. In tuberculosis the mass is greyish and necrotic, discharging thin pus, and there will be evidence of tuberculous disease in the underlying testis and other genital organs. Tubercle bacilli very rarely may be found in the discharge. A distinctive feature of the gummatous hernia testis is found in the appearance of the cutaneous opening; if the fungating mass is pushed aside the opening in the scrotal skin will be seen to be cleanly cut and to encircle the protruding tissue tightly. The fungating hernia testis of tubercle or syphilis must also be diagnosed from other conditions producing a raised tumour on the scrotum. An epithelioma of the scrotum has raised borders, but the centre is excavated, and there is rarely any enlargement of the testis. A sloughing papilloma of the scrotum may more nearly reproduce the appearance, but the tumour and the skin are freely movable on the underlying testis, while in hernia testis the mass is connected with the testicle, and the tubular structure of the latter is often apparent on picking up a small fragment of the fungating tumour.

New growths of the testis seldom cause ulceration of the scrotum because they have generally been removed by operation before so late a stage is reached; any variety, however, whether seminoma or teratoma, may cause local recurrence in the scar, with ulceration; the diagnosis depends upon histological examination, either of the tumour previously removed or of a biopsy from the edge of the recurrence. Occasionally fungation of the tumour is seen through the scar of the biopsy site in the scrotal skin when there has been delay in carrying out definitive treatment, a state of affairs which should never be allowed to happen.

5. Cysts of the scrotum

A sebaceous cyst in the scrotal skin may suppurate and leave an open sore. The areas remaining present raised borders, and are easily mistaken for an early epithelioma. An accurate history of the previous swelling in the skin is of little assistance in these cases, but microscopical examination of a piece removed from the margin of the ulcer will exclude malignancy. A suppurating cyst in the scrotum is less common than epithelioma.

6. Haematocele

A haematocele which becomes infected may form an abscess which bursts through the scrotal coverings. It may have a superficial resemblance to a gumma.

7. Mustard gas

Mustard gas caused most troublesome ulceration of the scrotum, as of other parts, during the war of 1914–18; but the diagnosis is easy if the correct history of exposure to this or some other irritant is available.

8. Behçet's syndrome

Behçet's syndrome causes painful ulcerative lesions of the scrotum as well as the penis, unlike the lesions in the vulva and vagina, which are often painless and therefore often missed. Behçet's may be accompanied by abscess or herpes-like lesions of the scrotum. Herpes simplex, both types I and II, may cause vesicular lesions less commonly, and very rarely candidiasis.

Harold Ellis

Skin tumours

Cutaneous tumours are growths on the skin. They may be firm, fleshy, cystic, multilobulated or ulcerated. The chief causes are neoplasms, both benign and malignant (*see Table* S.2).

Malignant tumours

a. *Secondary deposits* commonly occur late, as multiple, hard, fleshy nodules of any colour. Subcutaneous secondaries can masquerade as benign lesions and a high level of suspicion should be maintained. Even infectious lesions can be simulated, for example by carcinoma erysipeloides on the chest of a patient with breast cancer. Certain areas are predisposed to metastases, including the scalp (breast, lung and genitourinary tract carcinoma), the chest wall (breast cancer), and

Table S.2. Skin tumours

Malignant
a. Secondary deposits
b. Kaposi's sarcoma
c. Primary malignant tumours
   i. Squamous-cell carcinoma (*Fig.* S.7)
   ii. Malignant melanoma (*Fig.* S.8)
   iii. Rodent ulcer (basal-cell carcinoma) (*Fig.* S.9)
   iv. Mycosis fungoides (cutaneous T-cell lymphoma) (*Fig.* S.10)
   v. Xeroderma pigmentosum (*Fig.* S.11)

Benign
Sebaceous cyst
Lipoma
Seborrhoeic keratosis (basal-cell papilloma)
Cutaneous horn (*Fig.* S.12)
Pyogenic granuloma (*Fig.* S.13)
Adnexal tumours

the abdominal wall especially around the umbilicus (carcinoma of the stomach and the colon). The skin is sometimes infiltrated by leukaemia or lymphoma.

b. *Kaposi's sarcoma* is a malignant proliferation of vascular endothelial cells giving rise to superficial, subcutaneous or deeper vascular tumours. These tumours do not metastasize but are multi-site in origin. They are probably due to infection with an as yet unidentified viral strain. Tumours flourish when immunity is depressed, e.g. HIV, post-transplant, old age. Classical lesions first described in patients of Jewish or Italian descent living in Vienna in the 1880s are probably acquired on the genome and expressed in old age. Endemic Kaposi's sarcoma was first recognized in the 1950s as a common tumour in sub-Saharan Africa, in younger patients and following a much more aggressive course. The epidemic Kaposi's sarcoma was described in New York in the 1980s. It seemed to spread by sexual intercourse (usually but not exclusively in HIV-positive homosexual men).

Individual lesions begin as pink vascular macules, often in multiple sites, which gradually enlarge and become palpable. They darken with time. Draining oedema is often prominent. The vascular lesions can simulate granulomata, histiocytomata or haemangiomata. Internal lesions can occur chiefly in the gastrointestinal tract and lungs. If immunity improves tumours may shrink.

c. *Primary malignant skin tumours*
i. *Squamous-cell carcinoma* (*Fig.* S.7) is usually single and as a rule fairly slow growing, extending peripherally and infiltrating deeply while ulcerating at its centre. Sooner or later the lymphatic nodes draining the affected area become involved and enlarged. The usual sites for squamous-cell carcinoma are the lips, especially the lower lip and sun-exposed areas, as well

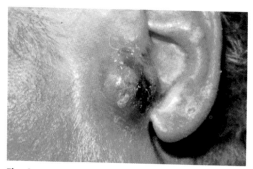

Fig. S.7. Squamous-cell carcinoma. (*Westminster Hospital.*)

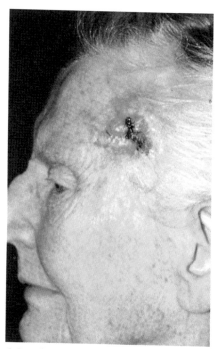

Fig. S.9. Rodent ulcer, basal-cell carcinoma.

as glans penis and vulva. Solar keratoses, X-ray scars and lupus vulgaris may all undergo malignant squamous change. The main diagnostic features are its origin as a single growth, its craggy hardness, its slow development and the metastases to neighbouring lymph nodes.

ii. *Malignant melanoma* (*Fig.* S.8) can arise anywhere on the skin surface at any age, often in a simple pigmented or non-pigmented mole. It is rare in blacks and increases in frequency with the fairness of the skin and the amount of previous sun exposure. Interestingly, cutaneous melanoma in black people when it does occur is usually found on the non-pigmented sole of the foot. Patients with a history of severe sunburn in childhood, more than 50 moles on their skin, more than five unusually large moles or a family history of malignant melanoma, are at increased risk.

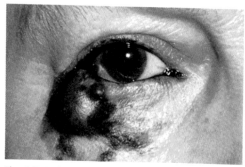

Fig. S.8. Malignant melanoma. (*Addenbrooke's Hospital.*)

It may occur on the scalp, under a nail or on anogenital skin.

Occasionally melanomas lose the capacity to produce pigment—amelanotic melanoma. The characteristics of malignant melanoma are its rapid development and growth, its deepening colour, its ulceration, areas of depigmentation, bleeding and crust formation

and its rapid metastases. Sometimes multiple metastases occur in the skin itself. The disease is highly malignant but early diagnosis and excision is curative. Prognosis depends on the thickness of the primary at the time of excision.

iii. *Rodent ulcer* (*basal-cell carcinoma*) usually affects the face (*Fig.* S.9) and is dealt with on p. 113. These are the commonest primary skin malignancies. They do not metastasize though local invasive destruction can be extensive if lesions are neglected.

iv. *Mycosis fungoides* (cutaneous T-cell lymphoma) is a rare, chronic, slowly fatal disease which is characterized in its final stage by tomato-like neoplasms which may ulcerate. For many years a 'pre-mycotic' non-specific red, scaly rash is present, later (sometimes 30 years plus) forming red plaques of differing hue, and finally neoplasms (*Fig.* S.10).

v. *Xeroderma pigmentosum* is an extremely rare disorder of nuclear protein repair inherited as a recessive trait. It presents in childhood as a proneness to sunburn and early gross sun damage with elastosis, atrophy, telangiectasia and finally multiple skin tumours (squamous-cell carcinoma, rodent ulcer, malignant melanoma, kerato-acanthoma) (*Fig.* S.11).

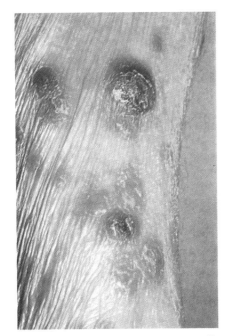

Fig. S.10. Mycosis fungoides. (*Westminster Hospital.*)

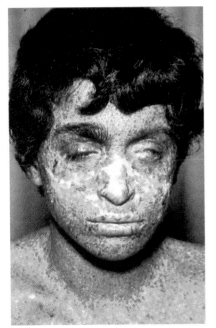

Fig. S.11. Xeroderma pigmentosum. (*Westminster Hospital.*)

Benign cutaneous tumours

Sebaceous cysts, commonest on the back, face, scalp and scrotum, are of variable size, cystic on palpation, and with a minute orifice (punctum) to be found somewhere on their surface. They do not occur on the palms of the hands or soles of the feet, where sebaceous glands are absent. *Lipomas* are usually multiple subcutaneous nodules which may be lobulated, and found on any part of the body apart from the scalp, the palms of the hands and soles of the feet. They occur as a familial trait but can often not be discerned until adulthood. *Seborrhoeic keratosis* (basal-cell papillomas) are extremely common and start as papules in middle age, growing into larger, flat, greasy, warty pigmented neoplasms. They are sometimes unkindly called senile keratoses.

A *cutaneous horn* is a peculiar cutaneous neoplasm surmounted by a spectacular horny overgrowth (*Fig.* S.12). The nature of the underlying neoplasm can only be safely diagnosed by examining the histopathology, e.g. actinic keratosis, squamous-cell carcinoma, viral wart, keratoacanthoma and seborrhoeic wart (basal-cell papilloma).

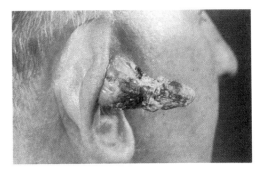

Fig. S.12. Cutaneous horn: keratoacanthoma.

A *pyogenic granuloma* (granuloma telangiectaticum) is a fairly common skin neoplasm (*Fig.* S.13). It often develops at the site of a recent injury and is composed of proliferating capillaries in a loose stroma. This produces a rapidly growing vascular neoplasm which bleeds easily when traumatized. It is distinctive,

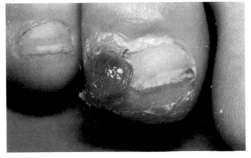

Fig. S.13. Pyogenic granuloma. (*Westminster Hospital.*)

being bright red, 0.5–1 cm in diameter, often pedunculated and surrounded by a collar of thickened epidermis. The common sites are the fingers, upper chest, lips and toes. It must be differentiated from amelanotic melanoma, and glomus tumour. Kaposi's sarcoma in HIV-infected patients can accurately mimic pyogenic granuloma and for this reason histological analysis after curettage or excision is advisable.

Adnexal tumours. The superficial dermis contains many specialized tissues, some of ectodermal and some of mesodermal origin, forming the various adnexal structures, e.g. hair, sebaceous glands, sweat glands, etc. Benign, or rarely malignant, neoplasms of all these specialized tissues can occur, for example *leiomyoma, hydradenoma, neurofibroma, sebaceous adenoma, tricho-epithelioma* and *glomus neoplasm.* The diagnosis of these rare neoplasms requires many years' experience and is often first made by the pathologist.

Richard Staughton

Spine, curvature of

An abnormal curve in *flexion* is called a 'kyphosis' and where this presents as an acute angle the hump of bone is called a 'gibbus' or a 'kyphus'. The extension curve constitutes a 'lordosis'. The lateral spinal curve is called a 'scoliosis' in the thoracic and lumbar regions and in the neck the wry neck is described as a 'torticollis'. The scoliosis is designated 'left' or 'right' according to the direction of the convexity of the curve. There is often a combination of curves and a kyphoscoliosis is often seen. A scoliosis or lateral curvature of the spine is always associated with some rotational deformity.

Scoliosis

There are two fundamental types of scoliosis: postural and structural.

POSTURAL SCOLIOSIS

A postural scoliosis disappears when the patient is observed from behind and asked to flex forward to touch his toes. The spine then reverts to its straight position and there is no associated rotation or rib hump. This postural scoliosis is seen in a variety of conditions—the short lower limb will produce a functional compensatory scoliosis convex to the side of the short leg. The poor stance of a child frequently produces this postural scoliosis which is of little importance and can always be corrected by appropriate instruction and discipline.

STRUCTURAL SCOLIOSIS

There are many causes of a structural scoliosis, both congenital and acquired. The major classification is divided into (1) osteopathic; (2) neuropathic and (3) myopathic.

With a structural scoliosis there is always rotation of the spine in association and this produces the characteristic rib rotation or hump. The scapula may be elevated on one side and the hip may project on the concave side of the curve (*Fig. S.14*).

Types of structural scoliosis

CONGENITAL

A wedge-shaped hemi-vertebra is present. This produces a kypho-scoliosis which is seen at birth and continues through life. There may be some increase in the curvature around the congenital deformity in the teenage years. Spina bifida will also produce abnormal curves seen at birth and is progressive through the first decade.

INFANTILE SCOLIOSIS

This scoliosis develops before the age of three. It is differentiated from congenital scoliosis by the absence of abnormalities of the vertebral bodies or the ribs at birth. In most cases it resolves spontaneously and only in a few will the curve progress. There is associated plagiocephaly and sometimes a postural adduction contracture of one hip.

IDIOPATHIC ADOLESCENT SCOLIOSIS

This refers to the structural scoliosis whose aetiology is unknown. It constitutes 80 per cent of patients with a structural scoliosis and occurs from the age of 10 years to the end of skeletal growth.

This type of scoliosis is familial. The child usually presents with a high shoulder or prominant hip and it is rare to complain of associated pain or fatigue. Later in life pain may be present from the degenerative changes which occur in the curved segment. In severe scoliotic curves the pressure of the ribs against the iliac crests may produce some discomfort. Respiratory and later cardiac abnormalities may occur in the patient with a severe curve.

The examination of the child with a scoliosis must include the general posture, the alignment of the spinous processes and the level of the shoulders. Rotation producing deformity of the rib cage is best observed in the patient bending forwards and the 'rib

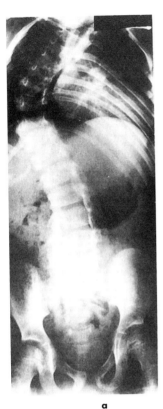

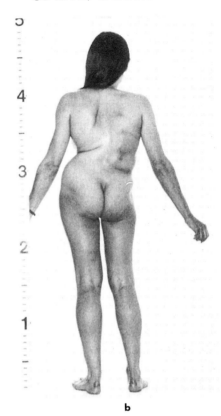

Fig. S.14. Scoliosis with rib rotation and hump. *a*, X-ray. *b*, Clinical photograph.

hump' then becomes apparent. General and neurological examination of the patient must also be undertaken, for the differential diagnosis between an idiopathic adolescent curve and that present in neurofibromatosis or neurological deficit is important in assessing the prognosis.

Causes of scoliosis

Neuromuscular causes of scoliosis
Neurofibromatosis
Cerebral palsy with spastic paralysis
Poliomyelitis
Syringomyelia
Intraspinal tumour
Friedreich's ataxia
Muscular causes of scoliosis
Muscle dystrophies
Arthrogryphosis multiplex congenita
Other myopathies
Scoliosis due to other abnormalities of the spinal column
Osteochondrodystrophies
Osteogenesis imperfecta
Fracture-disclocations
Tumours such as osteoid osteoma

Kyphosis

This indicates a forward flexion deformity of the spine producing a hump-back or a hunch-back. It may be diffuse over the whole spine or angular in which a gibbus or kyphus is present. The kyphosis may be congenital or acquired.

CONGENITAL CAUSES (*Fig.* S.15)

There may be a generalized abnormality of the skeleton such as a mucopolysaccharidosis. In Morquio's disease and also Hurler's disease (gargoylism) a kyphosis is present frequently with a gibbus.

ACQUIRED CAUSES

Tuberculosis of spine or Pott's disease (*Fig.* S.16)

The child is ill and holds the spine stiffly. The dorsal spine is most commonly affected and an angular prominence is felt when the infection has produced bone destruction and wedging of the vertebral bodies. An abscess frequently occurs around the diseased

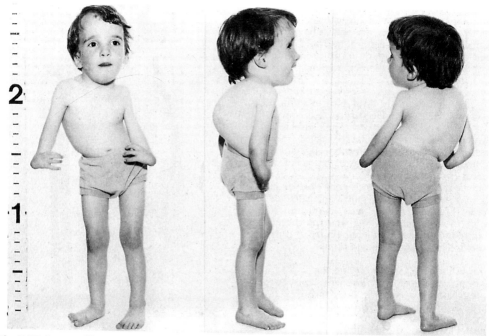

Fig. S.15. Congenital kyphoscoliosis. Note the radial club hands due to absence of the radii.

vertebrae and later may present in the lumbar triangle or in the groin as a cold abscess in the psoas sheath. Spinal cord compression may occur—Pott's paraplegia.

Crush fracture of the vertebral body
An angular kyphosis may be present at the site of a wedge crush fracture. In the osteoporotic, osteoma-lacic or rachitic patient, multiple wedge-shaped crush fractures may occur producing a smooth kyphosis in the thoracic region.

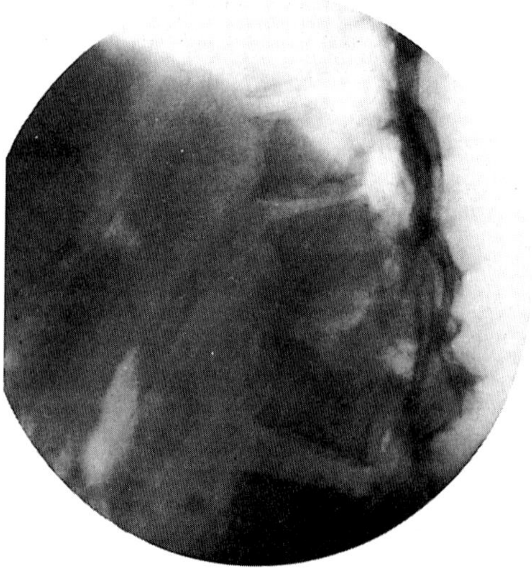

Scheuerman's disease or adolescent kyphosis
There is a fixed kyphosis developing at about the time of puberty. A wedge-shaped deformity of one or more vertebrae occurs. The cause is not known and the diagnosis is confirmed radiologically where there are multiple wedge-shaped vertebrae and excessive fragmentation of the vertebral end plate epiphyses.

The patient presents with poor posture and there may be aching and pain especially after exercise. The condition is seen in the thoracic spine in 75 per cent (*Fig.* S.17) and the thoracolumbar region in most of the remainder. A purely lumbar Scheuermann's disease is rare.

Paget's disease (osteitis of deformans)
This produces a uniform curve with consequent stooping without a compensatory lordosis (*Fig.* S.18). It is irreducible and the curvature first makes its appearance after middle age. There is usually evidence of the disease in other parts—progressive increase in the size of the head and thickening and bowing of the tibias and femurs. The disease may be pronounced in long bones long before the spine is affected.

Fig. S.16. Old tuberculous osteomyelitis.

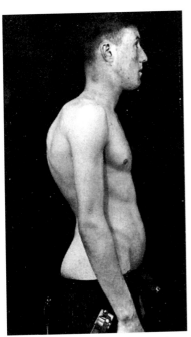

Fig. S.17. Smooth thoracic kyphosis due to longstanding Scheuermann's disease.

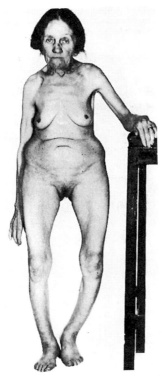

Fig. S.18. Paget's disease showing the kyphosis, bowing of the legs and apparently over-long arms, with increase in the size of the head. (*Dr. C. Baker.*)

Ankylosing spondylitis

In this condition some patients have a straight, stiff spine, but others are bent forwards with greater or lesser degrees of kyphosis, sometimes associated with scoliosis (*see Fig.* B.7). The neck is frequently flexed and the hips and shoulders may become involved. It is most common in the younger man and usually starts in the twenties.

Osteoarthritic changes

These occur in the vertebral bodies with advancing age. A fixed stoop occurs and the whole spine including both dorsal and lumbar regions becomes affected.

Porters carrying heavy weights may develop a kyphosis with osteoarthritis in the upper thoracic region. There is frequently a bursa over the 7th cervical spinous process ('Porter's bursa' or 'Porter's hummy').

Lordosis (hollow-back)

A lordosis occurs in the lumbar region and the lower dorsal area. It is an exaggeration of the normal lumbar contour and it usually occurs in compensation for some fixed flexion deformity of the hips. This is frequently seen in untreated bilateral congenital dislocation of the hips.

General muscle weakness as seen in muscle dystrophy frequently produces a lordosis.

SPONDYLOLISTHESIS

The slipping forwards of one vertebral body on the next is seen most commonly at the L5/Sl level. The spondylolisthesis is usually due to trauma and to a fracture through the pars interarticularis. The gradual slip of one vertebral body on the next may produce an increasing hollow of the lumbar region and in severe slips a step may be palpated at the unstable level.

Torticollis (wry neck)

CONGENITAL MUSCULAR TORTICOLLIS

Unilateral contracture of the sternomastoid muscle results in a deformity of the head and neck in which the head is tilted to the side and the chin rotated to the opposite side (*Fig.* S.19). The cause of this deformity is within the sternocleidomastoid muscle in which there is contracture and shortening. It may be due to birth trauma with a bleed into the muscle within its closed compartment and subsequent infarction and then fibrosis of the muscle belly. In the neonate the sternomastoid muscle may present a lump in its mid

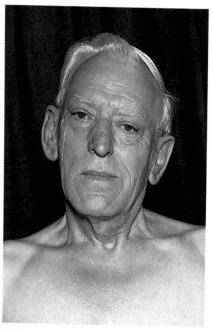

Fig. S.19. Congenital torticollis, with contracture of the sternocleidomastoid muscle. Note the associated hemi-atrophy of the left side of the face.

zone (sternomastoid tumour). This is the site of the developing fibrosis and gradually the sternomastoid muscle contracts and as the torticollis continues the face and the facial skeleton become flattened on the affected side.

KLIPPEL–FEIL SYNDROME

This is a rare cause of a torticollis in which there is a congenital fusion of two or more vertebrae in the cervical region. There is also hemi-vertebral malformations of the cervical vertebral bodies. The curvature may be severe and fixed and the facial asymmetry is often less than that seen in the congenital muscular type. Klippel–Feil syndrome may be associated with other deformities such as a congenital high scapula (Sprengel's deformity).

Paul Aichroth

Spine, tenderness of

(*See also* BACK, PAIN IN)

Tenderness of the spine is usually due to local disease of or injury to the tissues at the site of tenderness. Such tenderness is always deep, but may be associated with cutaneous hyperalgesia as well. In a second and less important group the tenderness is partly or entirely cutaneous, and is a referred phenomenon found in visceral disease. In testing for spinal tenderness it is therefore desirable to differentiate between cutaneous and deep tenderness and, in the case of the latter, between tenderness elicited by pressing upon the spinous processes and tenderness in the adjacent muscles, since spinal disease is usually accompanied by local muscular spasm and the muscles thus affected become tender although they are not themselves the site of the disease. Failure to allow for this fact is the usual explanation of the mistakes — sometimes serious — which are so often made in attributing muscle tenderness to a strain or to a rheumatic condition when in reality it is due to local spasm in response to disease of the vertebrae, intervertebral discs, or to the spinal cord and its membranes.

The chief conditions in which spinal tenderness occurs are summarized in *Table S.3.*

Table S.3. Chief conditions in which spinal tenderness occurs

1. **Diseases of the overlying skin and subcutaneous tissue**
   These are rare and clinically obvious

2. **Diseases of the vertebral column**

   a. INFLAMMATORY

Pott's disease	Ankylosing
Staphylococcal	spondylitis
spondylitis	Actinomycosis
Typhoid spine	Hydatid cyst
	Paget's disease

   b. DEGENERATIVE

Spondylosis	Herniation of nucleus
Osteochondritis	pulposus
(rare)	

   c. NEOPLASTIC

Secondary deposit	Myelomatosis
Sarcoma	Leukaemic deposits

   d. TRAUMATIC

Fracture	Disc herniation
Dislocation	Spondylolisthesis

   e. EROSION BY AORTIC ANEURYSM

3. **Diseases of the spinal cord and meninges**

Metastatic epidural	Meningitis serosa
abscess or tumour	circumscripta
Meningioma	Tumour of the spinal
Neurofibroma	cord
Herpes zoster	Syringomyelia

4. **Hysteria and malingering:**
   Compensation neurosis

5. **Metabolic disorders: osteoporosis, osteomalacia, hyperparathyroidism**

The investigation of spinal tenderness requires an exhaustive case history, a careful examination and certain special investigations. The history is of particular importance, because not only will it disclose the duration, site and severity of the spinal symptoms, but it will also indicate whether the spinal cord or nerve roots are involved (root pain, girdle sensations, paraesthesiae in the limb, muscular weakness or stiffness, sphincter disturbances). A systematic interrogation as to general health, previous diseases, and symptoms referable to the other systems of the body may bring out facts relevant to the spinal condition. There is no laboratory procedure which can give this information, and a further advantage of the historical approach is that it provides a guide to the patient's mental and emotional conditions which is invaluable in assessing the reality and severity of the spinal symptoms.

The second step, physical examination, must cover the whole body in a search for factors which may throw light on the spinal tenderness. Reference has already been made to the need for care in determining that the tenderness is really in the spine itself, and not in the adjacent muscles or the overlying skin. The extent of the tenderness and the presence or absence of limitation of movement must be established. Acute tenderness of organic origin is always associated with limitation of movement in one or more directions. The examination of sensation, power, and reflexes below the level of tenderness is important, for significant neurological abnormalities may be found in the absence of any subjective symptoms. Attention must be paid to the chest, cardiovascular system, abdomen and prostate. The long bones should receive attention, and the skull must not be forgotten, because in carcinomatosis painless secondary deposits may be found in the latter. Of the special investigations, X-ray examination of the spine takes the first place, but evidence of local disease may be long delayed and it is dangerous to assume that a negative finding is conclusive; further radiographs, taken at a later date, may tell a different tale, CT or MRI scanning of the spine give very accurate delineation of the spinal anatomy. X-ray examination of the chest, aorta, skull and long bones may be necessary. The cerebrospinal fluid should be examined, not only to see whether there is a raised protein and presence of leucocytes such as may be present in disease within the spinal canal, but also to exclude the possibility of a spinal block (Queckenstedt's test). A rise in the prostate specific antibody acid phosphatase of the serum will suggest the presence of a secondary growth from the prostate, and a high alkaline phosphatase is found in Paget's disease. A raised serum calcium will suggest hyperparathyroidism.

Pain and tenderness in the spine are sometimes functional. There is usually an organic nucleus to this either in the form of a long-past injury to the back or some minor physical abnormality. Marked spinal tenderness, especially in the thoracic spine, is frequently associated with current stress. Patients with spinal osteoarthritis and ankylosing spondylitis, for instance, are seldom tender over the spine unless anxiety or other mental overtones become superimposed.

Tenderness in the spine due to disease in other parts of the body

Superficial tenderness over the spine is a common association of visceral disease, and the tenderness is situated over the portion of the spine corresponding to the segmental innervation of the affected viscus. The tenderness is not associated with local rigidity, and there is invariably well-marked evidence of the visceral disease, so that such tenderness is unlikely to be taken for a manifestation of spinal disease. On the other hand, spinal disease which gives rise to local tenderness and to a root pain in the chest or abdomen is easily mistaken for visceral disease.

Harold Ellis

Splenomegaly

The normal sized spleen fits comfortably into the cupped hand and is impalpable on clinical examination. If splenic enlargement is detected the organ must be at least two or three times its normal size. As the spleen enlarges, its sharp anterior edge moves downwards and medially from below the left costal margin and the mass moves freely with respiration. Its edge is notched, but a 'palpable notch' is more often in the mind of the enthusiastic examiner than in clinical reality. A minor degree of splenomegaly may be detected by bimanual palpation. The right hand is passed around the lower left rib cage, which is lifted forward as the patient takes a deep breath. This lifts the spleen forwards, enabling it to be felt by the right hand anteriorly. The enlarged spleen is dull to percussion, in contrast to an enlarged left kidney (often a difficult differential diagnosis), which has resonant stomach and bowel in front of it.

An enlarged spleen may present because it is causing pressure symptoms or it may be found on examination of a patient who is generally unwell. Occasionally splenomegaly may be found on routine medical examination, in an individual who is asymptomatic, e.g. pre-employment or for insurance purposes. In this instance, particularly in a young person without other abnormal physical signs and a normal blood count, it can sometimes be extremely difficult to reach a diagnosis. A mass in the left hypochondrium, apart from a spleen may be an enlarged kidney, tumour of the splenic flexure of the colon or of the stomach or may arise from a retroperitoneal structure. Good medical practice dictates that an explanation should be found in all individuals for the splenomegaly; on occasions it will be necessary to proceed to laparoscopy or even laparotomy in an attempt to make a diagnosis.

The causes of splenomegaly are set out in Table S.4 and the most likely diagnosis varies considerably with the age, geographical location and social habits of the patient. Almost all causes of lymphadenopathy may be associated with splenomegaly and failing positive findings in other investigations, biopsy of an enlarged lymph node often renders a diagnosis possible.

Patients with splenomegaly may present with the symptoms and signs of pancytopenia due to hypersplenism which may occur with only a modest enlargement of the organ. There is usually an approximately parallel reduction in erythrocytes, leucocytes and platelets although on occasions there may be a more marked reduction of only one cell line. In the presence of such haematological abnormalities it is important to demonstrate normal or hyperplastic bone marrow morphology. In addition to the cellular elements being pooled and preferentially destroyed in the spleen the cytopenias are often exacerbated by a consistent increase in plasma volume.

Many diseases may result in enlargement of the spleen by several different mechanisms. For example in schistosomiasis the spleen may be enlarged because of chronic infection as well as portal hypertension secondary to portal fibrosis. A grossly enlarged spleen has a vastly increased blood supply and portal hypertension may result from high blood flow. In myelofibrosis with gross splenomegaly, for example, such a high flow of its own accord may cause portal hypertension such that ascites develops. When this is observed the prognosis is usually poor and splenectomy should be considered.

Investigation

A careful history and examination along with a full blood count and liver function tests will often provide a short differential diagnosis. If an infection is suspected appropriate microbiological tests will need to be carried out. When difficulty is encountered it is usually necessary to undertake fairly wide-ranging investigations. These should start by confirming that the mass palpated is spleen and not another pathology. Although traditionally a plain abdominal X-ray may delineate the splenic outline, other more recently developed techniques are now more informative. An

ultrasound examination will confirm the presence of a mass and also provide accurate dimensions; it is usually possible to distinguish between spleen and the other causes of a left hypochondrial mass, e.g. enlarged kidney. Furthermore, it may be valuable for detecting

Table S.4. Causes of splenomegaly

Infections
Viruses
  Glandular fever
Bacterial
  Typhus
  Typhoid
  Septicaemia ('septic spleen')
Protozoal
  Malaria
  Kala-azar
  Egyptian splenomegaly (schistosomiasis)
Parasitic
  Hydatid

Congestion (portal hypertension)
Hepatic cirrhosis
Portal vein obstruction
Splenic vein obstruction
Budd–Chiari syndrome
Cardiac failure

Haemolytic anaemias
Haemolytic anaemia
Hereditary spherocytosis
Thalassaemias
Red cell enzyme defects
Immune-mediated haemolysis

Haematological malignancies
Chronic myeloid leukaemia
Acute leukaemias
Chronic lymphatic leukaemia
Macroglobulinaemia
Polycythaemia rubra vera
Myelofibrosis
Essential thrombocythaemia
Lymphomas
  Hodgkin's disease
  Non-Hodgkin's disease
Hairy-cell leukaemia

Connective-tissue disorders
Systemic lupus erythematosus
Felty's syndrome

Storage disorders
Gaucher's disease
Niemann–Pick disease
Histiocytosis X

Space-occupying lesions
Abscess
Metastatic tumour
Cysts
  Hydatid
  Haemangioma
  Dermoid

space-occupying lesions, e.g. cysts or abscesses. An isotope liver and spleen scan will confirm splenomegaly and this investigation is particularly useful for detecting diffuse parenchymatous disease in the liver which may be causing portal hypertension, e.g. cirrhosis, or may be due to an infiltrate which could also be affecting the spleen. An abdominal CT scan will delineate the size and consistency of the spleen and is the investigation of choice if a lymphoma is suspected as it is useful for delineating retroperitoneal and mesenteric lymph nodes.

C. A. Ludlam

Stomach, dilatation of

(*See also* ABDOMINAL SWELLINGS)

Dilatation of the stomach presents itself clinically under two totally different aspects: (1) *Acute*; (2) *Chronic*.

1. Acute dilatation of the stomach

This is generally a serious complication or even a fatal catastrophe arising in the course of some other condition, especially after operations (notably laparotomy), or after abdominal injury.

The diagnosis is generally easy. The abdomen is distended and tympanitic; there is constant effort to bring up wind, sometimes in vain, sometimes with copious and recurrent eructations, often with intractable hiccoughs. Sometimes immense quantities of blackish-brown of greenish-brown fluid flow effortlessly from the mouth and nostrils. The dilatation itself is of the nature of an acute paralysis of the stomach. Diagnosis is confirmed, and indeed treatment initiated, by the passage of a stomach tube which deflates the gastric dilatation.

2. Chronic dilatation of the stomach

This is due to conditions which cause stenosis at, or more commonly on either side of, the pylorus.

CAUSES OF STENOSIS

Peptic ulcer, particularly of the duodenum although much less commonly a benign gastric ulcer at the pylorus or in the antrum may be responsible

Carcinoma of the pylorus or antrum

Other tumours in this region; these include leiomyoma, leiomyosarcoma, infiltration with Hodgkin's disease or lymphosarcoma or invasion from an adjacent carcinoma of pancreas or gallbladder

Congenital pyloric septum

Adult hypertrophy of the pylorus

Heterotopic pancreatic tissue

Adhesions of the duodenum to the liver bed following cholecystectomy

The history in an established case of pyloric stenosis may be absolutely typical. In the case of a peptic ulcer there may be a long preceding story of ulcer pain. Vomiting is an important symptom and occurs in at least 9 out of every 10 patients. Typically copious amounts of vomitus are produced in a projectile manner and the patient will recall (but often only on direct questioning) that he has noticed fragments of food, particularly vegetable or fruit debris, which had been ingested one day and vomited up the next, or even two or three days later. There is really no condition other than obstruction to the gastric outlet in which this state of affairs obtains. Obstruction due to carcinoma, in contrast, often has a shorter history, perhaps of only a few months, and pain is completely absent in about one-third of patients. Examination of the patient often reveals features of importance. There may be evidence of dehydration and loss of weight; indeed the classic 'ulcer facies' applies only rarely to uncomplicated examples of peptic ulcer but is perfectly mirrored in the usual appearance of the victim of long-standing stenosis (*Fig.* S.20). A gastric splash which is present 3 or 4 hours after a meal or drink is elicited in two-thirds of patients with benign stenosis. Often the patient when asked directly will agree that he himself has noticed a splashing sound when walking or moving about. Visible gastric peristalsis, passing from left to right, is present much less frequently, and still less often the loaded and hypertrophied stomach may actually be palpable as well as audible and visible (*see* PERISTALSIS, VISIBLE). About half the patients with malignant obstruction will reveal a palpable tumour at the pylorus. Such a mass may, it is true, be felt rarely in the benign case, when a large inflammatory mass is present around the first part of the duodenum. Because of the more rapid progression in the malignant case, gross dilatation of the stomach is much less often seen than in benign obstruction, so that a gastric splash and visible peristalsis may not be elicited.

Radiological investigation in these cases is mandatory. The findings can be divided into two groups: the first confirms the presence of an obstruction at the gastric outlet and the second indicates its pathology. A plain radiograph of the abdomen may itself be at least suggestive of pyloric stenosis by demonstrating a large gastric gas bubble with considerable quantities of retained food particles as demonstrated by patchy translucent areas. A sign of obstruction at the gastric outlet on the barium meal is the large residue of food within the stomach shown after taking a few mouthfuls of barium. Instead of the normal appearance of the barium running down the lesser curvature, the particles of barium can be seen to sink through a layer of fluid and then to rest at the bottom of the greater curve

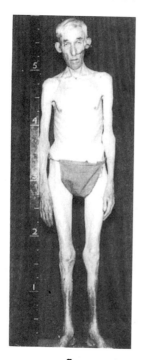
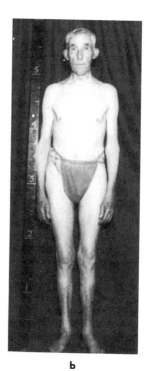

a
b

Fig. S.20. a, Typical appearance of a patient with longstanding pyloric stenosis due to a duodenal ulcer. The patient demonstrates the drawn, anxious facies, gross dehydration and wasting. b, Note the dramatic change following vagotomy and pyloroplasty.

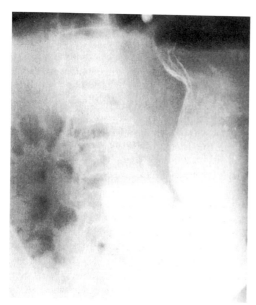

Fig. S.21. Pyloric stenosis due to chronic duodenal ulcer. Note three layers: air, gastric juice and barium.

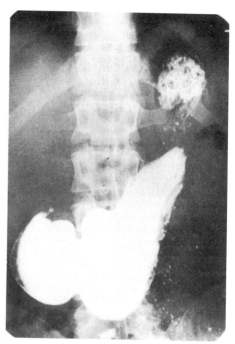

Fig. S.22. Pyloric stenosis due to chronic duodenal ulcer. The picture was taken 3 hours after a barium meal; note the considerable residium of barium. (Dr Keith Jefferson.)

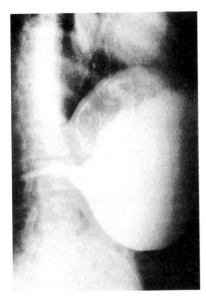

Fig. S.23. Pyloric obstruction due to extensive antral carcinoma.

like a saucer. In the erect position three layers can be seen; the air bubble above, then the layer of gastric juice, and finally the lowermost layer of barium (*Fig. S.21*). In the early phase of pyloric stenosis giant peristaltic waves may be seen passing along the gastric wall, but in late decompensated obstruction the stomach is a large atonic bag. Obstruction of the gastric outlet is confirmed by taking further films at 4–6 hours when it will be seen that a large residium of barium remains in the stomach (*Fig. S.22*). Under normal circumstances the stomach is all but empty at the end of 2 hours. It is not always easy to tell the exact cause of the pyloric obstruction. Radiological evidence that a duodenal ulcer is responsible is given by the presence of an active ulcer crater or severe scarring in the duodenal cap. If the obstruction is situated in the antrum of the stomach it is most probable that the diagnosis is cancer (*Fig. S.23*) but occasionally a similar appearance is given by a penetrating benign gastric ulcer. A further sign of duodenal bulb obstruction that we have found to be useful is abnormal dilatability of the pyloric canal which may be seen on screening to dilate up to 2.5 cm or more in width and then contract down again to its usual size proximal to the point of stenosis.

Gastroscopy by means of a fiber-optic endoscope may visualize the obstructing ulcer and allow a biopsy to be performed, but often adherent gastric contents obscure the view.

The less common causes of pyloric obstruction mentioned above which may be associated with chronic dilatation of the stomach are rarely diagnosed before laparotomy. However, since obstruction of the gastric outlet almost invariably requires surgical intervention the elucidation of the exact cause preceding operation is a luxury rather than a necessity for the experienced surgeon.

Harold Ellis

Stools, mucus in

Mucus in the stools is not pathognomonic. It occurs in *malignant disease of the colon* as a clear glairy substance, often bloodstained, and it has the same character in *intussusception*; the obstruction in both these conditions accounts for the absence of faecal colouring. Large amounts of mucus may be secreted by extensive *benign papillomatous tumours* of the colon and rectum. Since mucus is rich in potassium, profound potassium depletion may occur in this condition, leading to weakness, paraesthesiae and even paralysis and vascular collapse. The volume of fluid passed may amount to 2 or 3 litres daily. Mucus is often seen with *constipated motions*, the hard faeces having led to irritation of the large bowel with consequent increased secretion of mucus as a defensive mechanism against misguided therapy, especially intestinal lavage. In severe cases a motion may consist almost entirely of coagulated shreds with little faecal matter. In other cases, complete casts of the bowel formed of coagulated mucus are passed; they may be a foot or more in length. They may have become broken into fragments which the patient describes as skins, looking not unlike segments of tape-worm for which indeed they are on inadequate examination easily mistaken. Patients passing this variety of mucus are said to have *membranous* or *spastic colitis*, an incorrect term, for no inflammatory process occurs. The term 'irritable colon syndrome' is also used for this disorder, which is characterized by colonic abdominal pain, abnormal stools and alteration in bowel habits. It is more common in females aged 15–45 years but may occur in either sex under conditions of emotional tension. The patients on examination often appear anxious and tense and perspire excessively. Curiously enough, this hypersecretion of mucus has almost disappeared during the past 30 years, although the general symptomatology is still recognized. It may be added that the popular treatment of lavage to remove the mucus will be responsible for its continued secretion as a protest against irritation of the mucosa.

In the more acute varieties of inflammation of the bowel the mucus passed is jelly-like and semi-liquid, of varying colour according to the amount of faecal staining. In *polyposis coli* and severe cases of *ulcer-*

ative colitis, Crohn's colitis, enteritis and *dysentery* the motions consist of nothing but mucus and blood. One cannot differentiate between the numerous varieties of enteritis and colitis upon the basis of the mucus in the stools alone.

Harold Ellis

Stools, pus in

Pus in the stools in sufficient amount to be recognizable by the naked eye indicates the rupture of an abscess into the intestinal tract. Such recognition is, however, unusual; for even when a large appendicular abscess perforates into the caecum the pus becomes indistinguishable either from admixture with the faeces, the patient believing he simply has diarrhoea, or on account of digestion and decomposition. The less the pus is mixed with other intestinal contents, the nearer to the anus must the size of rupture have been; but the diagnosis of the source of the abscess needs to be determined upon other grounds, particularly the history and the results of examination, including that of the rectum and vagina. Abscesses most apt to cause a discharge of pus with the stools are of the appendicular, pericolic, pelvic or other local peritoneal types; of prostatic or perirectal origin; or a pyosalpinx.

Microscopical quantities of pus in the stools may be due to any of the causes already mentioned and, in addition, to affections of the mucous membrane itself. These comprise acute or chronic ulcerative colitis, Crohn's colitis; dysentery; cholera; dengue; malignant, tuberculous, typhoidal, carcinomarous or venereal ulceration of the bowel. The pus cells may be recognizable as such under the microscope. Examination with the signoidoscope, followed by a barium enema X-ray, is invaluable in deciding the diagnosis.

Harold Ellis

Strangury

Strangury differs somewhat from mere pain on micturition, in that, in addition to severe pain before, during or after the act, the patient is troubled constantly by urgent and repeated necessity to pass his urine, sometimes as often as every few minutes, yet without satisfactory relief to his discomfort. The condition is also spoken of as 'vesical tenesmus'. Very little urine is passed each time; sometimes the desire and the necessity are urgent when there is no urine in the bladder at all. The causes resolve themselves into five groups, as follows:

1. Nervous conditions, especially:

Hysterisa
Anxiety state
Tabes dorsalis (vesical crises)

2. Obstruction to the urine outflow

Urethral stricture
Enlarged prostate
Prostatic calculus
Carcinoma of the prostate
Retroverted gravid uterus
Uterine fibroid ⎫
Ovarian cyst ⎬ impacted in the pelvis
Ovarian carcinoma ⎭
Extreme prolapse of the uterus and bladder
Calculus impacted in the urethra
Inflamed urethral caruncle
Gonorrhoea
Urethritis other than gonococcal
Periprostatic abscess
Ischiorectal abscess

3. Local affections of the bladder wall

Injury
Acute cystitis
Chronic cystitis
Interstitial cystitis (Hunner's ulcer)
Tuberculous cystitis
Calculus irritating the trigone
Carcinoma
Bilharziasis
Infiltration by—
  Carcinoma of the uterus
  Carcinoma of the rectum
Acute vesiculitis

4. Reflex conditions

Inflamed haemorrhoids
Tuberculous kidney, before the bladder is involved
E. Coli bacilluria ⎫ even before there is infection of
Pyelitis ⎬ the bladder wall

5. The effects of certain drugs, especially:

Cantharides
Oxalic acid
Turpentine
Hexamine and its derivatives

Most of the conditions mentioned above, and the methods of distinguishing between them, are discussed in the Section on MICTURITION, FREQUENCY OF.

Interstitial cystitis (Hunner's ulcer) is probably not an infectious disease. Histologically there is inflammatory infiltration of the bladder wall, unifocal or multifocal with mucosal ulceration and scarring, leading to contraction of smooth muscle, diminished capacity and frequent painful micturition with haematuria. The patients are usually middle-aged women.

Another point that merits attention is the strangury produced by certain drugs. *Cantharides* is familiar in this respect, but more from its prominence in textbooks upon forensic medicine than from its occurrence in actual practice. The same applies to *oxalic acid* and to *turpentine*. Hexamine and similar drugs derived from it are important. These have been employed in the treatment of pyuria, as well as other conditions, but have now been largely replaced by sulpha drugs and antibiotics. If given for pyuria, when there may have been frequent and painful micturition already, the increased frequency and pain that sometimes ensue when any of the above drugs are administered are apt to be attributed to an increase in the cystitis or other genitourinary lesion, and the dose of the drug may be increased instead of diminished. The important point is that hexamine and other drugs of like nature may be responsible for such strangury as may simulate local disease of the bladder, and unless this is borne in mind an erroneous diagnosis is liable to be made.

Harold Ellis

Succussion sounds

Succussion sounds may be heard when a viscus or cavity that contains both liquid and air or gas is shaken whilst the ear or the stethoscope is applied over it. The sounds may be loud enough to be audible at a distance from the patient. A good example of succussion is often afforded by the normal stomach after a quantity of liquid has been swallowed. Gastric succussion sounds are not necessarily evidence of abnormality, they merely indicate that the viscus contains liquid and gas. Succussion sound may be heard in the chest in cases of *hydropneumothorax* when the patient oscillates his trunk to and fro. Less often, succussion sounds may be produced by a pyopneumothorax or a haemopneumothorax, the difference between these being decided by a pleural tap. Other succussion sounds are uncommon.

The following is a list of all possible causes:

1. Causes of succussion sounds in the thorax

Hydropneumothorax
Pyopneumothorax
Haemopneumothorax
Diaphragmatic hernia
Subdiaphragmatic abscess communicating with the stomach or duodenum, or infected with E. coli: in either case, gas and pus are present
Hydropneumopericardium
Pyopneumopericardium

2. Causes of succussion sounds in the abdomen

The normal stomach
Dilatation of the stomach
Gross dilatation of the caecum
Gross dilatation of the colon
Pneumoperitoneum due to: (*a* Perforated gastric ulcer; (*b*) Perforated duodenal ulcer; (*c*) Perforated typhoid ulcer of the intestine; (*d*) Perforated carcinoma of the colon; (*e*) Production of gas by E. coli, either in a local abscess (e.g. appendicular or subdiaphragmatic) or in the general peritoneum
Subdiaphragmatic abscess communicating with the interior of the stomach
Air and urine in the bladder (*see* PNEUMATURIA)
Gas-production by E. coli in a large pyonephrosis
Infection by a gas-producing micro-organism of an ovarian cyst or other collection of fluid.

Succussion sounds in the chest

It is almost unknown for a *tuberculous cavity* to give succussion sounds. Should it do so, the situation would be subapical rather than basal, and thus distinguishable from most cases of hydro-or pyopneumothorax. *Hydro-* and *pyopneumopericardium* are also rare: they are identified by the churning sounds made by the heart beating within the mixture of air and liquid. The cause is generally a tumour of the oesophagus or bronchus opening the pericardium from behind, a foreign body such as dental plate ulcerating through from the oesophagus, the opening of an air-containing subdiaphragmatic abscess through the diaphragm into the pericardium or infection of the pericardial sac by a gas-producing organism.

A *subdiaphragmatic abscess* containing air due to communication with a hole in a gastric or duodenal ulcer may elevate the diaphragm so high that the condition may be mistaken for hydro- or pyopneumothorax. Decision may be impossible until the position of the diaphragm is ascertained by X-rays and ultrasonography. When the pathology is subdiaphragmatic the tendency is to displace the heart upwards rather than towards the opposite side of the chest; the contrary is usual in the case of pneumothorax.

Diaphragmatic hernias, if large and if the stomach is herniated into the thorax, will show the effect of eating and drinking upon the physical signs and may point to the diagnosis. X-rays will demonstrate the condition on barium meal.

Most cases of *hydropneumothorax* present little difficulty in diagnosis although it may not be easy to ascertain its cause. If the onset has been sudden with acute pain in the affected side of the chest, cyanosis and dyspnoea, the most likely cause is *tuberculosis*. In some instances, an injury or a ruptured emphysematous bulla may have been responsible, but injury seldom produces hydropneumothorax unless a tuberculous or other lesion in the lung was present at the time of the accident. Hydropneumothorax may result from *paracentesis thoracis*; if bleeding occurs during the puncture, *haemopneumothorax* will be produced. This too is common after bullet wounds of the chest. Either a hydro- or a haemopneumothorax may become infected with pyogenic organisms and converted into a *pyopneumothorax*. Pyopneumothorax may develop in cases of gangrene of the lung, obstruction of a bronchus by a foreign body or a tumour, the breaking down of an infective bronchopneumonia or pulmonary infarct, or the conversion of a pleural haematoma into a mixture of pus and gas as the result of infection by gas-gangrene organisms after gunshot or other wounds of the chest. Fluid often collects in the pleural cavity when an artificial (therapeutic) pneumothorax has been induced, giving succussion sounds.

Succussion sounds in the abdomen

The first point in the differential diagnosis of succussion sounds in the abdomen is to decide whether the sounds are or are not of gastric origin. This is usually obvious but any doubt can be at once resolved by a barium meal. Dilatation of the stomach has three causes, namely atony, non-malignant pyloric or duodenal obstruction, especially by a healed simple ulcer, and malignant pyloric obstruction by primary gastric carcinoma (*see* PERISTALSIS, VISIBLE; STOMACH, DILATATION OF). The presence of visible peristaltic waves or the occurrence of vomiting will indicate some degree of pyloric obstruction. Such obstruction will usually result in periodic vomiting, when the particles of food eaten a day or more previously can be recognized. Visible peristaltic waves corresponding to the stomach are another confirmatory feature. The most certain method of detecting gastric outflow obstruction is by means of a barium meal examination.

If there are well-marked abdominal succussion sounds that can be definitely shown to be of non-gastric origin there are generally other signs and symptoms to assist the diagnosis. Succussion sounds in the peritoneal cavity are exceedingly rare, for even though this cavity should contain both gas and liquid — for instance after perforation of a typhoid ulcer — the coils of bowel prevent the sounds from being readily produced. The most common cause is iatrogenic, occurring when air is introduced into the peritoneum, when ascites is tapped or when carbon dioxide is introduced at laparoscopy in the presence of ascites. It would clearly be next to impossible to diagnose most of the conditions listed above unless the previous state of the patient was known or without a laparotomy. *E. coli* produces gas so that intra-abdominal abscesses, appendicular and otherwise, are occasionally resonant; the occurrence, however, of marked non-gastric succussion sounds in the abdomen of a patient who is not acutely ill will support the conclusion that there is distension with gas and liquid of some part of the large bowel, especially the caecum or the sigmoid colon. This distension is generally the result of either chronic constipation or intestinal stenosis. In cases of idiopathic dilatation of the colon, volvulus of the sigmoid colon or Hirschsprung's disease, the sigmoid dilatation may be so extreme that this part of the intestine bulges up as far as the diaphragm.

Ian A. D. Bouchier

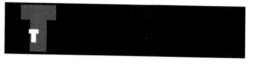

Testicular pain

Pain in the testicle of varying degree may be present in many conditions, which may be discussed under separate headings as follows: (A) *Diseases of the body of the testis or epididymis*; (B) *Affections of the coverings of the testicle*; (C) *Affections of the spermatic cord*; (D) *A retained or misplaced testicle*; (E) *Pain from lesions remote from the testis*.

A. Diseases of the body of the testis or epididymis

Inflammatory lesions

Inflammatory lesions may attack the testis proper, or, as is more common, may begin in the epididymis. The investing tunica vaginalis distends with inflammatory exudate to form a secondary hydrocele. This tender mass may be mistaken for a swelling of the testis proper and the condition is frequently labelled an 'acute epididymo-orchitis'. However, surgical exploration and histological study reveal that the testis proper is rarely implicated and it is accurate, therefore, to speak of 'acute epididymitis'. An inflammatory affection of the testicle may be acute, subacute or chronic, the last often being the terminal result of the others.

An acute epididymitis arises most commonly by spread of infection to the organ from the urethra via the vas deferens or by the lymphatics accompanying the vas. When any inflammation has reached the prostatic portion of the urethra the orifices of the vasa deferentia may become infected, and inflammation spreads along the duct to the epididymis.

CAUSES OF ACUTE EPIDIDYMITIS

Causes of urethral origin
Urethritis due to *N. gonorrhoeae*
Urethritis due to *C. trachomatis*
Septic urethritis
Passage of catheters
Urethral instrumentation
Infection behind a stricture
Ulceration about an impacted calculus
Injections into the posterior urethra
After operations on the prostate
Urinary infections
Non-specific epididymitis

CAUSES OF ACUTE ORCHITIS

Fevers:
  Parotitis (mumps)
  Typhoid
  Scarlet fever

CAUSES OF CHRONIC EPIDIDYMITIS

Tuberculosis
Resolving acute epididymitis

SYPHILITIC DISEASE OF THE TESTIS

Diffuse interstitial orchitis
Gummatous orchitis

OTHER DISEASES

Malignant tumours of the testis
Torsion of the testis
Cysts of the epididymis

Acute epididymitis

Acute epididymitis begins as a painful thickening of the epididymis associated with febrile symptoms. Before any actual pain is noticed in the testis there is often a sense of discomfort and weight over the external abdominal ring and inguinal canal due to the inflammatory process extending along the vas deferens. The swelling of the epididymis increases, and with it there is a secondary effusion of exudate into the tunica vaginalis (secondary hydrocele), causing swelling of its body and increase of pain. The whole organ thus becomes enlarged, and it is often exquisitely tender, the touch of the clothes or the most gentle examination causing pain. The swollen gland is often flattened on the outer and posterior aspect from pressure against the adductor muscles of the thigh; the vas deferens and tissues of the spermatic cord are thickened.

By far the most common cause of an acute epididymitis was formerly an *acute gonorrhoeal urethritis*; under the more effective modern antibiotic treatment of gonorrhoea it occurs much less often. During the disease the prostatic portion of the channel frequently becomes infected, when the orifices of the ejaculatory ducts may share in the inflammation, and infection be conveyed by the vas deferens to the testicle. Infection may also arise following an attack of non-specific urethritis, acquired as a result of sexual intercourse with a partner suffering from non-specific genital infection. Non-specific urethritis today is the commonest sexually transmitted disease in the Western world and at least 1 per cent of all male cases develop epididymitis. *C. trachomatis* is commonly found and appears to be the cause in around 50 per cent of cases. The gonorrhoeal form of acute epididymitis usually resolves slowly, and shows little liability to suppurate, whereas the inflammation resulting from a staphylococcal or streptococcal infection may break down into a testicular abscess.

Acute epididymitis may also arise from septic processes in the urethra following the *passage of catheters*, of *instruments* for vesical operations, transurethral prostatic resection or lithotrity for example, from infection behind a *urethral striction* or about a *calculus* in the prostatic urethra, occasionally after the *instillation of strong solutions* into the posterior urethra in the treatment of a chronic urethritis, or after operations on the prostate, especially prostatectomy, or as a complication of a urinary infection by *E. coli* or other organisms. It may follow prostatic massage. In any case the onset of pyrexia with pain and rapid swelling of the testis should lead to suspicion of a urinary tract infection. Bacteriological examination of any urethral discharge and of the urine is essential (*see* URETHRAL DISCHARGE).

In *non-specific epididymitis* there may be no evidence of urethral infection and bacteriological studies are entirely negative; the condition sometimes arises after unaccustomed exercise and has been attributed to a reflux of urine down the vas. The testicle becomes painful, and enlarges rapidly in the same manner as in acute inflammation from urethral infection, and under appropriate conservative treatment by means of a scrotal support gradually resolves. Less frequently testicular inflammation may occur after a direct injury to the organ, such as a *blow* or *squeeze*.

The pain in an acute inflammation is generally of an aching character at first, felt not only in the testis but also at the external abdominal ring, and often as a heavy dragging pain in the inguinal or iliac areas of the affected side. As the testis enlarges the local pain becomes more severe, so that the swollen gland is exquisitely tender to pressure or to the touch. After a few days the pain subsides to a large extent, but remains as a dull ache until the swelling becomes greatly reduced, and it usually does not disappear entirely until the organ returns to the normal size. In a few cases in which a fibrous scar remains in the epididymis pain may remain and cause some difficulty in the diagnosis from an incipient tuberculous lesion, but the earlier history of acute inflammation will help in forming an opinion. In other cases the persistence of the pain and swelling may indicate the formation of an abscess in the testicle, when, after decreasing at first, the swelling increases, the skin covering it becomes reddened and oedematous, and a soft area becomes evident in one aspect of the organ.

Acute orchitis

Acute orchitis may complicate *acute specific parotitis* (mumps), especially when this occurs in adolescents or adults. Both testes may be affected and the result may be testicular atrophy. Much less often the testis may be affected in *typhoid*, *scarlet fever* or *influenza*.

Tuberculosis of the testicle

Tuberculosis of the testicle is comparatively common today in many parts of the world, including India and the Far East, but is now quite rare in Great Britain. It arises with extreme rarity as a primary disease but more commonly as secondary to tuberculous disease of the kidney, bladder, prostate or seminal vesicles. It is most frequently seen in young adults. It begins as a localized deposit in almost all cases, causing a rounded, firm nodule in the epididymis, usually in the lower pole. This nodule may remain unaltered for many months, or may enlarge, soften, become adherent to the skin and coverings of the testicle, or actually ulcerate through them to form a discharging sinus in the scrotum. The small nodule in the epididymis is usually painless at first and may be found by accident, but later, as it gradually enlarges, it causes an aching pain in the organ. There may be an associated hydrocele of the tunica vaginalis. Other nodules may be formed in the epididymis, or the body of the testis may become involved, while commonly small shot-like thickenings may be felt in the course of the vas deferens, or a progressively increasing thickening as it

is traced down to the epididymis. In the more advanced stages nodules may be felt upon rectal examination in the seminal vesicles or prostate, or there may be some in the epididymis of the other side.

Tuberculous disease of the testicle usually presents some difficulty in its diagnosis from non-specific epididymitis, particularly when it has an acute onset, as sometimes happens. In an early case the occurrence of one or more nodules in the epididymis, which are painful on pressure and which have not resulted from a preceding acute epididymitis, should always suggest a tuberculous focus, and a careful search should be made for other tuberculous lesions in the body. The urine is examined for acid-fast bacilli and cultured for *M. tuberculosum* and intravenous pyelography performed. If no evidence of tuberculosis is found the gradual subsidence of the lesion under careful observation will indicate that it was a non-specific epididymitis. In later stages the diagnosis is less difficult; the gradual enlargement of the nodules, their craggy or bossy feel, the infection of the vas or other genitourinary organs with tuberculosis, and above all the tendency of the focus in the epididymis to soften and to become adherent to the scrotal coverings and to produce an indolent sinus, are points to be looked for.

Syphilitic disease of the testis

Syphilitic disease of the testis, once common, but now a rarity, causes very little pain in the organ, but there is often a sense of dragging or heaviness. Syphilis may attack the testicle in several different ways, producing:

IN ACQUIRED SYPHILIS

Diffuse interstitial orchitis
Localized gummatous orchitis

IN CONGENITAL SYPHILIS

interstitial orchitis
localized gummatous orchitis

The outstanding feature of syphilitic disease of the testicle is that it affects the body of the testis rather than the epididymis, thus differing in a marked degree from tuberculous disease. in the interstitial form there is thickening of the intertubular connective tissue, with an infiltration of spindle cells, which, forming young connective tissue, yield fibrous tissue. the subsequent contraction of this fibrous tissue may cause atrophy of the testis. the testis may, on section, show small gummas in addition to the diffuse orchitis, or if the inflammation is more localized, gummas may be the main feature, these varying in size from that of a pea to that of a walnut, or larger. the epididymis is affected but rarely, though cases are on record of a nodular swelling in the epididymis during the secondary stage of syphilis which disappears rapidly under anti-syphilitic treatment.

In congenital syphilis, both the interstitial and gummatous forms exist; they usually occur in childhood or in young adult life, and in many cases the affection is bilateral. syphilitic inflammation of the testicle may be accompanied in either the acquired or the congenital form by a vaginal hydrocele. a gummatous testis may ulcerate through the scrotum, usually in front, producing a circular 'punched-out' ulcer with a slough in the base.

There is a sense of weight in the scrotum rather than pain, and often an aching or dragging feeling in the inguinal or lumbar region. on palpation, the body of the testis feels enlarged and nodular with the gummatous deposits, but the epididymis can usually be distinguished from the testis and found to be unaffected. testicular sensation is lost. the tissues of the cord remain unthickened. tertiary syphilitic lesions of the testicle give rise to very little tenderness on palpation.

The diagnosis of syphilitic disease of the testis is usually simple. there may or may not be a history of syphilis, but other signs of the disease should be looked for—thus, in the acquired form, any scar of previous ulceration or periosteal thickening, or, in the congenital variety, signs in the teeth, eyes or ears. syphilitic disease is distinguished from *tuberculous disease* of the testis by the fact that the epididymis is usually free; that the cord, prostate and vesicles remain normal; and that pressure applied directly to the testicle gives little or no pain. Tuberculous deposits tend to soften and to involve the scrotal coverings in spite of treatment. From haematocele it is differentiated by the history of injury or by the absence of the history or signs of syphilis. From *malignant tumours of the testis* it is distinguished by the history of syphilis, the tendency of syphilitic disease to be bilateral, the slow enlargement, and positive serological tests. In malignant disease, the increase in the size of the testicle is more rapid, while the tumour often shows areas of varying consistence; the cord is often thickened in malignant or in tuberculous cases, but seldom in syphilitic.

It should be pointed out that gumma of the testis is so rare in Great Britain today, compared with its former frequency, that it is safer to regard any solid swelling in the testicle itself as the much more common and more likely malignant tumour of the testis, and treat it as such by orchidectomy. In the unlikely event that a gumma is thus removed, the surgeon can comfort himself with the fact that a functionally useless organ has been excised.

Malignant tumours of the testis

Malignant tumours of the testis may give rise to pain in the organ, but as a rule pain is experienced only in the later stages of the disease. Although benign tumours of the epididymis may occur, nearly all tumours of the testis are highly malignant. They fall into two main pathological varieties, *seminoma* and *teratoma*, the latter including the subgroups of *chorionepithelioma*, *dermoid* and *fibrocystic disease*. The *seminoma* (*Fig.* T.1) is a soft vascular solid growth composed of large spheroidal cells derived from the germinal epithelium of the seminiferous tubules. It occurs at about the age of 30–40 and is less malignant but more radiosensitive than teratoma. It tends to retain the shape of the testis as it enlarges.

The *teratoma* (*Fig.* T.2) or mixed tumour is a solid or multilocular cystic growth in which one or other of the germinal layers may preponderate. Dermoids, containing hair or teeth, are less common than in the ovary but sometimes occur in childhood and are relatively benign.

Fibrocystic disease pursues an even more benign course and may be present for 10 or more years before exhibiting its malignant characteristics by sudden rapid

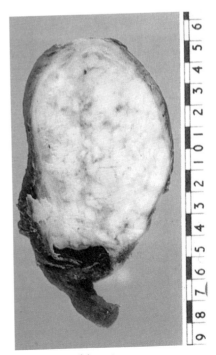

Fig. T.1. Seminoma of the testis.

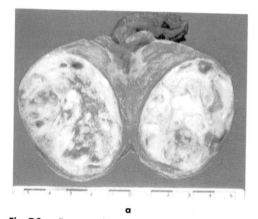

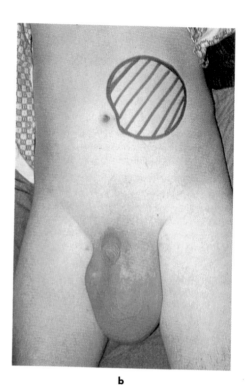

Fig. T.2. *a,* Teratoma of the testis. *b,* Teratoma of the left testis with a large mass of para-aortic nodes.

growth and the formation of metastases. Most cases of teratoma occur at the age of 25–30; they give a short history, are more resistant to X-ray treatment, and show early metastases. There may be enlargement of the breasts and chorionic hormone may be present in the urine; in seminoma the pituitary gonadotrophic hormone is sometimes found in the urine. Either type may follow injury in a significant proportion of cases although it is likely that trauma merely draws attention to the testicular mass. The undescended testis is more prone to develop malignant disease than is the normally placed one. The testis which has been initially undescended and subsequently brought down into the scrotum maintains this higher tendency to malignant change, estimated at about ten times that of the normal organ.

A testicle that is the seat of a malignant growth enlarges slowly or rapidly, but as pain is at first absent there may be nothing to arouse the patient's suspicions. As long as the tunica albuginea remains intact the swelling retains the shape of the testis, but when perforation of the fibrous covering takes place nodular projections appear and render the tumour irregular. These projections are softer than the remainder of the growth, and form a valuable point in the diagnosis. A rapidly growing malignant tumour of the testis may be so soft as to appear to be a fluid collection in the tunica

vaginalis. Generally, however, although a growth may be accompanied by a small amount of fluid in the tunica vaginalis, the more solid mass can be felt through the fluid on careful examination; this fluid is often blood-stained. The epididymis may become incorporated in the growth so that it cannot be distinguished, and the tissues of the cord become thickened. The coverings of the testis become stretched over the tumour; the mass does not become adherent to the scrotal skin until late in the disease. Clinically it is impossible to distinguish between a teratoma and a seminoma. In both types the para-aortic lymph nodes become enlarged, and may be felt in a thin subject to one or other side of the epigastric area, and pain due to the pressure of these nodes upon nerve structures may become marked (*Fig.* T.2b). The inguinal nodes are usually not enlarged unless the scrotal skin is affected; retrograde spread may then occur to the iliac nodes which may be felt at the brim of the pelvis. In advanced cases, the left supraclavicular lymph nodes are involved and become palpably enlarged. Mediastinal or pulmonary metastases are frequent, the latter giving the characteristic radiological appearance of 'cannon-ball' secondaries. The diagnosis of malignant disease of the testis may be quite easy in the case of rapidly growing tumours, but in others, especially in the early stages, it may present great difficulty. Rarely an *interstitial-cell tumour* occurs in a child and produces sexual precocity. Differential diagnosis must be made between malignant tumours and the following:

Gummatous orchitis may be confused with the more slowly growing forms of tumour. In both the swelling may have followed an injury, and in both there may be a syphilitic history. Gummatous orchitis is, however, either more acute or more chronic; it retains more the oval shape of the testis, and does not present the rounded, slightly raised bosses which are commonly present in a malignant testis. In orchitis the epididymis is usually distinguished more easily, and the cord is not so thickened as with a growth. In any case of doubt it is a wise course to advise exploration. (*See above.*)

Tuberculous disease is usually diagnosed easily from malignant disease by the tendency of tubercle to attack the epididymis, to caseate, suppurate and to become adherent to the scrotal skin comparatively early. Tuberculosis occasionally attacks the body of the testicle first, however, forming an oval, smooth tumour of the organ; the epididymis and vas deferens may be unaffected for a time, and if no deposit is found in the prostate or vesicles the differential diagnosis between tubercle and growth may be far from easy before operation. Tuberculosis most frequently occurs in young adults.

The diagnosis between a *haematocele* and a malignant tumour of the testis may present considerable difficulty. In both, the swelling may date from an injury, while the indistinct fluctuation obtained in the soft areas of a growth, accompanied sometimes by some fluid in the tunica vaginalis, may simulate a haematocele. The latter feels heavy to the hand, but is usually softer in its whole mass and more regular than a growth. Care must be taken not to place too much reliance upon the withdrawal of a few drops of blood from the tumour by means of needle aspiration, a result which may happen equally with growth or haematocele. A haematocele may cease to enlarge, or even diminish in size, whereas, in growth, increase in size is progressive. The cord remains unaffected with haematocele, and testicular sensation is more likely to be lost in growth.

Ultrasonography of the testis can be very useful in localizing the exact site of the mass and in differentiating between a solid and a cystic mass. If any doubt exists it is advisable to excise the testis, dividing the cord at the internal ring. Incision into a testis which is the seat of a growth is almost invariably followed by rapid recurrence. If necessary, a radical operation can be done after the histology is known, or radiotherapy can be given. (*See also below.*)

A *hydrocele* of very long standing with an irregular, nodular surface, and absence of translucency due to the thickened tunica vaginalis and the thick contents of the sac, may simulate a new growth, but the long history of the case, and the absence of progressive increase in size of the swelling, will prevent a mistake of this kind. (*See also below.*)

Torsion of the testis

Torsion of the testis on its vascular pedicle may occur in a testis which has a mesorchium or in one which is ectopic. It occurs most commonly in youths soon after puberty, or in infants; the exciting cause may be some mild exertion or movement such as crossing the legs or turning over in bed. There may be a history of repeated minor attacks before complete torsion takes place, and the other testis may have suffered similar incomplete attacks or be found to be unduly mobile or horizontally placed. At the moment of torsion there is severe sickening pain which may be felt at first in the abdomen but is quickly localized to the testis; the boy may even say that his testicle has twisted. There is usually nausea and sometimes vomiting. The testis forms a tense tender swelling in the upper part of the scrotum or at the external abdominal ring, and the scrotum below is empty. This sign serves to distinguish the condition from a strangulated hernia or an inflamed lymph node. In acute epididymitis the testis is in its normal position and there may be evidence of urethral discharge or of a urinary tract infection. Because of the initial abdominal pain and vomiting the condition has been mistaken for acute appendicitis, but adherence to the rule of examining the scrotal contents in all abdominal cases should prevent this error.

Cysts of the epididymis

Cysts of the testis occur most frequently in connection with the epididymis, very rarely with the body of the testis. These cysts are quite different from hydrocele of the tunica vaginalis, and are often spoken of as a spermatocele, although all do not contain spermatozoa and the term is thus better avoided. They cause a swelling of varying degree in the scrotum, and there may be an aching in the testicle, groin or lumbar region. They may arise as retention cysts of the tubules of the epididymis or from one of the fetal remains which occur about the globus major of the epididymis. These cysts are usually placed above and to the outer side of the testis, occasionally behind it. They move with the organ, and can usually be distinguished from the latter by the test of translucency. They may be multiple and are frequently bilateral. Their increase in size is very slow, but they may cause aching pain in the testicle by pressure upon, or stretching of, the tissues of the epididymis. They can be distinguished from hydrocele of the tunica vaginalis by the position of the swelling relative to the testicle, and by the fact that the fluid contained in them is colourless or slightly opalescent from the contained spermatozoa, in distinction from the straw-coloured clear fluid of a vaginal hydrocele.

A separate clinical entity is a cyst of the appendix testis (a small globular swelling on the superior pole of the testis) or a similar cyst, the appendix epididymis, on the upper pole of the epididymis (a hydatid of Morgagni). Rarely these cysts undergo torsion and produce acute pain in the testis.

B. Affections of the coverings of the testis causing pain in the organ

The only common lesions of the coverings of the testis are *hydrocele* and *haematocele*: new growths of the testicular tunics are so rare as to render them surgical curiosities and they rarely cause pain.

Hydrocele

Hydrocele may occur occasionally as an acute affection accompanying an acute epididymitis, injury to the scrotum or in the course of acute specific fevers such as mumps. Acute hydrocele has been described in conjunction with acute lesions of other serous membranes, e.g. polyserositis. The more usual form of hydrocele is the chronic variety, which may be due to some disease of the testicle, but for which, in the majority of cases, no ascertainable cause can be found (primary or idiopathic hydrocele).

A hydrocele may cause some aching in the testicle, but more frequently it causes a dragging sensation in the inguinal or iliac areas from the mechanical effect of its weight. It forms a swelling on one side of the scrotum, oval with smooth uniform surface; it gives a distinct sense of fluctuation. The swelling is limited above from the cord or external abdominal ring, and gives no sense of impulse on coughing; with a good light it can be found in most cases to be translucent, the testicle occupying a posterior and low position in the swelling. The diagnosis of hydrocele is usually easy, but difficulty may be experienced in old-standing cases in which the walls are much thickened. A hydrocele must be diagnosed from: (1) A scrotal hernia; (2) Haematocele; (3) New growth and; (4) A cyst of the epididymis.

Scrotal hernia. Usually a hernia gives an impulse on coughing, can be reduced into the abdomen with a sudden slip or gurgle, and varies in size with the position of the patient. A hernia comes from above and descends into the scrotum. In a large irreducible hernia, some part of it is usually resonant from the contained intestine, the swelling is not limited above, and the testis can be distinguished at the bottom of the scrotum. A hydrocele is distinctly limited above so that the examining fingers can meet above it, gives no impulse on coughing, is translucent, and the spermatic cord can be distinguished easily. The testis in a hydrocele cannot usually be distinguished in the scrotum as in a hernia. Difficulty may arise between the two conditions when the hydrocele extends along the funicular process in the inguinal canal and thus gives an impulse on coughing, or if the translucency is lost owing to the thickness of the walls of the sac. A scrotal hernia in an infant may be translucent.

Haematocele is distinguished from hydrocele by the absence of translucency and the rapidity of the onset, usually after an injury or puncture (*see also below*).

New growths of the testis. A hydrocele is of much slower rate of increase in size, of smooth surface and uniform consistence, and is translucent.

Cyst of the epididymis. (*See above*.)

In cases of doubt, **ultrasonography** of the swelling usually enables accurate anatomical delineation of the mass to be made and distinguishes between a cystic and a solid swelling.

Haematocele

Haematocele may occur from puncture of a vein in the sac or of the testicle as the result of tapping a hydrocele, or by the occurrence of bleeding into a hydrocele. It may occur quite independently of a hydrocele, usually after direct injury. As a rule there is a rapid onset of swelling in the scrotum following the injury, with ecchymosis of the scrotal skin; the resulting tumour resembles a hydrocele in its clinical symptoms, save that it is not translucent. In other cases the swelling arises more slowly, when a pyriform or oval swelling is present in one side of the scrotum covered by normal skin; the surface of the swelling is smooth, and gives a sense of fluctuation and elasticity. There is no translucency, and on tapping, dark blood-stained fluid is withdrawn.

The diagnosis in the less acute cases often presents a difficulty, especially with regard to *malignant disease of the testicle (see above)*; this is particularly so when the haematoma is organized. From *hydrocele* it is distinguished by the absence of translucency; from *hernia* by the same points, except translucency, mentioned above in the diagnosis between hydrocele and hernia.

C. Affections of the spermatic cord causing testicular pain

An inflammatory affection of the cord secondary to urethral infection is not uncommon. Tuberculous infection of the cord is practically never present without corresponding infection of the epididymis. New growths of the cord, lipomas, sarcomas (extremely rare) and hydroceles of the cord cause no pain in the testis. A *varicocele*, especially if large, in a pendulous scrotum, is a frequent cause of a dull, aching pain in the testicle; it is nearly always left-sided, although the reason for this is obscure. The characteristic feel of the enlarged veins in the erect position, and the slight impulse and thrill on coughing, will readily point to the correct diagnosis.

D. Retained or misplaced testis

This, in its various situations, may give rise to pain. A testis may be arrested in its descent at the external abdominal ring, in the inguinal canal, may remain inside the abdomen, or may pass upwards and outwards from the external abdominal ring into the superficial inguinal pouch where it can be felt readily. It is doubtful if a testis retained within the inguinal canal is ever palpable. Occasionally it passes into the perineum after traversing the inguinal canal, to the upper part of the thigh via the crural ring, or to the root of the penis in front of the pubis. In one fifth of all cases, the undescended testes are bilateral.

In the various situations in which an undescended or ectopic testicle is placed it may be attacked by the several diseases which affect the normally placed organ, and thus give rise to pain; but in addition, owing to the effect of recurrent muscular strains and the comparative immobility of the organ, it is particularly liable to attacks of inflammation, especially when the testis is retained in the inguinal canal; in the intra-abdominal position it remains protected from muscular injury, while ectopic testicles have a greater range of mobility than has one that is retained in the inguinal canal and are thus especially prone to torsion. The inflammation of an undescended testicle may be so acute as to lead to gangrene of the organ, with or without torsion of the cord. The pain may be complained of first when the testes begin to enlarge at puberty, at which time an undescended right testicle may produce symptoms which can be easily mistaken for appendicitis.

The diagnosis of undescended testicle rests upon the following points: the fact that one side of the scrotum is empty; the outline and situation of the swelling in the superficial inguinal region or elsewhere; the testicular sensation upon pressure; and the recurrent attacks of pain. An undescended testicle may give rise to acute pain from inflammatory lesions or from acute torsion of the organ, and may if it is in the inguinal canal give rise to symptoms suggesting a strangulated hernia. A partially descended testicle is often accompanied by an inguinal hernia. The misplaced testis is especially liable to become the seat of malignant disease.

It should be remembered that an imperfectly descended testis is a small and poorly developed organ and the spermatogenesis from the gland may be absent or only last for a short time after puberty.

E. Testicular pain from lesions other than in the testicle

Complaint may be made of testicular pain when on clinical examination the testis is found to be normal. After an acute inflammation of the organ, even when no palpable nodule remains, the resulting cicatrization may cause aching in the organ, especially after *sexual excitement* or prolonged desire. Apart from former testicular disease pain may be felt in the organ if a *calculus* is present *in the pelvis of the kidney* or *upper ureter*, or from stimulation of the peripheral nerves by *secondary deposits in the bodies of the lumbar vertebrae*, pressure from an *extramedullary intraspinal tumour* such as a neurofibroma, meningioma or ependymoma, or the pressure of an *aneurysm* in this situation. Pain in the testicle is occasionally present in *appendiceal inflammation* when the appendix turns down into the pelvis. Finally when no organic cause of any sort is present the condition is usually called *neuralgia testis*; this is pain of an aching character which may occur in patients of a neurotic tendency.

Harold Ellis

Testicular swelling

(*See also* TESTICULAR PAIN)

It is first essential to prove that the swelling is really testicular. This is done by grasping the root of the scrotum between the thumb and index fingers to determine whether any of the swelling extends along the cord into the inguinal region. True scrotal swellings may arise in: (1) skin; (2) the various connective-tissue coverings of the testicle; (3) tunica vaginalis; (4) testicle; (5) epididymis; (6) the lower end of the spermatic cord; (7) the urethra; (8) the bones of the pubic arch. Of these the swellings in the cord, testicle, epididymis and tunica vaginalis are the commonest and most important.

1. Swellings affecting the skin

The nature of these is usually obvious. The only common ones are sebaceous cysts. Much less common are soft sores, chancre, warts and epithelioma. The last-named soon ulcerates and was once commonly seen in sweeps or in those who work in tar, tar products or petroleum. It is now relatively rare (*see also* SCROTUM, ULCERATION OF).

2. Swellings of the various connective-tissue coverings

These are rare, but occasionally a fibrosarcoma may occur. These swellings are movable upon the testicle. The symmetrical enlargement called *elephantiasis scroti* (*Fig.* T.3), due to *Wuchereria bancrofti*, is limited to the tropics, though sometimes a similar state of scrotal distension and overgrowth results in Great Britain from lymphatic obstruction due to pelvic cellulitis or to congenital abnormality. The enlarged scrotum resulting from acute generalized oedema in acute or chronic renal disease is seldom difficult to recognize; the penis and prepuce are generally distended by oedema at the same time as are the legs,

loins, eyelids and other parts, and the diagnosis is confirmed by the albumin and tube-casts in the urine.

Gross oedematous scrotal swelling also occurs with ascites or inferior vena caval thrombosis, and may accompany the abdominal swelling of pellagra and infantile kwashiorkor.

Neurodermatitis affecting the scrotum may produce a considerable amount of scrotal oedema, as does moniliasis (candidiasis).

3. The tunica vaginalis

The tunica vaginalis may become distended with serous fluid, blood or pus: distension with fluid may be primary, the ordinary vaginal hydrocele, or secondary to disease of the testis or epididymis. *Vaginal hydrocele* usually arises slowly, though some follow injury and give a short history. The patient is well, with no pain or urinary complaint, and merely complains of the lump or of the drag it causes. The swelling is large, heavy, ovoid, tense and elastic rather than fluctuating, though fluctuation can be proved if the swelling is fixed by an assistant or the patient; neither testis nor epididymis can be felt apart from the swelling. A hydrocele can be transilluminated, but it needs a dark room and a strong light (*Fig.* T.4). When transilluminated the testicular shadow will be noticed at one edge of the swelling, usually behind. Tapping withdraws a golden fluid of soapy feel, with a specific gravity of about 1030, that coagulates solid on boiling. *Secondary hydrocele* follows disease of the testis or epididymis: the amount of fluid is usually small, and the swelling lax, so that the finger can be passed through it to touch the testis. The complaint is of the causative disease rather than of the hydrocele, which is usually discovered on examination. Transillumination will confirm the presence of fluid. A *haematocele* has the physical characters of a hydrocele except that it is not translucent. Vaginal hydroceles vary very much in this respect, for their wall becomes thicker from fibrosis or deposition of fibrin, particularly after repeated tapping, and the fluid becomes stained with blood-pigment and hazy with cholesterol crystals, so that the strongest light may only just be perceptible across them. Tapping may be required to establish the presence of blood. *Haematocele* is due to injury, torsion or growth of the testis, and its discovery is therefore the indication for exploration, unless the history of trauma is recent and definite, for example, as the result of tapping a hydrocele. A *pyocele* is merely part of a suppurative process arising in the testis or the epididymis. The differential diagnosis of hydrocele is from translucent swellings in the epididymis and cord—cyst of the epididymis and encysted hydrocele.

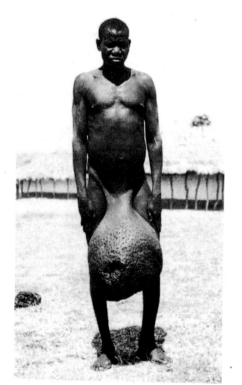

Fig. T.3. Elephantiasis of the scrotum due to filariasis. (*Dr C. J. Hackett, Wellcome Museum of Medical Science.*)

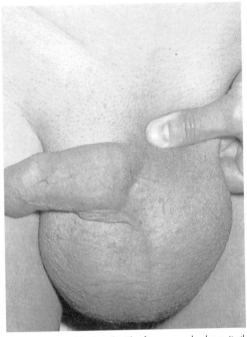

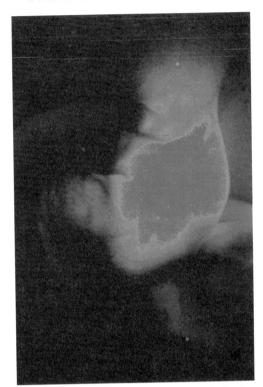

Fig. T.4. Vaginal hydrocele. The fingers reach above it, thus excluding inguinoscrotal hernia. It transilluminates brilliantly.

Ultrasonography has proved to be invaluable in the investigation of at testicular mass, in particular in determining whether or not there is underlying testicular disease in a patient with hydrocele.

4. Swellings of the testicle

These usually affect either the body or the epididymis, rarely the two together. The first group includes torsion, mumps, gumma and new growth; the second tuberculosis, gonorrhoea, *E. coli* infection and cysts. Determination of the anatomical site of the swelling will therefore go some way towards settling its pathological nature.

SWELLING OF THE BODY OF THE TESTICLE

Torsion is met with as an acute condition accompanied by abdominal pain and vomiting, and it often occurs in the undescended testis (*see* INGUINAL SWELL-ING). Torsion of a fully descended testis, giving rise to a scrotal swelling, is seldom seen except in small boys; the local signs, in addition to the abdominal pain and vomiting, are moderate enlargement of the testicle, tenderness, the presence of a small haematocele and the appearance after a few hours of oedema of the scrotal wall on the affected side. Recurring

subacute torsion of the testicle is not uncommon, and in these cases the signs and symptoms are less pronounced than in the acute variety into which they eventually pass.

The main points of distinction between the less acute enlargements of the corpus testis may be tabulated as in *Table* T.1.

It is often difficult to distinguish syphilitic enlargement of the testicles from that due to growth; but a course of anti-syphilitic therapy and the serological reactions may settle the matter. Gumma of the testis, once common, is now a clinical rarity in Western communities, so that today a solid mass in the testis is highly suspicious of a neoplasm. Malignant new growth nearly always grows steadily, and being entirely within the tunica albuginea it maintains the shape and smooth surface of the testicle until it reaches a size much larger than that of a syphilitic testicle.

The pathology of malignant tumours of the testicle has proved a fertile ground for debate, but nothing can be gained by discussing their classification since the differentiation depends upon examination of sections from the removed specimen and is impossible on clinical grounds. Both the teratomas, which may contain structures representing the three layers of the embryo, and the seminomas, supposedly derived from the germinal elements, may give rise to metastases in

Table T.1. Swellings of the body of the testicle

	Mumps	*Syphilis*	Tumour
Age	Puberty or adolescence	Any age, but usually 18 to 30	Any age, commoner after 20
History and other symptoms	Short history with pyrexia. Previous contact with mumps. Parotids enlarged	Previous history of exposure to venereal disease; usually has had chancre and rash. Gumma or tertiary rashes may be found elsewhere	Onset insidious. History of months
Scrotum	Normal or red and hot	Normal or adherent in front. Later, ulcer with sharp edges and slough at base, or hernia testis	Normal or merely stretched till growth is size of tennis ball, when it may be invaded
Testis Size and shape	Moderately enlarged, shape normal	Enlarged up to two or three times normal. May be nodular	Increases steadily and may reach diameter of 10–13 cm. First smooth, later nodular
Sensation	Tender and painful. Testicular sensation present	Not tender or painful. Testicular sensation lost	Painful, but not tender. Testicular sensation lost late in disease
'Weight'	This test is hoary with tradition, but it is quite valueless. It will be found that the specific gravity of a cubic centimetre of each of the pathological tissues is identical		
Tunica vaginalis	Slight hydrocele in most	Hydrocele in 60 per cent	Hydrocele in early stages: later haematocele
Epididymis	Unaltered	Usually unaltered	Flattened
Cord	May be tender	Normal	Usually normal, but may have nodules of growth in lymphatics
Nodes	Not characteristically enlarged	Not characteristically enlarged	Drainage to para-aortic nodes at kidney level. These may form very large mass. Eventually left supraclavicular nodes involved. Inguinal nodes not enlarged unless scrotal skin is invaded

the lymphatics to the para-aortic nodes and the bloodstream. (*See Figs.* T.1 and T.2.)

5. The epididymis

The epididymis may become enlarged as the result of inflammation, new growth or cystic degeneration. Primary new growth of the epididymis is excessively rare and need not give rise to much concern in differential diagnosis; it will generally be regarded as tubercle until after operation and microscopical examination of the tissue excised.

Inflammatory swellings are characterized by being elongated in a vertical direction; by their relation to the testicle, which they overlap at its posterior border and its upper and lower poles; and by being flattened from side to side. Inflammatory swellings may be: (*a*) tuberculous; (*b*) due to *Escherichia coli*

(certain cases of epididymitis, indistinguishable clinically from *E. coli* infection, are of very obscure aetiology: some say that they are due to irritation by urine passing by reflux up the vas, others that a virus is responsible; they are grouped as 'non-specific' epididymitis, and they tend to settle spontaneously in about three to four weeks); (*c*) *C. trachomatis*; (*d*) gonorrhoeal; (*e*) septic, secondary to some infection of the urethra. The main points of the distinction are shown in *Table* T.2.

It will be seen that *E. coli* epididymitis may bear a close resemblance to a tuberculous lesion, particularly when the acute infection has been partially aborted by antibiotic therapy, but lacks any distant or constitutional evidence of the disease. Support of the testicle in a suspensory bandage and the administration of suitable antibiotic therapy will cause marked improvement in a few days and thus settle the

Table T.2. Inflammatory swellings of the epididymis

	Tuberculosis	E. coli and 'non-specific'	Gonorrhoeal	Septic
History	Previous tuberculous infection, especially urinary	Usually none	Recent infection, with gleet, and pain on micturition	Recent catheterization or operation on bladder or prostate
Other signs and symptoms	? Cough, wasting. ? Evidence of phthisis in lungs. ? Tubercle bacilli in urine	Usually none. Urine may smell fishy and contain E. coli	Urethral discharge. Gram-negative diplococci: other manifestations such as joints	Pus in alkaline urine
Scrotum	May be adherent behind. May have sinus discharging thin pus	Normal	Red, hot, swollen and tender	Red, hot, swollen and tender. May suppurate
Testes	Usually normal	Normal	Normal, but outline obscured by surroundings	Normal, but outline obscured by surroudings
Tunica vaginalis	Hydrocele in 30 per cent	Normal	Small hydrocele usually present	Hydrocele or pyocele
Epididymis	Nodular enlargement of globus minor, less commonly globus major or whole epididymis. Nodules, hard and very tender. Later break down to abscess, with sinus	No local nodules or much enlargement, but affected part hard and tender. Changes usually involve globus minor or whole epididymis. Does not break down	Whole epididymis large, hard and broad; hot and tender	Globus minor or whole epididymis enlarged and broad; hot and tender
Cord	Oedema of cord. Vas may be thickened. Beading of vas excessively rare	Normal	Whole cord tender and swollen	Whole cord tender and swollen
Prostate and seminal vesicles	Vesicle on affected side may be hard and tender	Normal	Prostate may be hot and tender. Tenderness along vesicles	Swollen and tender. Vesicles may be felt

diagnosis. Apart from the history and an increased liability to suppuration in septic epididymitis, there is little to distinguish the latter from the gonococcal variety.

Cysts of the epididymis may be solitary or multiple, and may be bilateral. A cyst of the epididymis is placed above and behind the testicle, from which it is distinct; though attached to the epididymis, it is rounded, but being thin-walled it does not feel as tense as a hydrocele; it tends to have several rounded projections rather than a simple surface; and the fluid withdrawn by tapping is milky or opalescent, of low specific gravity, containing little albumin but showing numerous cells under the microscope, some of which may be spermatozoa. *Multiple cysts* occur in men past middle age, and are probably analogous to cystic degeneration of the breast. They are painless and increase in size very slowly. These swellings are usually strikingly translucent.

6. Swellings of the lower end of the cord

The most important swelling of the lower part of the spermatic cord is *varicocele*. It is apt to be mistaken for an inguinal hernia, but this mistake should never be made because of the characteristic feel of the varicocele (like a bag of worms), and the reappearance of the swelling after it has been completely reduced by elevation of the scrotum and the finger is firmly pressed on the external abdominal ring. Varicocele is far commoner on the left than the right.

7. **Urethral conditions**

Occasionally a *peri-urethral abscess* may form a swelling in the scrotum. Tenderness, oedema and fluctuation, together with the history and evidence of urethral disease, serve to make the diagnosis clear. *Primary epithelioma of the urethra*, which is rare, is distinguished by the great pain and urethral obstruction that it engenders.

8. **Diseases of the pubic bones**

Inflammatory products may travel into the scrotum from diseases of the bones of the pubic arch, especially from the neighbourhood of the symphysis pubis. *Acute necrosis* of these bones is sufficiently indicated by the grave constitutional symptoms which always accompany it.

Harold Ellis

Throat, sore

Sore throats are common and affect all age groups but are most common in children and young adults. Most sore throats are part of the spectrum of viral upper respiratory infections but they may be caused by bacterial infections in younger patients. Prolonged pain in the throat in middle-aged or elderly adults is cause for concern, especially if they are heavy smokers or drinkers. In this situation one must consider the presence of a neoplasm. The complaint of a sore throat demands a thorough physical examination of the oral cavity, oropharynx, hypopharynx, larynx, thyroid gland and neck. Pain is sometimes referred to the throat from the oesophagus, stomach or heart.

When the diagnosis is not immediately obvious on physical examination, routine cultures for bacteria and viruses, routine haematological studies, lateral X-rays of the neck, barium studies of the pharynx, oesophagus and stomach and CT scanning of the neck may be required. If pain in the throat is initiated or accentuated by exertion, then cardiac assessment is needed. Frequent recurrent infections of the pharynx may be an expression of immunodeficiency as seen in the diGeorge syndrome or AIDS. It is also seen in subclass deficiencies of immunoglobulins.

The causes of sore throats are shown in *Table T.3*.

The present thinking about tonsillitis is that there is a resident Epstein–Barr virus in the tonsil which is activated by physical factors. There then occurs a viral tonsillitis which causes a mild malaise and mild sore throat but its importance lies in the fact that the tonsil no longer secretes immunoglobin A and is, thus, prone

Table T.3. Causes of sore throats

Tonsillitis
  Bacterial—streptococcal
  Viral—mononucleosis
Viral pharyngitis
  Rhinovirus
  Coxsackie
  Epstein–Barr
  Adenovirus
  Herpes, Type I and II
Vincent's angina
Fungal pharyngitis
  Candida
  Phycomycetes
  Blastomyces
Syphilis
AIDS
Aphthous ulcers
Pemphigus
Erythema multiforme
Eagles's syndrome
Glossopharyngeal neuralgia
Carotidynia
Cervical spine pain
Blood dyscrasias
Thyroiditis
Reflux oesophagitis
Lymphoma
Carcinoma
  Tonsil
  Tongue base
  Soft palate
  Supraglottic larynx
Minor salivary gland tumours

to secondary opportunistic bacterial infections. This may cause a bacterial tonsillitis, which presents with an elevation of temperature, pain in the throat, trismus, difficulty in eating and speaking, and is often accompanied by cervical lymphadenopathy (*Fig.* T.5). There is usually a good response to antibiotics. Tonsillitis may go on to spread outside the capsule of the tonsil, resulting in a peritonsillar abscess or even

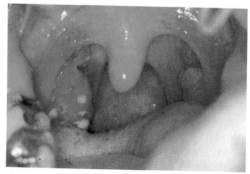

Fig. T.5. Acute tonsillitis on the right side showing the tonsillar crypts filled with pus.

into the parapharyngeal space in the neck causing a parapharyngeal abscess.

Viral pharyngitis can be caused by the influenza virus, herpes simplex virus, adenovirus, rhinovirus, Coxsackie virus and the Epstein–Barr virus. The patient usually complains of severe pain with comparatively mild clinical findings. There will probably be redness and oedema of the pharynx, especially along the pillars of the tonsil and the posterior pharyngeal wall. Lymphoid aggregates in the pharyngeal mucosa swell, causing a nodular appearance on the posterior pharyngeal wall.

Vincent's angina, or trench mouth, is a contagious disease of the oral cavity and pharynx which is more frequent in young adults and is caused by *Treponema microdentium* and a fusiform bacterium. There is extensive smelly, painful bleeding ulceration covered in grey, nectrotic membrane along the margins of the gum.

Fungal pharyngitis due to candida infection is not uncommon in debilitated adults or in diabetic or immunosuppressed patients. Less common is infection with the phycomycetes and blastomyces fungi and it is usually confined to selected geographic areas.

Aphthous lesions are painful superficial ulcers occurring on the mucosa of the oral cavity. They occur episodically and may be recurrent. They are often associated with regional ileitis (Crohn's disease) and the patient must be investigated for this coexisting condition.

Eagle's syndrome, or stylalgia, is a controversial symptom. It consists of pain in the tonsillar fossa which is usually unilateral and is presumed due to an elongated styloid process. It is difficult to distinguish between this and glossopharyngeal neuralgia.

Acute or subacute thyroiditis can cause pain in the neck or throat (*see* THYROID, PAIN IN). In the acute phase of the disorder, the patient has no difficulty in localizing the problem to the neck. Patients with subacute thyroiditis, however, frequently complain of a persistent soreness in the throat. Discomfort is constant and is aggravated by swallowing and is associated with the sensation of a lump in the throat. Patients are intolerant of constriction of the neck by shirt collars, etc.

Reflux oesophagitis usually causes vague symptoms of soreness in the throat or a sensation of a lump in the throat. The patient may have chronic hoarseness or a constant feeling of wanting to clear his throat. The pain may be aggravated after meals or at night-time when the patient is recumbent.

Lymphoma rarely causes pain in the throat and usually presents as enlargement of one tonsil. *Carcinoma* in the area of the base of tongue, tonsil, soft palate, or upper part of the larynx produces a deep

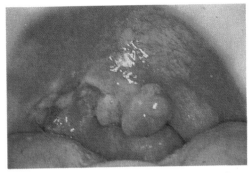

Fig. T.6. Adenoid cystic carcinoma arising in a minor salivary gland of the soft palate.

pain in the throat which is quite often difficult to diagnose because it remains hidden and is usually of an ulceral infiltrative variety. Most minor salivary gland tumours in this area are malignant, the adenoid cystic variety being the commonest (*Fig.* T.6).

A. G. D. Maran

Thyroid enlargement

(*See also* NECK, SWELLING OF; THYROID, PAIN IN)

An enlarged thyroid gland gives rise to a swelling in the front of the neck, medial and deep to the sternomastoid muscles and medial to the carotid vessels, which, if the swelling is large enough, are displaced laterally and backwards. The gland is connected intimately with the larynx so that it rises and falls with the larynx and trachea during deglutition. This sign alone is generally sufficient to establish the diagnosis of enlarged thyroid gland. The only other lump in the neck which moves on swallowing is a thyroglossal cyst, which characteristically, and in addition, moves upwards when the patient protrudes the tongue. This is because of the attachment of the cyst by a fibrous strand extending to the foramen caecum of the tongue. (*See Fig.* N.12.)

Inspection with the patient at rest and on swallowing may alone be enough to render a diagnosis of thyroid swelling extremely likely. Palpation will confirm this, and is usually best performed while standing behind the patient. The lateral lobes are palpated with the appropriate sternomastoid muscle relaxed, and, if the enlargement is only slight, help may be obtained by displacing the trachea towards the side being examined, when it is possible to introduce the fingers under the relaxed sternomastoid to feel the posterior border of the lobe. The trachea and larynx may of course already be the subject of pathological displacement by pressure of the enlarged gland and this should be determined at the time of palpation. The larynx should also be examined with a mirror for paralysis or asymmetry of the vocal cords. Vocal cord paresis will usually be accompanied by alteration in the voice and, if both cords are affected, possibly with dyspnoea and stridor as well.

The possibility of pressure effects always requires investigating, and these may be enumerated as follows:

(i) Pressure on the trachea causing deviation or compression or both, with varying degrees of dyspnoea and stridor.

(ii) Pressure on the oesophagus causing dysphagia.

(iii) Pressure on nerves, usually the recurrent laryngeal nerves, producing various forms of vocal cord palsy with or without alteration in the voice, dyspnoea, stridor and 'brassy' cough. The cervical sympathetic is occasionally involved, as shown by contracted pupil and ptosis (Horner's syndrome). Such nerve palsies are almost invariably associated with invasive tumours of the thyroid gland.

(iv) Pressure on veins, giving rise to engorgement and setting up of anastomotic channels, as a result of superior mediastinal obstruction from a large retrosternal extension of the gland.

Acute pressure symptoms may arise, or those already present may become acutely aggravated, by haemorrhage into a cystic space in a goitre.

Retrosternal prolongation of the thyroid should not be forgotten, and may be recognized by dullness on percussion over the manubrium, but this sign is unreliable. When the patient is asked to swallow or cough it is sometimes possible to feel the lower limit of the gland as it rises; at the end of deglutition it slips back behind the sternum ('plunging goitre'). The thyroid in the neck may occasionally appear of normal size in the presence of a retrosternal enlargement, and in a few rare cases the whole gland lies behind the sternum. Pressure symptoms are liable to be great when part or the whole of the gland is in this position, and sometimes the result of pressure on the great veins is seen in the presence of dilated anastomotic skin veins over the upper anterior part of the thorax.

Radiographic examination is a most useful adjunct in the diagnosis of thyroid enlargement, showing both the presence of retrosternal prolongation and tracheal displacement and compression. Ultrasonography is valuable in differentiating between a solid or cystic nodule. Histological confirmation of the diagnosis can usually be made by fine needle aspiration although larger amounts of material may be required for histological examination and can be obtained using a Tru-cut biopsy trocar. Other aids may be apparent with individual cases.

Varieties of enlargement and their differential diagnosis

PHYSIOLOGICAL ENLARGEMENT

Occurs at puberty and during menstruation and pregnancy, usually symptomless

INFLAMMATORY ENLARGEMENT

1. Acute

Acute thyroiditis, symptoms include the usual signs of acute inflammation; the condition is rare

2. Chronic

Tuberculosis, syphilis, Riedel's disease; all rare; lymphadenoid goitre (Hashimoto's disease)

SIMPLE GOITRE

(Endemic and sporadic.) Parenchymatous goitre, colloid goitre, nodular goitre, solitary (fetal) adenoma

HYPERTHYROID (THYROTOXIC) GOITRE

Primary hyperthyroidism (*Fig.* T.7)
Secondary hyperthyroidism

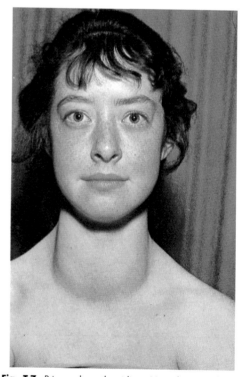

Fig. T.7. Primary hyperthyroidism. Note the even thyroid swelling and exophthalmos. (*Courtesy of the Gordon Museum, Guy's Hospital.*)

GOITRE OF THYROID DEFICIENCY

Cretinism
Myxoedema
Drugs, e.g. resorcinol, phenylbutazone

MALIGNANT GOITRE

Carcinoma
Sarcoma (rare)

These conditions can be regrouped for diagnostic purposes as follows:

THYROID ENLARGEMENT WITH HYPERTHYROIDISM

Primary hyperthyroidism (enlargement general)
Secondary hyperthyroidism
  Localized enlargement—Toxic adenoma (rare)
  Generalized enlargement—Nodular goitre in which one nodule may be so large as to suggest a solitary adenoma, occasionally parenchymatous or even malignant goitre.

THYROID ENLARGEMENT WITH SIGNS OF DEFICIENT SECRETION

Congenital

Cretinism

Acquired

Myxoedema (mild deficiency may be exhibited by colloid or malignant goitre), Hashimoto's disease

THYROID ENLARGEMENT UNCOMPLICATED

Localized enlargement

One large nodule in a small nodular goitre, cyst, adenoma, Riedel's disease (early stages), malignant disease (early stages)

Generalized enlargement

Parenchymatous goitre, colloid goitre, nodular goitre, lymphadenoid goitre, Riedel's disease (late stages), malignant goitre (late stages)

The thyroid gland is in a continual state of fluctuating activity and the structure varies not only at different times but in different parts of the same gland. When enlarged, even more diversity of structure may be present. This may render clinical distinction of the various pathological types of simple goitre impossible. Parenchymatous, colloid and diffuse nodular goitre will therefore be grouped together.

Thyroid enlargement with hyperthyroidism

Primary thyrotoxicosis or hyperthyroidism is characterized by the presence of symptoms of hyperthyroidism from the onset of the disease; in secondary thyrotoxicosis these symptoms develop after a simple goitre has been present for a variable period, often many years. The diagnostic points of each condition are tabulated below (and *see Table* T.4).

Table T.4. Diagnostic points of hyperthyroidism

	Primary hyperthyroidism	*Secondary hyperthyroidism*
Age of onset	Young	Middle aged
Onset	Acute	Insidious
Thyroid swelling	Not present before onset. Generalized soft elastic and vascular swelling; the enlargement not gross. May harden if iodine has been given	Present before onset. Enlargement may be considerable; frequently nodular
Exophthalmos	Generally present, often gross	Rare, and if present slight
Heart	Tachycardia, but fibrillation and heart failure not common except in late or severe cases	Tachycardia. Cardiovascular failure most prominent symptom. Atrial fibrillation fairly common
Tremor and general excitability	Marked	Slight
Loss of weight	Marked	Present, not so marked
Increased perspiration	Marked	Present, not so marked
Results of iodine medication	Often striking improvement	Improvement, but of a lesser degree
Thyroid function tests	Raised	Raised
Radio-iodine uptake	Raised	Raised

Various eye signs are described in connection with exophthalmos, of which the following are the best known:

von Graefe's sign—Lagging behind of the upper lid as the patient looks downward
Dalrymple's sign—Retracted lids causing a wide palpebral opening
Stellwag's sign—Diminished frequency of blinking
Moebius' sign—Inability to maintain convergence for close vision

Dalrymple's sign is fairly constantly present, but may be found in other conditions, while the other signs are neither constantly present nor confined to exophthalmic goitre. Indeed, lid retraction alone may be found without true exophthalmos.

Cretinism

Usually the thyroid is atrophic in this condition, but a goitre is occasionally present, especially in a long-standing case. An untreated patient is easily recognizable, but one seldom seen nowadays (see Fig. F.2). Slow development, either physical or mental, should rouse a suspicion of thyroid deficiency, remembering other possible causes of backward development such as rickets, renal rickets, achondroplasia, etc. The diagnosis of cretinism will not be detailed more as it is barely relevant.

Myxoedema

As in cretinism, the thyroid is only occasionally enlarged, and here again a detailed account will not be given (see Fig. F.3). The characteristic symptoms of hypothyroidism include slowed mentality, coarse features, dry skin, brittle nails and sparse coarse hair, and a gain in weight, often gross.

Certain drugs, e.g. resorcinol as an external application and phenylbutazone by mouth, may occasionally be associated with thyroid enlargement with signs of hypothyroidism reversible on stopping drug administration. Occasionally a moderately enlarged gland may increase in size during treatment with an antithyroid agent, e.g. neomercazole.

Lymphadenoid goitre (Hashimoto's disease)

In this disorder the thyroid gland becomes infiltrated with lymphoid tissue as a result of an auto-immune reaction. It is a disease occurring in women in middle life and usually produces a uniform, firm enlargement of the thyroid with evidence of hypothyroidism. The gland is often H-shaped. Laboratory tests for thyroid function show low levels. There is an increased serum cholesterol, a raised erythrocyte sedimentation rate, and auto-immune thyroid antibodies are present in the blood. Occasionally, lymphadenomatous goitre will occur with normal thyroid function and, very exceptionally, with hyperthyroidism. In the past, diagnosis has often been made after operation as a result of histological section of the tissue removed, but with careful investigation this should not be necessary in a typical case.

Carcinoma of the thyroid may cause confusion, but this condition is practically never associated with hypothyroidism in an untreated case.

Riedel's disease

This is an interesting and rare condition where an intense sclerosing fibrosis starts in one area of the gland and spreads first to the whole gland and then to surrounding structures. The progress is slow as a rule, but gradually the trachea, the oesophagus, and the great vessels all suffer from constriction while the recurrent laryngeal nerves are affected early. The diagnosis from malignant disease is very difficult, but the condition should be suspected when an intensively hard goitre with pressure symptoms out of all proportion to its size is found in a young adult. Diagnosis is confirmed by histological examination of biopsy material.

Uncomplicated thyroid enlargement

A true adenoma is an uncommon condition, but a particularly large nodule in an otherwise small nodular goitre forming an asymmetrical swelling in the thyroid tissue is common (Fig. T.8). It may be cystic or solid but palpation is not always reliable in determining this. Nodular goitre may give rise to a uniform enlargement, as also may colloid goitre. This last condition may present a smooth surface, as it is usually the case in parenchymatous enlargement. A simple cyst is quite common and may suddenly enlarge from haemorrhage into it.

Malignant disease starts in one area and spreads to involve the whole gland, finally breaking through the capsule to invade surrounding structures. Movement on deglutition may be lost, the recurrent laryngeal nerve is involved early, and the growth tends to surround the carotid bundle rather than push it back, as is the case with large simple goitres, so that pulsation of these vessels may be impalpable in the middle of the neck. The sympathetic chain is often involved late in the disease, with a resultant Horner's syndrome. The swelling is usually hard, as in Riedel's disease, but tends to be much greater in size and more rapid in growth.

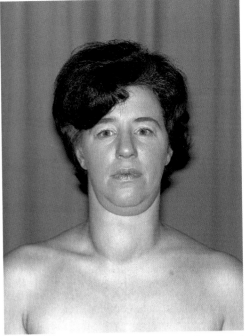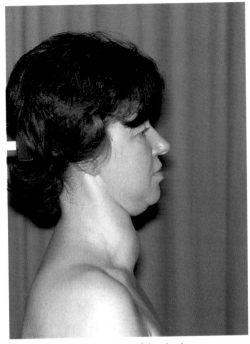

Fig. T.8. Large colloid mass in right lobe of the thyroid producing an asymmetrical enlargement of the gland.

Pressure symptoms are early and pain is often a marked feature, particularly on swallowing. Bone and lung metastases are not uncommon. One type of thyroid carcinoma, namely the papillary carcinoma, deserves special mention. This typically occurs in the 4th and 5th decades and metastasizes to the lymph nodes. The secondary deposits may be much larger than the primary which cannot be detected, so that these cases often present with soft lumps in the side of the neck which used to be called, erroneously, 'lateral aberrant thyroids'. Thyroid tissue so situated is always a secondary deposit from a small primary in the thyroid which has completely replaced the lymphoid tissue in which it metastasized.

Harold Ellis

Thyroid, pain in

A painful thyroid swelling is not a common clinical situation. The following conditions may give rise to this symptom:

1   Inflammatory:
     Acute (suppurative) thyroiditis
     Subacute thyroiditis (De Quervain's disease)
     Inflammation of a thyroglossal cyst or fistula
2   Haemorrhage into a cyst of the thyroid
3   Hashimoto's disease (rarely)
4   Carcinoma of the thyroid in its late stages

Acute (suppurative) thyroiditis

This is a rare condition which is nearly always bacterial in origin. Fungal and parasitic causes can be regarded as medical oddities. The usual organisms producing this condition are *Staphylococcus aureus, haemolytic Streptococcus, Pneumococcus*, and occasionally *Salmonella* and *E. coli*. In two-thirds of cases, there is pre-existing thyroid disease. The sexes are equally affected.

The source of the bacterial invasion is either extension from an adjacent infection or bacteraemia secondary to a distant focus. Commencing as an acute inflammation, the condition usually progresses to suppuration.

The clinical features are a sudden onset with severe pain in the neck which may be referred to the ear, the lower jaw or the occiput and which is aggravated by swallowing and movement of the neck. There is associated malaise and fever.

Examination reveals a febrile patient (the temperature in the range 38–40°C), and tachycardia. Swelling, tenderness and redness in the region of the thyroid generally appears later; more characteristically, only one lobe of the thyroid is involved. Regional lymphadenopathy is variable. The neck is held flexed and neck movement is painful. Fluctuation is not usually elicited because of induration of the surrounding tissues. There is leucocytosis and, untreated, the mass progresses to the formation of an obvious abscess.

Subacute (non-suppurative) thyroiditis (De Quervain's thyroiditis)

This is probably viral in origin. Any age may be affected, ranging from 3–76 years, although the fifth decade is commonest. Females are far more often affected than males. Usually the condition involves a previously normal gland.

The illness is preceded frequently by an upper respiratory infection and the thyroid symptoms are often anteceded by muscular aches and malaise with fever (in the region of 39°C) and weight loss. Pain then develops in the thyroid gland and the pain may radiate to the ears. It is aggravated by movement of the neck and by swallowing. Usually both lobes are enlarged, although in one-third of cases one lobe is involved first and the inflammation then spreads to the opposite side. Examination of the neck reveals a tender, firm or hard enlargement of the thyroid gland.

Quite often there are accompanying symptoms and signs of hyperthyroidism.

Laboratory tests reveal a raised white count and ESR. Usually the T_4 is raised and this elevation lasts for 1 to 3 months.

The condition runs a variable course of weeks or months and even if untreated usually subsides without sequelae. Rarely it is followed by clinical hypo-thyroidism. As its name implies, it does not proceed to frank suppuration.

Inflammation of a thyroglossal cyst or fistula

The typical thyroglossal cyst lies in the midline of the neck, usually at the cricothyroid space, less commonly at a higher or lower level, although it may deviate somewhat to one or other side of the midline. It usually presents in children or young adults and character-istically moves upwards on protrusion of the tongue as well as on swallowing (see NECK, SWELLING OF). Infec-tion of the cyst is not uncommon and then presents as an obvious inflammatory mass above the anatomical region of the thyroid gland. A thyroglossal fistula is occasionally congenital but may follow infection or inadequate removal of a thyroglossal cyst. The fistula discharges mucus and is frequently the site of recur-rent attacks of inflammation.

Thyroid cyst

Haemorrhage into a pre-existing thyroid cyst produces a sudden, painful enlargement of a lump in the thyroid

gland which may or may not have already been noted by the patient. Its danger is that it may also produce sudden and dangerous compression of the trachea with respiratory obstruction. The symptoms may require urgent surgical treatment but, if less severe than this, the swelling gradually subsides over the succeeding few days.

The cystic nature of the swelling can be con-firmed by ultrasound examination of the mass.

Hashimoto's disease

This condition (see p. 376) is usually painless, but from time to time the thyroid enlargement may be painful and tender.

Carcinoma of the thyroid

Poorly differentiated (anaplastic) carcinomas of the thyroid usually occur in elderly patients. In their advanced stages, they produce a tender and painful infiltrating mass in the neck, usually with local lymphadenopathy (Fig. T.9). Clinical diagnosis is not usually in doubt but can be confirmed by needle biopsy.

Harold Ellis

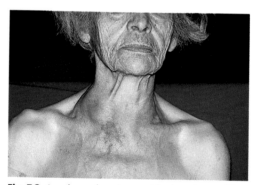

Fig. T.9. An advanced carcinoma of the thyroid in an elderly lady. The right sternocleidomastoid muscle and regional nodes are involved. The gland is painful and tender.

Tinnitus

Tinnitus is a term which denotes a ringing or whistling sound in the ears but is customarily applied to other sounds described by patients such as hissing, throb-bing, buzzing or roaring. It has been known since the time of Hippocrates and is one of the most irritating auditory sensations. Some patients can cope with it but, in many others, it represents a severe strain and in some may even cause severe psychological disorders and suicide. It seems to be a symptom that is on the increase and, in the 1980s and 1990s, tinnitus has been in the position of fever a century ago. It is something which can now be reasonably quantified and there are a plethora of treatments advocated. As with fever, however, it is essential not to consider the entity in itself but rather the underlying cause. Most subjective tinnitus is considered to arise in the cochlea—one of the most inaccessible parts of the human body. Determination of the underlying cause, therefore, is inevitably by indirect methods and by extrapolation. It has been shown that the sensitive hair cells, which change sound waves into electrical impulses in the cochlea, are in constant mechanical vibration. The reason for this is probably because a completely passive system would not be sensitive enough to pick up the very quietest sound the normal ear can hear. Experiments with normal hearing adults show that everyone can hear this background hair cell vibration if they are in quiet enough surroundings (e.g. an anechoic chamber). One might refer to this as the 'sound of silence' or 'physiological tinnitus'. The normal vibration of hairs on these hair cells in the inner ear can be measured using a sensitive microphone placed in the outer ear canal. In some cases of low-frequency tinnitus, extra loud hair cell vibrations, or cochlear emissions as they are called, can be detected by this method. On many occasions, however, the tinnitus experienced by the patient is quite different to the cochlear emissions which can be recorded so this is not the whole answer. In addition, these cochlear emissions cannot at present be recorded from those with a hearing loss greater than 40 dB, so a different explanation has to be found for those with deafness and tinnitus.

One explanation could be that the hearing centres in the brain control, to some extent, the function of the internal ear. Cochlear efferents act as a gain control, constantly adjusting the function of the inner ear. In a noisy environment the gain control would be turned down, resulting in less spontaneous vibration, and this might explain why tinnitus is often less noticeable in the presence of environmental noise.

Another theory is that certain forms of tinnitus are related to abnormal phase locking of discharges in groups of auditory nerve fibres. The normal nerve, in situations of total quietness, transmits random messages which are interrupted as the absence of external noise. The ear responds to sound by synchronizing with firing of adjacent fibres in the auditory nerve and this, together with the change of pattern of firing, is interpreted by the brain as a sound from the outside.

The character of the sound may give some clue to the cause. Thus a pulsatile or rhythmical sound may be produced by the flow of blood through an ather-omatous internal carotid artery, which in its course through the carotid canal is separated from the tympanum only by a thin plate of bone. Internal carotid thrombosis should be suspected if the pulse in one carotid artery is absent or greatly diminished. The noise in the ear may be heard on the opposite side on account of compensatory dilatation. Other symptoms of this condition may be intermittent headache, often over one eye, transitory hemiparesis, transitory loss of vision in one eye, temporary aphasia and fits. Digital compression of the carotid on the sound side may precipitate such phenomena, which also include hemiparaesthesia. A carotid arteriogram (*Figs* T.10, T.11) is diagnostic.

Tinnitus is common in cases of arteriosclerosis, and conditions associated with high blood pressure: it may also occur when there is severe anaemia; the noises heard may be variously described by patients as humming, hissing, rhythmic thumping, roaring, whistling or musical. A crackling noise may be produced by cerumen, or a foreign body, in the external auditory canal. A bubbling noise may be due to catarrhal exudation in the middle ear. A crackling or clicking sound may be caused by spasmodic contraction of the dilator tubae and salpingopharyngeus muscles which are attached to the Eustachian tube. A clicking sound may be caused by intermittent contraction of the tensor tympani. In rare cases the tinnitus may be associated with a carotid artery murmur, which is detected on examination of the neck with the stethoscope.

Though tinnitus is very common in diseases of the ear, yet serious lesions of the middle ear, internal ear or auditory nerve may be present without this symptom. There is no constant relation between tinnitus and deafness. The former may be present with good hearing, but when long continued the hearing tends to become impaired. The sounds may persist when a patient has become totally deaf.

Tinnitus may occur from the following diseases of the ear:

1. The presence of *cerumen, aural polyps* or *a foreign body* in the external auditory meatus coming in contact with the drum. Removal of the offending body leads to the cessation of the tinnitus.

2. In any *inflammatory disease, acute or chronic, suppurative or non-suppurative, of the middle ear*. In catarrhal inflammation of the middle ear, the noise frequently has the character of bursting bubbles, and is due to movements of the viscid exudation in the ear itself. Low-frequency vibratory clicks, pops and roaring noises arise almost always from the middle ear and Eustachian tube. Chronic sinusitis may be the underlying cause. In *otosclerosis*, tinnitus is a very prominent and usually early symptom.

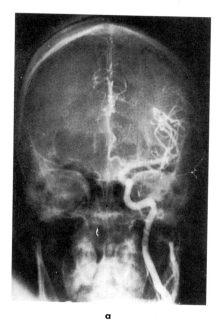

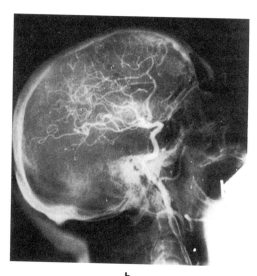

a

b

Fig. T.10. Normal left-sided cerebral arteriogram. *a*, Anterior view. *b*, Lateral view. (Dr R. D. Hoare.)

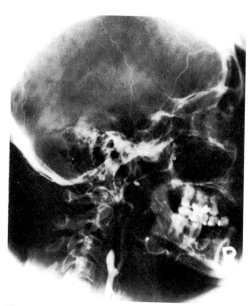

Fig. T.11. Arteriogram showing occlusion of internal carotid artery. (Dr R. D. Hoare.)

It may occur before any alteration in hearing is present.

3. In diseases of the *internal ear* tinnitus may be severe and intractable; especially in *Ménière's disease, syphilitic disease* of the internal ear, and in those lesions of the internal ear which may arise in the course of *typhoid* and other *specific fevers. Extension of suppuration to the labyrinth* from the middle ear is

also an important cause; and tinnitus, usually associated with deafness, may persist after *fracture of the base of the skull.*

Perhaps the commonest cause of an inner ear tinnitus is from the cochlear damage caused by exposure to excessive noise.

Paget's disease of the skull may be associated with tinnitus, often intermittent, and sound may be conducted to the ear from a congenital intracranial aneurysm, an arterial angioma or a carotico-cavernous fistula.

Persistent unilateral tinnitus with progressive internal-ear deafness and vertigo raises suspicion of *acoustic nerve tumour.* Unilateral tinnitus with a ringing or bell-like quality and reduced hearing suggests cochlear involvement. High-pitched tonal non-vibratory tinnitus strongly suggests disease of the cochlea and 8th nerve.

'Noises in the ears' are complained of in many general diseases with or without a lesion of the ear; thus, they are frequent in *anaemia, leukaemia*; some *cardiac lesions*, especially aortic regurgitation, may be found in the pulsatile variety of tinnitus. *Chronic nephritis, uraemia* and *arteriosclerosis* with high blood pressure may also be responsible for tinnitus, and it may occur during attacks of *neuralgia* or of *migraine.* Quinine, salicylates and streptomycin may cause tinnitus.

Tinnitus masking remains by far the best treatment for those patients who have any useful hearing.

The masking noise is usually quite different to the tinnitus and may well be at a much lower intensity. Since it is an external noise it is often easy to adapt to, rather like the noise of passing traffic in the street. The sort of noise used in maskers has also been used for producing sleep, relaxation and even anaesthesia under different circumstances. So, far from being irritating, many tinnitus sufferers find this noise soothing as well as effective in masking their tinnitus. In about half of those who are effectively masked, there will be the phenomenon of residual inhibition. This means that the tinnitus is turned 'off' or turned 'down' for a period of time after the masker is removed.

There are no medical drugs that will make tinnitus disappear. Those who are getting psychological problems from their tinnitus are best treated with antidepressants.

A. G. D. Maran

Tongue, discoloration of

The mucous membrane of the tongue is covered mainly by filiform papillae which cover the major portion of the tongue and vary in length from 1–3 mm. Fungiform papillae are found at the apex and along the lateral aspect of the tongue. They are barely visible but on occasions even in the normal patient may be red, large, smooth and round.

Discoloration of the tongue has much less of a diagnostic role in gastrointestinal disease than in the past. Changes that are thought to take place with constipation, appendicitis and other gastrointestinal diseases are insignificant and unreliable. On the other hand, there are more important changes which are associated with infectious diseases, deficiency states and metabolic disorders.

The tongue surface may be dry, brown and slightly furred in patients who are *mouth breathers* or who are *dehydrated*. A brown, dry tongue is common in *tobacco smokers*. Furring of the tongue is due to heaping up of the squamous epithelium on the filiform papillae probably from inadequate cleansing of the tongue which ordinarily occurs during chewing. The term '*geographic tongue*' is used when an area of filiform papillae, is lost from the dorsum of the tongue (*see Fig*. T.15). Smooth, pink mucosa is seen which contrasts sharply against that mucosa which is covered with normal papillae. A feature of the condition is that the appearance of the tongue will change from day to day, creating a 'wandering rash' across the surface of the tongue. This condition can be regarded as a variant of normal.

Very marked overgrowth of the filiform papillae produces a *black, hairy tongue (see Fig*. M.5). This rare condition is encountered in patients on antibiotic therapy and some smokers. Hypertrophy of the fungiform papillae in *scarlet fever* produces the classic 'strawberry' or 'raspberry' tongue.

Leucoplakia describes white patches on the surface or lateral aspect of the tongue (see *Fig*. T.22). These, on histology, show hyperkeratosis, acanthosis and dyskeratosis. The white areas may be seen as a patch or a raised plaque and are usually painless. Leucoplakia is regarded as a precancerous lesion as is the asymptomatic red, velvety lesion which may sometimes be seen on the ventrolateral aspect of the tongue. 'Hairy' leucoplakia is unique to *HIV infection* and is found particularly along the side of the tongue, although it may occur anywhere in the mouth. The lesions are slightly raised, poorly demarcated, and show a corrugated white 'hairy' surface which does not rub off and which is asymptomatic. Histology is distinctive showing keratin projections, parakeratosis, acanthosis, and a characteristic ballooning change in the pickle-cell layer. The significance of this lesion is that it is a strong predictor of AIDS, for 80 per cent of patients will develop the full syndrome within 1 year.

Mucosal infection with the yeast *Candida albicans* produces the clinical picture of *moniliasis*, or candidosis or thrush. Creamy white curd-like patches occur on the tongue and other areas of the buccal mucosa. When scraped they reveal a raw bleeding area. The lesion can be quite painful and is found particularly in sick infants, debilitated patients, or those receiving broad spectrum antibiotics or high doses of corticosteroids. Candidiasis is a common manifestation of *immunodeficiency* and over 50 per cent of HIV antibody positive patients with this infection will develop the AIDS syndrome within 2 years. In infants thrush is distinguished from milk curds by the difficulty with which the former are removed leaving an underlying patch of inflamed mucosa.

The tongue will appear blue in patients who are centrally *cyanosed* and pale in *anaemic* patients. Many anaemic patients however have a red, painful, bald tongue. This is the consequence of complete atrophy of the papillae which may occur in *pernicious anaemia*, severe *iron-deficiency anaemia*, and/or *deficiency states involving other B vitamins*. The red, painful tongue may be associated with other evidence of mucosal atrophy in the mouth and fissuring at the corner of the lips known as angular stomatitis. The mucosal lesions of folic acid deficiency are often more marked than those encountered in vitamin B_{12} deficiencies. Other terms which have been used to describe the colour changes taking place in vitamin B deficiencies are the 'beefy red' tongue of *pellagra* and the 'magenta' tongue of *riboflavin deficiency*. The *Plummer–Vinson* (or *Patterson–Kelly*) syndrome describes the iron-deficiency state in which the tongue is painful, reddened and smooth. There is cheilitis, postcricoid webs and koilonychia.

Pigmentation of the tongue may be found in *Addison's disease* and *acanthosis nigricans* in which the tongue undergoes hypertrophy of the filiform papillae to produce a shaggy, papillomatous dorsum. *Acrodermatitis enteropathica* is a rare autosomal recessive disorder related to zinc deficiency. Intraoral features include a white coating to the tongue and buccal mucosa with marked halitosis. There is chronic diarrhoea, hair loss, severe dermatitis and failure to thrive. The condition may also occur in patients on maintained hyperalimentation who become deficient in zinc.

In *hereditary haemorrhagic telangiectasia* (Osler–Weber–Rendu syndrome) telangiectasia occur throughout the gastrointestinal tract. The most commonly occur in areas of the oral cavity, including lips, gingiva, buccal mucosa and tongue. The lesions are dilated capillary vessels and small arterioles. The pigmentary changes involving *Peutz–Jeghers syndrome* and *pseudoxanthoma elasticum* do not normally involve the tongue. Granulomatous involvement of the tongue and buccal mucosa in *Crohn's disease* produces raised, smooth, red nodules and hyperplastic ridges on the tongue. These may appear erythematous. A number of dermatological diseases may affect the mouth, including *erythema multiforme, lichen planus, pemphigus* and *pemphigoid*, but involvement of the tongue in these conditions is rare.

Ian A. D. Bouchier

Tongue, pain in

(*See also* Tongue, Swelling of)

Pain in the tongue may be attributable to some obvious lesion, usually with breach of surface such as an epithelioma. Such conditions are discussed under the heading of Tongue, Ulceration of. On the other hand, pain in the tongue or soreness of the tongue may be an insistent complaint when there is no superficial evidence of abnormality. The conditions that have to be considered include the following:

1 *When the pain complained of is not on the dorsum, tip or sides of the tongue but underneath or deeper:*
   Injury to the frenulum linguae
   Ranula
   Calculus in the duct of a submandibular salivary gland
   Foreign body in the tongue
   Myositis
   Trichinosis

2 *When the pain complained of appears to be upon the surface of the tongue, even if it also affects the tongue as a whole:*

Bitten tongue
After an anaesthetic (mouth-gag)
Injury by tooth or dental plate
Antibiotic glossitis, associated with lichen planus, Behçet's disease or pemphigus vulgaris
Congenital fissured tongue
Geographical tongue
Median rhomboid glossitis
Moeller's glossitis
Glossitis of deficiency disease
Smoking
The effects of over-hot beverages or foodstuffs
The effects of pungent condiments such as cayenne pepper
Minor viral diseases
Carcinoma

The differential diagnosis depends upon the following considerations:

1. Pain underneath the tongue or deeper

Injury to the frenulum linguae may cause visible abrasion or a definite ulcer. The most injured spot is tender as well as painful, the diagnosis depending on careful attention to the appearance and to the site of greatest tenderness. The cause may be injury by a fishbone or other sharp or puncturing object. In violent coughing bouts as in whooping cough the protruded tongue may be forced against the lower incisor teeth with such violence that the frenulum becomes abraded, inflamed or ulcerated.

Ranula is not painful unless it becomes inflamed. It is an asymmetrical red smooth cystic swelling in the floor of the mouth under the tongue on one or other side of the fraenum. It may result from obstruction of the duct of one of the sublingual salivary glands but more often it is a retention cyst arising in one of the many mucous glands in the floor of the mouth.

Calculus in the duct of a submandibular salivary gland is not necessarily painful. It may produce discomfort or more or less severe pain recurrent or constant according to the degree of inflammation. The stone may be very small and difficult to detect either with a probe or by X-rays, but its existence may be suspected by the situation of the discomfort, or by the corresponding salivary gland swelling when the patient begins to eat, the stone interfering with the free passage of the increased flow of saliva. The calculus can frequently be palpated bimanually in the floor of the mouth and is occasionally seen to protrude through the duct orifice. An X-ray will confirm the diagnosis.

Foreign body in the tongue is uncommon, though a fish-bone may become impacted in it. More often the foreign body injures the tongue, itself escaping but leaving pain behind. The diagnosis depends on the accuracy of the story obtained or the discovery of the foreign body by palpation or by radiography.

Myositis of the tongue is seldom if ever a localized condition; it may, however, be a prominent feature in *polymyositis* or in *trichinosis*, in which the embryo trichinellae have a special predilection for the muscles at the base of the tongue which become stiff, painful and tender. The diagnosis of trichinosis is difficult especially as it will hardly be thought of unless there is an epidemic at the time. The blood exhibits eosinophilia, but the only way of clinching the diagnosis is by demonstrating the trichinellae embryos microscopically in portions of the muscles excised.

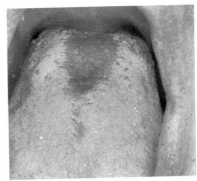
Fig. T.12. Glossitis due to oral antibiotic. (*Professor Martin Rushton.*)

2. Pain upon the surface of the tongue

Bitten tongue will usually present an obvious lesion but pain may persist after a tongue-bite even when no obvious bruising or breach of surface can be detected. The patient may be unaware of having accidentally inflicted the bite, if the accident occurred during sleep or during an epileptic seizure. Indeed, the occurrence of a local painful area in the tongue suggesting the effect of tongue-bite may be the first indication that the patient is an epileptic. In tetanus, traumatic glossitis is common and may cause airways obstruction.

After general anaesthetics, patients often complain of soreness of the tongue resulting from the use of tongue forceps or of a mouth-gag.

Injury by a tooth or *dental plate* may cause a local painful place upon one side of the tongue, often fairly far back, the pain being increased by movements of the tongue in speaking, eating or swallowing. Fear of cancer is usual until the cause is found in the jagged edge of the adjacent tooth, or of the dental plate at the corresponding site. The condition needs to be watched carefully to be certain that the lesion disappears after the offending irritant is smoothed down or removed, and to allay any anxiety that the jagged tooth or plate may have initiated an epithelioma. Tuberculosis of the tongue, presenting as a painful deep persistent ulcer, is now rarely seen.

Antibiotic glossitis. A common cause of diffuse soreness of the tongue is the taking of antibiotics by mouth. The pain is sometimes due to infection with *Monilia albicans* which can be grown from the surface. Its preponderance is favoured by the wide-spectrum antibiotics. In other cases of antibiotic glossitis no such cause can be found and the change is attributed to vitamin deficiencies arising from suppression of normal gut flora. The tongue is clean, red and very sensitive to heat (*Fig.* T.12). Glossitis occurs in deficiency of vitamin B_{12}, and folic acid, in pellagra, malabsorption syndrome and the Plummer–Vinson

syndrome but seldom causes acute pain in these conditions.

Lichen planus affecting the tongue may be confused with monilia glossitis because both produce small whitish patches on the surface. The lichen tends to produce lines or a mesh of pearly dots and to favour the cheeks near the occlusal line of the molars.

The tongue may also become inflamed and painful in Behçet's disease, erythema multiforme or pemphigus vulgaris.

Congenital fissured tongue (*Fig.* T.13) or 'scrotal tongue' is thick, deeply fissured and usually symptomless. If food particles lodge in the fissures infection may arise and thus cause pain.

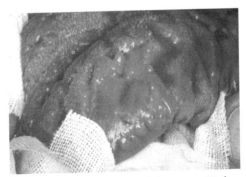
Fig. T.13. Congenital fissuring of the tongue. (*Professor Martin Rushton.*)

Geographical tongue (*Fig.* T.14) shows red denuded patches of irregular outline which often change their position. It causes anxiety rather than pain.

Median rhomboid glossitis (*Fig.* T.15) is a rare congenital abnormality due to persistence of the tuberculum impar between the two halves of the tongue. It occupies the middle third of the dorsum and is smooth, shiny and red. It carries no filiform papillae.

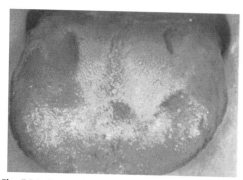

Fig. T.14. Geographical tongue. (*Professor Martin Rushton.*)

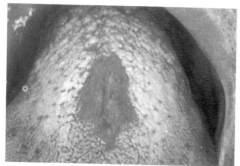

Fig. T.15. Median rhomboid glossitis. (*Professor Martin Rushton.*)

Opalescent nodules may be scattered over the surface. The area may become inflamed and thus cause soreness and often unfounded fear of cancer.

Moeller's glossitis (*Fig.* T.16), often confused with Hunter's glossitis of pernicious anaemia (q.v.), presents atrophic sharply defined red patches on the dorsum and sides: the atrophy in pernicious anaemia is evenly spread and the mucosa pale and dry. Spiced food causes pain. The condition may be met in allergic

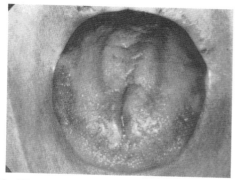

Fig. T.16. Moeller's glossitis.

states, nutritional deficiencies and with certain drug eruptions (e.g. reserpine).

Glossitis of deficiency disease occurs with avitaminosis, particularly of the B group, as in pellagra, but also with iron deficiency and pernicious anaemia.

Smoking and the effects of tea or other *hot liquid* or *food* may cause acute pain in the tongue lasting for days after the cause has ceased to act. *Pungent condiments* such as capsicum, cayenne pepper, ginger and the like may similarly be responsible.

Minor viral diseases. Foot-and-mouth disease may rarely be contracted by humans from infected farm animals or consumed milk or milk products from infected herds, vesicles appearing in the mouth and on the tongue. In the so-called 'hand-foot-and-mouth disease', probably due to Coxsackie A viruses, children are affected. Vesicular stomatitis contracted from horses, cattle and pigs occurs in North and South America.

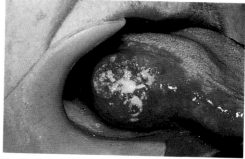

Fig. T.17. Carcinoma of the tongue.

Carcinoma of the tongue (*Fig.* T.17) starts as a nodule, fissure, or ulcer, usually on the lateral border of the organ. At first painless, it becomes painful as it invades and becomes grossly septic. The pain often radiates to the ear, being referred from the lingual branch of the trigeminal nerve supplying the tongue along its auriculotemporal branch. Ulceration is accompanied by bleeding; hence the typical picture of late disease is an old man spitting blood into his handkerchief with a plug of cotton-wool in his ear.

Harold Ellis

Tongue, swelling of

Swelling of the tongue is a condition the nature of which is generally obvious on inspection and palpation, if the history is taken into account at the same time. Many causes given in the following list need little detailed discussion:

1. Causes of acute swelling of the tongue

A bite or sting

Injury, for instance by a fish-bone, or by biting during an epileptic fit

Corrosives or acute irritant applications

Acute oedema, secondary to:

a.   Inflammatory conditions within the mouth–stomatitis (p. 388)

b.   The effects of certain drugs, e.g. mercury, rarely aspirin

c.   Erythema bullosum or pemphigus (p. 271)

d.   Variola

e.   Serum injections and other conditions liable to cause giant urticaria

f.   Angioneurotic oedema (angio-oedema)

Haemorrhage into the substance of the tongue, as in scurvy, leukaemia and other haemorrhagic states.

2. Causes of chronic or persistent swelling of the tongue

Where the swelling is general

Macroglossia

Cretinism

Myxoedema

Mongolism

Acromegaly

Primary amyloidosis

Where the swelling is local or asymmetrical

Irritation of a dental plate or decayed tooth

Epithelioma

Gumma

Leucoplakia (chronic superficial glossitis)

Tuberculous infiltration

Actinomycosis

Ranula

Calculus in a sublingual salivary gland

Suprahyoid cyst

Haemangioma or lymphangioma

Sarcoma

Lipoma

If the nature of the tongue enlargement is not obvious from the history and simple inspection and palpation—as will probably be the case when it is due to a *bite, sting, injury, corrosive* or *irritant* application, after the use of *serum, mercury, aspirin* or other drugs, *variola, pemphigus* or *erythema multiforme*— it may be so from the concomitant symptoms, as in the case of *cretinism, acromegaly, mongolism* or *myxoedema.*

Simple *macroglossia* is rare; when it does occur the history is that it dates from youth or childhood and the patient may otherwise be perfectly normal, unless

he also has some other congenital peculiarity, such as macrocheilia (blubber-lips).

The chronic local lesions associated with swelling are in many cases accompanied by superficial ulceration, and the difficulties, that may arise in distinguishing *simple, syphilitic* and *epitheliomatous* ulcers are discussed under Tongue, Ulceration of. *Tuberculous* and *actinomycotic glossitis* are both rare, and may be mistaken for malignant or syphilitic disease. Tuberculous lesions are usually painful and this cause should always be thought of when considering the possible causes of a painful swollen tongue, particularly as the manifestations of tuberculosis of the tongue may assume unusual and bizarre forms. *Ranula* and *sublingual salivary gland calculus* or *cyst* both cause swellings that are beneath the front part of the tongue rather than in its substance, generally bulging up one side of the floor of the mouth near the frenulum linguae. A ranula is a distended mucous gland, and after enlarging slowing to perhaps the size of a chestnut, it often ceases to grow further; it does not fluctuate in its dimensions in relationship to meals as a salivary gland swelling often does.

A *suprahyoid cyst* is situated in the root of the tongue posteriorly, where it arises from remains of the embryological thyroglossal duct. It is seldom large; its nature is suggested by its situation.

An *angioma* of the tongue is rare (*Fig.* T.18): sometimes, however, after remaining latent for years, it grows with rapidity and necessitates an operation. The diagnosis may be suggested by the colour of the tumour, but histological examination subsequent to removal may be required before one can be sure whether the tumour is a simple angioma, an angiosarcoma or a *sarcoma*.

A *lipoma* occurs not infrequently in the tongue and its lobulated form generally breaks surface and presents like a cluster of soft white cherries.

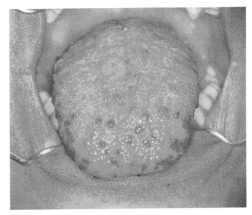

Fig. T.18. Angioma of the tongue.

Haemorrhage into the substance of the tongue, with swelling and inability to speak or eat, may result from certain blood disorders, such as acute leukaemia or primary or secondary thrombocytopenic purpura.

Acute oedema of the tongue may be due to *severe stomatitis, angioneurotic oedema of the tongue* and *Ludwig's angina.* This is an acute inflammatory condition, often streptococcal in origin, affecting the floor of the mouth and tongue, and spreading rapidly through the deeper structures of the mouth, throat and neck, causing extreme swelling of the adjacent tissues.

Angioneurotic oedema of the tongue is rare, but it is important because it may, rarely, prove fatal. As a rule there is a history of previous similar attacks in other parts of the body and other members of the family may have had similar episodes. Tracheostomy may, though very rarely, be necessary as a life-saving measure, the diagnosis becoming clear only when the oedema of the tongue and adjacent parts subsides almost as rapidly as it came on, and the patient develops similar (angio-oedema), probably in other parts, on subsequent occasions.

Harold Ellis

Tongue, ulceration of

(*See also* TONGUE, PAIN IN)
To enable a good view to be obtained of the affected part the patient should be seated in a good light and the protruded tongue gently dried with a piece of gauze. The presence of an ulcer being ascertained, its nature may be considered under the following heads: (1) *Carcinomatous*; (2) *Syphilitic*; (3) *Dental*; (4) *Tuberculous*; (5) *Ulcer in connection with stomatitis.*

1. Carcinomatous ulcer

Carcinomatous ulcer is much more common in men than in women. It is very unusual before the age of 30, and rarely starts before 45. The foul smell of the breath and the ill and wearied expression of the patient may awaken suspicion before the tongue is seen, for the sloughing ulcer is usually heavily infected, and the toxic absorption combined with pain and loss of sleep have a rapid and marked effect upon health. The tongue in a normal individual can be protruded from three to four centimetres beyond the teeth; if the protrusion is limited, or if the tongue is not protruded straight, it can generally be inferred, except in cases of paralysis, that there is some tumour binding it down (ankyloglossia). The position of the ulcer is to be studied and its relation to any sharp and carious tooth. An epithelioma is usually on the side of the tongue, but

it may be anywhere on the upper, lateral or undersurface or on the floor of the mouth, but is hardly ever exactly in the midline.

As regards the ulcer itself, the typical appearance when fairly developed may be described as irregular, deep, foul, sloughy, with raised nodular everted edges and a surrounding area of induration. Other types associated with minimal ulceration of the mucous membrane are the scirrhous, where there is an excessive fibroblastic reaction, and the affected part of the tongue is shrivelled up as in the similar atrophic scirrhous cancer of the breast; and the nodular, where the lesion is mostly buried within the substance of the tongue and, like an iceberg, broaches the surface over a deceptively small area. In addition, the papilliferous type and multiple ulceration are not uncommon. Lastly there is the fissure carcinoma associated with leucoplakia (*Fig.* T.19). Except in early cases some of the

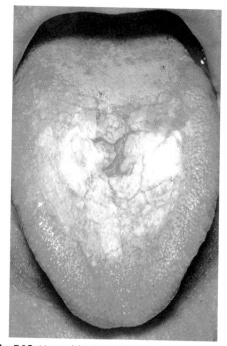

Fig. T.19. Non-syphilitic leucoplakia of the tongue.

lymphatic nodes are enlarged and hard, and they may be fixed. The submandibular group is generally the first affected, but the disease sometimes misses these and invades the jugular and even the supraclavicular nodes. Examination, therefore, should not be concluded before the whole of the neck has been palpated. The diagnosis should have been made, however, before the disease has developed thus far; in its earliest stages an epithelioma may be represented by a superficial ulcer no more than a sixteenth of an inch in diameter, by a crack or a small lump, without any enlargement of the nodes. In all these conditions, however, the ulcer is already hard and very resistant to any form of simple topical treatment. Any ulcer of the tongue occurring in a middle-aged man, and lasting for more than 2 or 3 weeks, should always awaken suspicion (*Figs.* T.20, T.21).

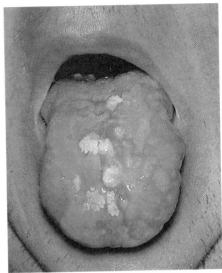

Fig. T.22. Leucoplakia of the tongue (syphilitic) with extensive carcinomatous charge.

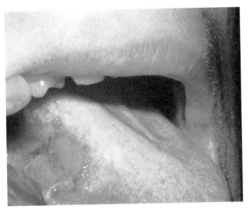

Fig. T.20. Carcinomatous ulcer of the tongue. Surprisingly, the patient was a girl of 17, with no demonstrable aetiology.

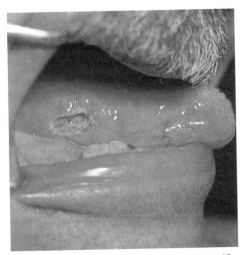

Fig. T.21. Ulceration from epithelioma of the tongue. (*Courtesy of the Gordon Museum, Guy's Hospital.*)

DIAGNOSIS FROM SYPHILITIC ULCER. This may be a very real difficulty, owing to the fact that the two conditions may exist side by side (*Fig.* T.22), and that the syphilitic leucoplakia may be the actual precursor of a cancer. Positive serological reactions, therefore, are not proof that an epithelioma is not present. If a well-formed gumma is present, antisyphilitic remedies soon make a great change in its appearance. Although a biopsy is necessary for a definite diagnosis, certain clinical criteria are characteristic and a putative diagnosis of gumma may be made when the ulcer is centrally situated, painless, serpiginous in outline, and has the steep-cut edges and wash-leather slough base typical of syphilitic ulcers elsewhere.

DIAGNOSIS FROM DENTAL ULCER. The ulcer in this case is caused by a carious or otherwise jagged tooth, and therefore is in a corresponding position on the tongue. Further, the ulcer is soft to the touch and heals rapidly when the offending tooth is stopped or extracted. There is seldom difficulty in differentiation except when the ulcer is of very long standing.

2. Syphilitic ulcer

This may be primary, secondary or tertiary.

PRIMARY SYPHILIS or CHANCRE is certainly rare on the tongue and, owing partly to its rarity and partly to the fact that it is unexpected, it is frequently missed. It is more common in men than in women, but it may occur even in children. It starts as a small pimple which ulcerates and becomes indurated, though the induration is not so marked as when it is situated on the glans penis. The appearance of a secondary rash with general enlargement of the lymphatic nodes would indicate the true diagnosis. Further proof is supplied by positive serological tests, and the detection of spirochaetes in serum from the sore. Furthermore, the sore heals rapidly under the influence of treatment.

SECONDARY SYPHILIS manifests itself by the formation of mucous patches and superficial ulcers. The latter are almost always multiple, and situated along the edges and tip of the tongue, and with them are also found similar sores on the mucous membrane of the cheek, lips, palate and tonsil, and at the edges of the mouth. The ulcers are small, round, painful, with sharply cut edges and a greyish floor. Other secondary symptoms will be present to make the diagnosis clear.

TERTIARY SYPHILIS or GUMMATOUS ULCERATIONS. These lesions, now extremely rare, are divided into superficial and deep. *Superficial* gummas begin as small round-celled infiltrations in the mucous and sub-mucous tissue. The ulcers are usually shallow, often irregular and associated with chronic glossitis, fissures and leucoplakia. Though rare today they are extremely important, for they may be followed by epithelioma. The ulcers themselves are not at first indurated, but if surrounded by interstitial fibrosis may appear hard; a histological examination is essential if there is the least doubt. A *deep* gumma starts as a hard swelling in the substance of the tongue. It is usually situated in the midline, and in the posterior half. Later it softens, breaks down and shows itself as a deep cavity with irregular soft steep-cut walls, and a wash-leather-like slough at its base. It is not painful, and does not increase progressively in size. The important thing is to distinguish it from epithelioma and tuberculous disease. Unlike epithelioma it does not infiltrate widely or fix the tongue, its history is short and it causes no pain. Furthermore, it yields rapidly to anti-syphilitic treatment.

3. **Dental ulcer**

Dental ulcer is due to repeated small injuries from the sharp edge of a decayed tooth or damaged denture and is situated opposite the tooth, generally on the side of the tongue. The ulcer is small, superficial and not indurated unless it is of long standing. It is therefore not easily mistaken for any other kind of ulcer, or if doubt arises it is allayed by the healing of the ulcer on appropriate dental treatment: failure to heal within a fortnight suggests that it is an epithelioma.

There is a form of dental ulcer which is found on the fraenum of the tongue in children suffering from whooping cough; during the violent expiratory spasms peculiar to the illness, the undersurface of the tongue may suffer from rubbing over the lower incisor teeth.

4. **Tuberculous ulcer**

This is rare in the Western world, but it occurs at that period of life during which tuberculous disease of the lung is common, between the ages of 15 and 35. It is due to infection with tubercle bacilli brought up into the mouth. The ulcer itself is usually on the tip of the tongue or the side in its anterior half and is generally painful, although sometimes entirely painless. The outline is irregular. The edges are usually thin and undermined, and the base is covered by pale granulations, or excavated clearly down to the underlying muscle-fibres; less commonly the edges are raised, though never everted or hard, and the base is nodular, sloughy or caseous. It has often been mistaken for epithelioma or gumma. The fact that it is not hard, that is usually painful, and that pulmonary tuberculosis is present should point to the true diagnosis. Negative serological tests exclude a syphylitic gumma, though histological proof may be necessary by biopsy, and cultures carried out for bacteriological confirmation. A further example of tuberculous ulceration is the so-called 'truncated tongue'. In this type there is an oedematous infiltration of the parenchyma of the tongue, causing it to become swollen and almost 'woody', and there is a shallow ulceration of the tip, giving an appearance as if part of the tongue had been amputated. In fact the clinical manifestations of tuberculosis of the tongue are so protean that this disease should always be suspected in unusual lesions, especially if associated with pain.

5. **Ulcers in connection with stomatitis (ulcerative stomatitis)**

Septic infection of the mouth due to a variety of causes, such as irritation from decayed teeth, alkalis, acids or mercury, may be accompanied by the formation of small vesicles which, on bursting, give rise to superficial ulcers (*Fig.* T.23). They are not limited to the tongue, but appear as well on the mucous membrane of the cheeks and gums. Aphthous stomatitis commonly occurs in conjunction with the febrile diseases of childhood. It is characterized by the formation of whitish spots on the buccal mucous membrane; and by

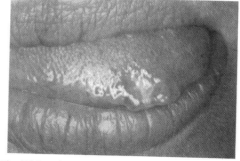

Fig. T.23. Aphthous ulcer. (*Professor Martin Rushton.*)

the shedding of epithelium small superficial ulcers may be formed. The ulcers of the tongue here occur in the course of a general inflammation of the mouth. One type that may be resistant to treatment is produced by Vincent's angina organisms; bacteriological tests give the diagnosis, but it may be suggested by the extreme foetor of the breath.

When ulceration of the tongue, and at the same time, very probably of the inside of the mouth generally, occurs in such conditions as *chickenpox, pemphigus* and other conditions that may affect the buccal mucosa as well as the skin, the diagnosis depends, not upon the appearances of the ulcers or the tongue, but upon the concomitant skin eruption.

Harold Ellis

Tonsils, enlargement of

The palatine tonsils consist of lymphoid tissue with minor salivary glands and a covering of squamous epithelium. They lie encapsulated between the anterior and posterior pillars of the pharynx and intermingle with the lymphoid tissue at the base of the tongue. There is a *physiological increase* in size between the ages of 4 and 6 and subsequently the tonsils shrink. At this age, the tonsil enlargement is usually accompanied by enlargement of the adenoids. This can lead to the sleep apnoea syndrome which can vary from snoring to respiratory obstruction. It is not thought to occur early enough to be accountable as a cause of cot death. These patients improve dramatically with removal of tonsils and adenoids.

Large tonsils in young adults, especially if accompanied by malaise, are due to a *glandular fever.* The types of fever that cause the most marked tonsillar swelling are mononucleosis and especially toxoplasmosis.

Bacterial tonsillitis make the tonsils enlarge. A peritonsillar abscess means the infection has passed through the capsule of the tonsil so that there is oedema between the superior constrictor muscle and the capsule of the tonsil. This pushes the tonsil medially on one side and causes trismus, difficulty in speaking and marked elevation in temperature and malaise. There is dramatic relief when the pus is evacuated.

Lymphoma also occurs in young adults and presents with unilateral enlargement of the tonsil. This may, or may not be, accompanied by enlargement of the cervical lymph nodes.

In adults, *salivary gland tumours* can cause tonsillar enlargement in two ways. Firstly, an ectopic pleomorphic adenoma can occur in a tonsil, causing unilateral tonsillar enlargement, as can a malignant minor salivary gland tumour such as an adenoid cystic carcinoma or a mucoepidermoid carcinoma. Secondly,

a tumour arising in the deep lobe of the parotid lies in the parapharyngeal space and can push the tonsil medially. Other lesions in the parapharyngeal space, such as chemodectoma, glomus vagale, schwannoma or a parapharyngeal space abscess, can cause the same tonsillar displacement and apparent enlargement of the tonsil.

A. G. D. Maran

Trismus (lockjaw)

(*See also* FACE, ABNORMALITIES OF APPEARANCE AND MOVEMENT)

Trismus, or lockjaw, signifies a maintained muscular spasm tending to closure of the jaws so that the mouth cannot be opened. The term does not include mechanical inability to open the jaws owing to such affections as mumps, alveolar abscess with surrounding inflammatory oedema, injury, Ludwig's angina, quinsy or severe tonsillitis, an odontoma, epithelioma of the mouth, myositis ossificans or cervicofacial actinomycosis. There are two conditions which may not at first sight be obvious, but may lock the jaws together and simulate true trismus—*impaction of a wisdom tooth* and *arthritic changes in the temporomandibular joint.* These are diagnosed by careful local examination of the teeth and of the joint respectively; in the latter case there may be arthritic changes in other joints also. X-ray examination may be required to detect the joint changes or the impacted wisdom teeth (*Fig.* T.24).

Circumstantial evidence will generally serve to distinguish trismus due to *hysteria* or to *facial neuralgia;* any doubt at first experienced is dispelled if the patient is watched for a while. Convulsive seizures in a hysterical patient with trismus can generally be distinguished from those due to tetanus or to strychnine poisoning by their polymorphous character, and by the fact that touching the patient, and other similar stimulation, does not bring them on so certainly as would be the case with strychnine or tetanus.

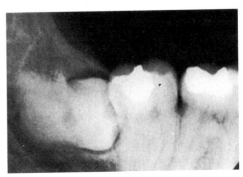

Fig. T.24. Radiograph showing impacted third molar.

In fits, for example epilepsy, the trismus is of short duration and offers no difficulty in diagnosis.

MALINGERING may sometimes take the form of lockjaw, and it may be a little while before the fraud can be detected. In sleep the malingerer's muscles relax completely.

TRICHINIASIS is rare, but if infected pork is eaten raw, or insufficiently cooked, the larvae of the parasites find their way to many different muscles, and they show predilection for those of the tongue, mouth and jaws. The resultant irritation, pain and stiffness can cause trismus, the origin of which may be difficult to determine unless the history points to pork. The patient is very ill in the earlier stages, with high fever, and the condition may be fatal. The malady may be epidemic. The blood exhibits eosinophilia. The final criterion of the diagnosis is the discovery of the typical parasites coiled up in their little oval cysts among the affected muscle fibres.

HYDROPHOBIA (RABIES) and TETANY seldom exhibit trismus as a prominent symptom. The former, though now almost unknown in Great Britain, would suggest itself if a convulsive illness developed after a bite by a dog, fox or other similar animal, particularly if the spasmodic muscular difficulty is markedly increased by efforts at swallowing. The symptoms may not develop for weeks or months after the bite, so that the patient may fall ill when he has come from a country overseas where rabies is endemic. *Tetany*, also rare, is at once distinguished by its typical carpopedal contractions; trismus, almost constant in tetanus, is nearly always absent in tetany.

STRYCHNINE POISONING gives rise to generalized twitchings and convulsions long before trismus, the lateness of the development of the latter serving to distinguish it from tetanus. Furthermore there is complete muscular relaxation between spasms. There may be evidence of strychnine having been taken or administered, either by the mouth or hypodermically; the symptoms develop very acutely, and are often rapidly fatal.

TETANUS is the cause *par excellence* of trismus. The diagnosis is often obvious if the illness develops in an otherwise healthy person, with stiffness starting usually in the neck muscles, spreading to those of the face and jaw, and thence to the rest of the trunk and limbs, with extremely painful exacerbations on the slightest stimulation even by a stroke with a feather or the banging of a door; dysphagia; risus sardonicus; opisthotonos; no complete relaxation of the stiff muscles unless an anaesthetic be given; a duration of days rather than hours; especially if all these things follow a few days, or a week or more, after a small penetrating wound which becomes septic. It may be possible to demonstrate the presence of the drum-stick bacilli in films prepared from the deeper parts of the wound. The chief difficulty arises when there is no clear history, or when the wound has been so small that it has healed or cannot be found; even then, most cases are so typical that they can be diagnosed as tetanus without difficulty. Unnecessary anxiety arises chiefly in cases of an impacted wisdom tooth, or of hysteria, where tetanus may be suspected at first; the subsequent course of the malady soon serves to exclude this. Involvement of the temporomandibular joint in a *serum reaction*, especially if prophylactic tetanus antitoxin has been given, may lead to the belief that tetanus has in fact set in.

Trismus may be simulated by *scleroderma* of the face. But here the condition is rather one of fixation of the skin than of the muscles; the skin becomes like parchment so that one cannot pick it up between the fingers, it feels firm or almost hard, and the patient becomes unable to open the mouth properly. The disease is of slow onset and gradual progress, so that there is seldom difficulty in diagnosis.

Ian Mackenzie

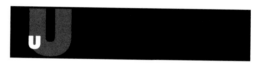

| **Urethral discharge**

The causes are as follows:

1. Gonorrhoea
2. Non-specific urethritis
3. Trichomoniasis
4. Bacterial:
   E. coli
   Ducrey's bacillus (*Haemophilus ducreyi*)
   Tuberculosis
5. Chemical
6. Traumatic:
   Instrumental
   Accidental
7. New growth
8. Foreign bodies

Any inflammatory process in the urethra causes a discharge. Although often the result of infection by the *gonococcus*, by no means every urethritis is of this nature, and bacteriological examinations show that other organisms besides the gonococcus may produce a urethral discharge and the same symptoms as gonorrhoea. Further than this, a purulent discharge may occur in which no micro-organisms can be found; for instance, when the urethra has been injured or subjected to irritation by the injection of strong solutions, or when it contains a foreign body, such as a calculus or a retained catheter.

There is no doubt that an acute *non-specific* urethritis may be caused by other organisms than the gonococcus, and is today more common than gonococcal urethritis. These cases may cause complications in the genito-urinary organs similar to those due to the gonococcus, such as prostatitis, epididymitis or cystitis. They may arise by the infection of the urethra by septic instrumentation, or after connection with a woman with trichomoniasis. A careful bacteriological examination should always be made in order to determine the causative organism. An acute urethritis may accompany a haematogenous urinary infection; for instance, an acute infection of the upper urinary tract due to *E. coli* may be followed by acute cystitis, prostatitis and urethritis, in which no other organism but *E. coli* can be found. *Non-specific (non-gonococcal) urethritis* is due probably to several infective agents, such as *Chlamydia trachomatis* and *Trichomonas vaginalis*. It is usually a venereal disease contracted in coitus. A watery, whitish penile discharge in males may be associated with mild dysuria and lower abdominal discomfort. The discharge may be so slight as to be overlooked, but there is a tendency for exacerbations and remissions to occur, and the urethral discharge is sometimes purulent, serous or mucopurulent. In Reiter's disease there is arthritis and sometimes conjunctivitis and uveitis in addition. In such cases although the urethritis may respond to tetracycline therapy, the arthritis does not. Reiter's disease, although commonly venereal in origin in Great Britain, may follow bacillary dysentery.

GONORRHOEAL URETHRITIS

This is due to the infection of the urethra by the gonococcus (*Neisseria gonorrhoeae*). The gonococcus is seen in a stained specimen to be *intracellular*, penetrating not only the leucocytes but also the epithelial cells found in a smear preparation, and, although the cocci may be found also between the cells, their appearance in the cells is strong evidence of their specific nature.

In any case presenting a purulent discharge from the urethra it is necessary, in order that appropriate treatment may be carried out, first to make a smear of the discharge for bacteriological examination, and secondly to make a culture of the discharge in order to determine drug sensitivity of the organisms, and also to confirm the smear test

A gonococcal complement fixation test (GCFT) is not useful in diagnosis of early cases as it is associated with many false-negative results.

It must be established that the pus comes from the urethra and not from beneath the prepuce. For the purposes of clinical investigation the urethra is divided into anterior and posterior portions, separated by the membranous urethra, the anterior comprising the bulbous and penile urethra, and the posterior the prostatic portion. A urethritis is also, according to its clinical aspect, acute or chronic, the acute form being characterized by a thick, creamy, purulent discharge, with pain, and the chronic by a thin, greyish, mucopurulent discharge. Acute gonorrhoea affects not only the superficial layers of the urethral mucous membrane, but also the subepithelial tissues and the glandular elements, causing a leucocytic infiltration. The tendency of the inflammation is to spread backwards along the canal so that the prostatic urethra may become infected even in the acute stage, though most frequently this occurs at a later period; the prostatic and the ejaculatory ducts may become infected, and the inflammation may spread to the seminal vesicles and epididymes. In the acute stages of the disease the infection of the anterior urethra is accompanied, as a rule, by redness of the external meatus, scalding pain during micturition, and painful emissions. These patients have described the pain on micturition as like passing red-hot fish-hooks through the urethra. Occasionally all pain is absent, especially in patients previously infected with gonorrhoea. If the anterior urethra alone is infected and the urine is passed into two glasses, the first portion will be turbid from admixture with the urethral discharge, whilst the second portion may remain clear.

When the posterior urethra becomes infected in the acute stages the symptoms are much more severe. Micturition is more painful and greatly increased in frequency, both by day and by night, the patient often being obliged to pass urine every half-hour. It may follow that a prostatic abscess develops to complicate posterior urethritis, in which case micturition becomes very painful, or a painful retention of urine may occur. There is usually an associated high fever and rigors. On rectal examination the prostate is found much swollen, hot to the touch, and extremely tender, while with an abscess a soft fluctuating area may be felt. An acute posterior gonorrhoea is only rarely accompanied by infection of the bladder, cystitis supervening on the urethritis.

With successful antibiotic treatment the purulent urethral discharge will disappear within 24 hours and the patient will be symptom-free in 2–3 days.

NON-SPECIFIC URETHRITIS

Non-specific urethritis (NSU) is now the commonest sexually-transmitted disease in the UK. The urethral discharge tends to be thinner and more mucopurulent than the thick creamy pus of the typical gonococcal urethritis. However, it may be clinically impossible to distinguish between gonorrhoea and NSU and, indeed, some patients may have a mixed infection with the gonococcus and one of the other organisms which may have caused NSU.

Among the causative organisms of NSU are:

1 *Chlamydia trachomatis*
2 *Ureaplasma urealyticum*
3 *Trichomonas vaginalis*
4 *Secondary bacterial infections* from coliforms, anaerobes, yeasts, etc.

Chlamydia trachomatis is the predominant cause of NSU infections and the organism can be seen on microscopy or isolated from something like half the patients with NSU. The organism proliferates within epithelial cells and this produces characteristic large intracytoplasmic inclusion bodies which stain with specific fluorescent antibody techniques.

Ureaplasma urealyticum (T strains of mycoplasma) are found in the genital tract of many sexually active individuals without clinical evidence of infection but occasionally clinical urethritis is probably caused by these organisms.

Trichomonas vaginalis may colonize the male urethra and may in some cases produce urethritis.

Reiter's syndrome may complicate NSU in a small proportion of patients. Symptoms include conjunctivitis, uveitis, arthritis and pustular hyperkeratosis on the soles of the feet.

A urethral discharge may in rare cases be gonorrhoea or non-specific urethritis, and as difficulty may arise if one of these cases is met with it is necessary to mention them.

Herpetic Urethritis. The mucous lining of the urethra may be affected by herpes in the same manner as other mucous membranes. There is irritation of the urethra during micturition, and a slight mucopurulent discharge from the meatus. The small vesicles may be seen by the endoscope, and may be associated with herpes of the prepuce or glans penis.

Soft sores in the urethra (**Chancroid**) are distinctly uncommon. They occur in the terminal portion of the urethra, and cause painful micturition and a profuse, thin, purulent discharge, which contains no gonococci; Ducrey's bacillus (Haemophilus ducreyi) may be found. There may be other sores on the glans penis, and an ulcerated surface will be seen on endoscopic examination. They occur within a few days of infection, and, if extensive, may produce narrowing of the urethra on healing. Lymph nodes in the groins may be enlarged and tender.

Syphilis may affect the urethra either as a hard chancre or as a gumma.

The *chancre* occurs in the terminal inch of the urethra, forming a firm indurated mass which can be felt readily on external palpation. The meatus is oedematous and swollen, so that the introduction of an endoscopic tube is impossible; there is a thin, purulent, and often blood-stained discharge from the meatus. A urethral chancre must be diagnosed carefully from peri-urethral infiltration due to urethritis; the period of incubation from time of infection, the presence of small, hard inguinal nodes, the occurrence of secondary lesions of syphilis, and positive serological tests will point to the diagnosis. The *Treponema pallidum (Spirochaeta pallida)* may be found in the fluid expressed from the surface of the sore

Gumma of the urethra is now extremely rare; it gives rise to a watery urethral discharge when it ulcerates. It may ulcerate through the canal and form fistulas, but may usually be recognized on careful examination.

PAPILLOMAS OF THE URETHRA

These may occur either in the anterior or posterior portion, as small, pedunculated tumours in the canal, and frequently as a sequel to a chronic gonorrhoea. They may arise, however, in the urethra of a patient who has never had urethritis. They cause a thin, scanty discharge together with spontaneous urethral bleeding; they are seen readily through the endoscope and some are often visible when the lips of the meatus are retracted.

CARCINOMA

Carcinoma of the urethra is very rare as a primary disease, and many of the cases recorded have been in association with stricture. It forms a tumour in the urethra palpable from the exterior, and causes painful micturition with a blood-stained discharge, and enlargement of the inguinal nodes. Suspicion of carcinoma should arise if a hard, irregular tumour is felt in the course of the urethra, without gonorrhoeal infection, in an elderly patient. Carcinoma of the urethra may also occur as an extension from carcinoma of the bladder or prostate or as a malignant change in urethral papilloma; the papillary type will not be palpable from the exterior. The final diagnosis depends on histological examination of a portion of the growth, removed for biopsy through an endoscope. An irrigating posterior urethroscope or panendoscope is the best instrument for this purpose.

TUBERCULOSIS OF THE URETHRA

This is always secondary to disease elsewhere in the genito-urinary tract, usually of the prostate or seminal vesicles; it is very rare. Tubercle bacilli may be found in the urethral smear.

FOREIGN BODIES IN THE URETHRA

These may cause a purulent urethral discharge if they remain for any length of time. They may be introduced through the meatus by intent—matches, pins, etc.; or a piece may be detached from a damaged catheter; or a small calculus may come down from the bladder and be arrested; in the latter case the history is usually clear—sudden stoppage of the stream of urine during micturition, with penile pain; a calculus may be felt from the exterior or seen through the endoscope.

Harold Ellis

Urethra, faeces passed through

Faeces or faecal fluid are passed per urethram only when the bladder is in fistulous communication with some part of the bowel, or with an abscess infected with *Escherichia coli*, PNEUMATURIA (q.v.) may occur at same time. The chief causes are as follows:

Diverticular disease of the sigmoid colon with a fistula into the bladder (the commonest cause).
Carcinoma of the bladder opening into the rectum or into some loop of bowel which has become adherent to the bladder.
Carcinoma of
  the rectum
  the sigmoid   } opening into the bladder either
  colon   } directly or through the medium of
  the caecum   } an intervening abscess
Carcinoma of the uterus opening both into the bladder and into the rectum.
Crohn's disease of large or small bowel with vesical fistula.
Prostatitis or prostatic abscess opening into the rectum.
Rectovesical fistula from injury and sloughing, particularly after childbirth.
Appendicular abscess opening into the bladder.
Pelvic actinomycosis.

The passage of faeces into the urine may be simulated by some cases of very foetid cystitis due to infection by *E. coli*, especially in diabetic subjects

If the symptom is due to carcinoma it matters little which viscus is the primary site by the time the growth has involved both bladder and bowel. The differentiation resolves itself, therefore, between malignant and non-malignant conditions. If malignant disease is not obvious it will nearly always be advisable to resort to surgical measures in the hope of discovering some curable primary condition—rectal, appendicular, prostatic or otherwise. The diagnosis will be suggested by the history and confirmed by local examination or exploration with appropriate biopsy.

Harold Ellis

Urine, abnormal colour of

(*See* HAEMATURIA)

The normal amber colour of urine is due mainly to urochrome; the depth of colour naturally varies with the concentration and very dilute urine is nearly colourless. In very concentrated urine the depth of colour may raise suspicions of biliuria. Several substances can alter the colour of the urine. This is usually of no pathological significance although a patient may seek an explanation; in a few conditions the colour is characteristic and of diagnostic significance. Discolouration due to blood, confirmed by 'Dipstick' test and beyond all doubt by microscopic examination, is, of course, the most significant finding and is considered under HAEMATURIA.

Bile pigment imparts a deep *orange* colour to the urine; in high concentration the appearance resembles beer. Senna and rhubarb ingestion can produce a similar colour.

A *red* colour in the urine can be due to a number of substances. Haemoglobin is the most important, either in intact red cells when the urine has a turbid or 'smoky' appearance or as free pigment when the urine is clear. If large amounts are present and, particularly, if some of the haemoglobin has been oxidized to methaemoglobin, the colour may be brownish-black. In porphyrinuria the colour is typically that of 'port wine' but it may be pink or red. Myoglobinuria may give a red or brown colour in the urine. Other substances causing red urine include beetroot, blackberries, phenolphthalein in purgatives (if the urine is alkaline) and certain aniline dyes in sweets. Eosin produces a pink colour with a green fluorescence and uro-erythrin often contributes to the red colour of abnormal urine; it is of no pathological significance and is mainly seen adsorbed on deposits of urate ('brick-dust' deposit).

Apart from methaemoglobin, a *dark brown* or *black* urine may be due to phenol (carboluria), melanin, homogentisic acid or p-hydroxy-phenyl pyruvic acid. In carboluria, due to phenol poisoning, the urine may be greenish-brown. Melanin or melanogen is found in the urine in some cases of disseminated malignant melanoma; the urine may be of normal colour when passed but turns black on standing, from above downwards. A similar colour change on standing occurs in the urine in alkaptonuria in which homogentisic acid is excreted. This substance also accumulates in the cartilage of the ear and in the sclera, which may become black, and in joint cartilage causing severe arthritis; this syndrome is known as ochronosis. The urine may also darken in air in the very rare tyrosinosis in which *p*-hydroxyphenyl pyruvic acid is excreted. The antimicrobial drug metronidazole also causes the urine to become dark brown.

Due to the presence in normal urine of urochrome, any blue compound in low concentration may produce a green colour. *Green* and *blue* urines are most commonly due to biliverdin in long-standing obstructive jaundice or to methylene blue in pills or sweets. Indigo-carmine and indigo-blue can also colour the urine. The former may rarely be present after exposure to industrial dyes and the latter is the consequence of oxidation of indican. Indicanuria is due to intestinal malabsorption of tryptophan which is metabolized to indole by intestinal bacteria in such conditions as coeliac disease and Hartnup disease.

Peter R. Fleming

Urine, incontinence of

Incontinence is the involuntary loss of urine from the bladder at times and in places which are inappropriate and inconvenient. Preservation of continence depends on the integrity of the lower urinary tract, both anatomically and physiologically. Incontinence secondary to an anatomical abnormality occurs congenitally, as in ectopic ureter, or is acquired, as in vesico-vaginal fistula; physiological disturbance occurs because of imbalance between the tone of the detrusor muscle and that of the external urethral sphincter.

Sphincter weakness results in genuine stress incontinence, sometimes called simply stress incontinence; detrusor incontinence occurs when detrusor activity is sufficiently enhanced to overcome the resistance offered by a normal sphincter mechanism. Overflow incontinence occurs when the detrusor is flaccid so that urine trickles out when the fully distended bladder can hold no more, in much the same way that water trickles over the lip of a dam.

The common causes of incontinence of urine can be divided into: (1) Sphincter damage; (2) Neurological lesions.

1. Sphincter damage

Mechanical damage to the sphincter is the commonest cause of genuine stress incontinence. Broadly speaking, the sphincter apparatus in both sexes consists of three components: the bladder neck, which is a muscle group derived from the detrusor muscle of the bladder wall; the intrinsic urethral apparatus, which consists of muscle components from both bladder neck and external sphincter together with fibrous and vascular components; and the external sphincter, which consist of the striated muscle of the pelvic floor.

In women, all three components can be affected by stretch or direct damage during the passage of the fetal head during labour, giving rise to stress incontinence.

In men, prostatectomy is a common cause of stress incontinence; the bladder neck has been ablated inevitably during prostatectomy itself, but there is additional damage to the intrinsic apparatus and even occasionally to the external sphincter. Prostatectomy inevitably implies internal sphincter ablation and considerable resection of the intrinsic apparatus but provided this procedure is limited to the zone proximal to the verumontanum the remaining intrinsic urethral mechanism and the external sphincter together will allow preservation of continence. Incontinence is almost inevitable following total prostatectomy carried out for carcinoma of the prostate. Sphincter involvement by malignant extension from prostatic carcinoma is rarely enough in itself to give rise to stress incontinence as the simultaneous obstruction produced by the enlarged malignant gland will compensate for loss of sphincter tone.

The pelvic floor can be injured by trauma, such as gun shot wounds, and is particularly vulnerable to injury when the pelvis is fractured. A dual mechanism is often responsible for incontinence in the latter as direct damage to the pelvic floor is compounded by damage to its nerve supply, particularly the pudendal nerves.

STRESS INCONTINENCE

Genuine *stress incontinence in women* is related to sphincter damage during childbirth and to the weakening of the supporting pelvic floor muscles. The sphincter apparatus falls below the level at which it can be protected by transmitted pressure during coughing and other activity so that the intra-abdominal pressure acts in an unopposed manner on the bladder dome. Increases in abdominal pressure produce a simultaneous leak of urine. The condition is usually associated with anterior and posterior vaginal wall prolapses, manifested as cystocele or rectocele respectively, but this is by no means invariable. Supporting the bladder neck by inserting the index and middle finger against the anterior vaginal wall and pushing upwards will control the leaking. This test mimics the effect of a successful surgical procedure. Genuine stress incontinence also occurs in some congenital abnormalities, such as the short urethra, the wide urethra and epispadias.

Some degree of *stress incontinence in men* is usual after prostatectomy but clears up as the prostatic cavity heals and infection is eradicated. If there has been sphincter damage as a result of the procedure, the resulting incontinence improves slowly with time. A period of some 12 months must elapse before the degree of remaining incontinence can be judged permanent.

URGE INCONTINENCE

Incontinence after prostatectomy also usually relates to the irritability of the bladder base related to the oedema of the healing zone. This incontinence is called urge incontinence, where the desire to micturate is so strong that it overrides all attempts of the sphincters to retain urine. urge incontinence is frequent in both sexes and is the major differential diagnosis from genuine stress incontinence. The detrusor contracts in an abnormal manner and, as it does so, it opens the bladder neck and thus decreases the outflow resistance. This kind of incontinence is sometimes called 'unstable bladder' incontinence. It is not related to any neurological factor but is seen in association with acute cystitis, chronic cystitis, post-radiotherapy, in tuberculous cystitis, interstitial cystitis, in the presence of a foreign body in the bladder, when a stone is impacted at the uretero-vesical junction, in outflow tract obstruction secondary to posterior hypertrophy and bladder neck stenosis. In most cases, no specific aetiological feature can be discovered. It is difficult to distinguish from genuine stress incontinence on clinical grounds as, during the circumstances of examination, the first cough may not precipitate incontinence but subsequent coughing on request may initiate a detrusor contraction which is strong enough to open the sphincter.

2. Neurological lesions

Incontinence related to neurological causes may be due to upper or lower motor neurone lesions. In upper motor neurone lesions the central inhibitory impulses to the micturition centre in the sacral segments are lost. Sudden contractions of the detrusor muscle occur, resulting in unheralded precipitate micturition. The volume of urine lost in upper motor neurone lesions is almost always greater than that lost in simple detrusor instability. The condition is associated with disseminated sclerosis, follows cerebrovascular accidents, is seen in some cases of Parkinson's disease, syringomyelia, and in fact any condition which affects the conducting pathways in the upper part of the spinal cord. The reflex centre in the cord is intact so that the stretching of the bladder wall causes reflex detrusor spasm and micturition. The difficulty arises because the sphincter mechanism is also subject to a similar degree of spasm. The result is bladder wall hypertrophy with trabeculation, formation of saccules and diverticula and the presence of a urine residue. If the patient is paraplegic, management becomes extremely difficult as sepsis, excoriation of the genitalia and perineum, and areas of pressure necrosis occur.

In lower motor neurone lesions which affect the afferent and efferent portions of the sacral reflex arc as well as the reflex centre itself, the bladder is cut off from this spinal regulatory centre. As the pathognomonic feature of an upper motor neurone lesion is spasticity, so is flaccidity the feature of a lower motor neurone lesion. The detrusor muscle becomes flaccid, often insensitive to stretch, and the bladder distends enormously. The concomitant weakness of the sphincter mechanism eventually leads to overflow incontinence where urine trickles through the urethra. The bladder is readily palpable, is asymmetrical, often enormous, not tender and relatively soft; from the side, the huge bulge above the symphysis pubic is readily apparent and unchanging, during respiration while the upper abdomen adopts a scaphoid shape.

Pressure on the bladder dome often results in the expression of urine, a diagnostic test which, in itself, can sometimes be adapted as a therapeutic technique to promote bladder emptying,

Lower motor neurone lesions are also associated with peripheral neuritis, as in diabetes or tabes. In diabetes, a selective peripheral neuropathy can affect bladder behaviour, and the mechanism of erection in the male, without any peripheral signs of such a neuropathy. Damage to the autonomic supply to the bladder also follows pelvic surgery, especially abdomino-perineal excision of the rectum and Wertheim hysterectomy. Operations which spare the autonomic supply to the pelvis and genitalia have been developed.

A similar picture of incontinence with overflow is also seen in chronic outflow obstruction, almost always secondary to prostatic enlargement or bladder neck stenosis. Enuresis is a pathognomonic clinical feature of this condition (*Fig*. U.1).

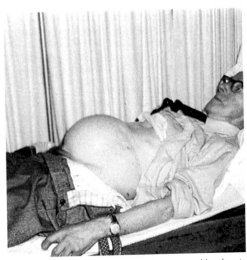

Fig. U.1. Swelling in the lower abdomen caused by chronic retention of urine due to an enlarged prostate.

All the conditions described so far present as incontinence of an intermittent variety. Continuous incontinence, day and night, is found in some congenital abnormalities. The most severe of these is *ectopia vesicae* (bladder extrophy) where there is failure of development of the abdominal wall and anterior wall of the bladder so that the mucosa of the bladder is exposed and the two ureteric orifices can be seen with urine dripping from them (*Fig.* U.2). There is wide separation of the two pubic rami (pubic diastasis).

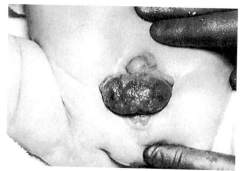

Fig. U.2. Ectopia vesicae in a boy of 6 months. The bladder mucosa protrudes and urine drips constantly from the ureters.

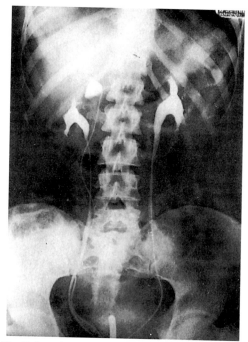

Fig. U.3. Pyelogram in a case of incontinence of urine in a woman. There is a duplex kidney on the right; the ureter from its upper segment drained into the vestibule.

An *ectopic ureter* occasionally opens into the vagina in the female or into the urethra beyond the sphincter apparatus in either sex. Urine leaks continually. The ectopic ureter usually drains a duplex kidney and when a pyelogram shows a duplex system in a case of incontinence an ectopic ureter should be sought. The opening is often extremely difficult to find, but the intravenous injection of indigo-carmine or methylene blue will facilitate its location. The rule in duplex kidneys is that the ureter of the lower moiety is orthotopic, the ureter of the upper moiety always heterotopic and opening inferior to the orthotopic ureter. The upper moiety ureter will always be the ectopic ureter and the affected moiety is usually hydronephrotic; it may drain only one calicine system (*Fig.* U.3).

Incontinence from a *fistula* is usually continuous, but if the abnormal opening is between the ureter and vagina leakage may appear to be intermittent. Fistula from the urinary tract may communicate with the uterus(in which case urine can be seen escaping from the cervical os), or with the vagina (when the fistula can usually be seen on speculum examination of the anterior vaginal wall). Uretero-vaginal fistula may arise in the female from erosion of a calculus into one of the vaginal fornices, and also after gynaecological surgery. Vesico-vaginal fistulae are secondary to malignant

processes within the upper vagina or in the posterior bladder wall, invading anteriorly or posteriorly respectively. They may follow surgery.

The investigation and diagnosis of incontinence when there is no overt cause such as fistula or congenital abnormality depends on urodynamic assessment of the patient. The study consists of three phases:

1. *Sphincterometry*, where the pressure exerted by the sphincter apparatus is measured and the configuration of the sphincter complex observed. When there is sphincter incompetence the pressure is low, and when the sphincter is in spasm, as in an upper motor neurone lesion, the pressure is high (*Fig.* U.4).

2. *Cystometry*, where bladder pressure is monitored during filling. Two parameters are measured, the intra-abdominal pressure through a vaginal or rectal transducer and the total bladder pressure through a bladder transducer. Electronic subtraction of the former from the later gives a reading of true or intrinsic bladder pressure.

The bladder is a perfectly compliant organ in that intrinsic bladder pressure does not rise as the bladder fills. The normal curve is observed in genuine stress incontinence. In enuresis and in minor degrees of bladder disturbance secondary to upper motor neurone lesions, a 'delayed voiding contraction' is seen,

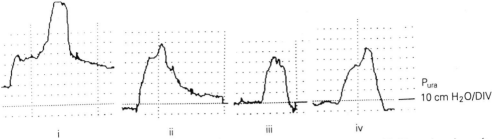

i   ii   iii   iv

P_{ura}
10 cm H_2O/DIV

Fig. U.4. Profilometry. i, Normal male urethral pressure profile (UPP). ii, Male UPP showing no bladder neck peak, as after prostatectomy or α-blockage. iii, Female UPP showing sphincter incompetence (predicted normal pressure = 100 fl patient's age). iv, Female UPP showing distal urethral stenosis. P_{ura} = urethral pressure.

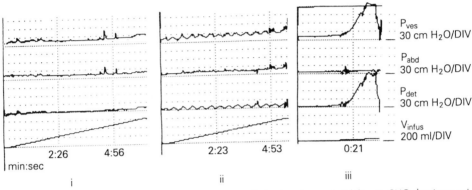

P_{ves}
30 cm H_2O/DIV

P_{abd}
30 cm H_2O/DIV

P_{det}
30 cm H_2O/DIV

V_{infus}
200 ml/DIV

2:26   4:56   2:23   4:53   0:21

min:sec

i   ii   iii

Fig. U.5. Cystometry. i, Normal cystometrogram (CMG). ii, CMG showing detrusor instability. iii, CMG showing a voiding contraction. P_{ves} = intravesical pressure; P_{abd} = abdominal pressure; P_{det} = detrusor pressure; V_{infus} = volume of infusion.

the bladder contracting vigorously near capacity. When the bladder is extremely irritable, as in acute cystitis, or when there is an upper motor neurone lesion affecting the bladder to a considerable degree, an uninhibited pattern of behaviour is seen. The 'unstable detrusor' is manifest as waves of contraction of a pressure which exceeds 10 cm H_2O. In lower motor neurone lesions, or in bladders affected by chronic retention, filling goes on and on with little alteration in intrinsic bladder pressure (*Fig.* U.5).

3. *Voiding pressure and flow rate.* During the void phase, the bladder voiding pressure and the flow rate are measured. When there is sphincter incompetence voided pressure is low while flow rate is often abnormally high; in obstruction the voiding pressure will be high and the flow rate low.

Lynn Edwards

Urine, retention of

Retention of urine is the inability to empty the bladder completely; the end result is the acute or gradual accumulation of urine within the bladder. In *acute*

retention there is a sudden inability to pass urine. The condition is painful and presents as a surgical emergency. In **chronic retention** there is a gradual increase in bladder size; it can often reach enormous proportions, occasionally reaching as high as the xiphisternum (*see Fig.* U.1). Pressure effects on the upper tract are not uncommon and an elevation of the blood urea, in association with bilateral hydronephrosis and hydroureters, is observed; the condition is a medical emergency in that stabilization of the biochemical changes is a pre-requisite precursor to surgical correction of the cause. Retention of the urine must be distinguished from anuria, when the kidneys fail to secrete urine. In retention, whether acute or chronic, the kidneys still function and urine continues to collect in the distended bladder.

Acute retention

Acute retention produces severe pain. The bladder is palpable some two fingers' breadths above the symphysis pubis. It is central, tense and tender. The commonest cause is outflow tract obstruction in the male, secondary to *prostatic enlargement* or *bladder neck stenosis*. It should be noted that the severity of outflow tract obstruction bears no relation to the size of the prostate, a tiny prostate often being responsible for an acute retentive episode, the largest prostate often remaining asymptomatic.

Acute retention from *urethral stricture* alone is uncommon but secondary spasm and congestion proximal to the stricture, especially involving the sphincter apparatus, may result in retention.

Acute retention may be precipitated by exposure to *cold*, overindulgence in *alcohol*, the administration of *anticholinergic agents* in order to relieve the urinary frequency which the patient almost invariably has, and *bronchodilating agents*, thus explaining the increased frequency of acute retention in elderly men with chronic bronchitis in winter when their chests need treatment. Under some circumstances, particularly delay in the act of micturition beyond reasonable limits, a feat often accomplished while the patient is 'anesthetized' with alcohol, the prostate becomes acutely congested and retention follows. The retention is relieved by catheterization, the congestion subsides and normal micturition can be re-established, to recur with the next bout of excess.

Acute retention in women is sometimes associated with *pregnancy*, especially when the *gravid uterus is retroverted*, while large uterine *fibroids* may produce the same effect. In young women, *herpes genitalis*, acquired as a sexually transmitted disease, may also precipitate acute retention, not only because of the urethral oedema associated with the herpetic lesions, but also by neurological involvement of the sacral reflex arc in such a way that detrusor activity is lost. *Herpes zoster* may give rise to acute retention in both sexes; in this case the pathognomonic herpetic eruptions will be seen over the buttock area or the sacrum.

Chronic retention

Chronic retention is insidious in its onset and symptoms develop so slowly that the patient may deny urinary difficulty. It is only in retrospect and after surgical correction that the patient admits that there were significantly lower urinary track symptoms preoperatively. Enuresis (bed-wetting) is a frequent presenting feature.

Retention secondary to *urethral stricture* can be related to previous episodes of sexually transmitted diseases, *Chlamydia trachomatis* being a potent cause of extensive stricture formation.

The history in stricture is of a gradual increasing difficulty with micturition, slowing of the stream, and dribbling after micturition; this last symptom occurs because of the column of urine which is trapped between the sphincter apparatus and the stricture. An important distinction between stricture and prostatic obstruction is that straining assists urine flow in the former and reduces flow in the latter. The investigation of choice is urethrography (*Fig.* U.6), but if instrumentation is undertaken as a primary investigation direct vision urethroscopy is obligatory; the stricture may then be visualized before it has been traumatized and divided appropriately by direct vision urethrotomy.

Prostatic enlargement is unusual below the age of 50 but *bladder neck stenosis* can occur much earlier. The condition which has been recently recognized is that of *detrusor-sphincter dyssynergia*, where contraction of the detrusor is not accompanied by reflex relaxation of the bladder neck. The presenting features of both conditions are similar, the patient having increased frequency of micturition, especially at night, hesitancy, reduction in flow, dribbling post-micturition and sometimes urgency.

On rectal examination, prostatic enlargement may be found. The gland may be smooth, uniform in consistency, elastic and movable within the pelvis when the enlargement is benign. A nodular, hard, irregular prostate may indicate *carcinoma*, while fixation to either side of the pelvic walls implies malignant extension well beyond the confines of the capsule. With bladder neck stenosis and detrusor-sphincter dyssynergia, the prostate is of normal size.

When retention of urine follows *acute prostatitis* or a prostatic abscess, a history of recent urethral discharge will be obtained. The patient will be obviously ill, with a fever, rigors, frequency of micturition, pain on micturition, and perineal and pelvic discomfort.

Acute retention of urine secondary to urethral intra-luminal causes is most commonly caused by the *impaction of a calculus* in the urethra. A calculus may impact at the site of a stricture, when it can often be felt on examination of the penis, or at the external urethral meatus, in which case it can usually be seen. The history in such a case is dramatic in that a normal flow of micturition is quite suddenly interrupted, causing a sudden pain along the urethra, a feeling similar to receiving a blow in the bladder area and the dribbling of a few drops of blood.

As transurethral resection is now the favoured procedure for correction of prostatic enlargement, and the removal of all the resulting chips often difficult, especially if there are bladder diverticula, 'chip retention' is a relatively new but not uncommon phenomenon, having the same symptoms as retention secondary to impaction of a stone.

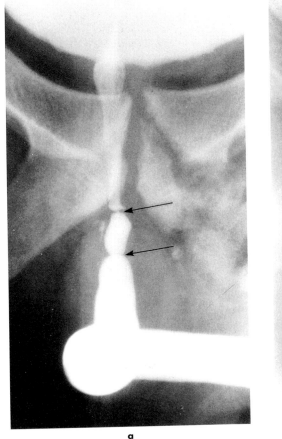

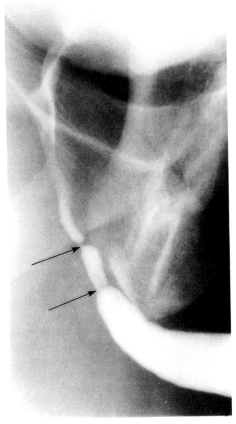

a

b

Fig. U.6. Urethral stricture. *a,* anteroposterior view of urethrogram showing two strictures (arrows) of a male urethra, one submembranous, one bulbar. *b,* Same strictures (arrows); lateral view.

Blockage of the bladder neck by the free-floating area of a *pedunculated bladder tumour* is rare; the growth is forced into the orifice during micturition, causing obstruction.

Complete *traumatic rupture of the urethra* leads to acute retention of urine. It almost always follows rupture of the pelvis but may follow a blow to the perineum, for example from a boot or from falling astride a bar. There will be history of injury and blood will appear at the external urethral meatus; perineal haematoma may not be too evident in pelvic fracture but will certainly indicate local urethral trauma. If urethral rupture is incomplete, the patient should be encouraged not to pass urine as extravasation may occur and cause a haemato-urinoma in the perineum (*Fig.* U.7).

Prolapse of an intervertebral disc will occasionally cause acute neurological urinary retention from direct pressure on the nerve roots. Retention may

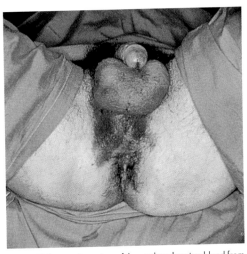

Fig. U.7. Traumatic rupture of the urethra showing blood from meatus and perineal haematoma limited by attachment of Colles' fascia.

occasionally be the presenting feature of the condition which, from the spinal point of view, remains asymptomatic.

Acute retention is a fairly common complication of *operations on the rectum* and pelvic organs. It may also follow operations on the hip (in both sexes) and hernia repairs. The mechanism in these cases must be reflex spasm of the sphincter apparatus. When there is dual pathology, for example, hernia or haemorrhoids in the presence of benign prostatic enlargement, it may be as well to combine the two surgical procedures to avoid the acute retention that the hernia or haemorrhoid operation may cause. It is particularly important to record prostatic size in all male patients with rectal carcinoma requiring abdomino-perineal excision of the rectum. If acute retention follows such as procedure it is no longer possible to assess prostatic size accurately and inform the patient regarding the prostatectomy technique that will be employed, in that a large gland will be beyond the reasonable range of resection (limit of some 80 gm). This failure to give the patient full information may, of course, change as abdominal ultrasound assessment of prostatic size becomes more accurate. (Transrectal ultrasound assessment is impossible, of course, after excision of the rectum).

Acute retention of urine may be a manifestation of *hysteria*, but in common with all other diagnoses, medical and surgical, an organic cause should be sought and excluded before any psychogenic element is ascribed to the diagnosis. Hysterical retention usually occurs in children and in young women. Retention due to psychiatric illness is more usually a complication of therapy as tricyclic antidepressants are powerful anticholinergic agents which suppress detrusor activity to the extent that retention, either acute or chronic, may occur.

Acute retention in female children is unusual but it not infrequently occurs in males. While the male infant is still wearing nappies, *ammoniacal ulceration* of the foreskin, or of the meatus if circumcised, can give rise to acute retention because micturition is so painful that the child refuses to allow the act to continue. Retention in the presence of a tight *phimosis* is unusual but the pathognomonic feature will be ballooning of the foreskin during micturition. *Meatal stenosis* following ulceration secondary to circumcision can occasionally lead to acute retention in young males; when micturition is attempted, the urethra can be often felt as a distended and rigid band on the ventrum of the penis. Retention may also follow the inadvertent insertion of a *foreign body*, such as a beam or screw, into the anterior urethra.

Lynn Edwards

Vagina and uterus, prolapse of

Prolapse is essentially a condition in which the supports of the vagina fail to hold it in place, with the result that it tends to turn inside out and to bulge externally at the vulva. Because the uterus is inserted into the vaginal vault, if the upper part of the vagina descends the uterus comes down with it as a uterine prolapse or vaginal vault prolapse. The vagina is normally held in place by the transverse cervical ligaments (of Mackenrodt), the pubo-cervical and the utero-sacral ligaments. At a lower level the vagina is supported by the pelvic floor or levator ani muscle. During pregnancy the supporting ligaments are softened and stretched and during childbirth the opening in the pelvic floor is enlarged. Prolapse therefore occurs mainly in women who have had children, but the vaginal vault may prolapse with projection of the cervix through the vulva in nulliparous women.

Prolapse does not usually occur until the menopause and the patient complains of a swelling at the vulva giving rise to a feeling of bearing down and discomfort on walking or straining. The swelling and the symptoms disappear when the patient lies down. If the patient is examined in the left lateral or Sims' position, with a Sims' speculum holding back first the posterior and then the anterior vaginal wall, it is possible to determine which part of the vagina is prolapsing. Low down anteriorly is a *urethrocele*, which is associated with stress incontinence of urine. At a higher level prolapse of the anterior vaginal wall contains the bladder to give rise to a *cystocele*. Straining may cause kinking of the urethra with inability to micturate. The bladder does not empty completely and basal cystitis with urinary frequency is common. *Uterine (or vaginal vault) prolapse* occurs in three degrees. In the first degree the cervix descends to the vulva; in the second it protrudes through the vulva; and in the third, which is a *procidentia*, the whole of the uterus is outside the vulva. Sometimes there is much elongation of the supravaginal portion of the cervix, the vagina is turned completely inside out, but the body of the uterus remains within the pelvis. If the vagina in relation to the posterior fornix prolapses it is related to the pouch of Douglas to give rise to an *enterocele* containing loops of small gut or a *pouch of Douglas hernia*. Lower down the vagina posteriorly is the rectum and prolapse of this part gives rise to a *rectocele*. It is possible to hook the finger into the rectocele through the anus. Patients often find difficulty in emptying the rectum because the faeces tend to go forward into the pouch of the rectocele.

Prolapse of the vaginal wall has to be differentiated from other swellings which protrude at the vulva. These include: a *fibroid polyp* which has a pedicle passing through the hard rim of the cervix into the uterine cavity where it is attached; *chronic inversion of the uterus*, a rare condition in which the uterus turns inside out, the fundus passing through the cervical rim leaving a cup-shaped depression where the uterine body should be; a long tongue-shaped *endometrial polyp*; a large *mucous polyp of the cervix*; a *vaginal cyst* and a *malignant growth* of cervix of vagina.

N. Patel

Vagina, discharge from

The normal discharge from the vagina is a mixture of secretions from the uterine body, cervix, and vaginal wall; that from the uterine body is watery and small in amount; that from the cervix is thick and mucoid, but clear and transparent, like unboiled white of egg; that from the vagina is merely a transudation of plasma from the vessels, mixed with desquamated vaginal epithelium, and in virgins looks like unboiled starch mixed with water; it is small in amount. The bulk of the discharge found in the vagina comes from the cervix; there are more glands there than in any other part of the genital tract; there are no glands in the vagina. The cervical secretion is alkaline, consisting of mucus with a pH of 6.5. The secretion varies during the menstrual cycle, being abundant, clear, and almost free from leucocytes at the time of ovulation. At this time its elasticity is greater than one inch (*Spinbaarkeit*) and it is more easily penetrated by the spermatozoa. At other times of the month the cervical mucus is scanty, opaque, and tenacious. The secretion from Bartholin's gland, thin and mucoid, may be copious under sexual excitement, but under normal conditions it is scanty, and so does not contribute to a vaginal discharge. The vaginal mixed secretion is acid in reaction, owing to the presence of lactic acid produced by Doderlein's bacillus from the glycogen in the basal cells of the vaginal epithelium. This bacillus is normally found in the vagina from puberty to the menopause. The pH of the vagina is 4.5, the vaginal acidity being a bar to vaginal infection; unmixed uterine secretion is alkaline.

Normally, the amount of mixed vaginal discharge should do no more than just moisten the vaginal orifice; when the amount is so great as to moisten the vulva and consequently stain garments, the discharge is pathological. *Excess of the normal discharge (leucorrhoea)* may be due to (1) such conditions as anaemia, tuberculosis, chronic nephritis, indeed any debilitating state; (2) any condition causing increased pelvic congestion, such as constipation, provoked but unsatisfied sexual desire, masturbation; (3) chronic passive congestion of heart disease or cirrhosis of the liver; (4) endocrine disorders resulting in hypersecretion of the cervical glands, the result of excessive oestrogen stimulation. This is not uncommonly found in those suffering from functional uterine bleeding; (5) no abnormality may be found. In many normal women a premenstrual mucoid discharge is seen, and in pregnant women leucorrhoea, the result of passive congestion or endocrine factors, is commonly encountered. Occasionally a congenital erosion may be responsible.

Girls before puberty and women after the menopause do not have the protection of an acid secretion in the vagina. Non-specific infection is liable to occur and discharge results. A foreign body may be the precipitating factor in young girls. Oestrogen withdrawal is the cause in post-menopausal women, when the condition is referred to as *atrophic (or senile) vaginitis*.

The composition of an abnormal discharge varies according to the source from which it comes and the acuteness of the inflammation; a frankly purulent discharge indicates acute inflammation, whereas a mucopurulent discharge indicates chronic inflammation involving the cervix.

1. The mucopurulent discharge

This, the commonest type, is a thick, white or yellow discharge. It contains much mucus, many leucocytes, masses of epithelium from the vagina (squames) and various bacteria: diphtheroids, streptococci, staphylococci, *Streptococcus faecalis*, *E. coli*. Doderlein's bacillus will not be found. This discharge is typically produced by endocervicitis and cervical erosions. When endometritis is present as well, which is uncommon, the discharge becomes thinner and white, yellow, brown or even bloodstained. Microscopically, the films made from the mixed cases show proportionally less mucus, but otherwise the constituents are the same.

2. The frankly purulent discharge

This discharge occurs in:

A.   ACUTE CERVICITIS

Due to gonorrhoea or sometimes following puerperal or post-abortal infections; the cervix is red, swollen and oedematous, being bathed in pus. There is nothing characteristic of gonorrhoeal discharge visible to the naked eye. The detection of the gonococcus can alone decide the question. This is often a matter of difficulty, because it is only in the few days immediately after infection that the organism can be found in the discharge. In chronic cases the gonococcus must be looked for in one of three places—in the interior of the cervical canal, in the urethra and Skene's tubules, which open posterolaterally at the entrance to the urethra, or in discharge squeezed from the orifices of Bartholin's glands. Discharge from the cervical canal should be taken on a platinum loop after carefully wiping away discharge from the os uteri with sterile wool, using a vaginal speculum to display the area. This discharge should be spread on to two glass slides and put by to dry. Two other films should then be made by massaging the urethra from above downwards and collecting any discharge thus made to appear at the urinary meatus. It is important that micturition should not have taken place for several hours beforehand. Finally two films should be taken from the orifices of Bartholin's glands after squeezing the glands between the finger and thumb. After drying in the air the films should be fixed by passing through a flame and then stained by Gram's method, followed by neutral red as a counter stain. In films thus prepared gonococci are strained red (Gram-negative) while organisms which retain Gram's stain appear deep violet or black (Gram-positive). The gonococci are found as diplococci in the cytoplasm of the polymorphonuclear leucocytes and epithelial cells. Cultures of the discharge should also be taken and grown on a suitable medium such as chocolate agar.

B.   GRANULAR VAGINITIS

The discharge is copious and purulent. It is associated with trauma of the vagina from the irritation of rubber, or poorly fitting ring pessaries, or actual ulceration as in decubitus ulcers on prolapsed portions. Practically no mucus is found in such discharge unless the cervix shares in the inflammatory process.

C.   TRICHOMONAS VAGINITIS

Due to a flagellate parasite, this produces a frothy purulent discharge causing local pain and soreness and being extremely irritating to the external genitalia. The discharge is green or greenish-yellow with small bubbles of gas in it and has a characteristic odour. The protozoon is to be found by diluting some of the vaginal discharge with normal warm saline and examining under the microscope with a high-power lens, when the parasite, which is about the size of a leucocyte, will be found actively mobile, being pro-

pelled by its flagellae. The trichomonas live in the vagina in symbiosis with the micrococcus *Aerogenes alcaligenes*, which organism forms the froth or bubbles so characteristic of the discharge, It is a Gram-negative micrococcus, smaller than the gonococcus. The vaginal walls have a typical red stippled appearance.

D.   MONILIA VAGINITIS

Common during pregnancy, giving rise to white patches of thrush on the vagina walls. It is a common cause of pruritis vulvae. It may complicate diabetes and the urine should always therefore be tested for sugar. If the white patches are scraped off the vaginal walls they leave raw bleeding areas. Vaginitis rarely exists alone, but when it does occur the discharge is thick and pasty if it is a simple catarrhal condition—pasty on account of the large admixture of vaginal squamous epithelium. Specimens of the discharge should be taken for recognition of the mycelium and spores of *Candida albicans* in stained smears and for culture.

E.   NON-SPECIFIC VAGINITIS

Some patients with a purulent and offensive discharge who do not have trichomoniasis have large numbers of *Gardnerella vaginalis* (*haemophilus*) and anaerobic bacteria in the vagina. The pH is 5.0 or more and the treatment similar to that of a trichomonas infection.

1.   Offensive-smelling vaginal discharge

This discharge is associated with decomposition; the discharge itself may decompose because it cannot escape fast enough from the passage, or the source of the discharge may be a decomposing substance like a *sloughing fibroid* or necrotic *carcinoma of the cervix*; in the two latter cases the discharge is copious, water and bloodstained, with a horribly fetid smell. When the discharge itself is decomposing it is usually thick and purulent as when a retained foreign body such as a ring pessary, an internal tampon or contraceptive cap is the cause. Infected retained gestation products, a faecal fistula or a pelvic abscess rupturing into the vagina may occasionally by responsible. In elderly women a foul discharge may come from the interior of the uterus, a *pyometra*; in which case pus can be made to flow from the os uteri by squeezing the uterus or passing a sound; it is due to *senile endometritis*, or it may be associated with carcinoma of the uterine body or cervix.

4. Watery blood-stained discharge

Watery blood-stained discharge, which is not offensive occurs with *carcinoma of the body of the uterus* in early *carcinoma of the cervix*, with *mucous polyps, placental polyps, hydatidiform mole* and *new growths of the Fallopian tubes*. Other causes such as endometrial hyperplasia, rupture of the membranes in early pregnancy, or an intermittent hydrosalpinx may be responsible. The differential diagnosis of these conditions cannot be made from the discharge alone, but must rest upon physical examination combined with the use of the microscope upon materials removed from the uterus. The use of vaginal smear tests (Papanicolaou) may help in the diagnosis, as in some cases cancer cells may be found in the discharge, but if malignancy is suspected reliance should not be placed on this test alone. Whenever there is any blood in the discharge the patient should be examined under anaesthesia and biopsies taken of the endometrium and cervix in case of malignancy.

Smears of the cervix and vagina may be taken with a wooden spatula for cytology. Malignant cells may be found in symptomless women with apparently normal cervices. Colposcopy and cervical biopsy is used to make the decision of cervical intra-epithelial disease. This condition is found in about 5 in every 1000 women examined over the age of 30 years. Its discovery and removal from the population may lead to the reduction in incidence of invasive carcinoma of the cervix but the hoped-for abolition has not been realized due to failure of screening programmes and the fact that a small proportion of invasive growths seems not to pass through a carcinoma-in-situ phase.

Vaginal casts may be composed of coagulated surface epithelium, the result of astringent injections or applications, and are recognized easily with the microscope. Membranous flakes may be passed with discharge in cases of *membranous vaginitis*; they consist of vaginal epithelium entangled in coagulated blood plasma, and present quite a different appearance from casts of coagulated epithelia layers. These membranous masses may be seen lining the whole vagina, and are generally due to special organisms. The *diphtheria bacillus* has been found to be the causal agent in some; in others the *Escherichia coli*.

N. Patel

Vagina, swelling in

Vaginal swellings may be classified thus:

Inflammatory

Gonorrhoeal
Non-specific; (*a*) streptococcus; (*b*) staphylococcus;
(*c*) E. coli

Trichomonas
Monilia
Senile
Chemical

New growth

1 Innocent:
   a. Cystic: (i) cysts of Gartner's duct; (ii) implantation cysts; (iii) endometriomas
   b. Solid: (i) fibroma; (ii) adenomyoma
2 Malignant
   Primary carcinoma, primary sarcoma, secondary carcinoma

Inflammatory causes

The vagina is resistant to infection because of its lining of stratified epithelium and the absence of glands; further protection is brought about by the action of Doderlein's bacillus on the glycogen in the vaginal cells, producing lactic acid which keeps the pH of the vagina at about 4.5. This acidity inhibits the growth of most organisms during the menstrual life of a woman; before puberty and after the menopause this protection is non-existent.

Trichomonas vaginitis is very common and gives rise to a typical red stippling of the vaginal walls, particularly in the fornices. The discharge is frothy, greenish-yellow in colour, and has a rather characteristic unpleasant smell. A discharge of sudden onset with soreness of the vulva is often due to trichomonas vaginitis. Sometimes *Gardnerella vaginalis* (*haemophilus*) and anaerobic bacteria are found.

Monilial infection may occur in the debilitated subject, but is most typically seen in diabetes. The discharge is thick, white, curdy and adherent to the vaginal walls. An accompanying vulvitis that has the appearance of raw beef steak with a rather abrupt edge is characteristic; pruritus is the leading symptom.

Gonorrhoeal vaginitis is most frequently seen in the young child. It is not common in the adult because of the vaginal resistance to infection.

The non-specific forms of vaginitis, due to *E. coli*, *Staph. aureus* and streptococci, are usually associated with the retention of some foreign body, such as a tampon, or a ring pessary. It may also occur before puberty or following childbirth or abortion.

Chemical. Occasionally a too-hot vaginal douche or the use of strong chemicals, such as potassium permanganate, may be responsible. The characteristic signs of inflammation, with vaginal discharge, are present.

Senile vaginitis. This is a common condition occurring after the menopause when the protective mechanism of the vagina is lost. The vaginal epithelium is thinned, and, in places, minute areas become completely denuded of epithelium, and appear as red points, giving a somewhat spotted appearance to the vagina. These areas may adhere and cause vaginal adhesions; they also cause a thin blood-stained watery discharge. On breaking down the adhesions with the finger, frank bleeding may take place. Senile vaginitis is most marked in the upper part of the vagina.

Cause from new growths

Cysts of Gartner's duct are cystic growths of the remains of the Wolffian mesonephric duct, which has failed to be obliterated. They are always found in the anterolateral wall of the vagina. They may be small but sometimes grow to a large size, protruding outside the vaginal orifice and occluding the vaginal cavity. The characteristic position and cystic feel serve to differentiate them from the various types of vaginal prolapse. *Small implantation cysts* may be seen at the vaginal orifice posteriorly; they are small, and may follow operations on the perineum, or lacerations at childbirth. Occasionally an *endometrioma* may burrow through into the posterior vaginal fornix from the floor of the pouch of Douglas, forming nodular growths which tend to bleed at the time of menstruation. This condition may be confused with a primary carcinoma of the vagina, but it is not friable. Microscopic section will settle its nature.

Benign tumours. Sessile and pedunculated swellings arise in the vaginal wall which on histology are found to be a papilloma, fibroma or lipoma. They are uncommon.

Primary carcinoma of the vagina is rare. It occurs in the posterior fornix, often following the retention of a pessary which has been forgotten for a number of years. It usually takes the form of a typical epitheliomatous ulcer, eventually producing a rectovaginal fistula. Its friability and vascularity make the diagnosis clear, which should be confirmed by biopsy. A rare form of adenocarcinoma occurs in the vagina of teenage girls whose mothers took large doses of stilboestrol during their pregnancies. It has to be differentiated from benign adenosis vaginae in which there are numerous small swellings in the mucosa with a profuse discharge of mucus.

Secondary carcinoma usually spreads to the upper part of the vagina from the cervix. Occasionally metastases spread from carcinoma of the body of the uterus; they occur constantly at the lower end of the vagina in the midline anteriorly about half an inch behind the urethral meatus. Curettage reveals the uterine growth and biopsy the nature of the metastasis. Secondary growths have been described as occurring at the same site from primary carcinomas in the ovary and colon and also from hypernephroma (clear cell carcinoma) of the kidney. They may ulcerate, causing bleeding. Microscopical examination will reveal their true nature.

Sarcoma of the vagina is rare, but occasionally the grape-like tumour sarcoma botryoides (or embryonal rhabdomyosarcoma) may appear to originate in the vagina rather than in the cervix. It occurs in infants and young children and is one of the causes of vaginal bleeding before puberty. It has a characteristic appearance, like a bunch of grapes, and microscopic section proves its nature.

In the normal adult the healthy vaginal transudation will be found to contain many cornified cells and few, if any, leucocytes. This is due to the normal circulation of oestrogen. Excessive oestrogen stimulation leads to a multiplication of the layers of the vaginal epithelial cells with an increase in their glycogen content. At the menopause, due to lack of oestrogen stimulation, the transudation contains few cornified cells but many nucleated cells and leucocytes. It is thus possible, by examining a smear of vaginal cells obtained from the pool of discharge in the posterior vaginal fornix and rolled on to a slide with a swab-stick, to obtain some idea of the excess or deficiency of oestrogen. The healthy vaginal walls take on a deep brown colour if painted with Lugol's iodine solution, due to the abundance of glycogen in the vaginal cells. This is also an indication of oestrogen sufficiency.

As carcinoma is an exfoliative disease cancer cells can be found in preparations of vaginal and cervical smears in some cases of carcinoma of the cervix or corpus uteri. The taking of smears is simple but the correct interpretation of the findings requires experience. It can be of the greatest use, however, as a positive smear test for cancer cells, in the absence of any symptoms or obvious signs of carcinoma of the uterus, calls for a thorough examination of the cervix with a colposcope and the uterine cavity by curettage. In about 5 cases per 1000 women examined the biopsy shows disease of the cervix. Invasive cancer can be prevented in these cases by cauterization, laser treatment or cone biopsy. If the disease persists after treatment and positive smears are obtained, a cone biopsy or hysterectomy is indicated.

N. Patel

Veins, varicose abdominal

The point at which distension of a vein becomes a varicosity is arbitrary; most conditions that produce undoubted varicosity of the veins of the abdominal wall in some cases merely dilate them in others. When this dilatation is considerable (*Fig.* V.1) it nearly always has much diagnostic significance, particularly if the direction of blood flow is reversed.

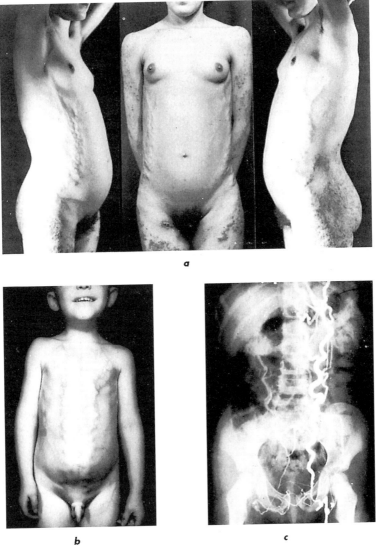

Fig. V.1. Inferior vena caval obstruction showing greatly dilated collaterals by means of surface and infrared photography and by venography. (Dr R. G. Ollerenshaw, Manchester Royal Infirmary.)

Veins, however, may seem to be dilated when they are but unduly visible owing to wasting of the subcutaneous fat; or they may, in rare cases, be simply varicose, like veins in the leg, owing to idiosyncrasy or hereditary predisposition. In neither of these cases however, is the blood current in them reversed. To test the direction of blood flow, part of a vein should be chosen where there are no side branches, and the blood should be expressed from it by means of two fingers pressed gently down on the vein close together and then drawn apart whilst pressure over the vein is maintained by each; when a length of the distended vein has been emptied in this way, one of the two fingers is taken off, and the time taken by the vein in refilling is noted. The procedure is repeated, the other finger being taken off this time; it is then generally easy to decide whether the vein fills from below upwards or from above downwards. Normally, the blood flows from above downwards in the veins of the lower two-thirds of the abdominal wall; when the blood flow is from below upwards there is almost certainly obstruction to the inferior vena cava, the blood which is unable to return by it finding a collateral circulation via the abdominal parietes to the superior vena cava.

Obstruction to the inferior vena cava is due to one or other of three main groups of conditions, namely;

1   *Great general increase in the intra-abdominal tension*, owing to such conditions as: ascites, ovarian cyst, great splenic or hepatic enlargement.
2   *Thrombosis* without external obstruction.
3   *Obstruction by local compression*, especially by secondary deposits in the retroperitoneal lymph nodes.

When the obstruction of the inferior vena cava is due not to the vein itself being thrombosed or invaded by new growth but to the *general intra-abdominal pressure* becoming so great that the vein is, so to speak, flattened out, the varicosity of the veins upon the abdominal wall is but a late symptom, and the diagnosis of the cause of the great abdominal distension, generally ascites or a large tumour, will already have been made. If there is marked varicosity of the superficial veins early in a case of ascites the probability is that both are due to malignant disease.

When the inferior vena cava is obstructed by 'simple' thrombosis, the clotting will probably have started, not in the inferior vena cava itself, but below it, either in the legs or in the pelvis; oedema of the legs will be pronounced, and it may be ascertained that one leg became oedematous and painful before the other; when this is so it suggests thrombosis starting in the calf or femoral vein of one side, the other leg becoming affected later when the clot has spread up through the iliac veins of the one side to the inferior vena, and thence down the iliac veins of the other side. The higher the thrombosis extends the higher up the back will the oedema spread; and when the renal veins have been reached, albuminuria, with tube casts, haematuria and ascites, may ensue, and acute nephritis may be simulated. Distension or varicosity of the veins of the abdominal wall assists in distinguishing such a case from one of acute or sub-acute nephritis; besides which there will be no oedema of the eyelids or face.

If there is no very tense distension of the abdomen; if the way the case began does not suggest thrombosis in one leg, or in the pelvis, extending upwards; and if, nevertheless, there is marked varicosity of the veins of the lower part of the abdominal wall, with the blood flow in them reversed, so as to be from below upwards, the history being a relatively short one—the probability is that the inferior vena cava is being obstructed by something that is in immediate contact with it. There will very likely be symmetrical oedema of the legs, and possibly albuminuria and haematuria. It is remarkable how seldom an aortic aneurysm or other non-malignant mass obstructs a large vein sufficiently to produce this collateral varicosity; hence, the presumption is that such varicosity

indicates *malignant disease*. It is worthy of note that carcinoma of the kidney is prone to extend into the renal veins and thus into the inferior vena cava by direct extension—sometimes the malignant clot reaches as far as the right atrium, and may produce therein a pedunculated polyp. In such cases there has generally been haematuria or other renal symptoms before evidence of inferior vena caval obstruction arises, whereby cases of growth in the kidney invading the inferior vena cava may be distinguished from cases of secondary growth in the retroperitoneal nodes, which if they produced haematuria at all, would do so by first obstructing the inferior vena cava, and thence involving the renal veins. In such cases there are often other symptoms pointing to primary growth in some organ from which lymphatics drain into the retroperitoneal nodes; the testes and ovaries should not be overlooked in this respect.

It is said that *cirrhosis of the liver* leads to varicosity of the veins around the umbilicus—the *caput medusae*; most cases of cirrhosis of the liver cause no distension of the superficial abdominal veins until the general intra-abdominal tension has been greatly increased by the tenseness of the ascites which occurs late. Not even the telangiectases that occur so commonly in men past middle age around the lower part of the chest, in a line with the attachment of the diaphragm, indicate cirrhosis; they are quite as common in cases of emphysema without cirrhosis.

Varicosity of the superficial abdominal veins generally indicates either thrombosis of the inferior vena cava, secondary to direct spread of thrombosis up to it from veins in the pelvis or in the leg, or else stenosis of the vena cava by secondary malignant disease.

Harold Ellis

Vertigo

The term 'vertigo' implies by derivation a subjective sense of rotation, either of one's self or of the surroundings, but it is helpful to include within the term simply a feeling of being off-balance, without any sense of rotation, which some patients with Menière's disease experience between the more usual spinning attacks. Likewise the sensation which some people experience when looking down from a height or in the presence of diplopia might also be described as vertigo. It can then be concluded that vertigo, as more broadly defined, must always mean some involvement of the vestibular apparatus, either in its peripheral pathways or central connections.

Vertigo due to affections of the *external auditory meatus* must be very rare, if indeed it occurs at all, but removal of wax is said to have cured vertigo on occasion. *Disease of the middle ear and blockage of the Eustachian tubes by catarrh or new growth* may be accompanied by vertigo but probably the labyrinth is affected too in all such cases. Thus otitis media can cause either a serous or a purulent labyrinthitis, and otosclerosis may spread to involve the inner ear. If infection has caused a fistula into the internal ear, vertigo can occur either spontaneously or by increasing the pressure in the external meatus (the fistula sign), or even by the pressure changes within the Eustachian tubes during swallowing. These conditions of the middle ear are usually accompanied by deafness and tinnitus, and by auroscopic evidence of disease.

Disease of the internal ear is the most common source of paroxysmal vertigo. Labyrinthine causes may be listed under six subheadings:

1   *Spread of disease* from the middle ear as described above.
2   *Ototoxicity* with salicylates, quinine, streptomycin and acute alcoholism.
3   *Allergy* to foods, a very rare cause.
4   *Haemorrhage* into the semicircular canals, as in any disease accompanied by purpura or by a bleeding diathesis.
5   *Menière's disease*: a common affection due to degenerative changes in the membranous labyrinth with hydrops of the endolymph and characterized by paroxysms of vertigo which last minutes or hours and are often accompanied by pallor, prostration, vomiting, slight mental confusion and pain behind the ear or a more generalized headache. Vestibular nystagmus occurs during the vertigo but is not present between attacks. Tinnitus and nerve deafness ultimately supervene but are often slight or absent in the early stages of the disease.
6   *Positional* vertigo, which may arise when the head is placed in a particular position, can result either from a peripheral or from a central lesion.

If peripheral, the condition is commonly attributed to disease of the otolith organ and severe vertigo is experienced when the head is lowered so that the affected otolith organ is undermost. The vertigo will eventually pass off if the head is maintained in this position and there will be increasingly less vertigo as the manoeuvre of lowering the head with the affected otolith organ undermost is repeated. The vertigo may or may not be accompanied by nystagmus. This condition may develop after head injury, possibly as a result of nearby infection or for no apparent reason.

Positional vertigo may also arise, however, from central lesions such as multiple sclerosis or cerebellar neoplasm, often metastatic, and in such cases there is no adaptation but the vertigo is present and persists for as long as the head is held in the critical position.

Affections of the vestibular component of the 8th nerve are an infrequent source of vertigo so far as is known at present. In vestibular neuronitis there is intense vertigo with which a patient may waken and which may be accompanied by vomiting unless he lies absolutely still. There is no associated deafness or tinnitus but the caloric responses are abnormal in one or both ears. The intense vertigo usually passes off within a few days but there remains a liability to brief vertigo on head movement which may persist for weeks or even months. In many cases there is evidence of infection in the nose, sinuses; or tonsils. There is no pathological evidence as to its nature, but the term 'vestibular neuronitis' serves as a convenient label pending further clarification of the subject. In some cases the discomfort falls short of obvious vertigo, amounting to no more than an intermittent sense of inequilibrium which is aggravated by moving the head or by walking.

Less common than the above are *gross lesions of the 8th nerve*, notably *acoustic tumours, syphilitic and other inflammatory affections of the cerebellopontine recess, tumour of the petrous temporal bone, and gliomas and haemangioblastomas at the point where the nerve enters the pons*. The most important of these is the *neuroma*, a benign tumour which is easy to remove when small but which constitutes a formidable surgical hazard once it has grown large enough to produce the 'classic' signs — deafness, loss of the corneal reflex, facial weakness, homolateral cerebellar signs, and raised intracranial pressure with papilloedema. Fortunately, early diagnosis is now practicable in many cases at the stage of moderate deafness, with or without vertigo, and long before the facial or trigeminal nerves are affected, intracranial pressure is raised or the internal auditory meatus is expanded by the growth. In cochlear lesions the deafness is characterized by the fact that once the threshold of hearing is reached, sounds are heard as well as in the normal ear — and may even appear louder. This phenomenon is called *recruitment* and it is absent in deafness due to affections of the nerve itself. That is to say, in an 8th nerve tumour the affected ear will hear less than the normal side at all ranges of sound intensity. The best test, however, is the MRI scan with gadolineum enhancement. It is essential, therefore, to have tests carried out in all cases of vertigo and deafness for which no satisfactory explanation can be found.

Affections of the *medulla and lower pons* can cause vertigo. It may be paroxysmal or continuous, but generally speaking the diagnosis depends less upon the quality of the giddiness than on satellite symptoms and signs arising from simultaneous involvement of structures adjacent to the vestibular fibres and Deiter's vestibular nucleus. There is seldom tinnitus or deafness, because the auditory and vestibular pathways diverge after the 8th nerve enters the pons, but long tracts may be involved and nystagmus is present even when the patient is not actually feeling vertiginous; in labyrinthine and vestibular nerve lesions it usually ceases between attacks. Moreover, the nystagmus changes character: in labyrinthine and nerve lesions the quick component is always towards the affected side, whereas in central affections it is towards the left when the patient looks to the left and to the right when he looks to the right. (This is an oversimplification of a complicated subject, but it is a useful working rule, valid for most cases.) The diseases which produce vertigo in this situation include *multiple sclerosis*, thrombosis of the *posterior inferior cerebellar artery*, atheromatous *stenosis* of the basilar artery, *tumours* and *syringobulbia*. A condition notable for its extreme rarity and for its popularity amongst collectors of the recondite is *cysticercosis of the 4th ventricle*, which has been known to cause vertigo when the head is moved.

Cerebellar disease and injury can give rise to vertigo, more especially if the lesion is acute, as in penetrating injuries and infarction, but generally speaking chronic lesions cause a sense of disequilibrium rather than a sense of movement. In the case of tumours, however, a true vertigo may occur either through direct pressure on the vestibular centre in the brain-stem, or from *a rise of intracranial pressure* (which is communicated to the labyrinth through the ductus endolymphaticus), or perhaps from traction on the 8th nerve. It is apposite to remark that *transient vertigo can be caused by any rise of intracranial pressure*, irrespective of the nature or position of the lesion.

Disease of the cerebral hemispheres seldom causes vertigo. It can occur as the aura of an *epileptic fit*, and is occasionally seen in *migraine*, but it is uncommon in supratentorial tumours unless the intracranial pressure is high.

The relationship between 'giddiness' and *head injuries* requires separate treatment, because it is seldom possible to ascertain the anatomical seat of the trouble. Following either minor or major cerebral contusion, the patient is apt to complain of dizziness on quick movements of the head or movements of the head in space. Occasionally it amounts to a true vertigo, but more often it falls short of this and is described as dizziness or giddiness. In a minority of cases there is evidence of damage to the labyrinth, or to the 8th nerve, but usually there is no such evidence and the patient comes to the doctor with complaints not only of dizzy spells but of nervousness, irritability, incapacity for mental and physical effort, and dislike of loud noises—a story liable to be mistaken for neurosis by the uninformed. There is evidence that such cases react abnormally to labyrinthine tests, but it is not clear whether the site of the damage is in the semicircular canals or in the afferent conducting system. The main interest of this work is to confirm what neurologists have believed for many years, viz. that there is an organic basis for 'dizziness' and vertigo after head injury. The fact that patients are sometimes encouraged by circumstances to prolong these symptoms for gain does not invalidate this view.

Vertigo also occurs in *anaemias*, in *hypertension* and in *hypotensive states*. Anaemia, whether acute or chronic, can not only aggravate vertigo due to other processes but can also cause either lightheadedness or transient mild attacks of vertigo. With regard to hypertension, the position is confused by the circumstance that hypertension, atheroma and labyrinthine disease are all found in the same age-group. While it is true that hypertensives sometimes complain of vertigo, there is no evidence that the raised blood pressure is directly to blame and it is wiser to avoid this facile diagnostic alibi. The 'giddiness' of which so many hypertensives complain often resolves itself, on cross-examination, into a sense of confusion or faintness or lightheadedness rather than a true vertigo, and of those whose testimony survives interrogation some turn out to have labyrinthine disease and other are clearly suffering from focal or diffuse vascular lesions of the brain. Atheromatous stenosis of the basilar artery is frequently accompanied by vertigo presumably from reduction of blood supply to the brain-stem.

A further interesting cause of vertigo is the 'subclavian steal syndrome' (*Fig. V.2*). In this there is severe stenosis or occlusion of the subclavian artery before the origin of the vertebral artery and the blood pressure in that arm is considerably reduced. Characteristically, when the arm is used the distal part of the subclavian artery is supplied by reverse flow by the vertebral artery, thus rendering the hind brain ischaemic and causing vertigo.

Vertigo induced by turning the head in a particular way, sometimes known as 'cervical vertigo', can occur in subjects suffering from atheromatous stenosis of the carotid artery, or a similar narrowing of the vertebral arteries. It is thought that the flow of blood to the brain is obstructed by the movement of the head, and there is some evidence that the vetebral artery may also be compressed within its bony canal by the bulging intervertebral discs of spondylosis. Unlike positional vertigo, it is a movement of the neck, and not the position of the head, which determines the symptoms. In place of vertigo there may be syncope or merely a feeling of lightheadedness.

Hypertensive encephalopathy, i.e. cerebral symptoms of brief duration accompanying an exacerbation of an already high blood pressure, is said to include vertigo amongst its protean manifestations; this may be so, but it is always difficult to be sure of this diagnosis. Any sudden fall or cardiac output, whether from a

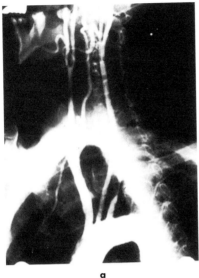 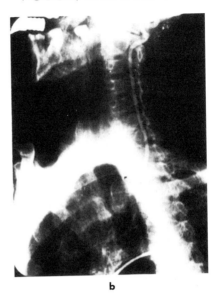

a   b

Fig. V.2. Subclavian steal syndrome. Aortogram showing (a) occlusion of the left subclavian artery and (b) some 6 seconds later showing filling of the distal portion of the subclavian artery by means of retrograde flow in the left vertebral artery.

haemorrhage, cardiac infarction, cardiac arrhythmia, or a prolonged fit of coughing (laryngeal vertigo), can cause vertigo, either by itself or as a prelude to complete syncope. The common faint is often preceded by vertigo, but it is usually coupled with sensations of lightheadedness, nausea, and tinnitus.

Hypotensive drugs used in the treatment of hypertension may produce faintness and occasional vertigo, particularly after sudden changes of posture from recumbency to the erect position.

Finally, there is no evidence whatsoever that true vertigo, as defined here, can be 'psychogenic'. On the other hand, vertigo is a frightening and unsettling experience which, when persistent or recurrent, can cause anxiety and loss of morale even in the most stable of persons, and its effect on neurotic subjects can be cataclysmic. Indeed, the emotional and visceral disturbances may come in time to overshadow the organic nucleus of the illness.

A. G. D. Maran

Voice, disorders of

The larynx consists of an outer skeleton and an inner mucosal framework. The skeleton consists of the hyoid bone, the thyroid cartilage and the cricoid cartilage. The arytenoid cartilages sit on top of the lamina of the cricoid cartilage and the vocal cords are attached to both the arytenoid cartilage and the prominence of the thyroid cartilage. Males have a longer vocal cord than females and the extra length is made up by the

development of the laryngeal prominence or Adam's apple. The vocal cords are supplied by the recurrent laryngeal nerves. On the left, the nerve is long and has an intrathoracic component, while on the right it is short.

To understand how sound is produced, it is necessary to understand the Bernoulli effect. This principle states that during the steady flow of a fluid or a gas, the pressure is less when the velocity is greater. In other words, when air passes from one large space to another (i.e. from lung to pharynx) through a constriction (the glottis), the velocity will be greatest and the pressure least at the site of the constriction.

When we wish to phonate, the recurrent laryngeal nerves set the vocal cords into the adducted position but, because the vocal processes are slightly bulkier than the membranous cord, a slight gap exists between the membranous cords. The lungs then expel air and the airstream passes through this chink between the vocal cords. According to the Bernoulli principle, therefore, there is a drop of pressure at this site and this causes the mucosa of the vocal cords to be drawn into the gap, thus blocking it. At this time the subglottic pressure rises, causing another stream of air to flow through the cords with another resultant pressure drop and closure of the gap. As this process is repeated, a vibratory pattern develops at the vocal cords and the resulting sound is what we appreciate as voice. The change of this sound into speech is accomplished by the tongue, teeth, lips and palate.

There are, thus, only two vocal symptoms, namely dysphonia or hoarseness and aphonia or loss of voice. Dysphonia is caused when the cords meet with an abnormality of the mucosa which causes a roughness in the voice and aphonia occurs when the cords do not meet and air flows between the edges of the vocal cords without voice being produced. In some circumstances when there is a large lesion on the vocal cord, there can be a mixture of dysphonia and air wastage.

The conditions causing abnormalities of the voice are shown in *Table V*.1.

Because of the relative simplicity of the two symptoms, some idea of the cause of the voice disorder can be gained while taking the history from the patient. The next stage is to carry out laryngoscopy. This can be done with a mirror and a headlamp or with a rigid Hopkin's rod attached to a fibreoptic light source. It can also be performed with a flexible laryngoscope although this is very uncomfortable for the patient since it needs to be passed through the nasal cavity. Since carcinoma of the larynx is relatively common and since the results of treatment are so good, it is essential that any patient who is hoarse has the larynx visualized so that carcinoma can be diagnosed early if it is, indeed, present.

Carcinoma of the larynx is a disease of smokers. It is not as common as carcinoma of the lung in Northern Europe but in Southern Europe it is commoner than carcinoma of the lung in smokers. The presenting symptom is hoarseness and this will occur when the tumour is only a few millimetres in size. This is why it is very important to examine the larynx and visualize the vocal cords in anyone who is hoarse. The tumour will gradually expand along the length of the cord but even when it occupies the whole length of one vocal cord, it will only be 2 cm long. Once it spreads into the tissues of the vocal cords then the prognosis is not nearly so good. Most early carcinomas can be cured with radiotherapy but when they are larger, the patient

Table V.1. Causes of voice disorders in adults

Inflammatory	**Traumatic**
Acute	Foreign bodies
Acute laryngitis following an upper respiratory	Intubation damage
infection	Burns
Herpetic laryngitis	Chemical, from inhalation
Acute epiglottitis	External injury with oedema and haematoma
Chronic	**Neurological**
NON-SPECIFIC	Recurrent laryngeal nerve (especially the left side as
Vocal abuse	this nerve has the longer course through neck and
Tobacco and alcohol	chest)
Pachydermia	
Polypoid degeneration (Reinke's oedema)	Palsy due to
Vocal nodules (Singer's nodes)	Surgical injury
SPECIFIC	Peripheral neuritis
Tuberculous	Diphtheria
Lupus vulgaris	Viral
Syphilis	Chemical. Lead
Leprosy	Vitamin B deficiency (beriberi)
Scleroma	'Idiopathic'
Mycoses	Carcinoma of thyroid or upper oesophagus
Actinomycosis	Carcinoma of lung—primary or lymph nodes (left)
Candidiasis	Aneurysm of subclavian artery or aorta
Coccidioidomycosis	Cardiac enlargement
Rhinosporidiosis	
Sarcoid	*Vagus nerve*
Wegener's granuloma	Poliomyelitis
	Ascending polyneuritis
Tumours	Vascular accidents in brain-stem
Benign	Aneurysm of cartoid artery
Vocal polyps	Malignant disease of nasopharynx
Retention cysts	Syphilis
Single papilloma	
Fibroma, haemangioma and neurofibroma	**Various**
	Allergic oedema (Quinke's oedema or 'angio-neurotic
Neoplastic	oedema')
Leucoplakia	Rheumatoid arthritis of crico-arytenoid joints
Carcinoma of the larynx (*Figs*.V.3, V.4)—growth on the	Myxoedema
cord	Myasthenia gravis
Growths of the laryngo-pharynx	Functional aphonia

will need either a partial or a total laryngectomy (*Figs V.3, V.4*).

Vocal cord nodules occur in people who abuse their voice. These are virtually 'corns' on the vocal cords and are caused by abnormal vibratory patterns.

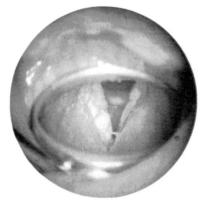

Fig. V.3. Carcinoma of the vocal cord.

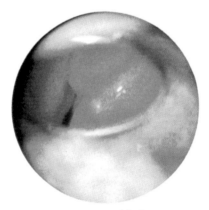

Fig. V.4. Advanced carcinoma of the larynx.

The patient who gives a loud shout or who has the vocal cords traumatized by intubation, can develop a vocal cord polyp on the edge of the cord. Polyps can also be the way that benign tumours such as neurilemomas, myoblastomas, etc. can present. Tuberculosis and sarcoid look like carcinoma in presentation. Myxoedema looks like gross oedema of the vocal cords and can look like a large polyp. A similar condition known as Reinke's oedema can occur sometimes related to myxoedema but often times not.

Depending on the cause, vocal cord paralysis may be unilateral or bilateral, complete or incomplete, giving four possible combinations, namely: (*a*) unilateral abductor; (*b*) unilateral adductor; (*c*) bilateral abductor; (*d*) bilateral adductor. Each of these presents a different clinical picture and each requires different management (*Fig.* V.5).

The conditions that affect either vagus nerve are: (*a*) tumours of the base of the skull, e.g. glomus jugulare tumours and nasopharyngeal carcinoma; (*b*) bulbar paralysis; (*c*) peripheral neuritis due to influenza, herpes or Epstein–Barr virus; (*d*) high neck injuries; e.g. trauma or surgical complication of radical neck dissection; (*e*) metastatic node involvement; (*f*) basal meningitis; (*g*) vagal tumours, e.g. glomus vagale or neurilemoma.

Lesions affecting the left recurrent laryngeal nerve (which has an intrathoracic course) include: (*a*) carcinoma of the bronchus; (*b*) carcinoma of the cervical or thoracic oesophagus; (*c*) carcinoma of the thyroid gland; (*d*) operative trauma from thyroidectomy, radical neck dissection, pharyngeal pouch removal, cricopharyngeal myotomy, ligation of a patent ductus, and other cardiac and pulmonary surgery; (*e*) mediastinal nodes or tumour, e.g. Hodgkin's disease; (*f*) any enlargement of the left side of the heart; (*g*) peripheral neuritis; (*h*) aortic aneurysm.

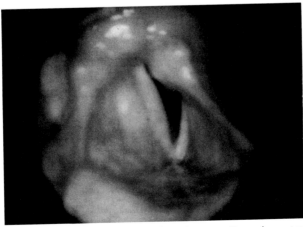

Fig. V.5. Right sided adductor paralysis. The right cord lies in the cadaveric position and cannot reach the midline when the patient attempts to phonate.

The lesions affecting the right recurrent laryngeal nerve are: (*a*) carcinoma of the thyroid gland; (*b*) operative trauma from thyroidectomy, pharyngeal pouch removal or myotomy procedures; (*c*) carcinoma of the oesophagus; (*d*) carcinoma of the apex of the right lung; (*e*) peripheral neuritis; (*f*) subclavian aneurysm.

In unilateral adductor paralysis, the cord lies in the cadaveric position and cannot reach the midline. Normal voice cannot be produced unless the vocal cord is brought towards the midline, either by surgery to medialize the cord or by a Teflon injection. Unilateral abductor paralysis means that the cord is in the midline and the good cord comes across to meet it and so the patient has a voice and no treatment is usually required. In bilateral adductor paralysis, the cause is usually a fatal neurological condition and the patient often dies from aspiration.

Bilateral abductor paralysis is when both vocal cords lie in the mid-position. This is sometimes seen after nerve injury, subsequent to thyroid gland surgery. The patient will have a normal voice but will have stridor. The treatment of this condition is either a permanent tracheostomy or an arytenoidectomy which allows one cord to be pulled laterally. The patient then has a breathy voice but does not have the inconvenience of a tracheostomy.

A. G. D. Maran

Vomiting

Vomiting is the forceful ejection of gastric contents through the mouth. It results from a forceful, sustained contraction of the abdominal muscles and pelvic floor against a closed glottis. The pylorus is contracted and the open cardia is herniated through a contracted diaphragm.

A vomiting centre is present in the medulla oblongata and is stimulated by raised intracranial pressure, brain lesions, hydrocephalus, posterior fossa lesions and vestibular disorders. The vomiting centre is also stimulated via a chemoreceptor trigger zone in the floor of the fourth ventricle which is responsive to drugs and metabolic abnormalities including electrolyte disorders, ketoacidosis or high fever. It is possible that other centres in the brain may be sensitive to emetic drugs or metabolic disturbances. While vomiting of a non-psychogenic mechanism is usually reflex, pathological vomiting of a voluntary nature can take place. Dopamine and opiate neurotransmitters may influence from both a central effect and also a peripheral effect. Thus brain gut peptides which influence gastric motility and emptying include motilin, cholecystokinin and neurotensin (increased motility) and secretin (decreased motility). Gut motility is also influenced by disorders of the autonomic nervous system at either peripheral or central levels. Stimuli carried to the brain by the somatic nerves can also elicit vomiting, for example, if there is severe pain such as in myocardial infarction or colic of one kind or another or pancreatitis.

Vomiting must be distinguished from *regurgitation* which is the effortless expulsion of food from, or the return of food to the mouth (*see* REGURGITATION). In a restricted sense it describes the expulsion of contents from the oesophagus only; but patients are often unable to distinguish between regurgitation, gross oesophageal reflux and vomiting. The absence of a bitter or acid taste helps to distinguish regurgitation from vomiting. *Rumination* is the repeated return of small quantities of food to the mouth where it is chewed and swallowed again. It is uncommon and usually occurs in patients who are psychiatrically disturbed. In order to ruminate the patient increases intra-abdominal pressure, thereby regurgitating food into the mouth. In *retching* there is forceful contraction of the stomach wall muscle, of the diaphragm, and the abdominal muscles similar to that which takes place in vomiting. There is, however, no relaxation of the cardiac sphincter and no food returns to the mouth. Retching is also known as 'dry heaves' and is seen most characteristically in the gastritis associated with alcohol abuse when the patient complains of early morning nausea and dry heaves. The causes of vomiting are listed in *Table* V.2. below.

Investigation of vomiting may include some or all of the procedures in *Table* V.3.

Vomiting is one of the commonest symptoms in clinical medicine. It may represent the beginning of a minor illness or herald a severe disease process. It may be associated with significant complications. The cause of the vomiting is helped if a number of associated features are questioned and elucidated.

1. THE NATURE OF THE VOMITUS: Bright red or altered blood suggests bleeding anywhere from the mouth to the duodenum. The quantity varies according to the speed of bleeding but it must be remembered that the volume of blood is often overestimated by the patient for the red blood is diluted with the volume of gastric contents. 'Coffee-ground' is usually taken to indicate blood altered by gastric juice. A coffee-ground appearance to the vomit is therefore taken to indicate that there is blood in the material but sometimes this is not so and a coffee-ground appearance can be given by altered food mixed with bile. Vomiting of bile occurs after *gastric surgery* and in *high small bowel obstruction*. Repeated vomiting in the absence of bile, particularly in children, suggests that the obstruction is proximal to the second part of the duodenum. The presence of food taken hours or days previously

Table V.2. Causes of vomiting

Gastrointestinal diseases
Gastritis, alcoholic, campylobacter and other causes
Peptic ulceration
Colic, biliary and renal
Cholecystitis
Appendicitis
Pancreatitis, acute and relapsing
Gastric outflow obstruction
Intestinal obstruction, small and large
Gastric cancer
Postgastrectomy syndrome
Acute liver failure
Amyloidosis
Hollow visceral myopathy
Chronic intestinal pseudo-obstruction

Acute infections
Urinary tract infections
Viral gastroenteritis
Viral hepatitis
Measles
Whooping cough
Pneumonia

Drugs
Aminophylline
Aspirin
Cytotoxic agents
Digoxin
General anaesthetic agents
Iron preparations
Metronidazole
Narcotic analgesics
Oestrogens
Sulphasalzine
Sulphonamides

Metabolic/endocrine
Pregnancy
High fevers
Diabetic ketoacidosis
Uraemia
Hyperparathyroidism and other causes of
hypercalcaemia
Addison's disease
Acute intermittent porphyria

Neurological
Meningitis
Raised intracranial pressure
Migraine
Menière's disease
Labyrinthine disorders
Autonomic neuropathy or diabetic
Gullaine–Barré syndrome
Chaga's disease
Tabetic crisis
Autonomic epilepsy
Paraneoplastic neuropathy

Psychogenic
Bulimia
Functional
Anorexia nervosa

Other
Cardiac failure
Myocardial infarction
Hypertensive encephalopathy
Irradiation
Food intolerance
Diffuse malignant disease
Acute glaucoma

Table V.3. Tests that may be necessary in unexplained vomiting

Full history and physical examination
Haematological and biochemical screen
Drug screen
Hormone tests
Protein electrophoresis
Plain X-ray abdomen
Gastric intubation
Endoscopy
Upper and lower GI tract barium examination
Intravenous urography
Computed tomography
Gastric emptying tests
Oesophageal manometry
Psychiatric assessment
Laparotomy with full thickness muscle biopsy

suggests that *gastric statis* is present. This may be due to reflect atony or may reflect long-standing gastric outflow obstruction such as in *pyloric stenosis*. Vomit which has a faecal smell suggests that there is *small bowel obstruction* or an *ileus*, or the presence of a *gastro-colic fistula*. Occasionally faecal-smelling vomit is seen in patients with *bacterial overgrowth* in the proximal small bowel.

2. TIMING OF THE VOMIT: Vomiting occurring during or soon after a meal can occur in patients with a *peptic ulcer* in the pyloric channel but it is also a feature of *psychoneurotic vomiting*. Early morning vomiting before breakfast occurs characteristically in *pregnancy, alcoholic gastritis* and *uraemia*. Patients who have *postnasal drip* or who have *chronic bronchitis* and who swallow their sputum may also vomit at this time. Patients with chronic bronchitis who cough a great deal in the early morning may follow a bout of coughing with vomiting.

3. RELIEF OF PAIN BY VOMITING: This is a feature of *peptic ulcer* disease particularly.

4. PROJECTILE VOMITING: This term is used to describe vomit which is ejected forcefully from the mouth. It is said to occur in *raised intracranial pressure* and also in patients who have *gastric outflow obstruction*. The description is however a poor one as many other causes of vomiting may be of a projectile nature while not every patient with raised intracranial pressure or gastric outflow obstruction will have vomiting. Most patients who vomit will have preceding nausea but in the case of projectile vomiting this is often absent.

MEDICAL HISTORY

It is very important to take a complete history in attempting to elucidate the cause of vomiting. Details of previous surgery are important as is information relating to childhood health, details of medication, alcohol consumption and any psychiatric disease. A social history is also of significance. Information is required about the patient's marriage, occupation, work satisfaction, and other issues relating to his personal life. This is the opportunity to explore phobias and fears and inappropriate anxiety situations.

PHYSICAL EXAMINATION

This is of importance not only to attempt to identify the underlying cause but also to elucidate whether or not complications of the vomiting have developed. A succussion splash and visible peristalsis, particularly when it passes from left to right in the anterior abdomen, is of value in indicating pyloric obstruction with gastric dilatation. Increased bowel sounds will be observed if there is small or large bowel obstruction. The features to observe are abdominal distension, an abdominal mass, the presence of weight loss and evidence for disease in other body systems.

COMPLICATIONS OF VOMITING

These can be considered under two headings, those related to damage to the gastrointestinal tract and those associated with metabolic disorder. Movement of the stomach through the oesophageal hiatus can cause damage to the mucosa resulting in severe haemorrhage. These tears at the gastro-oesophageal junction are known as the *Mallory–Weiss syndrome*. Rupture of the oesophagus can take place, the *Boerhaave's syndrome*. Aspiration of the vomitus can cause a *chemical pneumonitis*. This topic has received prominence as a complication of women who vomit as they go into labour with consequent severe pulmonary oedema due to the chemical pneumonitis. Prolonged vomiting may be associated with the following electrolyte changes, potassium deficiency, alkalosis, hyponatraemia, decreased blood volume and haemoconcentration. Subsequently renal failure may develop, paralysis due to potassium depletion may occur and malnutrition may become severe.

1. Gastric causes

Most *corrosive* and *irritant poisons* cause vomiting immediately after swallowing, accompanied by intense burning pain in the epigastrium. The vomit contains food, blood, mucus and may have the characteristic odour of the poison. With some irritant poisons, e.g. arsenic or phosphorus, the vomiting may be delayed and resemble that of an acute gastritis. The diagnosis

depends on chemical analysis of the vomit, as well as the associated signs and symptoms. Shreds of gastric mucosa may be seen or even a large portion of the mucosa forming a partial or complete cast of the interior of the stomach (*gastritis membranacea*). Many drugs medicinally employed may cause vomiting if administered in excess, and, in the case of susceptible persons, even in ordinary pharmacopoeial doses, iron preparations being a good example.

In *acute viral gastroenteritis* repeated vomiting is usually very severe and attended by abdominal pain. It occurs shortly after taking food and leads to some relief of pain. The vomited matter consists at first of food ingested, later of mucus and bile. There are often accompanying diarrhoea and febrile disturbances, especially in children.

In *chronic gastritis* pain is of variable degree. The vomited matter consists of partially digested food, mucus, and a considerable quantity of sour-smelling liquid. Hydrochloric acid is usually reduced, or entirely absent. When *dilatation* of the stomach is present, the quantity of liquid ejected is often very large; portions of food taken many hours previously may be recognized.

'Hour-glass' contraction is a rare condition and is due to transverse constriction of the stomach by fibrous tissue, may be a cause of vomiting which resembles in most respects that associated with dilatation. Examination with a barium meal will generally establish the diagnosis.

In adults, the vomiting due to *gastric outflow obstruction* presents no characteristics other than those associated with the dilatation of the stomach which it usually produces. The cause of the obstruction may be either irreversible fibrosis and stenosis (*pyloric stenosis*) or remedial oedema of the pyloric canal. Radiographic evidence that there is a large residuum in the stomach 8 hours after the intake of the barium is the most direct method of demonstrating pyloric stenosis. The absence of free hydrochloric acid and the presence of blood in the vomit would favour the diagnosis of carcinoma. Persistent vomiting in young male infants, especially if breastfed, attended by wasting and constipation, arouses suspicion of *hypertrophic stenosis of the pylorus*. The vomiting in these cases is very forcible, usually shortly after a feed. Visible gastric peristalsis and the presence of a small tumour in the epigastrium would complete the diagnosis.

Vomiting is by no means universal in cases of non-malignant *gastric ulcer*. Pain as a rule occurs within an hour of taking food and is relieved by vomiting. The vomit consists of food more or less digested, a variable but generally at least normal quantity of free hydrochloric acid, and sometimes blood.

2. Intestinal, peritoneal and general visceral causes

In *intestinal obstruction* vomiting sets in after an interval the length of which may depend on the situation of the obstruction. The higher this is situated in the intestinal canal the earlier and more severe the vomiting. The contents of the stomach are returned first, and later mucus, bile and intestinal contents, often of a dull brown colour and thin fluid consistence; obvious pieces of faecal matter are rarely distinguishable. Faecal vomiting should be recognizable by its odour.

Vomiting is an early symptom in *appendicitis* and may persist to resemble that met with in intestinal obstruction.

Intestinal worms may cause vomiting in children, probably owing to reflex irritation. A round-worm is sometimes found in the vomit.

Enemas induce vomiting in certain individuals and rare cases have been described where liquid injected per rectum has been returned by the mouth.

Vomiting is a common symptom in the condition known as *Henoch-Schönlein purpura*. The vomit may contain blood from the mucous membrane of the stomach. It is usually accompanied by abdominal pain, sometimes of an acute and agonizing character closely simulating that occurring with intestinal obstruction, in consequence of haemorrhage into the intestinal wall or the mesentery, occasionally simulating or even giving rise to intussusception. Recurrent attacks of vomiting and abdominal pain associated with arthropathies affecting one or more joints for a few days at a time, haematuria and a purpuric eruption particularly on the buttocks in a child would point to this not uncommon disease.

In *acute peritonitis*, vomiting is an early symptom; rarely the vomit may have a faecal odour. The history, together with the rigidity and immobility of the abdominal wall, generally indicates the need for early laparotomy.

Epidemic vomiting is caused by a number of viruses including the Norwalk virus. Characteristically there is sudden onset of severe vomiting, headache, dizziness, aches and pains, sweating and fever. In *biliary* and *renal colic* the vomiting accompanying the attacks of agonizing pain presents no special features. The pain in the upper right part of the abdomen distinguishes biliary colic from that due to renal calculus in which the pain is in the loin or the lower abdomen shooting down towards the groin and testicle and often followed by haematuria. True biliary colic results from a stone obstructing the cystic duct. Jaundice is absent if the gallstone is in the cystic duct. A gallstone in the common bile duct causes more prolonged pain rather than the waves of colic which accompany cystic duct obstruction.

Acute pancreatitis may closely simulate intestinal obstruction in that it is attended by nausea and vomiting, constipation and severe abdominal pain. The vomit is, however, not faecal in character; there is usually localized tenderness over the pancreas. There may be bluish discoloration of the skin of the abdominal wall as described by Grey Turner. If laparotomy is performed (on account of the urgency of the symptoms), fat necrosis is usually found in the omentum and mesentery.

Severe nausea and vomiting may occur with acute myocardial infarction. It may be caused by the drugs administered for pain.

3. Affections of the central nervous system

In all cases of vomiting with the least suspicion of an intracranial lesion a full examination of the central nervous system with X-ray of the skull, ophthalmoscopy for papilloedema or optic atrophy, and compured tomography are necessary. Instances occur when attacks of vomiting may be the only symptom of an intracranial tumour long in advance of any other symptom or sign of increased intracranial pressure.

Cerebral haemorrhage may be attended by vomiting especially when the cerebellum is the part affected or when the haemorrhage is subarachnoid.

Menière's syndrome is characterized by recurrent paroxysms of vertigo, vomiting, tinnitus and progressive nerve deafness. Vomiting tends to follow the attack of vertigo. Characteristically there is rotatory nystagmus and unsteadiness of stance and gait during an attack. *Vestibular neuronitis* and *benign recurrent vertigo* describe a clinical syndrome commonly occurring in the middle-aged associated with abrupt onset of vertigo, nausea and vomiting without any impairment of hearing. The attack lasts only for a few days and is followed by a brief period of mild positional vertigo (*see* VERTIGO).

Functional or *hysterical vomiting* may not be attended by nausea or pain, and although the vomiting may be a frequent occurrence the general state of nutrition often remains good. It is by no means unusual for a subject to vomit, and return to complete a meal. Other hysterical manifestations are generally present in these patients and detailed interrogation may elicit a psychological cause to encourage the conclusion that the act symbolizes a (possibly subconscious) feeling of disgust. Some people are prone to vomit on the slightest psychological disturbance as a means of expressing their emotions. In *bulimia* there is gorging followed by self-induced vomiting. Vomiting can also occur in *anorexia nervosa* but failure to eat is the prominent feature of the disease.

The *gastric crises* in tabes dorsalis are attacks of vomiting usually accompanied by severe epigastric pain. Occasionally, vomiting may be an isolated symptom. The attacks usually last for several days, and tend to recur at irregular intervals. During the intervals alimentary functions may be completely normal. The diagnosis would be supported by the characteristic Argyll Robertson pupil and the loss of the knee-jerks, but, in some cases, visceral crises are the only manifestation of tabes and a mistaken diagnosis of an abdominal catastrophe is by no means easily avoided. The absence of abdominal rigidity is an important feature. Blood and CSF tests are necessary for *Treponema pallidum* haemagglutination (TPHA) and a fluorescent test of treponemal antibody (FTA-ABS).

Disease of the labyrinth such as may be associated with drugs or viral infection is associated with nausea, vomiting and vertigo of the peripheral type. Hearing is almost invariably affected.

Disorder of the autonomic nervous system may alter gut motility and cause vomiting. Autonomic system degenerations occur in primary idiopathic hypotension and the Shy–Drager syndrome as well as diabetes mellitus. In the Shy–Drager syndrome, the basic lesion lies in the basal ganglia as well as degeneration of the autonomic nervous system. Neuromuscular disorders that cause vomiting require careful investigation of the central nervous system, the autonomic nervous system and an evaluation of gut smooth muscle. The latter may be achieved by manometry but frequently a full thickness biopsy is required.

Ian A. D. Bouchier

Vulva, swelling of

The differential diagnosis of vulval swellings includes not only tumours of the vulva itself, but also swellings which appear at the vulva as a result of the displacement of other structures as in cases of uterine prolapse and cystocele. Inflammatory lesions and ulceration of the vulva may be accompanied by swelling of the vulva due to oedema. These conditions are considered under VULVAL ULCERATION.

Vulval swellings may be tabulated as follows:

Inflammatory swellings

Warts
Condyloma acuminatum
Bartholin's abscess

Cystic swellings

Bartholin's cyst
Sebaceous cyst
Mucous cyst
Implantation cyst
Dermoid cyst
Hydrocele of the canal of Nuck
Vestigial (mesonephric) cyst (Gartner's cyst)

Blood cysts

Varicocele
Traumatic haematoma
Endometrioma

Benign new growths

Caruncle
Fibroma
Fibromyoma
Lipoma
Hidradenoma
Papilloma
Lymphangioma
Myxoma
Angioma
Melanoma
Neuroma

Malignant new growths

Squamous-cell carcinoma
Rodent ulcer
Adenocarcinoma
Sarcoma
Melanoma
Chorioncarcinoma

Hernia

Inguinal
Hernia of the pouch of Douglas (enterocele)

Displacement

Prolapse of the urethral mucosa
Prolapse of the vaginal vault and uterus
Cystocele
Rectocele
Chronic inversion of the uterus

INFLAMMATORY SWELLINGS. Warts on the vulva are usually multiple. They are caused by a virus of the papovirus group and may be transmitted sexually (*venereal warts*). They may spread up into the vagina and a careful inspection of the vaginal walls with the aid of a speculum should always be made in the presence of vulval warts. In pregnancy, or in the presence of much sweating, vulval warts proliferate and may become macerated. They are then referred to as *condyloma acuminata*.

BARTHOLIN'S ABSCESS presents as an extremely painful swelling in the region of the Bartholin (greater vestibular) gland. Pressure on the gland causes much pain, but a bead of pus can be seen escaping from the mouth of the Bartholin duct just below the lateral attachment of the hymen. If not incised, the abscess usually bursts through the skin of the posterior aspect of the labium majus with consequent relief of pain. Recurrence is common until the gland is removed surgically.

CYSTIC SWELLING. The commonest one is a Bartholin's cyst. This is usually a swelling in the duct of the Bartholin's gland producing a swelling in the posterior third of the labium majus which projects medially so as to encroach on the vaginal entrance and causing dyspareunia. It is not particularly tender unless it becomes infected to form an abscess. The cyst tends gradually to increase in size, causing local discomfort until marsupialization is performed.

Sebaceous cysts are fairly common affecting the labia majora as a rule. They may occur in groups. Mucous, inclusion and implantation cysts also occur, as do vestigial cysts of mesonephric duct (Wolffian duct) origin (Gartner's duct cysts). The true nature of these cysts is not usually known without histological examination.

VARICOCELE of the vulva occurs mainly in pregnancy giving rise to the characteristic 'bag of worms' feel to palpation. Since the veins are close to the skin, there is a bluish discoloration. The patient is conscious of an uncomfortable swelling on standing. The veins seldom rupture during delivery. Varicocele must be differentiated from an *inguinal hernia* extending into the labium majus and from a *cyst of the canal of Nuck* (the processus vaginalis which has failed to become completely obliterated). Both the latter tend to involve only the anterior parts of the labium majus, but all these conditions extend to the groin. Whereas a hernia is reducible as a rule, a cyst of the canal of Nuck is not. Inguinal hernias usually disappear as pregnancy progresses, but varicoceles become worse. If a hernia contains bowel, it is resonant to percussion. A strangulated hernia will not be reducible, but the accompanying acute symptoms and the history should make the diagnosis clear.

A *haematoma* of the vulva may follow delivery or occur as the result of direct trauma. It is recognized as a bluish swelling which is painful and tender and spreads up into the pelvis by the side of the vagina. The appearance is characteristic and the diagnosis is made on the history. An endometrioma is a rare cause of a blood-containing cyst on the vulva.

BENIGN NEW GROWTHS. Both *fibroma* and *lipoma* are seen in the vulva and may become pedunculated. They may occur at any age, are soft, oval or rounded and covered by vulval skin. They may grow slowly to reach the size of a fist. A lipoma is usually broader based than a fibroma. Several other benign swellings are found on the vulva. They are usually solitary and small (about 1 cm or so in diameter) and their nature is arrived at on histology. A *papilloma* is a sessile benign tumour of the skin of the labia in women of middle or old age. A *hidradenoma* is a tumour of sweat gland origin which may be solid or cystic and which may ulcerate to allow a red papillomatous growth to be extruded. When ulcerated it may suggest the diagnosis of carcinoma clinically. Biopsy solves the problem. Less commonly there are found fibromyoma, myxoma, angioma, lymphangioma, benign melanoma and neuroma, each distinguished by microscopic examination.

TUMOURS AT THE URETHRAL MEATUS. *Urethral caruncles* are frequent, especially in older women. A caruncle appears as a small reddish sessile growth arising from the posterior wall of the urethral meatus causing bleeding and painful micturition. It is often very tender but may be symptomless. It is usually granulomatous, but may be polypoidal and papillomatous. It has to be distinguished from *prolapse of the urethral mucosa* in which there is a ring of protruding red tissue all round the urethral opening.

MALIGNANT NEW GROWTH. *Squamous-cell carcinoma* (epithelioma) is the most important of these. It occurs mainly in elderly women over 60 or 70 years of age. In about half the cases, it is preceded by pruritus vulvae for several years due to hyperplastic vulval dystrophy. It commonly arises in the anterior part of the vulva in the skin of the labia majora, or is in the region of the clitoris. Usually there is a single lesion, but there may be two opposite each other, so-called 'kissing cancers'. It begins as a raised intracutaneous nodule which ulcerates to give rise to a hard-based ulcer with raised everted edges. The proliferative type presents with an irregular friable mass of growth. A biopsy and histology establish the true nature of the lesion. Spread occurs to the inguinal nodes which should always be felt for enlargement and hardness. In advanced cases the nodes ulcerate through the skin of the groin and become fixed to the deeper tissues.

Other malignant tumours found in the vulva include rodent ulcer (basal-cell carcinoma), forming a flat plaque with its characteristic rolled edge, malignant melanoma (pigmented and non-pigmented), adenocarcinoma arising in Bartholin's gland or in the urethra, and sarcoma. Metastatic tumours from primaries in the cervix, uterine body and ovary rarely occur. Chorioncarcinoma has also been described. The *displacements* given in the list above are dealt with under the heading VAGINA AND UTERUS, PROLAPSE OF.

N. Patel

Vulva, ulceration of

Ulceration of the vulva may be due to:

Squamous-cell carcinoma (epithelioma)
Rodent ulcer
Other malignant tumours (melanoma, sarcoma, adenocarcinoma, etc.)
Vulval dystrophy (hypoplastic and hyperplastic)
Carcinoma-in-situ (intra-epithelial carcinoma)
Bowen's disease
Paget's disease
Herpes genitalis
Behçet's syndrome
Soft sore (chancroid)
Granuloma inguinale
Lumphopathia (lymphogranuloma) venereum
Syphilis
Yaws
Tuberculosis
Furunculosis
Diptheria
Vincent's infection
Diabetic vulvitis
Mycotic vulvitis

MALIGNANT AND PREMALIGNANT ULCERATION

Malignancy of the vulva produces a localized swelling which becomes ulcerated. The various lesions are dealt with under VULVAL SWELLINGS. Vulval dystrophies are chronic conditions which cause intense itching of the vulva. Hyperplastic dystrophy with atypia seen under the microscope should be regarded as premalignant and excised. Intra-epithelial carcinoma (Bowen's disease) and Paget's disease also cause chronic pruritus. They give rise to thickening of the vulval skin which is dusky red in colour with patches of white due to hyperkeratosis and superficial ulceration from rubbing and scratching. Biopsies are needed for diagnosis, as they are both premalignant.

ACUTE MULTIPLE ULCERS

These may occur as the result of *herpes genitalis infection* transmitted sexually. Primary infection occurs 2–7 days after inoculation. Prodromal symptoms of tingling or itching are followed by vesicular eruptions which rapidly erode resulting in painful, shallow ulcers all over the vulva. They give rise to dysuria, bilateral inguinal lymphadenopathy, fever and malaise. Herpes virus can be obtained from the vesicular fluid in the early stages, 85 per cent being due to the herpes virus, type 2. The lesions, which are very painful, persist for 2–6 weeks before healing occurs and antibody appears in the blood. The ulcers tend to recur at intervals of weeks or months and the virus may be recovered from them. Coitus with a non-immune partner will pass on the infection. The disease is self-limiting in time and the lesions eventually heal spontaneously.

Behçet's syndrome is a rare disorder of unknown cause characterized by oral and vulval ulceration. Iridocyclitis, arthritis and nervous system involvement are complications of severe cases.

SEXUALLY TRANSMITTED INFECTIONS

Syphilis is the most important of these. Between 10 and 90 days after contact with an infectious lesion, the Hunterian chancre develops at the portal of entry. It is an indurated firm painless papule or ulcer with raised edges. In the case of a vulval lesion, the inguinal nodes are enlarged and firm and painless. Genital lesions in women often escape notice because they are hidden inside the vagina or on the cervix. The lesion has to be differentiated from an epithelioma. The serum from a chancre contains the spirochaete *Treponema pallidum* which can be seen under a microscope with the aid of dark ground illumination. If an epithelioma is suspected the ulcer and swelling should be excised and examined microscopically. The chancre persists for 1–5 weeks, but serological tests for syphilis do not become positive for about 4–6 weeks after the appearance of the chancre. The serological tests most commonly performed are the VDRL slide test and the FTA-ABS (fluorescent treponemal antibody absorption) test which have replaced the Wassermann, Kahn and TPI (treponemal immobilization test). To exclude primary syphilis, serological tests have to be done every week for 6 weeks after the appearance of the chancre. Untreated, two weeks to 6 months after the chancre has healed, the generalized cutaneous eruption of secondary syphilis appears. Numerous moist flat-topped papules occur on the vulva and round the anus. They are known as 'condyloma latum'. In only one-third of untreated cases does tertiary syphilis occur, but not until some years after the primary lesion. Spreading ulceration on the vulva is a rare manifestation which has to be differentiated from an epithelioma on histology.

Granuloma inguinale is a chronic venereal infection with a tendency to ulceration and massive granulation tissue affecting the vulva and groins. It is almost non-existent in Great Britain, but is seen in India, Brazil and the West Indies, islands of the South Pacific, Australia, China and Africa. It starts as a raised papilloma which soon ulcerates, the ulcer having a typical serpiginous outline. The granuloma in the groin rarely suppurates but much scarring develops. Scrapings from the ulcers reveal the causative organism, the Donovan body, a small bacterium encapsulated in mononuclear leucocytes with a curved rod-like nucleus.

Lymphogranuloma venereum is another sexually transmitted disease found in the tropical and subtropical regions of Africa, Asia and south-eastern USA. It is due to *Chlamydia trachomatis*. It begins with a vesicopustular eruption on the vulva which soon disappears but there follows painful suppuration in the inguinal nodes with hypertrophy and ulceration of the groins, vulva and perineum. Later scarring may cause anal stricture or severe dyspareunia. The diagnosis may be made by isolating the organism, by the intradermal injection of virus antigen when a cutaneous reaction develops (Frei test) or by a complement fixation test.

Chancroid (soft sore) occurs 3–5 days after coitus. It begins as a vesiopustule which becomes a punched-out ulcer with a red base or as a saucer-shaped, ragged ulcer. The lesion is extremely tender and produces a heavy foul discharge which is contagious. It contains the causative organism, Ducrey's bacillus (*Haemophilus ducreyi*) a Gram-negative rod. The lesion may be solitary or there may be several ulcers. Usually there is a painful inguinal adenitis which may break down and discharge. Syphilis, herpes, granuloma inguinale and lymphogranuloma venereum must be ruled out and attempts made to isolate the organism from the ulcers or from the buboes in the groin.

OTHER CONDITIONS

Yaws occurs in tropical countries and produces a lesion similar in appearance to the condyloma latum of secondary syphilis. *Tuberculous ulcers* are very uncommon on the vulva. They are very indolent and can only be diagnosed with certainty on microscopical section. *Furunculosis* (boils) due to staphylococcal infection of the hair follicles are common, affecting the labia majora in particular. *Diphtheria* produces ulceration with a characteristic membranous exudate. *Vincent's infection* of the vulva is the cause of indurated ulceration with an exudate containing fusiform bacilli and spirochaetes. *Mycotic and diabetic vulvitis* (thrush) cause soreness and pruritus of the vulva with redness, excoriation and oedema of the skin and a characteristic white curd-like discharge containing the mycelium of *Candida albicans*.

N. Patel

INDEX

References to figures are *italicized*; references to tables are in **bold type**